CURRENT PERSPECTIVES IN HIV INFECTION

Edited by **Shailendra K. Saxena**

Current Perspectives in HIV Infection
http://dx.doi.org/10.5772/46042
Edited by Shailendra K. Saxena

Contributors
Wan Majdiah Wan Mohamad, Rehana Basri, Osaro Erhabor, TEDDY ADIAS, Cagla Akay, Jennifer King, Brigid Jensen, Patrick Gannon, Claudia Colomba, Raffaella Rubino, Robert Muga, Arantza Sanvisens, Ferran Bolao, Daniel Fuster, Santiago Pérez-Hoyos, Jordi Tor, Marta Torrens, Gabriel Vallecillo, Inmaculada Rivas, José Miguel Azevedo-Pereira, Bakari Adamu Girei, Sani-Bello Fatima, Jose Castro, Maria Alcaide, Paula Freitas, Doris Wilflingseder, Wilfried Posch, Enrique Valdes, Joseph Ongrádi, Balázs Stercz, Károly Nagy, Mauro Pistello, Abdulkarim Alhetheel, Mahmoud Aly, Marko Kryworuchko, Gbemisola Agbelusi, Chi Dola, Amanda Johnson, Olivia Chang, Maga Martinez, Peter J. Jay Chipimo, Nitya Nathwani, Shailendra K. Saxena

Published by InTech
Janeza Trdine 9, 51000 Rijeka, Croatia

Publishing Process Manager Iva Simcic
Technical Editor InTech DTP team
Cover InTech Design team

Additional hard copies can be obtained from orders@intechopen.com

Current Perspectives in HIV Infection, Edited by Shailendra K. Saxena
p. cm.
ISBN 978-953-51-1057-6

For EU product safety concerns:
IN TECH d.o.o., Prolaz Marije Krucifikse Kozulić 3, 51000 Rijeka, Croatia,
info@intechopen.com or visit our website at intechopen.com.

Meet the editor

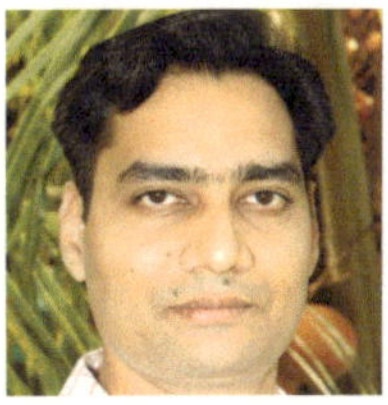

Dr Shailendra K. Saxena is a Medical Microbiologist at CSIR-Centre for Cellular and Molecular Biology (CCMB) in India. The main research interests of his group are to understand the epidemiology and molecular mechanisms of host-defense during human viral infections and to develop new predictive, preventive and therapeutic strategies for them using JEV and HIV as a model. His research work has been published in various high impact factor journals with high citation. He has received many awards and honors in India and abroad including various Young Scientist Awards, BBSRC India Partnering Award and named as "Global Leader in Science" by The Scientist magazine (USA).

Contents

Preface

During the past three decades, the world scientific community has witnessed major achievements understanding the pathogenesis of Human immunodeficiency virus (HIV) which leads to a deadly catastrophic disease acquired immune deficiency syndrome (AIDS). As per recent UNAIDS reports currently ~34 million adults and children are estimated to be living with HIV. Ever since the discovery of HIV, it has been an ultimate challenge to the health and scientific authorities. There is a constant research being done by scientists worldwide to find ways to combat with HIV. HIV has occupied place as a topmost health and social disaster. It is affecting several developing economies. Thus it becomes an urgency to find ways of management against HIV infection. To device a way, basic and thorough knowledge about HIV, stands as a priority. We need to understand viral morphology, functions, and mechanisms of viral replication, budding, cell signaling, pathogenesis, interaction with host factors, and various other important aspects. However many aspects of HIV infection are still poorly understood.

HIV-1, a retrovirus, attacks the T-lymphocytes of the hosts, and causes several multifaceted altered immune responses and finally leads to fatality. HIV-1 displays extraordinary genetic variation, leading to the classification of the viral strains into phylogenetically distinct groups and subtypes. Amongst the various subtype/clade (A to K) of HIV-1, subtype C is linked to ~48% of the infections globally and is associated with rapidly growing epidemics in Sub-Saharan Africa and parts of Asia, including India and China. In addition to genetic and demographic factors, biological properties unique to the subtype of HIV may also play a role in their exponential proliferation.

HIV is capable of being latent and hidden in various reservoirs in the body where drug targeting becomes impossible. HIV can enter brain and attack neuronal cells and deregulate there functioning which leads to neuropathogenesis. Hence drug targeting to viral reservoirs like brain stands as a big issue. Drugs capable of travelling across the Blood Brain Barrier (BBB) are an urgent need. Along with these genes specific targeting drugs are also important. These drugs can focus on one particular gene or a part of gene that is motif, which is conserved and is most stable. This stable part can be very well targeted by the designed drugs.

Henceforth, keeping in mind all the issues, this book gives a comprehensive overview of HIV and AIDS including NeuroAIDS. The book is divided into several parts which cover various topics deeply, explaining HIV and related pathology, immunity and immunopathology, altered immune responses, screening, diagnosis, manifestations, prevention, treatment, epidemiology and etiology to current clinical recommendations in management of HIV/

AIDS including NeuroAIDS, It also highlights the ongoing issues, recent advances and future directions in diagnostic approaches and therapeutic strategies.

The authors and editors of the book hope that this work might increase the interest in this field of research and that the readers will find it useful for their investigations, management and clinical usage. Also I would like to thank Council of Scientific and Industrial Research (CSIR-CCMB), Director CCMB Dr CM Rao, colleagues, family, and parents who gave me a lot of encouragement and support during the work on this book.

Shailendra K. Saxena, PhD, DCAP, FAEB,
CSIR-Centre for Cellular and Molecular Biology,
Hyderabad, India

Section 1

HIV and Altered Immune Responses

Chapter 1

Immune Responses and Cell Signaling During Chronic HIV Infection

Abdulkarim Alhetheel, Mahmoud Aly and Marko Kryworuchko

Additional information is available at the end of the chapter

http://dx.doi.org/10.5772/53010

1. Introduction

The immune response can be defined by the reaction of the immune system to a particular antigen to which it is exposed. In order to understand immune responses against an infectious agent such as human immunodeficiency virus (HIV) and their regulation during the course of chronic HIV infection, we will provide a brief overview of HIV and its proteins and attempt to shed light on this disease process. We will also review the immune system, its components and describe how these components interact at the molecular levels to fight an invading pathogen such as HIV.

2. Human immunodeficiency virus (HIV)

AIDS (Acquired Immuno-Deficiency Syndrome) in patients was discovered in 1981 and characterized by the appearance symptoms including persistent lymphadenopathy and opportunistic infections such as Kaposi sarcoma, *Pneumocystis carinii* pneumonia. In addition, it was found that all of these patients shared a common defect in cell-mediated immunity characterized by a significant decrease in CD4+T lymphocytes, later revealed to be a principal target of infection [1-3]. Three years later, the causative agent of AIDS was identified as HIV [4, 5]. HIV was classified under the *lentivirus* genus and the *Retroviridae* family. It is an enveloped virus with a size of about 100 nm in diameter. Its genome consists of two identical copies of positive-sense single stranded RNA (ssRNA) that are reverse transcribed into cDNA in infected cells [2, 5]. Each ssRNA is about 9,500 nucleotides in length, and encodes three structural genes called gag, pol, env, and a complex of several other nonstructural regulatory genes known as tat, rev, nef, vif, vpr, and vpu [2, 5]. The gag gene encodes the viral structural proteins including p24 (capsid), p17 (matrix), p7 (nucleocapsid). The pol gene, on the other hand, encodes viral enzymes including p32 (integrase), p66 and p51 (reverse transcriptase), and p10 (protease). The env gene encodes the coat glycoproteins gp120 (surface) and gp41 (transmembrane), which play a major role in viral attachment and fusion with host target cell membranes. The nonstructural genes including transactivator of transcription (Tat), regulator of virion protein expression (Rev), negative regulatory factor (Nef), viral infectivity factor (Vif), viral protein R (Vpr), and viral protein U (Vpu) proteins, respectively, are also essential for viral replication and pathogenesis [2, 5].

3. The immune system and its cellular components

The immune system is a very complex and dynamic network, which can be broadly divided into innate and adaptive components [4,6,7]. The cellular components of innate immunity include dendritic cells, natural killer (NK) cells, NK T cells, macrophages, and granulocytes, whereas, the adaptive immunity is mediated by B and T lymphocytes [4,6-8]. The components of both branches act in conjunction and are regulated by soluble mediator proteins known as cytokines and chemokines in order to fight, clear, and protect the host from a wide variety of pathogens [4,6-8].

3.1. The innate immune system

The innate immune system is the first line of defense against invading pathogens. Viral infections including HIV induce the interferon (IFN) response that is characterized by the production and secretion of pro-inflammatory cytokines including type-I IFN (IFN-α/β). These cytokines have antimicrobial and anti-proliferative properties and serve to propagate the adaptive immune responses [9]. In humans, cellular RNA molecules are short stem secondary structures. In contrast, RNA viruses produce long dsRNA molecules in the infected cells as a part of their life cycle. Thus, the long dsRNA can be recognized as a foreign molecule and triggers both cellular and humoral innate immune responses [10]. There are two well characterized ways in which a cell can recognize pathogens. Distinct extracellular pathogen components are recognized by different Toll- like receptors (TLR) expressed on the cell surface or in the endosome such as TLR2, TLR3, TLR4, TLR7, TLR8, and TLR9 [11]. Intracellular replicating pathogens however, are recognized by RNA helicases, which are encoded by the retinoic acid-inducible gene I (RIG-I) and/or melanoma differentiation-associated gene 5 (MDA5) [12]. Following viral recognition, the activation and translocation of the transcription factor nuclear factor κB (NFκB) and interferon-regulatory factor (IRF)-3 to the nucleus occurs and promotes the transcription of IFN type I [13]. Production of type-I IFN stimulates the surrounding cells to produce a wide range of antiviral proteins including protein kinase R (PKR), myxovirus resistance factor, 2'-5' oligoadenylate synthase/RNaseL and dsRNA adenosine deaminase 1, which subsequently leads to the activation of eukaryotic initiation factor (eIF)-2, and translation inhibition of both host and viral mRNAs [14].

Monocytes, which are the precursors of macrophages, as a part of the innate immune system, play a major role in controlling and clearing pathogens. They exhibit antimicrobial, antifungal, and antiparasitic properties [4,6-8]. They possess phagocytic and endocytic activity. In addition, they act as antigen presenting cells by uptaking, processing, and presenting antigen in the context of major histocompatibility complex (MHC) class II to CD4+ T cells. Moreover, they secrete inflammatory cytokines such as IFN type-I (IFN-α/β), interleukin (IL)-1, IL-6, IL-12, and chemokines such as IL-8 [4,6-8]. This stimulates the adaptive immune system and leads to the activation and differentiation of B and T lymphocyte populations. These important monocyte/macrophage (M/M) functions are largely driven and regulated by the responsiveness of these cells to numerous cytokines such as IFN-γ, IL-10, and Tumor Necrosis Factor (TNF)-α, and signals delivered to them via the TLR family through recognition of different microbial products such as bacterial lipopolysaccharide (LPS) and viral proteins and nucleic acids including those of HIV [4,6-8].

3.2. The adaptive immune system

B and T lymphocytes form the arm of the adaptive and antigen-specific immune response. B lymphocytes are antigen presenting cells, upon antigenic and cytokine stimulation they differentiate into plasma cells which produce antigen-specific antibodies. While T lymphocytes are divided into two distinct populations: helper and cytotoxic cells which are differ in their function T helper lymphocytes express the CD4 surface receptor, recognize antigens presented as peptide epitopes bound to MHC class II molecules expressed on the surface of antigen presenting cells, and function mainly as cytokine producing cells to 'help' the development of the immune response. Activated CD4+ T cells differentiate into T helper (Th)-1 and Th-2 effectors, and memory cell sub-populations. The Th-1 and Th-2 subsets of CD4+ T cells were originally defined by their polarized cytokine production patterns [15,16]. Th-1 cells produce IFN-γ, IL-2, IL-12 and lymphotoxin-α, which enhance antigen presentation, phagocytosis, and cell-mediated cytotoxicity. On the other hand, Th-2 cells secrete IL-4, IL-5, IL-9, IL-10, and IL-13, promoting more of an antibody response [16-18]. Cytotoxic T lymphocytes however, express the CD8 surface receptor, and recognize antigenic peptide epitopes presented on cell surface MHC class I molecules. Antigen-activated CD8+ T cells also proliferate and differentiate into effectors and memory cell populations, largely in response to cytokines that share the common γc receptor, such as IL-2, IL-15, and IL-7. Cytotoxic T cells secrete IFN-γ, which inhibits virus replication, as well as perforin, and granzymes in order to kill virus-infected cells.

3.3. HIV and the cellular immune response

HIV is commonly transmitted by sexual contact, and thus it initially interacts with and activates the innate immune system and antigen presenting cells including macrophages and dendritic cells at the mucosal surfaces [5,19,20]. Importantly, these cells then migrate to the lymphoid tissues and thereby also deliver the virus to other susceptible cells located at these sites. In the lymphoid tissues, HIV interacts and infects other cells such as CD4+ T cells and is able to disseminate to other areas such as the brain and gut [5,21]. Subsequently, inflammatory cells and cytokines accumulate during chronic infection and immune activation causing severe reactions and tissue pathology. This includes destruction of regulatory immune cells, mainly CD4+ T cells, and overall impairment of immune functions, which are the hallmarks of chronic HIV infection [5,22-24]. Studies have shown that M/M and T lymphocyte functions are impaired over the course of HIV infection, thus contributing to the overall immune dysfunction and appearance of the opportunistic infections observed in HIV-infected patients. Several *ex vivo* and *in vitro* studies have reported that many M/M defects arise during chronic HIV infection including poor phagocytic activity [25-27], altered cytokine and chemokine secretion [24,28-31], impaired antigen uptake and MHC class II molecule expression [32,33]. Other studies have shown defects in T lymphocyte effector functions including impairment of CD4 T lymphocytes to produce IL-2 and to proliferate in response to recall antigens (influenza, tetanus toxoid), alloantigens (mixed lymphocytes reaction), or exogenous mitogens (phytohemagglutinin) [34,35]. Also, CD8 T lymphocytes exhibit an altered differentiation and proliferative phenotype and impaired capacity to kill virus-infected cells and clear the virus [36]. However, the molecular mechanism by which HIV impairs these cellular functions remains unclear. One possible mechanism by which chronic HIV infection may adversely affect immune cell function is through the modulation of cell signaling molecules, as observed in several cell types including M/M, CD4+ and CD8+ T cells, and neuronal cells [37-42]. This may occur by the direct action of HIV and its different immunomodulatory proteins such as Gp120, Nef, Tat, and Vpr, or indirectly via its effects on the cytokine secretion profile induced during the course of the disease as discussed in more detail below [43-46].

4. Cytokines

As mentioned above, cytokines are small secreted proteins with molecular weights of about 10-40 kDa [18,47,48]. These proteins function as mediators to regulate both the innate and adaptive immune responses [4,6,7]. They transmit the biochemical message from the extracellular environment to the nucleus of the targeted cell via cytokine-cytokine receptor interaction and subsequent triggering of complex intracellular signal transduction [49,50]. They can affect cell function in a paracrine as well as an autocrine manner. There are many cytokines produced by the immune system. Certain cytokines are associated with the initial response to an infection or inflammation and are referred to as inflammatory cytokines. Other cytokines are induced according to the nature of the infectious agent and the type of immune responses produced against them. For instance, infection with *Influenza virus*, *Vaccinia virus*, or *Listeria monocytogenes* is known to induce a Th-1 immune response [51]. This type of immune response is associated with the production of cytokines such as IL-2, IFN-γ, and IL-12, which regulate cell-mediated immunity including delayed hypersensitivity reactions, activation of macrophages and leukocyte cytolytic processes, and result in the protection and elimination of intracellular pathogens [16,50,52]. On the other hand, infection with *Nippostrongylus barsiliensis* or *Leishmania major* is known to induce a Th-2 response [51]. This immune response is characterized by secretion of cytokines such as IL-4, IL-5, IL-9, IL-10, and IL-13 that predominantly regulate antibody-mediated immunity and generally lead to the protection and clearance of extracellular antigens/pathogens [16,50,52]. During chronic HIV infection, both types of immune response and their associated cytokines are dysregulated, which may result in altered M/M and lymphocyte functions and increased susceptibility to programmed cell death (PCD) [53-56].

The following section will focus on cytokines that play an important role in regulating M/M as well as T lymphocytes effector functions and cell survival. These cytokines include IFN-γ, granulocyte-macrophage colony-stimulating factor (GM-CSF), IL-10, IL-4, IL-2, IL-7, and IL-15 (summarized in Table 1).

Cytokine	Producer cells	Effects on M/M, T cells	STAT signaling in viremic patient
IFN-γ	Th1 lymphocytes, activated NK cells, and CD8 T cells	Upregulates the activation of MHC class I and II, and activates pathogen killing.	Increased STAT1 activation
IFN-α	Leukocytes, and virus-infected cells	Upregulates the activation of MHC class I.	Decreased STAT1 activation
GM-CSF	T cells, Macrophages	Stimulates growth and differentiation of myelomonocytic lineage cells. Enhances phagocytosis.	Not significantly affected
IL-10	T cells, Macrophages	Potent suppressor of monocytes/ macrophage function (e.g. inhibits MHC class II activation, antigen presentation, and phagocytosis).	Not significantly affected
IL-4	Th2 lymphocytes	Induces activation of MHC class II, induces endocytosis, and mannose receptor activation.	Not significantly affected
IL-2	Activated T lymphocytes and dendritic cells	Promotes T cell proliferation and T reg development	Decreased STAT5 activation
IL-7	Bone marrow and stromal cells in lymphoid organs	Maintains thymocytes survival.	Decreased STAT5 activation
IL-15	M/M, dendritic cells, mast cells, epithelial cells, and fibroblast	Induces survival and proliferation of CD8 T cells, NK cells and NK T cells.	Not significantly affected

Table 1. Cytokines and their effects on monocyte/macrophage and T lymphocyte functions

4.1. Cytokines that affect monocytes

Cytokines such as IFN-γ and GM-CSF affect mainly M/M, while, IL-10 and IL-4 act on both M/M and lymphocytes. IFN-γ is an 18-kDa potent pleiotropic cytokine produced by NK cells, NK T cells, Th-1, and CD8+ T cells. It has a critical role in the regulation of both innate and adaptive immunity [57,58]. It inhibits Th-2 and promotes Th-1 cell polarization and differentiation. Also, it inhibits viral replication and regulates cell death [57,58]. Moreover, it activates monocytes and macrophages, increases MHC class II expression, promotes antigen processing and presentation, and enhances their phagocytic, antimicrobial, and tumoricidal activities [59-64]. For instance, it has been shown that treatment of M/M with IFN-γ enhanced phagocytic activity against many pathogens including *Aspergillus fumigatus, Cryptococcus neoformans, Listeria monocytogenes, Mycobacterium avium, Toxoplama cruzi and gondii* [26,61,65]. Other studies have revealed that the lack of IFN-γ responses, such as in IFN- γ, IFN-γ receptor (IFN-γR), or STAT1-deficient mice, or in patients with mutations in the IFN-γ-R gene, lead to impaired immunity and increased susceptibility to infection [66-70]. GM-CSF is a 22-kDa protein secreted by macrophages and T cells. It facilitates growth and differentiation of monocyte and granulocyte lineages. It also enhances M/M effector functions including phagocytic, antimicrobial and antiparasitic activities [71,72].

IL-10 is a potent immunosuppressive and anti-inflammatory cytokine produced by macrophages and T cells. It downregulates MHC class II molecule expression and antigen presentation to CD4+ T cells [73,74]. It also inhibits the expression of co-stimulatory molecules, B7.1/B7.2, on monocytes and macrophages as well as the production of various cytokines such as TNF-α, IL-1, IL-2, IFN-γ, IL-3, and GM-CSF [73,75,76]. In addition, it suppresses macrophage nitric oxide production, and anti-fungal activity [77]. Moreover, it stimulates proliferation and differentiation of B cells, and polarizes T cells towards a Th-2 type response [17,78].

IL-4 is a 20-kDa cytokine secreted by Th-2 lymphocytes that promotes a Th-2 immune response. It has dual immunoregulatory functions [18]. It activates B cell differentiation and antibody production. Also, it enhances macrophage cytotoxicity and their expression of MHC class II and mannose receptor [79-84]. On the other hand, it inhibits cytokine secretion such as TNF-α, IL-1, IL-6, IL-18, GM-CSF and granulocyte colony-stimulating factor (G-CSF) [85-94]. It also suppresses cytokine-induced macrophage activation, oxidative burst, and intracellular killing [62,95]. Moreover, it downregulates monocyte adhesion and CD14 expression [96,97], monocyte-mediated cytotoxicity, nitric oxide production, and anti-fungal activity [77,98].

4.2. Cytokines that affect lymphocytes

Cytokines that share the γ-chain receptor, such as IL-2, IL-7, and IL-15, play a critical role in lymphocyte growth and differentiation [36,99]. IL-2 is a protein produced mainly by activated CD4 but also CD8 T lymphocytes and dendritic cells. It is a T cell growth factor and plays a critical role in regulating the immune response. It plays a major role in activating the immune system in the presence of antigenic stimulation, but also in downregulating this response following pathogen clearance. IL-2 stimulates T cell proliferation and is essential for developing regulatory T cells. In addition, IL-2 has been shown to upregulate expression of Tumor Necrosis Family death receptor ligand, FasL, in activated T cells thereby enhancing their susceptibility to activation-induced cell death [100,101].

IL-7 is a pleiotropic cytokine secreted by bone marrow and stromal cells of lymphoid organs. It stimulates the growth and maintains the survival of thymocytes (B and T lymphocyte progenitor cells) by increasing the expression of the anti-apoptotic molecule Bcl-2 and downregulating the expression of the pro-apoptotic molecule Bax [102-105]. Thus, it is an essential element for T cell survival, proliferation, and optimal effector function.

IL-15 is a cytokine that is produced by different cell types including M/M, dendritic cells, mast cells, epithelial cells, and fibroblasts. It plays an important role in growth and homeostasis. It provokes adaptive and innate immune responses. For example, it shares several biological effects with IL-2 such as mediating survival and proliferation of naïve and memory CD8 T cells. It also stimulates NK T cell expansion and regulates the development of NK cells and its cytotoxicity [36,99,106].

It has been reported that during the course of chronic HIV infection, many inflammatory and anti-inflammatory cytokines such as TNF-α, IFN-β, IFN-γ, IL-18, IL-2, IL-10, and IL-4 are increased in patients serum [77,107-115], and thus may play a role in the alteration of M/M and T lymphocyte functions and signaling pathways (Table 1) [38-42]. Several studies have also proposed and used cytokines such as IFN-γ, GM-CSF, IL-4, IL-2, IL-7 and IL-15 as therapeutics in clinical trials for diseases including HIV and myeloma in an attempt to compensate for impairments in the cytokine network [36,99,116-118].

4.3. Cytokine signaling pathways

Cytokine signaling pathways can be defined as biochemical signaling cascades that are triggered within minutes to relay the information required to mediate various cytokine-dependent cellular functions [119-123]. Most cytokines share general mechanisms of signal transduction in which cytokine-cytokine receptor binding causes the assembly of the specific receptor subunits. Subsequently, a number of tyrosine kinases from the Src and Syk families are activated leading to signal transduction through mainly three major signaling pathways: (i) Janus Kinase (JAK)/Signal Transducer and Activator of Transcription (STAT), (ii) Phosphoinositide 3-kinase (PI3K), and (iii) Mitogen-activated protein kinase (MAPK) [124-126]. These signaling pathways form a very complex and evolutionarily conserved network.

A general overview of these cascades is illustrated in Figure 1. Briefly, when the ligand-receptor interaction occurs, subsequent events are activated based on the nature of these ligands and receptors. For example, a receptor with intrinsic kinase activity (e.g. epidermal growth factor receptor) is usually autophosphorylated directly leading to the creation of a docking site for an adapter protein complex called Grb2/SOS (son of sevenless) [36]. As a result, SOS is recruited to the plasma membrane where it encounters and activates a small G protein named Ras [36,127,128]. Activated Ras induces the activation of several downstream signaling molecules, including a serine/threonine kinase called Raf, which in turn activates the MAPK and PI3K signaling pathways [36,127,129]. PI3K signaling molecules can also be activated directly via the p110α catalytic subunit of the PI3K [127]. A receptor with no intrinsic kinase activity (e.g. cytokine receptors) generally requires activation of receptor-associated kinases such as JAKs for its phosphorylation. Subsequently, activated JAKs can activate the STAT signaling pathway directly and also interact with and activate Grb2/SOS, which in turn activates PI3K and MAPK signaling [36,122,130,131].

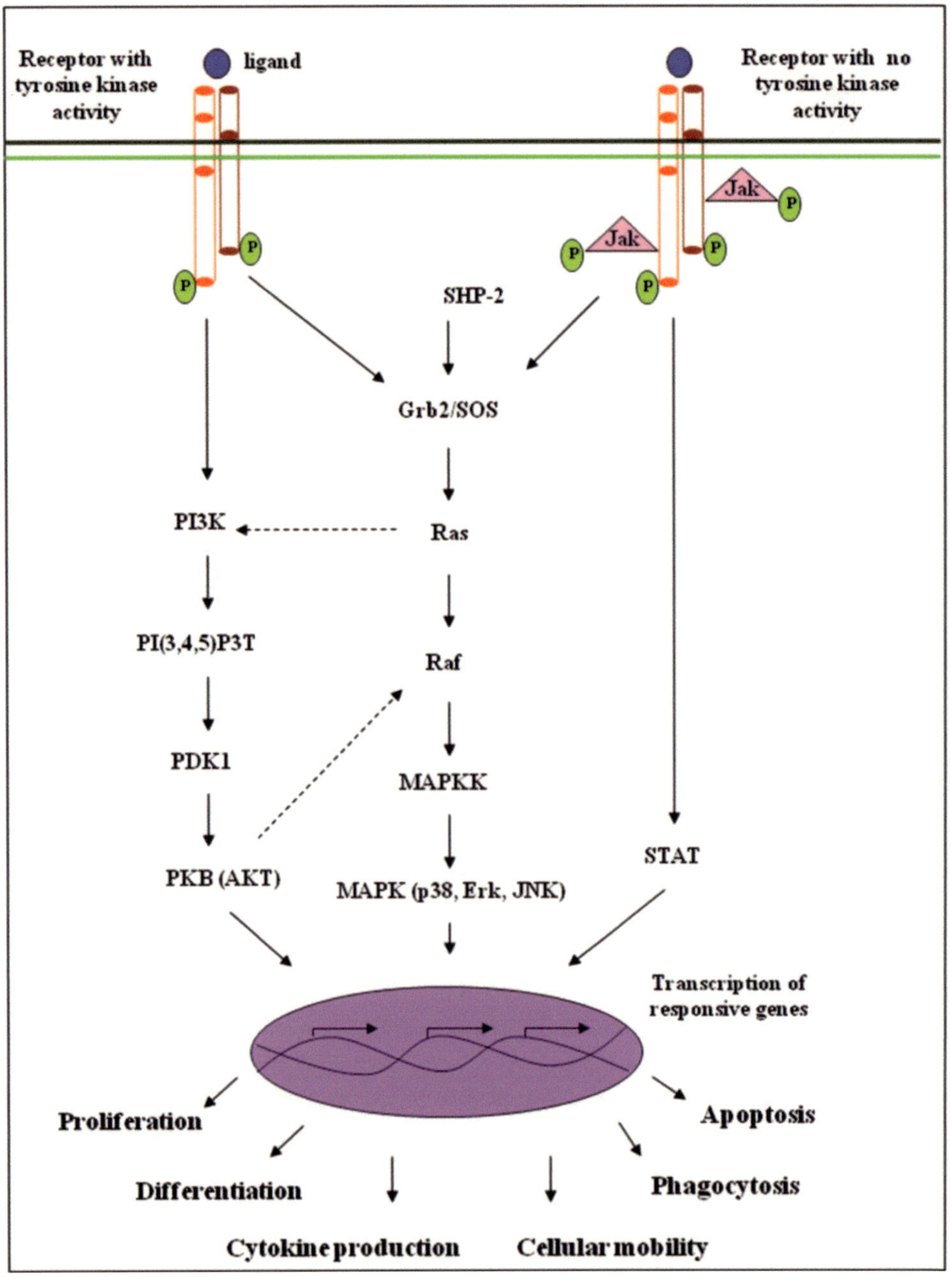

Figure 1. Overview of the major intracellular signaling pathways Upon ligand-receptor binding, signal transduction triggers takes place based on the type and nature of the receptor. If the receptor has intrinsic tyrosine kinase activity, autophosphorylation of the tyrosine residues of the receptor will occur and thus creates docking sites for a variety of different signaling molecules that have SH2 and PTB domains. Grb2/SOS complexes bind to docking sites and lead to recruitment of SOS (son of sevenless) to the plasma membrane where they interact with Ras. Subsequently, activated Ras molecules activate several downstream molecules including Raf, MAPKK, and MAPK. The PI3K signaling pathway can be activated directly via the p110α catalytic subunit of the PI3K. Phosphorylated receptors also

http://dx.doi.org/10.5772/53010

activate phospholipase Cγ (PLCγ), which activate Protein Kinase C (PKC) and calcium-dependent signaling pathways. If the receptor has no intrinsic kinase activity, activation of the Janus Kinase (Jak) or other receptor-associated kinase occurs. Subsequently, activated Jaks phosphorylate the receptor and thus create docking sites for various signaling molecules including members of the Signal Transducers and Activators of Transcription (STAT) family. Signal transduction culminates in the transcriptional activation of STAT responsive genes that influence cellular proliferation, differentiation, cytokine production, mobility, phagocytosis, and survival [modified from [187]].

Evidence has also demonstrated the presence of a complex crosstalk between these pathways. For instance, it has been shown that Jak2 is responsible for the activation of STAT, Erk MAPK, and Akt signaling pathways in response to growth hormone in hepatoma and preadipocyte cells [132]. Another report has demonstrated a role for Akt in serine phosphorylation of the STAT1 transcription factor and upregulation of gene expression in response to IFN-γ [133].

HIV-induced perturbation of the JAK/STAT, PI3K, and MAPK signaling pathways in immune cells including M/M and T lymphocytes has been documented (summarized in Table 1, 4) [41,134-146]. These effects appear to be to the advantage of the virus. On one hand, it may help the virus to replicate and establish infection. On the other hand, it may also help the virus to escape the immune system. In the following subsections, we will provide a brief overview of cytokine signaling and where HIV infection appears to target these cascades.

4.3.1. JAK/STAT signaling pathway

The JAK/STAT pathway is one of the major signaling pathways involved in cytokine responses. Studies have shown that many ligands such as epidermal growth factor (EGF), receptor tyrosine kinases (RTK), G protein-coupled receptors (GPCR) and several cytokine families including interferons and interleukins are the main triggers of the JAK/STAT signaling cascade [147-149]. An overview of the JAK/STAT signal transduction pathway is illustrated in Figure 1. Initially, cytokine-receptor interaction triggers tyrosine transphosphorylation of receptor-associated JAKs. This is followed by phosphorylation of receptor cytoplasmic domains by JAKs and recruitment of latent STAT proteins via their Src homology 2 (SH2) domains to the activated (tyrosine phosphorylated) receptor. This is followed by STAT tyrosine phosphorylation. Activated STATs form dimers via their SH2 domains and are translocated into the nucleus where they bind STAT responsive elements [119,120,123], and thus promote transcription of STAT responsive genes such as cytokine-inducible SH2-containing protein (CIS), members of the IRF family, and numerous other genes [150-153].

In mammalian cells, four JAKs (Jak1, Jak2, Jak3 and Tyk2) and seven STAT proteins (STAT1, 2, 3, 4, 5a, 5b, and 6) with their different isoforms have been identified. [147,154]. Through IL-6-induced signaling, Jak1 is the principal kinase in the downstream signaling cascade. It has been shown in many cell lines that down regulation of Jak1 would lead to impaired signal transduction. Activated JAKs lead to phosphorylation of STAT proteins. However, JAK kinases do not appear to show specificity for a particular STAT protein [147,154]. STAT proteins play an important role in regulating and maintaining both innate and adaptive immune responses (summarized in Table 2) [119-121,123]. For instance, studies have suggested that impairment of JAK/STAT signaling may increase susceptibility to many infections including HIV [65,67,70,155].

STAT gene	Activating cytokines	Examples of STAT responsive genes	Phenotype of knockout mice
STAT1	IFNs,IL-6,IL-10	IRF-1, ISG54, MIG, GBP, CIITA	Impaired IFN and innate immune responses, increase susceptibility to tumors, opportunistic and viral infections
STAT2	IFNs	IRF-1, ISG54	Impaired Type-1 IFN responses
STAT3	IL-2,IL-6,IL-10	JunB, SAA3, JAB, C-reactive protein, Bcl-xL	Embryonic lethal
STAT4	IL-12	IFN-γ, IRF-1, MHC class II, CD23, Fc-γRI	Defect in IL-4 and IL-12 responses, and impaired Th1 differentiation.
STAT5 a, b	Numerous (e.g. IL-2,IL-7,IL-15, GM-CSF)	CIS, IL-2R-α, β-casein, osm, pim1, p21	Impaired proliferation, growth and survival, defect in IL-2 responses, impaired growth.
STAT6	IL-4,IL-13	IL-4R-α, C-γ-1, C-γ-4	Defect in IL-4 responses, and impaired Th1 differentiation.

Table 2. STATs proteins and their role in the immune system

A number of reports have suggested that defects in cytokine responsiveness arise in different cell types during chronic HIV infection and these defects could be due to the direct effects of HIV and/or its proteins, or due to indirect effects associated with alterations of the host cytokine profile [38-42,139,141-143,156]. In M/M, it has been revealed that GM-CSF-induced STAT5 activation in monocyte-derived macrophages (MDM) is inhibited by *in vitro* HIV-1 infection [156]. Other *in vitro* reports have suggested that HIV and its Gp120 and Nef proteins are capable of activating STAT1 and STAT3 in monocytic cell lines and MDM [141-143]. Recently, the HIV matrix protein p17 has been shown to induce STAT1 and pro-inflammatory cytokines in macrophages [139]. Moreover, in *ex* vivo studies, we found that among the responses to cytokines tested (IFN-γ, IFN-α, IL-10, IL-4, and GM-CSF) in terms of STAT induction in monocytes, only IFN-γ showed a significant upregulation of STAT1 activation in HIV+ patients that were off antiretroviral therapy (ART) compared to HIV- controls and patients on ART [39]. Furthermore, this potentiation of IFN-γ-induced STAT1 activation was associated with increased total STAT1 expression levels and monocyte cell death [39]. Another *ex vivo* study has shown a defect in IFN-α induced STAT1 activation in monocytes obtained from a similar set of HIV patients, and this defect was due to the decreased IFN-α receptor expression levels on these cells [42].

In lymphocytes, we and others have shown that both IL-7Rα expression and IL-7-induced STAT5 activation was impaired in CD8 T cells from HIV+ patients [36,40,41]. STAT activation in response to IL-4 and IL-10 did not appear to be similarly impaired [40]. We also found that IL-2-induced STAT5 activation was inhibited in CD8+ T cells from a subset of HIV-infected patients naive to therapy, but was restored, at least in part, after ART [38]. Somewhat similar results have been observed in other *in vitro* studies in which activation of STAT5 in response to IL-2 was inhibited by HIV-1 infection through prior Gp120-CD4 interactions in CD4+ T cells [37,144].

http://dx.doi.org/10.5772/53010

4.3.2. PI3K signaling pathway

Phosphoinositide 3-kinases or phosphatidylinositol-3-kinases (PI3Ks) belong to a family of enzymes that have serine/threonine kinase activity. These enzymes can be activated by various stimuli including growth factors, antigens, cytokines [157,158], and are capable of phosphorylating the third position hydroxyl group of the inositol ring of phosphatidylinositol (PtdIns) [157,159]. This family is composed of four classes, which differ in their structure and functions (known as Ia, Ib, II, and III). However, all of them contain at least one catalytic domain and one regulatory domain [157,159]. Many PI3K cellular functions rely on the ability of PI3Ks to activate protein kinase B (PKB, also known as Akt) (Figure 1). In humans, three Akt genes have been identified named *akt1*, *akt2*, and *akt3*.

PI3-kinases have been shown to play a major role in diverse cellular functions, including cell growth, proliferation, differentiation, survival, and migration [160-163]. Thus, dysregulation of this pathway may influence different cellular responses that are associated with immunity as well as carcinogenesis (Table 3) [157,164]. It has also been reported that there is a basal activation of the PI3K/Akt pathways in macrophages that is required for their survival [165]. Certain reports have suggested a critical role for PI3K signaling in chronic immune activation by promoting cell survival [166]. For instance, an *in vitro* study has revealed that HIV infection and its protein Tat was sufficient to activate the PI3K/Akt pathway in macrophages [166]. Interestingly, PI3K/Akt inhibitors including Miltefosine, an antiprotozoal drug known to inhibit PI3K/Akt pathway, significantly reduced HIV-1 production from infected macrophages and increased susceptibility to cell death in response to extracellular stress, as compared to uninfected cells [166]. Another study has shown that inhibition of Akt phosphorylation is required for TNF related apoptosis inducing ligand (TRAIL)-induced cell death in HIV infected macrophages [167].

Target Gene	Phenotype
$p85^{\alpha}$	Decreased B cell development and activation, increased antiviral responses
$p85^{\beta}$	Increased insulin sensitivity
$p110^{\alpha}$	Embryonic lethal and defective proliferation
$P110^{\beta}$	Embryonic lethal
$P110^{\gamma}$	Decreased T cell development and activation, decreased inflammation, chemotaxis, and oxidative burst
PTEN	Embryonic lethal, autoimmune disease, decreased T cell development, increased T cell activation, and chemotaxis
SHIP1	Increased myeloid cell proliferation and survival, increased B cell activation, chemotaxis, and mast cell degranulation
SHIP2	Perinatal lethal

Table 3. Characteristics of PI3K knockout mice

Viral protein	Effects on M/M	Effects on lymphocytes
gp120	Stimulates STAT1 activation	Stimulates STAT1 activation
p17	Stimulates STAT1 activation	No report
Tat	Stimulates MAPK, Akt activation	Stimulates Akt, MAPK activation
Nef	Stimulates STAT1 & 3, MAPK activation	Stimulates Erk & p38 MAPK activation
Vpr	Stimulates MAPK activation	No report
HIV infection	Inhibits STAT5 activation, Stimulates STAT1, Akt activation	Inhibits STAT5 activation, Stimulates STAT1, MAPK activation

Table 4. HIV viral proteins and their effects on monocytes/macrophages and lymphocytes

4.3.3. MAPK signaling pathway

Mitogen-activated protein kinases (MAPKs) are also a family of enzymes that have serine/threonine kinase activity [168]. This family of kinases is generally activated in response to various extracellular stimuli such as growth factors and inflammatory signals, as well as cellular stress. They regulate different cellular processes including mitosis, proliferation, differentiation, and cell death [168]. The MAPK family is composed of three major subfamilies of kinases known as the extracellular receptor kinases (ERKs), the c-Jun N-terminal kinases/stress-activated protein kinases (JNK/SAPK) and the p38 MAP kinases [169]. Activation of a specific MAP kinase requires activation of a small GTP binding protein (e.g. Ras) which results in the phosphorylation of a series of downstream kinases (Figure 1) [128]. Activation of the MAPK kinase kinase (MAPKKK) (e.g. Raf) leads to the activation of downstream MAPK kinase (MAPKK), and finally, specific MAPK (p38, Erk or JNK) [170,171]. The Erk MAPK family is found in two isoforms called Erk1 and Erk2. Both isoforms are phosphorylated by members of the MEK family, which are often activated by extracellular stimuli such as growth factors, LPS and chemotherapeutic agents [129,172,173]. The JNK family is found in three isoforms named JNK1, JNK2, and JNK3 [174], while the P38 family is found in five different isoforms called p38 (SAPK2), p38β, p38β2, p38γ (SAPK3), and p38δ [175,176]. Both JNK and p38 MAPKs are phosphorylated by SAPK/Erk kinases (SEKs) and mitogen-activated protein kinase kinases (MKKs), which are usually induced by inflammatory cytokines as well as other stressors such as endotoxins, reactive oxygen species, protein synthesis inhibitors, and ultraviolet (UV) irradiation [174,177-179]. MAPKs have been shown to activate various downstream transcription factors such as activator transcription factor (ATF)-2, SP-1 (a member of Specificity Protein/Krüppel-like Factor family) and activator protein (AP)-1, and even STAT3 [178,180-182].

Several reports have shown that activation of the MAPKs resulted in phosphorylation of HIV Rev, Tat, Nef, and p17 proteins and enhanced viral replication [140,183]. Other studies have demonstrated a role for MAPK in regulating monocyte and lymphocyte functions and cell death during HIV infection. For example, in monocytes, it has been shown that the HIV Tat protein stimulates IL-10 production via activation of calcium/MAPK signaling pathways in human monocytes [134,135,184]. Another report has suggested that HIV Vpr is capable of inducing programmed cell death in primary monocytes and the monocytic cell line THP-1 cells [185]. Further, it has been shown that HIV and its protein nef induced FasL, Programmed Death-1 expression and apoptosis in peripheral blood mononuclear cells (PBMCs) and the Jurkat T cell line through activation of the p38 MAPK signaling pathway [138,186].

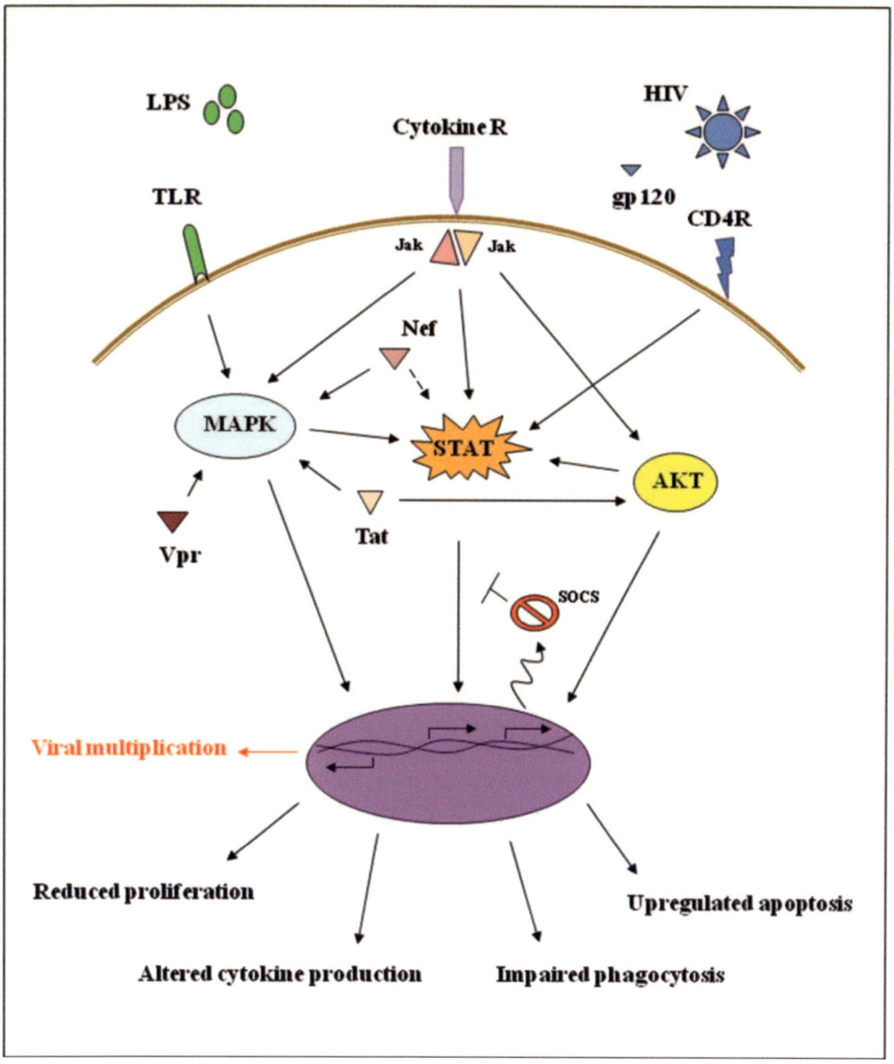

Figure 2. A model for the effect of chronic HIV infection on cellular signal transduction Cell signaling molecules may be regulated directly or indirectly during chronic HIV infection. In the direct setting, HIV and its proteins (Gp120, Nef, Tat, Vpr), through the binding of cellular receptors or internalization by endocytosis, alter signaling pathways including JAK/STAT, PI3K, and MAPK. In the indirect scenario, HIV infection may adversely affects the host cytokine network, which may in turn affect signal transduction. Both scenarios may thus promote viral replication and defective host immune effector functions and reduce immune cell survival [modified from [187].

5. Conclusion

It is well established that HIV targets the immune system and mainly immune cells that express the CD4 surface receptor, but the virus is not exclusive to these cells. Thus, through the course of chronic HIV infection the immune system becomes progressively impaired and unable to protect the body from opportunistic pathogens. This impairment not only includes CD4 T cell depletion, but also the dysregulation of immune cell effector functions, and a skewed cytokine/chemokine expression profile. These effects may be due to the disruption of the described signaling pathways as a result of direct HIV infection, through the action of numerous viral proteins and/or the chronic, but defective state of host immune activation, as summarized in Figure 2. Understanding the molecular mechanisms and identifying the key molecules involved in this impairment may provide important insight towards developing new therapeutic strategies aimed at prolonging the life span of HIV infected individuals and clearing HIV from the host.

Author details

Abdulkarim Alhetheel[1*], Mahmoud Aly[2] and Marko Kryworuchko[3]

*Address all correspondence to: abdulkarimfahad@hotmail.com or aalhetheel@ksu.edu.sa

1 Department of Microbiology, Faculty of Medicine, King Saud University, Riyadh, Saudi Arabia

2 King Abdullah International Medical Research Center, National Guard Hospital, Riyadh, Saudi Arabia

3 Department of Veterinary Microbiology, Western College of Veterinary Medicine, University of Saskatchewan, Saskatoon, Canada

References

[1] Barre-Sinoussi F, Chermann JC, Rey F, Nugeyre MT, Chamaret S, Gruest J, et al. Isolation of a T-lymphotropic retrovirus from a patient at risk for acquired immune deficiency syndrome (AIDS). Science 1983 May 20;220(4599):868-71.

[2] Chinen J, Shearer WT. Molecular virology and immunology of HIV infection. J Allergy Clin Immunol 2002 Aug;110(2):189-98.

[3] Levy JA, Hoffman AD, Kramer SM, Landis JA, Shimabukuro JM, Oshiro LS. Isolation of lymphocytopathic retroviruses from San Francisco patients with AIDS. Science 1984 Aug 24;225(4664):840-2.

[4] Chaplin DD. 1. Overview of the immune response. J Allergy Clin Immunol 2003 Feb; 111(2 Suppl):S442-S459.

http://dx.doi.org/10.5772/53010

[5] Levy JA. Pathogenesis of human immunodeficiency virus infection. Microbiol Rev 1993 Mar;57(1):183-289.

[6] Delves PJ, Roitt IM. The immune system. Second of two parts. N Engl J Med 2000 Jul 13;343(2):108-17.

[7] Delves PJ, Roitt IM. The immune system. First of two parts. N Engl J Med 2000 Jul 6;343(1):37-49.

[8] Medzhitov R, Janeway C, Jr. Innate immunity. N Engl J Med 2000 Aug 3;343(5): 338-44.

[9] Liu YJ. IPC: professional type 1 interferon-producing cells and plasmacytoid dendritic cell precursors. Annu Rev Immunol 2005;23:275-306.

[10] Cullen BR. Is RNA interference involved in intrinsic antiviral immunity in mammals? Nat Immunol 2006 Jun;7(6):563-7.

[11] Uematsu S, Akira S. The role of Toll-like receptors in immune disorders. Expert Opin Biol Ther 2006 Mar;6(3):203-14.

[12] Kato H, Takeuchi O, Sato S, Yoneyama M, Yamamoto M, Matsui K, et al. Differential roles of MDA5 and RIG-I helicases in the recognition of RNA viruses. Nature 2006 May 4;441(7089):101-5.

[13] Hornung V, Guenthner-Biller M, Bourquin C, Ablasser A, Schlee M, Uematsu S, et al. Sequence-specific potent induction of IFN-alpha by short interfering RNA in plasmacytoid dendritic cells through TLR7. Nat Med 2005 Mar;11(3):263-70.

[14] Schlee M, Hornung V, Hartmann G. siRNA and isRNA: two edges of one sword. Mol Ther 2006 Oct;14(4):463-70.

[15] Romagnani S. Regulation of the T cell response. Clin Exp Allergy 2006 Nov;36(11): 1357-66.

[16] Mosmann TR, Coffman RL. TH1 and TH2 cells: different patterns of lymphokine secretion lead to different functional properties. Annu Rev Immunol 1989;7:145-73.

[17] Itoh K, Hirohata S. The role of IL-10 in human B cell activation, proliferation, and differentiation. J Immunol 1995 May 1;154(9):4341-50.

[18] Paul WE. Interleukin-4: a prototypic immunoregulatory lymphokine. Blood 1991 May 1;77(9):1859-70.

[19] de Jong MA, Geijtenbeek TB. Human immunodeficiency virus-1 acquisition in genital mucosa: Langerhans cells as key-players. J Intern Med 2009 Jan;265(1):18-28.

[20] Iqbal SM, Kaul R. Mucosal innate immunity as a determinant of HIV susceptibility. Am J Reprod Immunol 2008 Jan;59(1):44-54.

[21] Sharma D, Bhattacharya J. Cellular & molecular basis of HIV-associated neuropathogenesis. Indian J Med Res 2009 Jun;129(6):637-51.

[22] Boasso A, Shearer GM. Chronic innate immune activation as a cause of HIV-1 immunopathogenesis. Clin Immunol 2008 Mar;126(3):235-42.

[23] Cadogan M, Dalgleish AG. HIV immunopathogenesis and strategies for intervention. Lancet Infect Dis 2008 Nov;8(11):675-84.

[24] Yoo J, Chen H, Kraus T, Hirsch D, Polyak S, George I, et al. Altered cytokine production and accessory cell function after HIV-1 infection. J Immunol 1996 Aug 1;157(3):1313-20.

[25] Baqui AA, Meiller TF, Zhang M, Falkler WA, Jr. The effects of HIV viral load on the phagocytic activity of monocytes activated with lipopolysaccharide from oral microorganisms. Immunopharmacol Immunotoxicol 1999 Aug;21(3):421-38.

[26] Kedzierska K, Azzam R, Ellery P, Mak J, Jaworowski A, Crowe SM. Defective phagocytosis by human monocyte/macrophages following HIV-1 infection: underlying mechanisms and modulation by adjunctive cytokine therapy. J Clin Virol 2003 Feb;26(2):247-63.

[27] Thomas CA, Weinberger OK, Ziegler BL, Greenberg S, Schieren I, Silverstein SC, et al. Human immunodeficiency virus-1 env impairs Fc receptor-mediated phagocytosis via a cyclic adenosine monophosphate-dependent mechanism. Blood 1997 Nov 1;90(9):3760-5.

[28] Amirayan-Chevillard N, Tissot-Dupont H, Capo C, Brunet C, Dignat-George F, Obadia Y, et al. Impact of highly active anti-retroviral therapy (HAART) on cytokine production and monocyte subsets in HIV-infected patients. Clin Exp Immunol 2000 Apr;120(1):107-12.

[29] Choe W, Volsky DJ, Potash MJ. Induction of rapid and extensive beta-chemokine synthesis in macrophages by human immunodeficiency virus type 1 and gp120, independently of their coreceptor phenotype. J Virol 2001 Nov;75(22):10738-45.

[30] Denis M, Ghadirian E. Alveolar macrophages from subjects infected with HIV-1 express macrophage inflammatory protein-1 alpha (MIP-1 alpha): contribution to the CD8+ alveolitis. Clin Exp Immunol 1994 May;96(2):187-92.

[31] Tartakovsky B, Turner D, Vardinon N, Burke M, Yust I. Increased intracellular accumulation of macrophage inflammatory protein 1beta and its decreased secretion correlate with advanced HIV disease. J Acquir Immune Defic Syndr Hum Retrovirol 1999 Apr 15;20(5):420-2.

[32] Polyak S, Chen H, Hirsch D, George I, Hershberg R, Sperber K. Impaired class II expression and antigen uptake in monocytic cells after HIV-1 infection. J Immunol 1997 Sep 1;159(5):2177-88.

[33] Shao L, Sperber K. Impaired regulation of HLA-DR expression in human immunodeficiency virus-infected monocytes. Clin Diagn Lab Immunol 2002 Jul;9(4):739-46.

[34] Clerici M, Hakim FT, Venzon DJ, Blatt S, Hendrix CW, Wynn TA, et al. Changes in interleukin-2 and interleukin-4 production in asymptomatic, human immunodeficiency virus-seropositive individuals. J Clin Invest 1993 Mar;91(3):759-65.

[35] Clerici M, Shearer GM. A TH1-->TH2 switch is a critical step in the etiology of HIV infection. Immunol Today 1993 Mar;14(3):107-11.

[36] Sirskyj D, Theze J, Kumar A, Kryworuchko M. Disruption of the gamma c cytokine network in T cells during HIV infection. Cytokine 2008 Jul;43(1):1-14.

[37] Kryworuchko M, Pasquier V, Theze J. Human immunodeficiency virus-1 envelope glycoproteins and anti-CD4 antibodies inhibit interleukin-2-induced Jak/STAT signalling in human CD4 T lymphocytes. Clin Exp Immunol 2003 Mar;131(3):422-7.

[38] Kryworuchko M, Pasquier V, Keller H, David D, Goujard C, Gilquin J, et al. Defective interleukin-2-dependent STAT5 signalling in CD8 T lymphocytes from HIV-positive patients: restoration by antiretroviral therapy. AIDS 2004 Feb 20;18(3):421-6.

[39] Alhetheel A, Yakubtsov Y, Abdkader K, Sant N, az-Mitoma F, Kumar A, et al. Amplification of the signal transducer and activator of transcription I signaling pathway and its association with apoptosis in monocytes from HIV-infected patients. AIDS 2008 Jun 19;22(10):1137-44.

[40] Benoit A, Abdkader K, Sirskyj D, Alhetheel A, Sant N, az-Mitoma F, et al. Inverse association of repressor growth factor independent-1 with CD8 T cell interleukin (IL)-7 receptor [alpha] expression and limited signal transducers and activators of transcription signaling in response to IL-7 among [gamma]-chain cytokines in HIV patients. AIDS 2009 Jul 17;23(11):1341-7.

[41] Vranjkovic A, Crawley AM, Patey A, Angel JB. IL-7-dependent STAT-5 activation and CD8+ T cell proliferation are impaired in HIV infection. J Leukoc Biol 2011 Apr; 89(4):499-506.

[42] Hardy GA, Sieg SF, Rodriguez B, Jiang W, Asaad R, Lederman MM, et al. Desensitization to type I interferon in HIV-1 infection correlates with markers of immune activation and disease progression. Blood 2009 May 28;113(22):5497-505.

[43] Westendorp MO, Frank R, Ochsenbauer C, Stricker K, Dhein J, Walczak H, et al. Sensitization of T cells to CD95-mediated apoptosis by HIV-1 Tat and gp120. Nature 1995 Jun 8;375(6531):497-500.

[44] Yang Y, Tikhonov I, Ruckwardt TJ, Djavani M, Zapata JC, Pauza CD, et al. Monocytes treated with human immunodeficiency virus Tat kill uninfected CD4(+) cells by a tumor necrosis factor-related apoptosis-induced ligand-mediated mechanism. J Virol 2003 Jun;77(12):6700-8.

[45] Zhang M, Li X, Pang X, Ding L, Wood O, Clouse K, et al. Identification of a potential HIV-induced source of bystander-mediated apoptosis in T cells: upregulation of trail in primary human macrophages by HIV-1 tat. J Biomed Sci 2001 May;8(3):290-6.

[46] Zhou D, Spector SA. Human immunodeficiency virus type-1 infection inhibits autophagy. AIDS 2008 Mar 30;22(6):695-9.

[47] Jang HR, Rabb H. The innate immune response in ischemic acute kidney injury. Clin Immunol 2009 Jan;130(1):41-50.

[48] Nadeen Ikram, Khalid Hassan, Samina Tufail. Cytokines. Int J Pathology 2004;2(1): 47-58.

[49] Aman MJ, Leonard WJ. Cytokine signaling: cytokine-inducible signaling inhibitors. Curr Biol 1997 Dec 1;7(12):R784-R788.

[50] Cohen MC, Cohen S. Cytokine function: a study in biologic diversity. Am J Clin Pathol 1996 May;105(5):589-98.

[51] Mueller SN, Hosiawa-Meagher KA, Konieczny BT, Sullivan BM, Bachmann MF, Locksley RM, et al. Regulation of homeostatic chemokine expression and cell trafficking during immune responses. Science 2007 Aug 3;317(5838):670-4.

[52] Lucey DR, Clerici M, Shearer GM. Type 1 and type 2 cytokine dysregulation in human infectious, neoplastic, and inflammatory diseases. Clin Microbiol Rev 1996 Oct; 9(4):532-62.

[53] Alfano M, Poli G. The cytokine network in HIV infection. Curr Mol Med 2002 Dec; 2(8):677-89.

[54] Clerici M, Sarin A, Coffman RL, Wynn TA, Blatt SP, Hendrix CW, et al. Type 1/type 2 cytokine modulation of T-cell programmed cell death as a model for human immunodeficiency virus pathogenesis. Proc Natl Acad Sci U S A 1994 Dec 6;91(25):11811-5.

[55] Estaquier J, Ameisen JC. A role for T-helper type-1 and type-2 cytokines in the regulation of human monocyte apoptosis. Blood 1997 Aug 15;90(4):1618-25.

[56] Sinicco A, Biglino A, Sciandra M, Forno B, Pollono AM, Raiteri R, et al. Cytokine network and acute primary HIV-1 infection. AIDS 1993 Sep;7(9):1167-72.

[57] Schroder K, Hertzog PJ, Ravasi T, Hume DA. Interferon-gamma: an overview of signals, mechanisms and functions. J Leukoc Biol 2004 Feb;75(2):163-89.

[58] Stark GR, Kerr IM, Williams BR, Silverman RH, Schreiber RD. How cells respond to interferons. Annu Rev Biochem 1998;67:227-64.

[59] Barrionuevo P, Beigier-Bompadre M, De La BS, Alves-Rosa MF, Fernandez G, Palermo MS, et al. Immune complexes (IC) down-regulate the basal and interferon-gamma-induced expression of MHC class II on human monocytes. Clin Exp Immunol 2001 Aug;125(2):251-7.

[60] Dellacasagrande J, Ghigo E, Raoult D, Capo C, Mege JL. IFN-gamma-induced apoptosis and microbicidal activity in monocytes harboring the intracellular bacterium Coxiella burnetii require membrane TNF and homotypic cell adherence. J Immunol 2002 Dec 1;169(11):6309-15.

[61] Kedzierska K, Paukovics G, Handley A, Hewish M, Hocking J, Cameron PU, et al. Interferon-gamma therapy activates human monocytes for enhanced phagocytosis of Mycobacterium avium complex in HIV-infected individuals. HIV Clin Trials 2004 Mar;5(2):80-5.

[62] Lehn M, Weiser WY, Engelhorn S, Gillis S, Remold HG. IL-4 inhibits H2O2 production and antileishmanial capacity of human cultured monocytes mediated by IFN-gamma. J Immunol 1989 Nov 1;143(9):3020-4.

[63] Griffith TS, Wiley SR, Kubin MZ, Sedger LM, Maliszewski CR, Fanger NA. Monocyte-mediated tumoricidal activity via the tumor necrosis factor-related cytokine, TRAIL. J Exp Med 1999 Apr 19;189(8):1343-54.

[64] Harris J, De Haro SA, Master SS, Keane J, Roberts EA, Delgado M, et al. T helper 2 cytokines inhibit autophagic control of intracellular Mycobacterium tuberculosis. Immunity 2007 Sep;27(3):505-17.

[65] Gavrilescu LC, Butcher BA, Del Rio L, Taylor GA, Denkers EY. STAT1 is essential for antimicrobial effector function but dispensable for gamma interferon production during Toxoplasma gondii infection. Infect Immun 2004 Mar;72(3):1257-64.

[66] Dalton DK, Pitts-Meek S, Keshav S, Figari IS, Bradley A, Stewart TA. Multiple defects of immune cell function in mice with disrupted interferon-gamma genes. Science 1993 Mar 19;259(5102):1739-42.

[67] Durbin JE, Hackenmiller R, Simon MC, Levy DE. Targeted disruption of the mouse Stat1 gene results in compromised innate immunity to viral disease. Cell 1996 Feb 9;84(3):443-50.

[68] Huang S, Hendriks W, Althage A, Hemmi S, Bluethmann H, Kamijo R, et al. Immune response in mice that lack the interferon-gamma receptor. Science 1993 Mar 19;259(5102):1742-5.

[69] Jouanguy E, Altare F, Lamhamedi-Cherradi S, Casanova JL. Infections in IFNGR-1-deficient children. J Interferon Cytokine Res 1997 Oct;17(10):583-7.

[70] Meraz MA, White JM, Sheehan KC, Bach EA, Rodig SJ, Dighe AS, et al. Targeted disruption of the Stat1 gene in mice reveals unexpected physiologic specificity in the JAK-STAT signaling pathway. Cell 1996 Feb 9;84(3):431-42.

[71] Armitage JO. Emerging applications of recombinant human granulocyte-macrophage colony-stimulating factor. Blood 1998 Dec 15;92(12):4491-508.

[72] Hamilton JA, Anderson GP. GM-CSF Biology. Growth Factors 2004 Dec;22(4):225-31.

[73] Moore KW, O'Garra A, de Waal MR, Vieira P, Mosmann TR. Interleukin-10. Annu Rev Immunol 1993;11:165-90.

[74] Moore KW, de Waal MR, Coffman RL, O'Garra A. Interleukin-10 and the interleukin-10 receptor. Annu Rev Immunol 2001;19:683-765.

[75] Akdis CA, Blaser K. Mechanisms of interleukin-10-mediated immune suppression. Immunology 2001 Jun;103(2):131-6.

[76] Redpath S, Ghazal P, Gascoigne NR. Hijacking and exploitation of IL-10 by intracellular pathogens. Trends Microbiol 2001 Feb;9(2):86-92.

[77] Cenci E, Romani L, Mencacci A, Spaccapelo R, Schiaffella E, Puccetti P, et al. Interleukin-4 and interleukin-10 inhibit nitric oxide-dependent macrophage killing of Candida albicans. Eur J Immunol 1993 May;23(5):1034-8.

[78] Levy Y, Brouet JC. Interleukin-10 prevents spontaneous death of germinal center B cells by induction of the bcl-2 protein. J Clin Invest 1994 Jan;93(1):424-8.

[79] Crawford RM, Finbloom DS, Ohara J, Paul WE, Meltzer MS. B cell stimulatory factor-1 (interleukin 4) activates macrophages for increased tumoricidal activity and expression of Ia antigens. J Immunol 1987 Jul 1;139(1):135-41.

[80] Littman BH, Dastvan FF, Carlson PL, Sanders KM. Regulation of monocyte/macrophage C2 production and HLA-DR expression by IL-4 (BSF-1) and IFN-gamma. J Immunol 1989 Jan 15;142(2):520-5.

[81] Raveh D, Kruskal BA, Farland J, Ezekowitz RA. Th1 and Th2 cytokines cooperate to stimulate mannose-receptor-mediated phagocytosis. J Leukoc Biol 1998 Jul;64(1):108-13.

[82] Stein M, Keshav S, Harris N, Gordon S. Interleukin 4 potently enhances murine macrophage mannose receptor activity: a marker of alternative immunologic macrophage activation. J Exp Med 1992 Jul 1;176(1):287-92.

[83] te Velde AA, Klomp JP, Yard BA, de Vries JE, Figdor CG. Modulation of phenotypic and functional properties of human peripheral blood monocytes by IL-4. J Immunol 1988 Mar 1;140(5):1548-54.

[84] Vercelli D, Jabara HH, Lee BW, Woodland N, Geha RS, Leung DY. Human recombinant interleukin 4 induces Fc epsilon R2/CD23 on normal human monocytes. J Exp Med 1988 Apr 1;167(4):1406-16.

[85] Cheung DL, Hart PH, Vitti GF, Whitty GA, Hamilton JA. Contrasting effects of interferon-gamma and interleukin-4 on the interleukin-6 activity of stimulated human monocytes. Immunology 1990 Sep;71(1):70-5.

[86] Donnelly RP, Fenton MJ, Kaufman JD, Gerrard TL. IL-1 expression in human monocytes is transcriptionally and posttranscriptionally regulated by IL-4. J Immunol 1991 May 15;146(10):3431-6.

[87] Hamilton JA, Whitty GA, Royston AK, Cebon J, Layton JE. Interleukin-4 suppresses granulocyte colony-stimulating factor and granulocyte-macrophage colony-stimulating factor levels in stimulated human monocytes. Immunology 1992 Aug;76(4): 566-71.

[88] Hart PH, Jones CA, Finlay-Jones JJ. Interleukin-4 suppression of monocyte tumour necrosis factor-alpha production. Dependence on protein synthesis but not on cyclic AMP production. Immunology 1992 Aug;76(4):560-5.

[89] Lee JD, Swisher SG, Minehart EH, McBride WH, Economou JS. Interleukin-4 downregulates interleukin-6 production in human peripheral blood mononuclear cells. J Leukoc Biol 1990 May;47(5):475-9.

[90] Standiford TJ, Strieter RM, Chensue SW, Westwick J, Kasahara K, Kunkel SL. IL-4 inhibits the expression of IL-8 from stimulated human monocytes. J Immunol 1990 Sep 1;145(5):1435-9.

[91] te Velde AA, Huijbens RJ, Heije K, de Vries JE, Figdor CG. Interleukin-4 (IL-4) inhibits secretion of IL-1 beta, tumor necrosis factor alpha, and IL-6 by human monocytes. Blood 1990 Oct 1;76(7):1392-7.

[92] Weiss L, Haeffner-Cavaillon N, Laude M, Cavaillon JM, Kazatchkine MD. Human T cells and interleukin 4 inhibit the release of interleukin 1 induced by lipopolysaccharide in serum-free cultures of autologous monocytes. Eur J Immunol 1989 Jul;19(7): 1347-50.

[93] Wong HL, Lotze MT, Wahl LM, Wahl SM. Administration of recombinant IL-4 to humans regulates gene expression, phenotype, and function in circulating monocytes. J Immunol 1992 Apr 1;148(7):2118-25.

[94] Yanagawa H, Sone S, Sugihara K, Tanaka K, Ogura T. Interleukin-4 downregulates interleukin-6 production by human alveolar macrophages at protein and mRNA levels. Microbiol Immunol 1991;35(10):879-93.

[95] Ho JL, He SH, Rios MJ, Wick EA. Interleukin-4 inhibits human macrophage activation by tumor necrosis factor, granulocyte-monocyte colony-stimulating factor, and interleukin-3 for antileishmanial activity and oxidative burst capacity. J Infect Dis 1992 Feb;165(2):344-51.

[96] Elliott MJ, Gamble JR, Park LS, Vadas MA, Lopez AF. Inhibition of human monocyte adhesion by interleukin-4. Blood 1991 Jun 15;77(12):2739-45.

[97] Lauener RP, Goyert SM, Geha RS, Vercelli D. Interleukin 4 down-regulates the expression of CD14 in normal human monocytes. Eur J Immunol 1990 Nov;20(11): 2375-81.

[98] Hudson MM, Markowitz AB, Gutterman JU, Knowles RD, Snyder JS, Kleinerman ES. Effect of recombinant human interleukin 4 on human monocyte activity. Cancer Res 1990 Jun 1;50(11):3154-8.

[99] Leone A, Picker LJ, Sodora DL. IL-2, IL-7 and IL-15 as immuno-modulators during SIV/HIV vaccination and treatment. Curr HIV Res 2009 Jan;7(1):83-90.

[100] Refaeli Y, Van PL, London CA, Tschopp J, Abbas AK. Biochemical mechanisms of IL-2-regulated Fas-mediated T cell apoptosis. Immunity 1998 May;8(5):615-23.

[101] Van PL, Abbas AK. Homeostasis and self-tolerance in the immune system: turning lymphocytes off. Science 1998 Apr 10;280(5361):243-8.

[102] Durum SK, Candeias S, Nakajima H, Leonard WJ, Baird AM, Berg LJ, et al. Interleukin 7 receptor control of T cell receptor gamma gene rearrangement: role of receptor-associated chains and locus accessibility. J Exp Med 1998 Dec 21;188(12):2233-41.

[103] Hare KJ, Jenkinson EJ, Anderson G. An essential role for the IL-7 receptor during intrathymic expansion of the positively selected neonatal T cell repertoire. J Immunol 2000 Sep 1;165(5):2410-4.

[104] Huang J, Muegge K. Control of chromatin accessibility for V(D)J recombination by interleukin-7. J Leukoc Biol 2001 Jun;69(6):907-11.

[105] Kang J, DiBenedetto B, Narayan K, Zhao H, Der SD, Chambers CA. STAT5 is required for thymopoiesis in a development stage-specific manner. J Immunol 2004 Aug 15;173(4):2307-14.

[106] Diallo M, Zheng Y, Chen X, He Y, Zhou H, Chen Z. Prospect of IL-2, IL-7, IL-15 and IL-21 for HIV immune-based therapy. Zhong Nan Da Xue Xue Bao Yi Xue Ban 2011 Nov;36(11):1037-45.

[107] Ameglio F, Cordiali FP, Solmone M, Bonifati C, Prignano G, Giglio A, et al. Serum IL-10 levels in HIV-positive subjects: correlation with CDC stages. J Biol Regul Homeost Agents 1994 Apr;8(2):48-52.

[108] Minagawa T, Mizuno K, Hirano S, Asano M, Numata A, Kohanawa M, et al. Detection of high levels of immunoreactive human beta-1 interferon in sera from HIV-infected patients. Life Sci 1989;45(11):iii-vii.

[109] Orsilles MA, Pieri E, Cooke P, Caula C. IL-2 and IL-10 serum levels in HIV-1-infected patients with or without active antiretroviral therapy. APMIS 2006 Jan;114(1):55-60.

[110] Pugliese A, Torre D, Saini A, Pagliano G, Gallo G, Pistono PG, et al. Cytokine detection in HIV-1/HHV-8 co-infected subjects. Cell Biochem Funct 2002 Sep;20(3):191-4.

[111] Reddy MM, Sorrell SJ, Lange M, Grieco MH. Tumor necrosis factor and HIV P24 antigen levels in serum of HIV-infected populations. J Acquir Immune Defic Syndr 1988;1(5):436-40.

[112] Sato A, Tsuji K, Yamamura M, Morita Y, Kanzaki H, Tada J, et al. Increased type 2 cytokine expression by both CD4+ CD45RO+ T cells and CD8+ CD45RO+ T cells in blood circulation is associated with high serum IgE but not with atopic dermatitis. J Invest Dermatol 1998 Dec;111(6):1079-84.

[113] Sindhu S, Toma E, Cordeiro P, Ahmad R, Morisset R, Menezes J. Relationship of in vivo and ex vivo levels of TH1 and TH2 cytokines with viremia in HAART patients with and without opportunistic infections. J Med Virol 2006 Apr;78(4):431-9.

[114] Srikanth P, Castillo RC, Sridharan G, John TJ, Zachariah A, Mathai D, et al. Increase in plasma IL-10 levels and rapid loss of CD4+ T cells among HIV-infected individuals in south India. Int J STD AIDS 2000 Jan;11(1):49-51.

[115] Stylianou E, Aukrust P, Kvale D, Muller F, Froland SS. IL-10 in HIV infection: increasing serum IL-10 levels with disease progression--down-regulatory effect of potent anti-retroviral therapy. Clin Exp Immunol 1999 Apr;116(1):115-20.

[116] de GM, Castrillo JM, Fernandez Guerrero ML. Visceral leishmaniasis in patients with AIDS: report of three cases treated with pentavalent antimony and interferon-gamma. Clin Infect Dis 1993 Jul;17(1):56-8.

[117] Squires KE, Brown ST, Armstrong D, Murphy WF, Murray HW. Interferon-gamma treatment for Mycobacterium avium-intracellular complex bacillemia in patients with AIDS. J Infect Dis 1992 Sep;166(3):686-7.

[118] Sabbatini F, Bandera A, Ferrario G, Trabattoni D, Marchetti G, Franzetti F, et al. Qualitative immune modulation by interleukin-2 (IL-2) adjuvant therapy in immunological non responder HIV-infected patients. PLoS One 2010;5(11):e14119.

[119] Ihle JN. The Stat family in cytokine signaling. Curr Opin Cell Biol 2001 Apr;13(2): 211-7.

[120] Imada K, Leonard WJ. The Jak-STAT pathway. Mol Immunol 2000 Jan;37(1-2):1-11.

[121] Levy DE, Darnell JE, Jr. Stats: transcriptional control and biological impact. Nat Rev Mol Cell Biol 2002 Sep;3(9):651-62.

[122] O'Shea JJ. Jaks, STATs, cytokine signal transduction, and immunoregulation: are we there yet? Immunity 1997 Jul;7(1):1-11.

[123] Ward AC, Touw I, Yoshimura A. The Jak-Stat pathway in normal and perturbed hematopoiesis. Blood 2000 Jan 1;95(1):19-29.

[124] Pokrovskaja K, Panaretakis T, Grander D. Alternative signaling pathways regulating type I interferon-induced apoptosis. J Interferon Cytokine Res 2005 Dec;25(12): 799-810.

[125] Rani MR, Ransohoff RM. Alternative and accessory pathways in the regulation of IFN-beta-mediated gene expression. J Interferon Cytokine Res 2005 Dec;25(12): 788-98.

[126] Wong CK, Zhang J, Ip WK, Lam CW. Intracellular signal transduction in eosinophils and its clinical significance. Immunopharmacol Immunotoxicol 2002 May;24(2): 165-86.

[127] Kolch W. Meaningful relationships: the regulation of the Ras/Raf/MEK/ERK pathway by protein interactions. Biochem J 2000 Oct 15;351 Pt 2:289-305.

[128] Scita G, Tenca P, Frittoli E, Tocchetti A, Innocenti M, Giardina G, et al. Signaling from Ras to Rac and beyond: not just a matter of GEFs. EMBO J 2000 Jun 1;19(11): 2393-8.

[129] Caunt CJ, Finch AR, Sedgley KR, McArdle CA. Seven-transmembrane receptor signalling and ERK compartmentalization. Trends Endocrinol Metab 2006 Sep;17(7): 276-83.

[130] Darnell JE, Jr., Kerr IM, Stark GR. Jak-STAT pathways and transcriptional activation in response to IFNs and other extracellular signaling proteins. Science 1994 Jun 3;264(5164):1415-21.

[131] Stepkowski SM, Kirken RA. Janus tyrosine kinases and signal transducers and activators of transcription regulate critical functions of T cells in allograft rejection and transplantation tolerance. Transplantation 2006 Aug 15;82(3):295-303.

[132] Jin H, Lanning NJ, Carter-Su C. JAK2, but not Src family kinases, is required for STAT, ERK, and Akt signaling in response to growth hormone in preadipocytes and hepatoma cells. Mol Endocrinol 2008 Aug;22(8):1825-41.

[133] Nguyen H, Ramana CV, Bayes J, Stark GR. Roles of phosphatidylinositol 3-kinase in interferon-gamma-dependent phosphorylation of STAT1 on serine 727 and activation of gene expression. J Biol Chem 2001 Sep 7;276(36):33361-8.

[134] Gee K, Angel JB, Ma W, Mishra S, Gajanayaka N, Parato K, et al. Intracellular HIV-Tat expression induces IL-10 synthesis by the CREB-1 transcription factor through Ser133 phosphorylation and its regulation by the ERK1/2 MAPK in human monocytic cells. J Biol Chem 2006 Oct 20;281(42):31647-58.

[135] Leghmari K, Bennasser Y, Tkaczuk J, Bahraoui E. HIV-1 Tat protein induces IL-10 production by an alternative TNF-alpha-independent pathway in monocytes: role of PKC-delta and p38 MAP kinase. Cell Immunol 2008 May;253(1-2):45-53.

[136] Mischiati C, Pironi F, Milani D, Giacca M, Mirandola P, Capitani S, et al. Extracellular HIV-1 Tat protein differentially activates the JNK and ERK/MAPK pathways in CD4 T cells. AIDS 1999 Sep 10;13(13):1637-45.

[137] Mishra S, Mishra JP, Kumar A. Activation of JNK-dependent pathway is required for HIV viral protein R-induced apoptosis in human monocytic cells: involvement of antiapoptotic BCL2 and c-IAP1 genes. J Biol Chem 2007 Feb 16;282(7):4288-300.

[138] Muthumani K, Choo AY, Hwang DS, Premkumar A, Dayes NS, Harris C, et al. HIV-1 Nef-induced FasL induction and bystander killing requires p38 MAPK activation. Blood 2005 Sep 15;106(6):2059-68.

[139] Renga B, Francisci D, D'Amore C, Schiaroli E, Mencarelli A, Cipriani S, et al. The HIV matrix protein p17 subverts nuclear receptors expression and induces a STAT1-dependent proinflammatory phenotype in monocytes. PLoS One 2012;7(4):e35924.

[140] Yang X, Gabuzda D. Regulation of human immunodeficiency virus type 1 infectivity by the ERK mitogen-activated protein kinase signaling pathway. J Virol 1999 Apr; 73(4):3460-6.

[141] Federico M, Percario Z, Olivetta E, Fiorucci G, Muratori C, Micheli A, et al. HIV-1 Nef activates STAT1 in human monocytes/macrophages through the release of soluble factors. Blood 2001 Nov 1;98(9):2752-61.

[142] Kohler JJ, Tuttle DL, Coberley CR, Sleasman JW, Goodenow MM. Human immunodeficiency virus type 1 (HIV-1) induces activation of multiple STATs in CD4+ cells of lymphocyte or monocyte/macrophage lineages. J Leukoc Biol 2003 Mar;73(3):407-16.

[143] Percario Z, Olivetta E, Fiorucci G, Mangino G, Peretti S, Romeo G, et al. Human immunodeficiency virus type 1 (HIV-1) Nef activates STAT3 in primary human monocyte/macrophages through the release of soluble factors: involvement of Nef domains interacting with the cell endocytotic machinery. J Leukoc Biol 2003 Nov; 74(5):821-32.

[144] Selliah N, Finkel TH. HIV-1 NL4-3, but not IIIB, inhibits JAK3/STAT5 activation in CD4(+) T cells. Virology 2001 Aug 1;286(2):412-21.

[145] Vyakarnam A, Matear P, Meager A, Kelly G, Stanley B, Weller I, et al. Altered production of tumour necrosis factors alpha and beta and interferon gamma by HIV-infected individuals. Clin Exp Immunol 1991 Apr;84(1):109-15.

[146] Herbein G, Gras G, Khan KA, Abbas W. Macrophage signaling in HIV-1 infection. Retrovirology 2010;7:34.

[147] Bromberg J, Darnell JE, Jr. The role of STATs in transcriptional control and their impact on cellular function. Oncogene 2000 May 15;19(21):2468-73.

[148] Calo V, Migliavacca M, Bazan V, Macaluso M, Buscemi M, Gebbia N, et al. STAT proteins: from normal control of cellular events to tumorigenesis. J Cell Physiol 2003 Nov;197(2):157-68.

[149] Hebenstreit D, Horejs-Hoeck J, Duschl A. JAK/STAT-dependent gene regulation by cytokines. Drug News Perspect 2005 May;18(4):243-9.

[150] Bach EA, Aguet M, Schreiber RD. The IFN gamma receptor: a paradigm for cytokine receptor signaling. Annu Rev Immunol 1997;15:563-91.

[151] Darnell JE, Jr. STATs and gene regulation. Science 1997 Sep 12;277(5332):1630-5.

[152] Lehtonen A, Matikainen S, Julkunen I. Interferons up-regulate STAT1, STAT2, and IRF family transcription factor gene expression in human peripheral blood mononuclear cells and macrophages. J Immunol 1997 Jul 15;159(2):794-803.

[153] Lehtonen A, Matikainen S, Miettinen M, Julkunen I. Granulocyte-macrophage colony-stimulating factor (GM-CSF)-induced STAT5 activation and target-gene expression during human monocyte/macrophage differentiation. J Leukoc Biol 2002 Mar; 71(3):511-9.

[154] Kohlhuber F, Rogers NC, Watling D, Feng J, Guschin D, Briscoe J, et al. A JAK1/JAK2 chimera can sustain alpha and gamma interferon responses. Mol Cell Biol 1997 Feb; 17(2):695-706.

[155] Bovolenta C, Lorini AL, Mantelli B, Camorali L, Novelli F, Biswas P, et al. A selective defect of IFN-gamma- but not of IFN-alpha-induced JAK/STAT pathway in a subset of U937 clones prevents the antiretroviral effect of IFN-gamma against HIV-1. J Immunol 1999 Jan 1;162(1):323-30.

[156] Warby TJ, Crowe SM, Jaworowski A. Human immunodeficiency virus type 1 infection inhibits granulocyte-macrophage colony-stimulating factor-induced activation of STAT5A in human monocyte-derived macrophages. J Virol 2003 Dec;77(23): 12630-8.

[157] Fruman DA, Meyers RE, Cantley LC. Phosphoinositide kinases. Annu Rev Biochem 1998;67:481-507.

[158] Rodriguez-Viciana P, Warne PH, Dhand R, Vanhaesebroeck B, Gout I, Fry MJ, et al. Phosphatidylinositol-3-OH kinase as a direct target of Ras. Nature 1994 Aug 18;370(6490):527-32.

[159] Wymann MP, Pirola L. Structure and function of phosphoinositide 3-kinases. Biochim Biophys Acta 1998 Dec 8;1436(1-2):127-50.

[160] Katso R, Okkenhaug K, Ahmadi K, White S, Timms J, Waterfield MD. Cellular function of phosphoinositide 3-kinases: implications for development, homeostasis, and cancer. Annu Rev Cell Dev Biol 2001;17:615-75.

[161] Koyasu S. The role of PI3K in immune cells. Nat Immunol 2003 Apr;4(4):313-9.

[162] Vanhaesebroeck B, Leevers SJ, Ahmadi K, Timms J, Katso R, Driscoll PC, et al. Synthesis and function of 3-phosphorylated inositol lipids. Annu Rev Biochem 2001;70:535-602.

[163] Deane JA, Fruman DA. Phosphoinositide 3-kinase: diverse roles in immune cell activation. Annu Rev Immunol 2004;22:563-98.

[164] Sasaki T, Suzuki A, Sasaki J, Penninger JM. Phosphoinositide 3-kinases in immunity: lessons from knockout mice. J Biochem 2002 Apr;131(4):495-501.

[165] Liu H, Perlman H, Pagliari LJ, Pope RM. Constitutively activated Akt-1 is vital for the survival of human monocyte-differentiated macrophages. Role of Mcl-1, independent of nuclear factor (NF)-kappaB, Bad, or caspase activation. J Exp Med 2001 Jul 16;194(2):113-26.

[166] Chugh P, Bradel-Tretheway B, Monteiro-Filho CM, Planelles V, Maggirwar SB, Dewhurst S, et al. Akt inhibitors as an HIV-1 infected macrophage-specific anti-viral therapy. Retrovirology 2008;5:11.

[167] Huang Y, Erdmann N, Peng H, Herek S, Davis JS, Luo X, et al. TRAIL-mediated apoptosis in HIV-1-infected macrophages is dependent on the inhibition of Akt-1 phosphorylation. J Immunol 2006 Aug 15;177(4):2304-13.

[168] Cowan KJ, Storey KB. Mitogen-activated protein kinases: new signaling pathways functioning in cellular responses to environmental stress. J Exp Biol 2003 Apr;206(Pt 7):1107-15.

[169] Zhang YL, Dong C. MAP kinases in immune responses. Cell Mol Immunol 2005 Feb; 2(1):20-7.

[170] Dong C, Davis RJ, Flavell RA. Signaling by the JNK group of MAP kinases. c-jun N-terminal Kinase. J Clin Immunol 2001 Jul;21(4):253-7.

[171] Dong C, Davis RJ, Flavell RA. MAP kinases in the immune response. Annu Rev Immunol 2002;20:55-72.

[172] Nishimoto S, Nishida E. MAPK signalling: ERK5 versus ERK1/2. EMBO Rep 2006 Aug;7(8):782-6.

[173] Sugden PH, Clerk A. Regulation of the ERK subgroup of MAP kinase cascades through G protein-coupled receptors. Cell Signal 1997 Aug;9(5):337-51.

[174] Gupta S, Barrett T, Whitmarsh AJ, Cavanagh J, Sluss HK, Derijard B, et al. Selective interaction of JNK protein kinase isoforms with transcription factors. EMBO J 1996 Jun 3;15(11):2760-70.

[175] Hale KK, Trollinger D, Rihanek M, Manthey CL. Differential expression and activation of p38 mitogen-activated protein kinase alpha, beta, gamma, and delta in inflammatory cell lineages. J Immunol 1999 Apr 1;162(7):4246-52.

[176] Ono K, Han J. The p38 signal transduction pathway: activation and function. Cell Signal 2000 Jan;12(1):1-13.

[177] Ashwell JD. The many paths to p38 mitogen-activated protein kinase activation in the immune system. Nat Rev Immunol 2006 Jul;6(7):532-40.

[178] Kyriakis JM, Banerjee P, Nikolakaki E, Dai T, Rubie EA, Ahmad MF, et al. The stress-activated protein kinase subfamily of c-Jun kinases. Nature 1994 May 12;369(6476): 156-60.

[179] Rouse J, Cohen P, Trigon S, Morange M, onso-Llamazares A, Zamanillo D, et al. A novel kinase cascade triggered by stress and heat shock that stimulates MAPKAP kinase-2 and phosphorylation of the small heat shock proteins. Cell 1994 Sep 23;78(6):1027-37.

[180] Chung J, Uchida E, Grammer TC, Blenis J. STAT3 serine phosphorylation by ERK-dependent and -independent pathways negatively modulates its tyrosine phosphorylation. Mol Cell Biol 1997 Nov;17(11):6508-16.

[181] Hibi M, Lin A, Smeal T, Minden A, Karin M. Identification of an oncoprotein- and UV-responsive protein kinase that binds and potentiates the c-Jun activation domain. Genes Dev 1993 Nov;7(11):2135-48.

[182] Zhang S, Liu H, Liu J, Tse CA, Dragunow M, Cooper GJ. Activation of activating transcription factor 2 by p38 MAP kinase during apoptosis induced by human amylin in cultured pancreatic beta-cells. FEBS J 2006 Aug;273(16):3779-91.

[183] Evans P, Sacan A, Ungar L, Tozeren A. Sequence alignment reveals possible MAPK docking motifs on HIV proteins. PLoS One 2010;5(1):e8942.

[184] Gee K, Angel JB, Mishra S, Blahoianu MA, Kumar A. IL-10 regulation by HIV-Tat in primary human monocytic cells: involvement of calmodulin/calmodulin-dependent protein kinase-activated p38 MAPK and Sp-1 and CREB-1 transcription factors. J Immunol 2007 Jan 15;178(2):798-807.

[185] Saxena M, Busca A, Pandey S, Kryworuchko M, Kumar A. CpG protects human monocytic cells against HIV-Vpr-induced apoptosis by cellular inhibitor of apoptosis-2 through the calcium-activated JNK pathway in a TLR9-independent manner. J Immunol 2011 Dec 1;187(11):5865-78.

[186] Muthumani K, Choo AY, Shedlock DJ, Laddy DJ, Sundaram SG, Hirao L, et al. Human immunodeficiency virus type 1 Nef induces programmed death 1 expression through a p38 mitogen-activated protein kinase-dependent mechanism. J Virol 2008 Dec;82(23):11536-44.

[187] Alhetheel A. HIV-induced dysregulation of IFN-gamma signaling and programmed cell death in human primary monocytes. Ph D Thesis, 2010.

Chapter 2

Role of Dendritic Cell Subsets on HIV-Specific Immunity

Wilfried Posch, Cornelia Lass-Flörl and
Doris Wilflingseder

Additional information is available at the end of the chapter

http://dx.doi.org/10.5772/52744

1. Introduction

DC are key regulators of immunity in view of the fact that they are involved in immune responses against infectious diseases, allergy and cancer [1, 2]. Ralph Steinman was awarded the Nobel Prize for Medicine 2011 for DC discovery in 1973 [3]. Steinman and Cohn [3] described a novel cell type in mouse spleen, which they named ′dendritic cell′ due to their tree-like shape. The major function of DC is the induction of adaptive immunity in the LN.Yet, DC can also interact with innate immune cells, for instance natural killer (NK) and NKT cells [1, 4].

Upon entry of HIV into the host, the virus has to be transported from mucosal surfaces to lymphatic tissues, where it is transmitted to its primary targets, $CD4^+$ T lymphocytes. This process is thought to be contrived by DC.

DC thereby play critical roles during HIV and SIV (simian immunodeficiency virus) infection.

The skin and mucosa are composed of two compartments, the epidermis and the dermis (skin) or stratified squamous epithelium and lamina propria (mucosa), each containing a major subset of DC - Langerhans cells (LC) reside in the suprabasal layers of the epidermis and epithelia [5], while dermal/interstitial DC are distributed throughout the connective tissue of the dermis [6, 7].

Both subsets represent immature DC that are very efficient in Ag uptake and processing. As immature DC (iDC), they reside in peripheral tissue, which they survey for invading pathogens. Upon encounter with antigen (Ag), DC mature (mDC) and migrate to the draining lymph nodes (LN). They pass through different maturation stages, which enable them to fulfill specific tasks such as the uptake, the processing and the presentation of Ag on major histocompatiblity complex (MHC) molecules to naïve T cells. In the T cell area of lymphatic tissue the mature DC stimulate Ag-specific CD4+ and CD8+ T cells to proliferate and develop effector function, such as cytokine production and cytotoxic activity. Effector T cells are recruited to inflamed peripheral tissue and participate in the elimination of pathogens and infected cells. This very particular life cycle illustrates why DC are called the ′sentinels of the immune system′ [8].

In humans, different DC subsets have been identified in blood, spleen and skin, but little is known respecting resident and migratory DC in human LN. This book chapter will review the major DC subsets found in humans and their role in HIV-pathogenesis. If data are available, also the role of the viral opsonization pattern and its impact on DC interaction will be discussed.

2. DC subsets and their role in HIV infection

DC are divided into two main groups: conventional myeloid DC (cDC) and non-conventional plasmacytoid DC (pDC) (Figure 1). As recently described byDoulatov et al. (2010) [9], human multi-lymphoid progenitors can bring forth all lymphoid cell types, including monocytes, macrophages and DC. Nonetheless, most DC in steady-state emerge from a common myeloid progenitor [10]. DC areheterogenous subtypes with distinct functions, properties and localization [11]. DC progenitors migrate from the bone-marrow through the blood to lymphoid organs and peripheral tissues. There, they give rise to different cDC subsets (Figure 1). LC display an exception within the cDC group since they maintain in the epidermis independent on circulating precursors [12]. Within cDC, migratory and lymphoid-resident DC are distinguished: migratory DC travel from peripheral tissues to lymphoid organs, whereas lymphoid-resident DC populate lymphoid organs during their whole lifespan and lack the migratory function. In humans cDC comprise Langerhans Cells (LC), dermal DC (CD103+ and CD103-), BDCA1+ (CD1c)- and BDCA3+ (CD141) DC, and the recently described CD56+ DC (Figure 1). They are localized in the skin, secondary lymphoid organs (spleen, tonsils) and blood. pDC develop in the bone-marrow and then they reside in lymphoid organs [13]. HLA-DR+CD123+pDC express BDCA2 and this cell subset is found in blood, secondary lymphoid organs as well as peripheral tissues, e.g. skin or lungs (Figure 1). The cDC subtypes and pDC express a different receptor repertoir and comprise distinct functions with respect to HIV spread, antiviral activity and transmission, which is reviewed below and shown in Figure 1 (Table adapted from Altfeld et al., [14]). Both cell types are resident in lymphoid tissues in the steady state, but during an inflammatory response, pDC and cDC are actively recruited to these tissues [15-17].

2.1. cDC

2.1.1. LC and HIV

LC survey the basal and suprabasal layers of the stratified squamous epithelium of the skin and oral and ano-genital mucosa for invading pathogens [18-21]. Due to their ideal

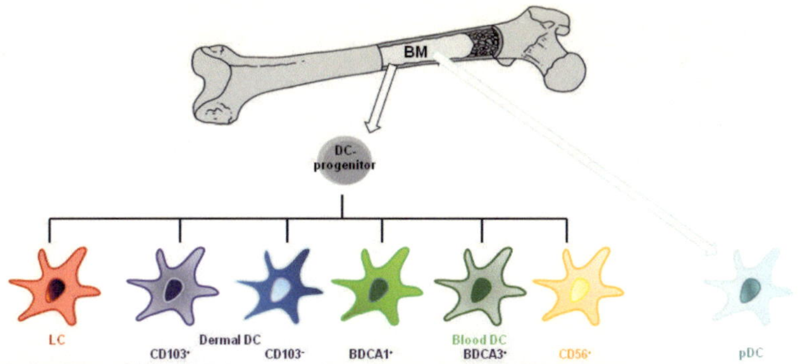

	LC	Dermal DC CD103+	Dermal DC CD103-	Blood DC BDCA1+	Blood DC BDCA3+	CD56+	pDC
C-type lectin expression	Langerin	Langerin DEC-205	DC-SIGN DEC-205	DEC205	CLEC9A	n.d.	BDCA-2
TLR expression	TLR2,3,5	TLR2,3,4,5	TLR2,3,4,5	TLR2,3,4,7,8	TLR2,3,8	n.d.	TLR7,9
Cytokine production	IL-1β, IL-6, IL-8, IL-12, IL-15, IL-23					IL-1β, IL-6	IFNα, IFNβ, IL-6, TNF
Function	•Prime Ag-specific T cells and B cells •NK cell activation by IL-12					• CD56+ γδ T cell activation • NK cell activation	• Treg induction • Plasma cell induction • NK cell activation by IFNs
Role in HIV infection	Degradation of HIV in Birbeck granules	HIV shuttle and transfer	HIV shuttle and transfer	Unknown	Unknown	Unknown	• Production of type I IFN: antiviral and induction of bystander T cell death • Induction of Treg cells by HIV-induced IDO up-regulation • Recruitment of T cells to sites of HIV-infection, thus facilitating viral spread
Pathology during HIV infection	•Reduced frequency in peripheral blood •Conflicting results respecting dysfunction and functionality						• Reduced frequency in peripheral blood • Conflicting results respecting dysfunction and functionality

Figure 1. DC-subsets and functions during HIV-infection (Table adapted from *Altfeld et al., 2011*; CD56+ DC added). HIV co-localizes with Langerin in LC to high extend as shown by confocal microscopic analyses (co-localization: yellow). CD1a+ LC were isolated from human skin, incubated with HIV for 2 hrs, fixed and permeabilized with Cytofix/-perm (BD Biosciences). The cells were then stained using an anti-human Langerin-PE mAb (red, Dendritics) and the anti-HIV-Ab KC57-FITC ((green, Beckman Coulter). The nucleus was stained using DRAQ5TM (blue, Invitrogen) (*Posch et al., unpublished*).

localization in mucosal tissues and their long dendrites to efficiently capture Ag, they comprise the first line defense against mucosal infections. After Ag acquisition, LC start to mature, as represented by up-regulation of co-stimulatory molecules (CD80, CD86, CD40), MHC class I and II molecules, CD83 and CCR7 and down-regulation of Langerin and E-cadherin [22].

Due to CCR7 up-regulation, the mature LC migrate to the LN along a CCL19 and CCL21-leu (leucine isoform of CCL21) gradient to efficiently prime T cells there [23]. Beside initiating an effective adaptive immune response, LC were illustrated by DeWitte et al. [24, 25] to also have important functions with respect to innate immune responses. Beside a specific set of TLRs (TLR2, 3, 5) and high expression of CD1a, LC express Langerin and contain Birbeck granules that might be crucial to their innate function [21, 26-29] (Figure 1). The C-type lectin Langerin interacts with non-opsonized HIV-1 (Figure 2) and other pathogens such as fungi and bacteria, via fucose or mannose residues. Thereby degradation of HIV-1 in Birbeck granules is promoted and HIV-1 dissemination is limited [24].

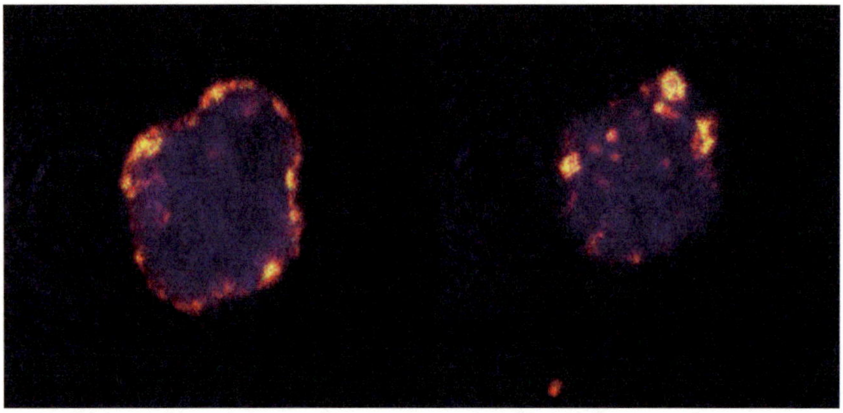

Figure 2. Co-localization of HIV and Langerin on CD1a+ Langerhans Cells isolated from human skin

Early investigations of HIV-LC interactions illustrated that LC are productively infected by HIV and that they efficiently transmit the virus to T cells [30-32]. These results suggested that HIV take advantage of the antigen-capturing properties of LC to reach the T cell zone in the lymphatic tissues and via this route, HIV can establish a productive infection of the host. However, *in vivo* only low percentages of LC are infected and despite abundant expression of the primary HIV-receptor CD4 and the chemokine co-receptor CCR5, high HIV-1 concentrations are required to infect LC *in vitro* [31, 32]. As shown by Wu and KewalRemani [33] the percentages to acquire HIV-1 after heterosexual contact with an HIV-positive individual are between 0.01 to 0.1%, which might be due to a restriction by LC.

Engagement of Langerin trimers on the surface of LC induces formation of Birbeck granules, which are part of the endosomal recycling system and uniquely found in LC (Figure 3, lower right panel) [34]. Upon capture of mycobacterial lipoproteins by Langerin, these were exposed to CD1a molecules in Birbeck granules [35], which suggests that Birbeck granule formation displays a non-classical antigen processing pathway [20]. Also HIV-1 attaches to Langerin on LC and is subsequently routed to Birbeck granules, which points to a role of the granules with respect to degradation of viruses.

Studies by Gejitenbeek´s laboratory [24] showed that under homeostatic conditions, Langerin expressed on LC and acts as restriction factor for HIV infection. They demonstrated that, if HIV-gp120 attaches to Langerin, the viral particle is internalized and subsequently degraded in Birbeck granules. Thus, LC are protected from infection with incoming, non-opsonized HIV particles and HIV-1 is not disseminated throughout the host [24]. The rapid internalization of HIV-1 into LC by Langerin impedes interactions and subsequent fusion with CD4 and CCR5 and also prevents transmission to the main target cells of the virus, CD4+ T cells. Thereby, Langerin acts as a protective anti-HIV barrier during the first steps of HIV-1 infection, if the virus is non-opsonized and if sexually transmitted pathogens are lacking.

As demonstrated, if the host system is facing other sexually transmitted infections, the anti-HIV-1-barrier of LC is abrogated and HIV-1 transfer to susceptible $CD4^+$ T cells is promoted [20, 36, 37]. Pathogens, such as Candida or Neisseria, directly interact with Langerin and compete with HIV-1-binding. Additional factors explaining the by-passing of the anti-HIV-1-barrier function of Langerin are that:

- by high viral loads the receptor becomes saturated,
- infections, e.g. Herpes simplex virus infection, down-regulate Langerin surface expression [20],
- the HIV-1 entry receptors CD4 and CCR5 are up-regulated during additional sexually transmitted infections [37],
- or the antiviral function of Langerin is reverted by inflammation-induced TNF-α (tumor-necrosis-factor α) production due to Candida albicans or Neisseria gonorrhoea [36].

These observations allow to conclude that during acute co-infection the anti-viral function of LC is significantly decreased.

Not only acute co-infection, but also opsonization of HIV with either complement fragments or specific Abs might result in reduction or abolishment of the anti-viral function mediated by Langerin (*Wilflingseder and Posch, unpublished data*). Upon entry of viruses into the body, immediate non-specific immune responses are triggered and within a short time the innate immune system is completely activated. During acute infection multiple humoral and cellular players, including cytokines, complement, acute-phase proteins, DC, macrophages, and natural killer (NK) cells, that co-operate to generate an efficient defense against infection, are activated. HIV-1 spontaneously triggers the complement system also in absence of specific Abs by interactions of gp41 with C1q [38-41]. Due to regulators of complement activation (RCAs) in the viral surface, HIV-1 is very efficiently protected against virolysis, which normally occurs due to MAC (membrane attack complex) formation and destruction of pathogens or infected cells. The incorporation of RCAs in the viral surface acts as protection mechanism and results in opsonization of HIV-1 with complement C3 fragments at the very initial steps following viral entry. After seroconversion, when HIV-1-specific Abs are established, the virus additionally is opsonized with specific IgGs. The different coating patterns of the virus change the receptor used on DC due to the density of complement fragments or Abs on the viral surface [42]. The C-type lectin-virus interaction becomes rather unimportant if the virus is opsonized and is substituted by complement or Fc receptor-virus interactions as already demonstrated using dermal DC [42]. After LC incubation using complement-opsonized HIV-1, we found that not only sexually transmitted diseases abrogate the antiviral barrier mediated via Langerin but also opsonization of HIV-1 (*Wilflingseder and Posch, unpublished data*).

In summary, during acute co-infection or by opsonization with complement fragments or Abs, the anti-viral function of LC is significantly reduced due to competition for Langerin or different receptor utilization. This facilitates HIV-1 infection of LC via CD4 and CCR5, intracellular uptake of the virus (Figure 3) and promotion of HIV-1 transfer to its targets, CD4$^+$ T cells.

On the other hand LC were implicated in establishment of infection due to their location in the foreskin and due to compelling evidence that male circumcision efficiently reduces the risk to become infected with HIV-1 [43]. It was furthermore shown *in vivo* in highly HIV-1-exposed but (IgG) seronegative individuals, that gp41-specific IgA Abs efficiently blocked transfer of sexually transmitted HIV-1 [44-46]. A very recent study by Tudor et al. [46] illustrated that monomeric 2F5 IgA2 bound to gp41 MPER (membrane proximal external region) and free virus with greater efficiency than IgG1 and interferred with the initial HIV-1 transmission via Langerhans Cells. 2F5 IgA2 and IgG1 monomers blocked HIV-1 transcytosis in monostratified or multilayered epithelia as well as in rectal tissue [46, 47]. These Abs decreased infection of CD4$^+$ T cells and transfer from LC to autologous CD4$^+$ T cells [46]. The 2F5 IgA2 monomer inhibited virus transcytosis and CD4$^+$ T cell infection more efficiently, while the 2F5 IgG1 monomer was superior in blocking the LC-CD4$^+$ T cell transmission. A synergistic effect of both, 2F5 IgA2 and IgG1, was observed with respect to LC-CD4$^+$ T cell transmission and decrease of CD4$^+$ T cell infection [46].

2.1.2. Dermal DC and HIV

Along with LC, HIV-1 firstly attaches to dermal (interstitial) DC upon entry at mucosal surfaces (Figure 1). Dermal DC are underlying the epithelium, do not contain Birbeck granules and express heterogenous amounts of CD1a [48].

Interstitial DC are localized in the dermis and oral, vaginal and colonic lamina propria [6, 49-52]. They are characterized by the expression of CD11c, high expression of various C-type lectin receptors (Langerin on CD103$^+$ DC, DC-SIGN on CD103$^-$ DC, DEC-205 on both subsets), TLR2, 3, 4 and 5 and they secrete various cytokines upon pathogenic stimulation (Figure 1). Since there are only 2 studies available on human CD103$^+$ DC and SIV [53, 54], the following chapter refers to CD103$^-$, DC-SIGN$^+$ dermal DC.

In vitro experiments showed that DC efficiently capture HIV-1 or SIV, independent on the maturation status of the cells (Figure 3 and [55]) and subsequently transfer the virus to CD4$^+$ T cells, which initiates a vigorous infection [41, 42, 56, 57]. These experiments imply that *in vivo* HIV exploits DC at mucosal sites as shuttles to CD4$^+$ T cells in the LN, but the exact events with respect to virus spread from mucosal sites to LN have not been enlightened yet. Thereby, DC seem to play a significant role in the spread of infection as well as in the induction of antiviral immunity.

As shown in Figure 3, dermal DC (left panel) and LC (right panel), which emigrated from whole skin explants, take up variable amounts of HIV-1 particles. As demonstrated by Frank et al. [55], human and macaque DC interacted similarly with SIV and ample amounts of virus were captured by DC. Transmission electron microscopic analyses revealed that iDC, which are endocytically highly active, captured few viral particles near the periphery of the membrane, while mDC, which down-regulate the endocytic capacity, retained high

http://dx.doi.org/10.5772/52744

amounts of virions in large vesicular compartments deeper within DC [55]. This points to a diverse entry and handling of virions within iDC and mDC.

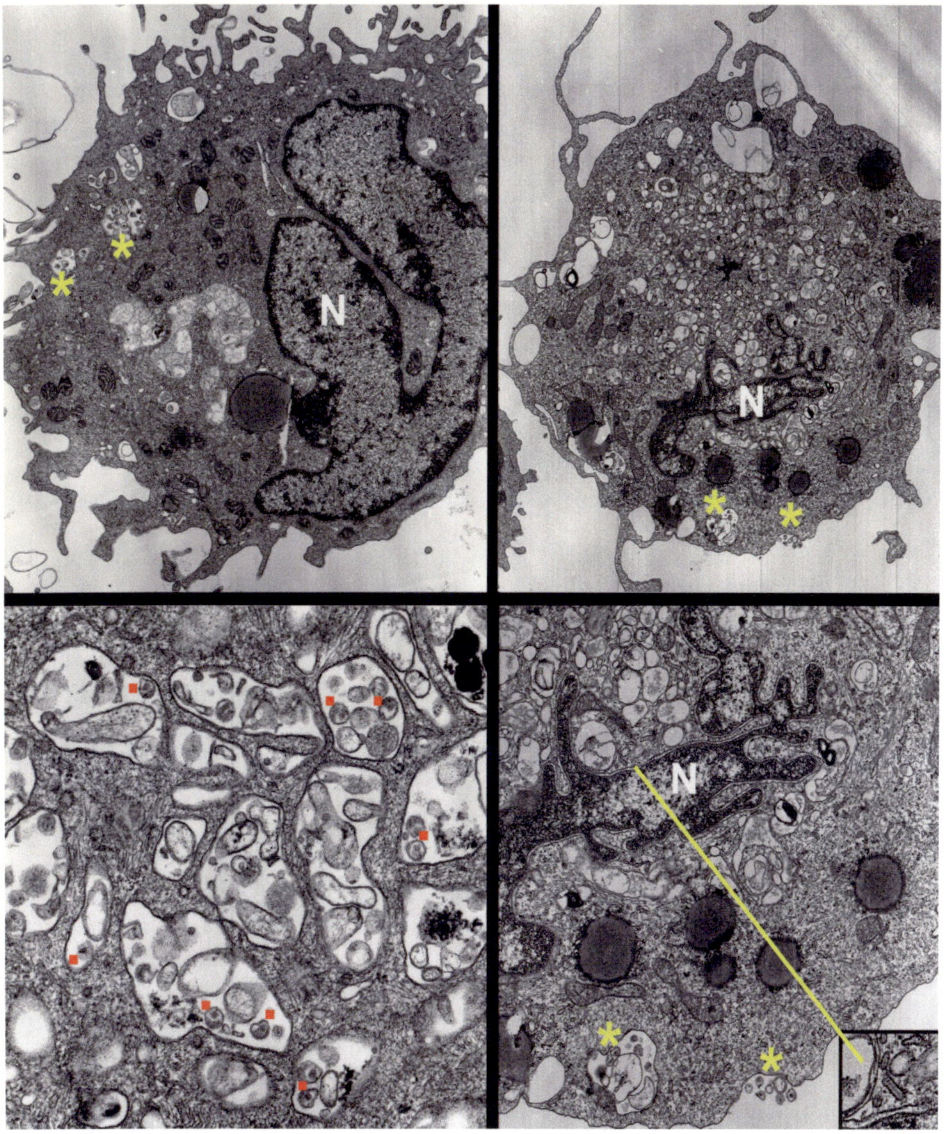

Figure 3. Uptake of HIV into dendritic cells from human skin. Dendritic cells emigrated from whole skin explants were incubated with HIV for 2h and then fixed and embedded for transmission electron microscopy. Variable amounts of viral particles are taken up by dermal dendritic cells (left panels) and epidermal Langerhans cells (right panels). Lower panels show higher magnifications of membrane-enclosed virus particles in a dermal dendritic cell (left panel; some viruses marked with red/black). In a Langerhans cell (lower right panel) viruses can be seen docking onto the surface membrane (right asterisk) and already taken up into vesicular structures (left asterisk). A Birbeck granule is depicted in the inset as the identifying structure for Langerhans cells. N, nucleus.(Photos courtesy of Hella Stössel and Nikolaus Romani).

Beside the different handling of HIV-1 or SIV within iDC and mDC, opsonization of the virus with either complement fragments and/or Abs significantly affects the binding mechanism, internalization and infection of DC as well as their T cell stimulatory capacity [41, 42, 58]. As shown by Pruenster et al. [42], the complement cloud around the virus significantly blocked the accessibility of gp120 and therefore interfered with C-type lectin interaction.

Similar amounts of HIV-1 bound to the surface of DC independent on the opsonization pattern of the virus (Pruenster et al., 2005). The attachment of the differentially opsonized HIV-1-preparations was found to be specific (Figure 4 [*Wilflingseder and Posch, unpublished data*]), since pre-incubation of the DC with blocking Abs against human DC-SIGN, CD11b (CR3-α chain) or CD32 (FcγRII) particularly blocked the interactions with the corresponding virus preparations:

- blocking α-DC-SIGN mAb inhibited interaction with non-opsonized HIV-1 (Figure 4, HIV),
- blocking α-CR3mAb (TMG6.5) significantly interferred with binding of complement-opsonized HIV (HIV-C) to DC (Fig.4, HIV-C) and
- blocking α-CD32mAb (AT10) inhibited binding of Ab-opsonized HIV-1 (Figure 4, HIV-Ig).

Additionally, we found variations respecting infection of DC with differentially opsonized HIV-1 preparations [41]. Productive infection of DC and LC with HIV-1 was described to be relatively inefficient compared to HIV-infection of $CD4^+$ T cells and HIV- or SIV-infected DC are rarely detected *in vivo* (rev. in Piguet and Steinman[59]). Our study using non-, complement-, complement-Ig- or Ig-opsonized HIV-1 uncovered that complement-opsonization of HIV-1 significantly enhanced DC-infection compared to non-opsonized HIV [41] and furthermore acted as an endogenous adjuvans for DC-mediated induction of HIV-specific CTLs [58].

In contrast, HIV-1 coated with specific, non-neutralizing Abs significantly impaired infection of and integration in DC and also *'trans'*-infection of $CD4^+$ T cells after delayed addition of T cells [41].

Despite the low-level productive infection of DC, non-opsonized HIV-1 is very efficiently transmitted to T cells either via de novo (*'cis'*-transfer) or without (*'trans'*-)infection [60]. This is also true for Ab-opsonized HIV-1, if $CD4^+$ T cells are added immediately to HIV-exposed DC [41]. Especially C-type lectins, such as DC-SIGN on dermal DC, were connected to transmitting HIV-1 to T cells in the LN [60, 61]. Similar to Langerin, DC-SIGN has high affinity for mannose and fucose structures, but despite sharing this feature these receptors exert completely different effects and functions regarding pathogen processing. Dermal $CD103^-$ DC express DC-SIGN, which captures low titres of HIV-1 by interaction with the envelope glycoprotein gp120 [62]. By complexing DC-SIGN via gp120, HIV-1 is protected from degradation within the DC in contrast to Langerin, which promotes degradation of the virus through Birbeck granules as described above [24, 62]. DC-SIGN-complexed HIV-1 remains stable and infectious over prolonged periods of time within non-lysosomal acidic organelles of DC [62, 63]. Thereby, DC-SIGN efficiently transfers HIV-1 to CD4⁺ T cells, enhances infection in DC-CD4⁺ T cell co-cultures and facilitates '*trans*'-infection of the T cells [62].

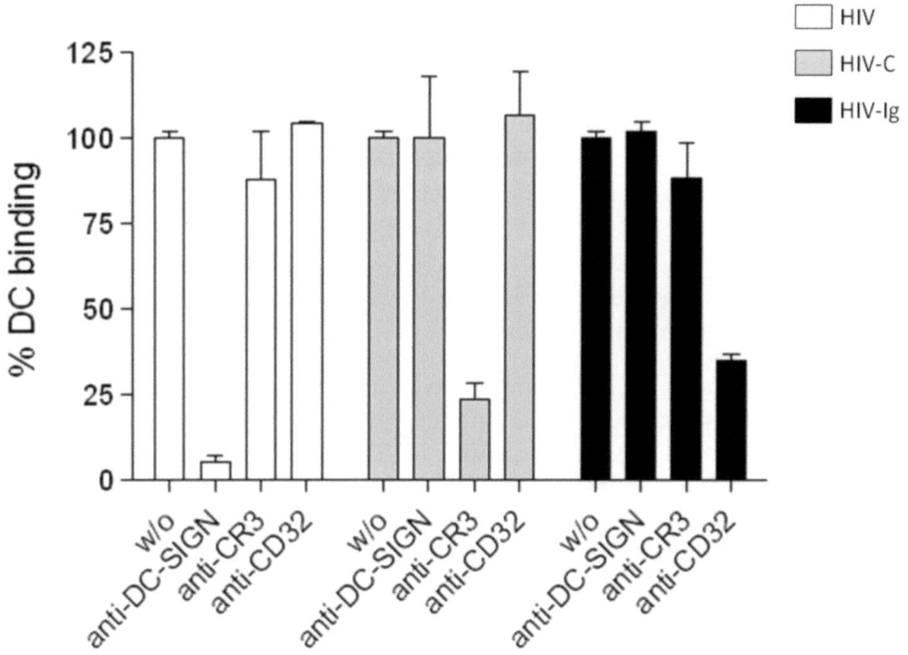

Figure 4. Binding of differentially opsonized HIV (non-opsonized HIV, HIV-C, HIV-Ig) in absence and presence of a blocking anti-human DC-SIGN, CR3 [CD11b] (TMG6.5) or CD32 (AT-10) antibodies. Binding of non-opsonized HIV was signficantly decreased in the presence of a blocking anti-DC-SIGN Ab, but not affected by pre-incubation of the cells with a blocking anti-CR3- or CD32-Ab (white bars). HIV-C-interaction with DC was inhibited using a blocking anti-CD11b (CR3)-Ab TMG6.5, but not by anti-DC-SIGN or CD32 (grey bars). Binding of IgG-opsonized HIV was inhibited by using a blocking anti-human CD32, but not DC-SIGN or CD11b-Ab (black bars).

Lastly, the antigen-presenting capacity of DC was also shown to be modulated by the opsonization pattern of the virus [58]. Earlier studies illustrated the role of complement opsonization respecting induction of effective CTL responses against viral infections, but the exact mechanism was not determined [64-66]. The exclusive role of DC in priming naïve CD8⁺ T cells in response to exogenous cell-associated as well as endogenously synthesized Ags has been shown [67, 68]. Endogenously synthesized antigens from DC infected with LCMV (choriomeningitis virus) mediated strong CTL responses, while macrophages and B cells infected with LCMV did not induce CTLs [68].

We recently found that opsonization of retroviral particles with complement fragments enhanced the ability of DC to induce CTL responses both *in vitro* and *in vivo* [58]. HIV-C-loaded DC mediated significantly higher CD8⁺ T cell expansion and signficantly better antiviral activity than DC exposed to non-opsonized HIV *in vitro*. This was further verified *in vivo* using the murine Friend virus model. These results indicated that 'complement acts as natural adjuvant for DC-induced expansion and differentiation of specific CTLs against retroviruses' [58].

Additionally, we demonstrated that in contrast to complement opsonization, antibody-coating of the viral surface attenuated the CTL-stimulatory capacity of HIV-exposed DC [69]. In some HIV-1-positive individuals, high levels of antibodies and low levels of complement fragments coat the HIV-1 surface and therefore we investigated the effects of the non-neutralizing Abs bound to the surface of HIV-1 on the CTL-stimulatory capacity of DC. We observed *ex vivo* and *in vitro* that DC loaded with IgG-opsonized HIV significantly impaired the HIV-1-specific $CD8^+$ T cell response compared to the earlier described efficient $CD8^+$ T cell activation induced by DC exposed to complement-opsonized HIV. These novel modulatory effects of the HIV-1-opsonization pattern on the CTL-activating capacity of DC might influence future vaccination strategies, since strong transient Ab responses subsequent to vaccination might weaken the CTL-induction by DC, which has to be considered [69].

Preferential expression of CCR5 on immature LC and DC restricts the transmission of X4-tropic isolates at the site of infection. Additionally, *ex vivo* analyses revealed that X4-tropic HIV replicate worse in DC and LC compared to R5-tropic viruses [31, 70, 71]. The relatively low susceptibility of DC to HIV-1-infection but efficient transfer of virus to CD4+ T cells was lately ascribed to an HIV-1 escape mechanism from innate recognition by DC [72, 73]. Manel et al. [72] showed that if DC by-pass resistance to HIV-1 infection [74, 75], they mature, exert a type I IFN response as well as adaptive immune responses. More recently, Laguette et al. [73] described the restriction factor SAMHD1 (SAM domain and HD domain-containing protein 1) to be responsible for inhibiting HIV-1 replication in DC and other cells of the myeloid lineage by degrading or preventing accumulation of HIV-1 DNA due to a putative nucleotidase activity. As shown by Lahouassa et al. [76], SAMHD1 depletes the pool of intracellular dNTPs and thus restricts HIV-1 infection in DC by blocking reverse transcription. These recent important findings respecting a formerly unknown cryptic innate sensor in DC, SAMHD1, and the induction of an efficient type I IFN and adaptive immune response due to DC infection might pave the way for novel therapeutical approaches to treat retroviral infections.

2.1.3. Blood DC and HIV

2.1.3.1. BDCA1⁺ DC, BDCA3⁺ DC, CD56⁺ DC and HIV

$BDCA1^+$ myeloid DC can be directly isolated from human blood. This population was described to be reduced in the blood of HIV-infected individuals [76-78]. We found that $BDCA1^+$ DC exerted a decreased transmission of HIV-1 to autologous $CD4^+$ T cells, when the virus was opsonized with specific IgGs in contrast to non- or complement-opsonized HIV-1 and when the T cells were added delayed [41]. When $CD4^+$ T cells were immediately added after washing the differentially loaded DC, the same infection efficiency was observed using HIV, HIV-C or HIV-Ig [41]. The two-phase transfer of HIV to DC as described above (*trans*-infection: by-passing of the virus from endolysosomal compartments, first 24 hrs; *cis*-infection: ′de novo′ HIV-1-infection of DC before transfer to T cells) was also observable in BDCA1$^+$ DC, because non- and complement-opsonized HIV-1, which cause productive infection of DC, efficiently infected autologous CD4$^+$ T cells in short- and long-term co-cultures. BDCA1$^+$ DC exposed to IgG-opsonized HIV-1, which were not productively infected by the virus, were not able to promote long-term transfer of HIV-1 to susceptible T cells [41].

BDCA3$^+$ DC represent the human equivalent to mouse CD8α^+ DC and they are the major producers of IFN-λ in response to dsRNA poly I:C [80].As recently described by Dutertre et al. [81] using an 11-color flow cytometric strategy, circulating BDCA1$^+$ DC and BDCA3$^+$ DC counts were reduced in 15 viremic, untreated patients compared to 8 HIV-1-positive individuals under treatment and 13 healthy donors. By using this method, they illustrated that both blood DC subsets expressed characteristic lineage markers: BDCA1$^+$ DC expressed CD14, while particularly BDCA3$^+$ DC displayed CD56 on their surface. BDCA3$^+$ DC were shown to be more significantly down-modulated in viremic patients compared to controls [82] and it remains to be investigated by longitudinal studies, if combined antiretroviral therapy can restore the pool of circulating myeloid BDCA1$^+$ and BDCA3$^+$ DC.

Blood CD56$^+$ DC were recently described by Gruenbacher et al. [83] and comprise intermediate-sized lymphocytes with an HLA-DR^{high}, CD80$^+$ and CD86$^+$ expression profile. Upon cultivation they acquire DC-like morphology with increased levels of above mentioned surface markers. Upon stimulation, they are able to efficiently stimulate CD56$^+\gamma\delta$ T cells, which results in secretion of IFNγ, TNF-α, and IL-1β [84]. The role of CD56$^+$ DC respecting HIV-1 infection and pathogenesis needs to be further investigated.

2.2. pDC and HIV

Plasmacytoid DC (pDC) (Figure 1) or type 1 IFN-producing dendritic cells are innate immune cells in blood, which are specialized in releasing massive amounts of IFNα and IFNβ upon viral challenge, including HIV-1 [83]. They constitute <0.2-0.5% of peripheral blood mononuclear cells (PBMC) [85] and in humans, pDC express the characteristic surface markers BDCA-2 (CD303, CLEC4C) and CD123 along with BDCA4 (CD304, NRP1), but they do not express CD11c, a marker of myeloid DC, or CD14 [86].

pDCs are key players of the innate immune response *in vivo* and they can prime adaptive immunity due to the afore mentioned production of high type I interferon levels, especially upon exposure to viral products [15, 83]. Upon stimulation with DNA or RNA viruses, they produce up to 1000-fold higher amounts of type I interferons than other cells [84, 87, 88]. The IFNα production in pDC by viruses represents a two-step process – uptake of viruses occurs due to recognition of envelope glycoproteins by C-type lectin receptors, e.g. mannose receptor or BDCA2, but induction of IFNα in fact starts in endosomal compartments by ligation of TLR9 or TLR7 [89-91]. Pathogenic single-stranded RNA or unmethylated DNA are mainly recognized by TLR7 and TLR9 expressed inside pDC [92]. Thus, the viruses have to be ingested by pDC into endosomes and NFkB- and MAPK signals through MyD88 must be stimulated [93]. Not only viruses, but also virus-infected cells can potently activate IFNα production from pDC [94]. Once activated, pDCs mature and produce large quantities of pro-inflammatory and antiviral cytokines [95-97]. pDC respond with high amounts of different IFNα subsets, IFNβ, IFNκ, IFNλ and IFNω on a wide range of enveloped viruses including HIV-1. They additionally produce pro-inflammatory cytokines TNFα, IFNγ and IL-6 as well as chemokines CXCL-10, CCL-5 and CCL-4 among others [98]. Thereby, pDC also act as a linker between innate and adaptive immunity.

Data by Zhou et al. [99] indicate that subsequent to HIV-1 challenge, signaling via TLR7 triggers autophagy and increased IFNα production from human pDC. The IFNα secretion mediated by an autophagy-dependent pathway may play an important role for T cell triggering during HIV-1 pathogenesis.

Beside acting as pro-inflammatory cells, pDC also provide negative regulatory signals and thus induce tolerance. pDC express IDO (indoleamine 2,3-dioxygenase) and PDL-1 (programmed death ligand; 1) which are associated with the negative modulation of T cell responses and regulatory T cell induction [100-102].

During acute HIV-1 infection, NK cells are recruited and activated by pDC to the sites of infection and to LN due to IFNα secretion [103, 104]. IFNα was demonstrated to increase the perforin levels in NK and $CD8^+$ T cells. At the sites of infection ′DC-editing′ occurs by NK cells, since activated NK cells delete immature pDC to select for the more immunogenic mature pDC [105-108].Beside NK cell recruitment and activation, pDC-secreted IFNα promotes maturation and migration of other DC subsets. Due to their localization, it is unlikely that pDC are involved in HIV-1 capture, transport and transmission, but they are supposed to control HIV-1 in the acute phase of infection due to their immediate antiviral and NK priming activity.

Chronic exposure to HIV-1 leads to hyperactivation of pDC resulting in simultaneous type I IFN secretion and IDO expression. Thus, pDC concurrently exert cytotoxic and suppressive effects on T cells during chronic HIV-1 infection [109].

HIV-1 infection not only disrupts DC homeostasis within myeloid DC subsets, but also pDC homeostasis is defective during chronic HIV-1 infection. cDC and pDC are lost from blood, which correlates with high viral loads and low $CD4^+$ T cell counts [76, 110-113]. Deficiencies in pDC function were among the earliest observations of immune dysfunction in HIV-1 infection and some of the earliest studies of the ′natural IFN-α-producing cells′ (i.e. pDC) illustrated that PBMC from AIDS patients were severely compromised in their ability to produce IFN-α *in vitro* after stimulation with the virus.

Cell death and/or a failure of bone marrow progenitors to differentiate into pDC might contribute to the loss of pDC from blood of chronically infected individuals. In non-pathogenic models of SIV infection, no depletion of blood pDC was observed [114, 115] and HIV-1-positive individuals, who are able to control infection (= long-term non-progressors) were also shown to have increased numbers of blood pDC [111].In contrast, it was described that during HIV-2 infection, which is highly attenuated compared to HIV-1 infection in humans, also the numbers of blood pDC is found reduced [116]. Thereby, the exact role of pDC depletion during HIV infection is not clear yet.

The depletion of cDC from the sites of infection was ascribed to a higher expression of CCR7 on the surface of cDC and a signficantly increased CCL19 expression in LN of SIV-infected animals, thus suggesting that inflamed LN lure cDC away from the sites of infection early during progressive SIV infection [117]. A similar mechanism can be imagined for pDC, which are recruited to inflamed LN via CXCL9 and E-selectin [16, 118], but the pDC loss could also be due to direct infection, enhanced apoptosis or CD95 up-regulation [119-123].

Not only pDC numbers are decreased during on-going HIV-1 infection, but also the quality of the cells is suffering. They exert a reduced ability to migrate towards the CXCR4 ligand CXCL12 [124], they stimulate Treg cells to dampen HIV-1 immunity and they furthermore shift the Treg-Th17 balance [125, 126]. So far, interactions of differentially opsonized HIV-1 preparations with pDC has not been investigated.

3. Outlook: Impact of the HIV-1 opsonization pattern on DC function

As follows of investigations on HIV-1 in the last 30 years, antibody responses against the virus are not effective and cellular immune responses not powerful enough to suppress or even control HIV-1. DC, the prime inducers and regulators of immunity and tolerance, are crucial in designing modern vaccines [127-130]. Therefore, nowadays vaccine science shall combine established classical vaccine approaches with new attempts based on the expanded immunological knowledge.

Innate and adaptive immune responses are needed to generate efficient, long-lasting protection. Immediate innate responses involve activation of the complement system, ligation of pattern recognition receptors e.g. TLRs, C-type lectins, activation of NK cells, cDC and pDC, and type I, II, as well as III interferons. For viral clearance, the optimal balance between $CD4^+$ and $CD8^+$ T cells is required during the adaptive immune responses. Current HIV-1 vaccination strategies include the use of peptides or monocyte-derived DC exposed to chemically inactivated HIV-1 and aim in designing a vaccine efficiently inducing both, cellular and humoral immune responses [131-133]. So far, disappointing results have been achieved in clinical trials targeting either cellular [134, 135] or humoral immunity [136, 137]. The most prominent AIDS vaccine trial so far was the RV144 in Thailand [138], which evoked strong, but transient Env-specific $CD4^+$ T cell and Ab responses, but only weak HIV-specific $CD8^+$ T cell responses [131, 138].

HIV-1 induces immediate responses of the immune system upon entering mucosal surfaces. There, the complement system constitutes a first line of defense against the virus. Recently, we illustrated an important role for complement opsonization of retroviruses as an endogenous adjuvant for DC-mediated CTL-induction [58].

Efficient early $CD8^+$ T cell responses are crucial in controlling HIV-1 replication and their key role in HIV-1 control is additionally substantiated by association of certain HLA class I alleles and an improved disease progression [139-141]. In view of our very recent observations ([58], [69]), we propose that $CD8^+$ T cells are efficiently primed by DC during acute viral infection, particularly by enhanced infection of DC with HIV-C [41]. Thus, more efficient presentation of endogenously synthesized viral Ags via HLA-ABC [41], and ore efficient cross-presentation from incoming complement-opsonized HIV-1 are mediated. In contrast, Ab-opsonization of HIV-1 weakens the CTL-induction by modulation of DC function and might influence future vaccination strategies [69].

As shown by Lu et al. [142-144] *in vitro* and *in vivo,* DC exposed to chemically (aldrithiol-2, AT-2)-inactivated HIV or SIV induced a virus-specific CTL response. This response was strong enough to kill HIV-1-infected CD4$^+$ T cells [142], to control the viral load in SIV-infected monkeys [143] and HIV-infected individuals [144].. The decrease of the viral load in the HIV-1-infected patients was associated with a higher amount of HIV-1-gag-specific CD8$^+$ T cells and HIV-1-specific CD4$^+$ T cells.

LC were described to allow more cross-priming of CD8$^+$ T cells, while dermal DC are more specialized in primingnaive CD4$^+$ T cells [145]. The finding that complement-opsonization of HIV prior loading of DC significantly enhanced the CD8$^+$ T cell-stimulatory capacity of the cells in combination with using specific DC subtypes might efficiently improve future vaccination strategies and there is good reason to address DC of the skin, especially Langerhans cells, for purposes of vaccination.

A greater understanding of the innate and adaptive processes and the different functions of DC subsets to HIV-1 infection will lead to development of an effective vaccine.

Acknowledgements

The authors would like to thank Nikolaus Romani and Hella Stössl for providing the transmission electron microscopic picture.

The work of the authors is supported by the Austrian Science Fund [FWF, P22165 and P24598 to DW], the Tyrolean Science Fund [TWF, project: D-155140-016-011 to WP] and the OeNB [project: 14875 to WP].

Author details

Wilfried Posch, Cornelia Lass-Flörl and Doris Wilflingseder

Innsbruck Medical University, Division of Hygiene and Medical Microbiology, Innsbruck, Austria

References

[1] Steinman RM, Hemmi H. Dendritic cells: translating innate to adaptive immunity. Curr Top Microbiol Immunol 2006; 311:17-58.

[2] Steinman RM, Idoyaga J. Features of the dendritic cell lineage. Immunol Rev 2010; 234:5-17.

[3] Steinman RM, Cohn ZA. Identification of a novel cell type in peripheral lymphoid organs of mice. I. Morphology, quantitation, tissue distribution. J Exp Med 1973; 137:1142-62.

[4] Fernandez NC, Lozier A, Flament C, et al. Dendritic cells directly trigger NK cell functions: cross-talk relevant in innate anti-tumor immune responses in vivo. Nat Med 1999; 5:405-11.

[5] Romani N, Holzmann S, Tripp CH, Koch F, Stoitzner P. Langerhans cells - dendritic cells of the epidermis. APMIS 2003; 111:725-40.

[6] McLellan AD, Heiser A, Sorg RV, Fearnley DB, Hart DN. Dermal dendritic cells associated with T lymphocytes in normal human skin display an activated phenotype. J Invest Dermatol 1998; 111:841-9.

[7] Dupasquier M, Stoitzner P, van Oudenaren A, Romani N, Leenen PJ. Macrophages and dendritic cells constitute a major subpopulation of cells in the mouse dermis. J Invest Dermatol 2004; 123:876-9.

[8] Banchereau J, Steinman RM. Dendritic cells and the control of immunity. Nature 1998; 392:245-52.

[9] Doulatov S, Notta F, Eppert K, Nguyen LT, Ohashi PS, Dick JE. Revised map of the human progenitor hierarchy shows the origin of macrophages and dendritic cells in early lymphoid development. Nat Immunol 2010; 11:585-93.

[10] Schlenner SM, Madan V, Busch K, et al. Fate mapping reveals separate origins of T cells and myeloid lineages in the thymus. Immunity 2010; 32:426-36.

[11] Heath WR, Carbone FR. Dendritic cell subsets in primary and secondary T cell responses at body surfaces. Nat Immunol 2009; 10:1237-44.

[12] Merad M, Manz MG. Dendritic cell homeostasis. Blood 2009; 113:3418-27.

[13] Randolph GJ, Ochando J, Partida-Sanchez S. Migration of dendritic cell subsets and their precursors. Annu Rev Immunol 2008; 26:293-316.

[14] Altfeld M, Fadda L, Frleta D, Bhardwaj N. DCs and NK cells: critical effectors in the immune response to HIV-1. Nat Rev Immunol 2011; 11:176-86.

[15] Cella M, Jarrossay D, Facchetti F, et al. Plasmacytoid monocytes migrate to inflamed lymph nodes and produce large amounts of type I interferon. Nat Med 1999; 5:919-23.

[16] Yoneyama H, Matsuno K, Zhang Y, et al. Evidence for recruitment of plasmacytoid dendritic cell precursors to inflamed lymph nodes through high endothelial venules. Int Immunol 2004; 16:915-28.

[17] Yoneyama H, Matsuno K, Toda E, et al. Plasmacytoid DCs help lymph node DCs to induce anti-HSV CTLs. J Exp Med 2005; 202:425-35.

[18] Katz SI, Tamaki K, Sachs DH. Epidermal Langerhans cells are derived from cells originating in bone marrow. Nature 1979; 282:324-6.

[19] Romani N, Stingl G, Tschachler E, et al. The Thy-1-bearing cell of murine epidermis. A distinctive leukocyte perhaps related to natural killer cells. J Exp Med 1985; 161:1368-83.

[20] de Jong MA, Geijtenbeek TB. Langerhans cells in innate defense against pathogens. Trends Immunol 2010; 31:452-9.

[21] Romani N, Clausen BE, Stoitzner P. Langerhans cells and more: langerin-expressing dendritic cell subsets in the skin. Immunol Rev 2010; 234:120-41.

[22] Merad M, Ginhoux F, Collin M. Origin, homeostasis and function of Langerhans cells and other langerin-expressing dendritic cells. Nat Rev Immunol 2008; 8:935-47.

[23] Villablanca EJ, Mora JR. A two-step model for Langerhans cell migration to skin-draining LN. Eur J Immunol 2008; 38:2975-80.

[24] de Witte L, Nabatov A, Pion M, et al. Langerin is a natural barrier to HIV-1 transmission by Langerhans cells. Nat Med 2007; 13:367-71.

[25] de Witte L, Nabatov A, Geijtenbeek TB. Distinct roles for DC-SIGN+-dendritic cells and Langerhans cells in HIV-1 transmission. Trends Mol Med 2008; 14:12-9.

[26] Valladeau J, Ravel O, Dezutter-Dambuyant C, et al. Langerin, a novel C-type lectin specific to Langerhans cells, is an endocytic receptor that induces the formation of Birbeck granules. Immunity 2000; 12:71-81.

[27] Liu YJ. Dendritic cell subsets and lineages, and their functions in innate and adaptive immunity. Cell 2001; 106:259-62.

[28] Flacher V, Bouschbacher M, Verronese E, et al. Human Langerhans cells express a specific TLR profile and differentially respond to viruses and Gram-positive bacteria. J Immunol 2006; 177:7959-67.

[29] Fahrbach KM, Barry SM, Ayehunie S, Lamore S, Klausner M, Hope TJ. Activated CD34-derived Langerhans cells mediate transinfection with human immunodeficiency virus. J Virol 2007; 81:6858-68.

[30] Blauvelt A, Glushakova S, Margolis LB. HIV-infected human Langerhans cells transmit infection to human lymphoid tissue ex vivo. AIDS 2000; 14:647-51.

[31] Kawamura T, Azuma M, Kayagaki N, Shimada S, Yagita H, Okumura K. Fas/Fas ligand-mediated apoptosis of murine Langerhans cells. J Dermatol Sci 2000; 22:96-101.

[32] Kawamura T, Qualbani M, Thomas EK, Orenstein JM, Blauvelt A. Low levels of productive HIV infection in Langerhans cell-like dendritic cells differentiated in the

presence of TGF-beta1 and increased viral replication with CD40 ligand-induced maturation. Eur J Immunol 2001; 31:360-8.

[33] Wu L, KewalRamani VN. Dendritic-cell interactions with HIV: infection and viral dissemination. Nat Rev Immunol 2006; 6:859-68.

[34] Birbeck MS. Electron microscopy of melanocytes. Br Med Bull 1962; 18:220-2.

[35] Hunger RE, Sieling PA, Ochoa MT, et al. Langerhans cells utilize CD1a and langerin to efficiently present nonpeptide antigens to T cells. J Clin Invest 2004; 113:701-8.

[36] de Jong MA, de Witte L, Oudhoff MJ, Gringhuis SI, Gallay P, Geijtenbeek TB. TNF-alpha and TLR agonists increase susceptibility to HIV-1 transmission by human Langerhans cells ex vivo. J Clin Invest 2008; 118:3440-52.

[37] Ogawa Y, Kawamura T, Kimura T, Ito M, Blauvelt A, Shimada S. Gram-positive bacteria enhance HIV-1 susceptibility in Langerhans cells, but not in dendritic cells, via Toll-like receptor activation. Blood 2009; 113:5157-66.

[38] 38. Ebenbichler CF, Thielens NM, Vornhagen R, Marschang P, Arlaud GJ, Dierich MP. Human immunodeficiency virus type 1 activates the classical pathway of complement by direct C1 binding through specific sites in the transmembrane glycoprotein gp41. J Exp Med 1991; 174:1417-24.

[39] Spear GT, Jiang HX, Sullivan BL, Gewurz H, Landay AL, Lint TF. Direct binding of complement component C1q to human immunodeficiency virus (HIV) and human T lymphotrophic virus-I (HTLV-I) coinfected cells. AIDS Res Hum Retroviruses 1991; 7:579-85.

[40] Stoiber H, Clivio A, Dierich MP. Role of complement in HIV infection. Annu Rev Immunol 1997; 15:649-74.

[41] Wilflingseder D, Banki Z, Garcia E, et al. IgG opsonization of HIV impedes provirus formation in and infection of dendritic cells and subsequent long-term transfer to T cells. J Immunol 2007; 178:7840-8.

[42] Pruenster M, Wilflingseder D, Banki Z, et al. C-type lectin-independent interaction of complement opsonized HIV with monocyte-derived dendritic cells. Eur J Immunol 2005; 35:2691-8.

[43] Auvert B, Taljaard D, Lagarde E, Sobngwi-Tambekou J, Sitta R, Puren A. Randomized, controlled intervention trial of male circumcision for reduction of HIV infection risk: the ANRS 1265 Trial. PLoS Med 2005; 2:e298.

[44] Mazzoli S, Trabattoni D, Lo Caputo S, et al. HIV-specific mucosal and cellular immunity in HIV-seronegative partners of HIV-seropositive individuals. Nat Med 1997; 3:1250-7.

[45] Tudor D, Derrien M, Diomede L, et al. HIV-1 gp41-specific monoclonal mucosal IgAs derived from highly exposed but IgG-seronegative individuals block HIV-1 epithe-

lial transcytosis and neutralize CD4(+) cell infection: an IgA gene and functional analysis. Mucosal Immunol 2009; 2:412-26.

[46] Tudor D, Yu H, Maupetit J, et al. Isotype modulates epitope specificity, affinity, and antiviral activities of anti-HIV-1 human broadly neutralizing 2F5 antibody. Proc Natl Acad Sci U S A 2012; 109:12680-5.

[47] Shen R, Drelichman ER, Bimczok D, et al. GP41-specific antibody blocks cell-free HIV type 1 transcytosis through human rectal mucosa and model colonic epithelium. J Immunol 2010; 184:3648-55.

[48] Bell D, Young JW, Banchereau J. Dendritic cells. Adv Immunol 1999; 72:255-324.

[49] Pavli P, Woodhams CE, Doe WF, Hume DA. Isolation and characterization of antigen-presenting dendritic cells from the mouse intestinal lamina propria. Immunology 1990; 70:40-7.

[50] Pavli P, Hume DA, Van De Pol E, Doe WF. Dendritic cells, the major antigen-presenting cells of the human colonic lamina propria. Immunology 1993; 78:132-41.

[51] Lenz A, Heine M, Schuler G, Romani N. Human and murine dermis contain dendritic cells. Isolation by means of a novel method and phenotypical and functional characterization. J Clin Invest 1993; 92:2587-96.

[52] Nestle FO, Zheng XG, Thompson CB, Turka LA, Nickoloff BJ. Characterization of dermal dendritic cells obtained from normal human skin reveals phenotypic and functionally distinctive subsets. J Immunol 1993; 151:6535-45.

[53] Klatt NR, Estes JD, Sun X, et al. Loss of mucosal CD103+ DCs and IL-17+ and IL-22+ lymphocytes is associated with mucosal damage in SIV infection. Mucosal Immunol 2012.

[54] Presicce P, Shaw JM, Miller CJ, Shacklett BL, Chougnet CA. Myeloid dendritic cells isolated from tissues of SIV-infected Rhesus macaques promote the induction of regulatory T cells. AIDS 2012; 26:263-73.

[55] Frank I, Piatak M, Jr., Stoessel H, et al. Infectious and whole inactivated simian immunodeficiency viruses interact similarly with primate dendritic cells (DCs): differential intracellular fate of virions in mature and immature DCs. J Virol 2002; 76:2936-51.

[56] Pope M, Gezelter S, Gallo N, Hoffman L, Steinman RM. Low levels of HIV-1 infection in cutaneous dendritic cells promote extensive viral replication upon binding to memory CD4+ T cells. J Exp Med 1995; 182:2045-56.

[57] McDonald D, Wu L, Bohks SM, KewalRamani VN, Unutmaz D, Hope TJ. Recruitment of HIV and its receptors to dendritic cell-T cell junctions. Science 2003; 300:1295-7.

[58] Banki Z, Posch W, Ejaz A, et al. Complement as an endogenous adjuvant for dendritic cell-mediated induction of retrovirus-specific CTLs. PLoS Pathog 2010; 6:e1000891.

[59] Piguet V, Steinman RM. The interaction of HIV with dendritic cells: outcomes and pathways. Trends Immunol 2007; 28:503-10.

[60] Turville SG, Santos JJ, Frank I, et al. Immunodeficiency virus uptake, turnover, and 2-phase transfer in human dendritic cells. Blood 2004; 103:2170-9.

[61] Geijtenbeek TB, van Vliet SJ, Engering A, t Hart BA, van Kooyk Y. Self- and nonself-recognition by C-type lectins on dendritic cells. Annu Rev Immunol 2004; 22:33-54.

[62] Geijtenbeek TB, Kwon DS, Torensma R, et al. DC-SIGN, a dendritic cell-specific HIV-1-binding protein that enhances trans-infection of T cells. Cell 2000; 100:587-97.

[63] Engering A, Geijtenbeek TB, van Kooyk Y. Immune escape through C-type lectins on dendritic cells. Trends Immunol 2002; 23:480-5.

[64] Kopf M, Abel B, Gallimore A, Carroll M, Bachmann MF. Complement component C3 promotes T-cell priming and lung migration to control acute influenza virus infection. Nat Med 2002; 8:373-8.

[65] Suresh M, Molina H, Salvato MS, Mastellos D, Lambris JD, Sandor M. Complement component 3 is required for optimal expansion of CD8 T cells during a systemic viral infection. J Immunol 2003; 170:788-94.

[66] Mehlhop E, Diamond MS. Protective immune responses against West Nile virus are primed by distinct complement activation pathways. J Exp Med 2006; 203:1371-81.

[67] Jung S, Unutmaz D, Wong P, et al. In vivo depletion of CD11c+ dendritic cells abrogates priming of CD8+ T cells by exogenous cell-associated antigens. Immunity 2002; 17:211-20.

[68] Probst HC, van den Broek M. Priming of CTLs by lymphocytic choriomeningitis virus depends on dendritic cells. J Immunol 2005; 174:3920-4.

[69] Posch W, Cardinaud S, Hamimi C, Fletcher A, Mühlbacher A, Loacker K, Eichberger P, Dierich MP, Pancino G, Lass-Flörl C, Moris A, Saez-Cirion A, Wilflingseder D. Antibodies attenuate the capacity of dendritic cells to stimulate HIV-specific CTLs. J All Clin Imm 2012; accepted

[70] Granelli-Piperno A, Delgado E, Finkel V, Paxton W, Steinman RM. Immature dendritic cells selectively replicate macrophagetropic (M-tropic) human immunodeficiency virus type 1, while mature cells efficiently transmit both M- and T-tropic virus to T cells. J Virol 1998; 72:2733-7.

[71] Ganesh L, Leung K, Lore K, et al. Infection of specific dendritic cells by CCR5-tropic human immunodeficiency virus type 1 promotes cell-mediated transmission of virus resistant to broadly neutralizing antibodies. J Virol 2004; 78:11980-7.

[72] Manel N, Hogstad B, Wang Y, Levy DE, Unutmaz D, Littman DR. A cryptic sensor for HIV-1 activates antiviral innate immunity in dendritic cells. Nature 2010; 467:214-7.

[73] Laguette N, Sobhian B, Casartelli N, et al. SAMHD1 is the dendritic- and myeloid-cell-specific HIV-1 restriction factor counteracted by Vpx. Nature 2011; 474:654-7.

[74] Mangeot PE, Duperrier K, Negre D, et al. High levels of transduction of human dendritic cells with optimized SIV vectors. Mol Ther 2002; 5:283-90.

[75] Goujon C, Jarrosson-Wuilleme L, Bernaud J, Rigal D, Darlix JL, Cimarelli A. With a little help from a friend: increasing HIV transduction of monocyte-derived dendritic cells with virion-like particles of SIV(MAC). Gene Ther 2006; 13:991-4.

[76] Lahouassa H, Daddacha W, Hofmann H, et al. SAMHD1 restricts the replication of human immunodeficiency virus type 1 by depleting the intracellular pool of deoxynucleoside triphosphates. Nat Immunol 2012; 13:223-8.

[77] Grassi F, Hosmalin A, McIlroy D, Calvez V, Debre P, Autran B. Depletion in blood CD11c-positive dendritic cells from HIV-infected patients. AIDS 1999; 13:759-66.

[78] Donaghy H, Pozniak A, Gazzard B, et al. Loss of blood CD11c(+) myeloid and CD11c(-) plasmacytoid dendritic cells in patients with HIV-1 infection correlates with HIV-1 RNA virus load. Blood 2001; 98:2574-6.

[79] Pacanowski J, Kahi S, Baillet M, et al. Reduced blood CD123+ (lymphoid) and CD11c + (myeloid) dendritic cell numbers in primary HIV-1 infection. Blood 2001; 98:3016-21.

[80] Luci C, Anjuere F. IFN-lambdas and BDCA3+/CD8alpha+ dendritic cells: towards the design of novel vaccine adjuvants? Expert Rev Vaccines 2011; 10:159-61.

[81] Dutertre CA, Amraoui S, Derosa A, et al. Pivotal role of M-DC8+ monocytes from viremic HIV-infected patients in TNFalpha over-production in response to microbial products. Blood 2012.

[82] Chehimi J, Campbell DE, Azzoni L, et al. Persistent decreases in blood plasmacytoid dendritic cell number and function despite effective highly active antiretroviral therapy and increased blood myeloid dendritic cells in HIV-infected individuals. J Immunol 2002; 168:4796-801.

[83] Gruenbacher G, Gander H, Rahm A, Nussbaumer W, Romani N, Thurnher M. CD56+ human blood dendritic cells effectively promote TH1-type gammadelta T-cell responses. Blood 2009; 114:4422-31.

[84] Siegal FP, Kadowaki N, Shodell M, et al. The nature of the principal type 1 interferon-producing cells in human blood. Science 1999; 284:1835-7.

[85] Tversky JR, Le TV, Bieneman AP, Chichester KL, Hamilton RG, Schroeder JT. Human blood dendritic cells from allergic subjects have impaired capacity to produce interferon-alpha via Toll-like receptor 9. Clin Exp Allergy 2008; 38:781-8.

[86] O'Doherty U, Peng M, Gezelter S, et al. Human blood contains two subsets of dendritic cells, one immunologically mature and the other immature. Immunology 1994; 82:487-93.

[87] Fanning SL, George TC, Feng D, et al. Receptor cross-linking on human plasmacytoid dendritic cells leads to the regulation of IFN-alpha production. J Immunol 2006; 177:5829-39.

[88] Fitzgerald-Bocarsly P, Dai J, Singh S. Plasmacytoid dendritic cells and type I IFN: 50 years of convergent history. Cytokine Growth Factor Rev 2008; 19:3-19.

[89] Milone MC, Fitzgerald-Bocarsly P. The mannose receptor mediates induction of IFN-alpha in peripheral blood dendritic cells by enveloped RNA and DNA viruses. J Immunol 1998; 161:2391-9.

[90] Dzionek A, Sohma Y, Nagafune J, et al. BDCA-2, a novel plasmacytoid dendritic cell-specific type II C-type lectin, mediates antigen capture and is a potent inhibitor of interferon alpha/beta induction. J Exp Med 2001; 194:1823-34.

[91] Krug A, French AR, Barchet W, et al. TLR9-dependent recognition of MCMV by IPC and DC generates coordinated cytokine responses that activate antiviral NK cell function. Immunity 2004; 21:107-19.

[92] Hemmi H, Kaisho T, Takeuchi O, et al. Small anti-viral compounds activate immune cells via the TLR7 MyD88-dependent signaling pathway. Nat Immunol 2002; 3:196-200.

[93] Gill MA, Bajwa G, George TA, et al. Counterregulation between the FcepsilonRI pathway and antiviral responses in human plasmacytoid dendritic cells. J Immunol 2010; 184:5999-6006.

[94] Beignon AS, McKenna K, Skoberne M, et al. Endocytosis of HIV-1 activates plasmacytoid dendritic cells via Toll-like receptor-viral RNA interactions. J Clin Invest 2005; 115:3265-75.

[95] Kadowaki N, Antonenko S, Lau JY, Liu YJ. Natural interferon alpha/beta-producing cells link innate and adaptive immunity. J Exp Med 2000; 192:219-26.

[96] Ito T, Amakawa R, Kaisho T, et al. Interferon-alpha and interleukin-12 are induced differentially by Toll-like receptor 7 ligands in human blood dendritic cell subsets. J Exp Med 2002; 195:1507-12.

[97] 97. Colonna M. Alerting dendritic cells to pathogens: the importance of Toll-like receptor signaling of stromal cells. Proc Natl Acad Sci U S A 2004; 101:16083-4.

[98] Fitzgerald-Bocarsly P, Jacobs ES. Plasmacytoid dendritic cells in HIV infection: striking a delicate balance. J Leukoc Biol 2010; 87:609-20.

[99] Zhou D, Kang KH, Spector SA. Production of interferon alpha by human immunodeficiency virus type 1 in human plasmacytoid dendritic cells is dependent on induction of autophagy. J Infect Dis 2012; 205:1258-67.

[100] Boasso A, Shearer GM. Chronic innate immune activation as a cause of HIV-1 immunopathogenesis. Clin Immunol 2008; 126:235-42.

[101] Boasso A, Vaccari M, Hryniewicz A, et al. Regulatory T-cell markers, indoleamine 2,3-dioxygenase, and virus levels in spleen and gut during progressive simian immunodeficiency virus infection. J Virol 2007; 81:11593-603.

[102] Chen W, Liang X, Peterson AJ, Munn DH, Blazar BR. The indoleamine 2,3-dioxygenase pathway is essential for human plasmacytoid dendritic cell-induced adaptive T regulatory cell generation. J Immunol 2008; 181:5396-404.

[103] Gerosa F, Baldani-Guerra B, Nisii C, Marchesini V, Carra G, Trinchieri G. Reciprocal activating interaction between natural killer cells and dendritic cells. J Exp Med 2002; 195:327-33.

[104] Megjugorac NJ, Young HA, Amrute SB, Olshalsky SL, Fitzgerald-Bocarsly P. Virally stimulated plasmacytoid dendritic cells produce chemokines and induce migration of T and NK cells. J Leukoc Biol 2004; 75:504-14.

[105] Portales P, Reynes J, Rouzier-Panis R, Baillat V, Clot J, Corbeau P. Perforin expression in T cells and virological response to PEG-interferon alpha2b in HIV-1 infection. AIDS 2003; 17:505-11.

[106] Portales P, Reynes J, Pinet V, et al. Interferon-alpha restores HIV-induced alteration of natural killer cell perforin expression in vivo. AIDS 2003; 17:495-504.

[107] Ferlazzo G, Tsang ML, Moretta L, Melioli G, Steinman RM, Munz C. Human dendritic cells activate resting natural killer (NK) cells and are recognized via the NKp30 receptor by activated NK cells. J Exp Med 2002; 195:343-51.

[108] Ferlazzo G, Munz C. NK cell compartments and their activation by dendritic cells. J Immunol 2004; 172:1333-9.

[109] Herbeuval JP, Shearer GM. HIV-1 immunopathogenesis: how good interferon turns bad. Clin Immunol 2007; 123:121-8.

[110] 110. Barron MA, Blyveis N, Palmer BE, MaWhinney S, Wilson CC. Influence of plasma viremia on defects in number and immunophenotype of blood dendritic cell subsets in human immunodeficiency virus 1-infected individuals. J Infect Dis 2003; 187:26-37.

[111] Almeida M, Cordero M, Almeida J, Orfao A. Different subsets of peripheral blood dendritic cells show distinct phenotypic and functional abnormalities in HIV-1 infection. AIDS 2005; 19:261-71.

[112] Killian MS, Fujimura SH, Hecht FM, Levy JA. Similar changes in plasmacytoid dendritic cell and CD4 T-cell counts during primary HIV-1 infection and treatment. AIDS 2006; 20:1247-52.

[113] Nilsson J, Boasso A, Velilla PA, et al. HIV-1-driven regulatory T-cell accumulation in lymphoid tissues is associated with disease progression in HIV/AIDS. Blood 2006; 108:3808-17.

[114] Mandl JN, Barry AP, Vanderford TH, et al. Divergent TLR7 and TLR9 signaling and type I interferon production distinguish pathogenic and nonpathogenic AIDS virus infections. Nat Med 2008; 14:1077-87.

[115] Campillo-Gimenez L, Laforge M, Fay M, et al. Nonpathogenesis of simian immunodeficiency virus infection is associated with reduced inflammation and recruitment of plasmacytoid dendritic cells to lymph nodes, not to lack of an interferon type I response, during the acute phase. J Virol 2010; 84:1838-46.

[116] Cavaleiro R, Baptista AP, Foxall RB, Victorino RM, Sousa AE. Dendritic cell differentiation and maturation in the presence of HIV type 2 envelope. AIDS Res Hum Retroviruses 2009; 25:425-31.

[117] Barratt-Boyes SM, Wijewardana V. A divergent myeloid dendritic cell response at virus set-point predicts disease outcome in SIV-infected rhesus macaques. J Med Primatol 2011; 40:206-13.

[118] Sallusto F, Schaerli P, Loetscher P, et al. Rapid and coordinated switch in chemokine receptor expression during dendritic cell maturation. Eur J Immunol 1998; 28:2760-9.

[119] Patterson BK, McCallister S, Schutz M, et al. Persistence of intracellular HIV-1 mRNA correlates with HIV-1-specific immune responses in infected subjects on stable HAART. AIDS 2001; 15:1635-41.

[120] Fong L, Mengozzi M, Abbey NW, Herndier BG, Engleman EG. Productive infection of plasmacytoid dendritic cells with human immunodeficiency virus type 1 is triggered by CD40 ligation. J Virol 2002; 76:11033-41.

[121] Lore K, Smed-Sorensen A, Vasudevan J, Mascola JR, Koup RA. Myeloid and plasmacytoid dendritic cells transfer HIV-1 preferentially to antigen-specific CD4+ T cells. J Exp Med 2005; 201:2023-33.

[122] Meyers JH, Justement JS, Hallahan CW, et al. Impact of HIV on cell survival and antiviral activity of plasmacytoid dendritic cells. PLoS One 2007; 2:e458.

[123] Brown KN, Wijewardana V, Liu X, Barratt-Boyes SM. Rapid influx and death of plasmacytoid dendritic cells in lymph nodes mediate depletion in acute simian immunodeficiency virus infection. PLoS Pathog 2009; 5:e1000413.

[124] Dillon SM, Robertson KB, Pan SC, et al. Plasmacytoid and myeloid dendritic cells with a partial activation phenotype accumulate in lymphoid tissue during asymptomatic chronic HIV-1 infection. J Acquir Immune Defic Syndr 2008; 48:1-12.

[125] Manches O, Munn D, Fallahi A, et al. HIV-activated human plasmacytoid DCs induce Tregs through an indoleamine 2,3-dioxygenase-dependent mechanism. J Clin Invest 2008; 118:3431-9.

[126] Favre D, Lederer S, Kanwar B, et al. Critical loss of the balance between Th17 and T regulatory cell populations in pathogenic SIV infection. PLoS Pathog 2009; 5:e1000295.

[127] Steinman RM, Banchereau J. Taking dendritic cells into medicine. Nature 2007; 449:419-26.

[128] Steinman RM. Dendritic cells in vivo: a key target for a new vaccine science. Immunity 2008; 29:319-24.

[129] Ueno H, Schmitt N, Klechevsky E, et al. Harnessing human dendritic cell subsets for medicine. Immunol Rev 2010; 234:199-212.

[130] Andrieu JM, Lu W. A dendritic cell-based vaccine for treating HIV infection: background and preliminary results. J Intern Med 2007; 261:123-31.

[131] McElrath MJ, Haynes BF. Induction of immunity to human immunodeficiency virus type-1 by vaccination. Immunity 2010; 33:542-54.

[132] Picker LJ, Hansen SG, Lifson JD. New paradigms for HIV/AIDS vaccine development. Annu Rev Med 2012; 63:95-111.

[133] Buchbinder SP, Mehrotra DV, Duerr A, et al. Efficacy assessment of a cell-mediated immunity HIV-1 vaccine (the Step Study): a double-blind, randomised, placebo-controlled, test-of-concept trial. Lancet 2008; 372:1881-93.

[134] McElrath MJ, De Rosa SC, Moodie Z, et al. HIV-1 vaccine-induced immunity in the test-of-concept Step Study: a case-cohort analysis. Lancet 2008; 372:1894-905.

[135] Flynn NM, Forthal DN, Harro CD, Judson FN, Mayer KH, Para MF. Placebo-controlled phase 3 trial of a recombinant glycoprotein 120 vaccine to prevent HIV-1 infection. J Infect Dis 2005; 191:654-65.

[136] Pitisuttithum P, Gilbert P, Gurwith M, et al. Randomized, double-blind, placebo-controlled efficacy trial of a bivalent recombinant glycoprotein 120 HIV-1 vaccine among injection drug users in Bangkok, Thailand. J Infect Dis 2006; 194:1661-71.

[137] Rerks-Ngarm S, Pitisuttithum P, Nitayaphan S, et al. Vaccination with ALVAC and AIDSVAX to prevent HIV-1 infection in Thailand. N Engl J Med 2009; 361:2209-20.

[138] McElrath MJ. Immune responses to HIV vaccines and potential impact on control of acute HIV-1 infection. J Infect Dis 2010; 202 Suppl 2:S323-6.

[139] Carrington M, O'Brien SJ. The influence of HLA genotype on AIDS. Annu Rev Med 2003; 54:535-51.

[140] Goulder PJ, Watkins DI. Impact of MHC class I diversity on immune control of immunodeficiency virus replication. Nat Rev Immunol 2008; 8:619-30.

[141] Streeck H, Jolin JS, Qi Y, et al. Human immunodeficiency virus type 1-specific CD8+ T-cell responses during primary infection are major determinants of the viral set point and loss of CD4+ T cells. J Virol 2009; 83:7641-8.

[142] Lu W, Achour A, Arlie M, Cao L, Andrieu JM. Enhanced dendritic cell-driven proliferation and anti-HIV activity of CD8(+) T cells by a new phenothiazine derivative, aminoperazine. J Immunol 2001; 167:2929-35.

[143] Lu W, Wu X, Lu Y, Guo W, Andrieu JM. Therapeutic dendritic-cell vaccine for simian AIDS. Nat Med 2003; 9:27-32.

[144] Lu W, Arraes LC, Ferreira WT, Andrieu JM. Therapeutic dendritic-cell vaccine for chronic HIV-1 infection. Nat Med 2004; 10:1359-65.

[145] Ratzinger G, Baggers J, de Cos MA, et al. Mature human Langerhans cells derived from CD34+ hematopoietic progenitors stimulate greater cytolytic T lymphocyte activity in the absence of bioactive IL-12p70, by either single peptide presentation or cross-priming, than do dermal-interstitial or monocyte-derived dendritic cells. J Immunol 2004; 173:2780-91.

Hematopoietic Stem Cell Transplantation in HIV Infected Patients

Nitya Nathwani

Additional information is available at the end of the chapter

http://dx.doi.org/10.5772/52686

1. Introduction

In the highly active antiretroviral therapy (HAART) era, the survival of HIV infected patients has improved. Opportunistic infections and AIDS related syndromes in these individuals have declined (Palella et al, 1998). HIV infected individuals have an increased tendency to develop malignancy. These include a number of non-AIDS defining malignancies, as well as the AIDS defining malignancies which are Kaposi sarcoma, invasive cervical cancer and non-Hodgkin Lymphoma (NHL). Among the NHL group, the incidence of systemic NHL, CNS Lymphoma and primary effusion lymphoma are increased in this population. Malignancies continue to be an important cause of mortality in these individuals.

The incidence of NHL increases with progressive immunosuppression in HIV-infected patients. The majority of these cases are intermediate or high-grade and almost all are diffuse large B cell (immunoblastic variant) or Burkitt-like lymphomas. The incidence of Hodgkin lymphoma (HL) is also increased in the HIV positive population (Bigar R et al, 2006) though it is not an AIDS defining illness. Acute myeloid leukemia may also occur with higher frequency in the setting of HIV infection (Grulich A et al, 2007). NHL and HL occurring in HIV infected individuals are characterized by an aggressive clinical course with an advanced stage at presentation (Levine AM, 2000).

In the pre-HAART era, the standard treatment for AIDS associated NHL was low dose chemotherapy. It was thought that they would be unable to tolerate intensive chemotherapy because of the underlying immunodeficiency. Randomized trials of standard doses of combination chemotherapy versus reduced doses revealed inferior results in the standard dose arm due to increased hematologic toxicity and infections (Kaplan LD et al, 1997). In the post-HAART era, patients were treated more aggressively due to improved hematologic reserve in patients on HAART. Patients are now treated similar to non HIV NHL patients.

Their remission rates and median survival with aggressive combination chemotherapy and HAART is similar to their HIV negative counterparts (Boue, F et al, 2006).

Consequently, more aggressive therapies such as high dose chemotherapy and stem cell transplantation have been explored in the HAART era with encouraging results. This chapter will go through autologous and allogeneic stem cell transplantation in HIV infected individuals and also highlight some of the recent developments in the field.

2. Autologous Stem Cell Transplantation (ASCT)

Autologous stem cell transplantation means transplantation with a person's own hematopoietic stem cells which are harvested ahead of time and cryopreserved for later use. Pluripotent hematopoietic stem cells are those which are capable of self renewal and of differentiation. These are the cells targeted for collection. The main advantage of this procedure is to enable the patient to receive myeloablative dose intense chemotherapy for a malignancy that has demonstrated a dose response to chemotherapy. Stem cells collected from the peripheral blood after priming with G-CSF (Granulocyte Colony Stimulating Factor) are generally preferred to stem cells from the bone marrow due to shorter engraftment times, thereby reducing morbidity and mortality. Stem cell apheresis is an outpatient procedure where cells are collected through large volume apheresis over approximately 4-6 hours. These stem cells are either cryopreserved with DMSO directly or can be manipulated by methods such as CD34 positive selection and transduction prior to cryopreservation.

There are various preparative regimens used for stem cell transplantation in patients with hematologic malignancy. The ideal regimen should be able to eradicate the malignancy, have no mortality and manageable side effects or toxicity. Alas, no such treatments exist. There are several treatment regimens in use. Selection of high dose chemotherapy regimens is based upon the use of chemotherapeutic agents that have a dose response in the hematologic malignancy. In addition, drugs are chosen that have nonoverlapping toxicities save for the hematologic toxicity. For example in NHL, typical agents include Cyclophosphamide, Etoposide, Carmustine (BCNU) and melphalan. In Hodgkin lymphoma, frequently utilized preparative regimens include the CBV regimen with Cyclophosphamide, Carmustine (BCNU), and Etoposide (VP-16) and the BEAM regimen with Carmustine (BCNU), Etoposide (VP-16), Cytarabine (Ara-C) and Melphalan.

Patients typically receive the conditioning regimen followed by infusion of thawed autologous stem cells approximately 24- 48 hours post completion of chemotherapy. Thereafter ensues a period of profound neutropenia, also often mucositis and GI toxicity such as nausea and diarrhea. During this period of neutropenia, the risk of infection is significantly increased. Hence patients are housed in hepa filtered rooms, and placed on low bacteria diets in addition to other infectious precautions. Nonetheless, fever and infection can be common. Mucositis is a risk factor for infection as it increases the likelihood of intermittent bacteremia from the GI tract. The use of peripheral blood progenitor cells harvested from apheresis instead of bone marrow stem cells led to a shortening of engraftment of white blood cell times.

http://dx.doi.org/10.5772/52686

This thereby reduced the period of neutropenia and mucositis, which improved survival in patients.

This procedure has been the standard treatment for HIV negative patients with relapsed NHL since the landmark PARMA trial published by Philip et al in the New England Journal of Medicine (1995). In this trial, patients with relapsed chemosensitive aggressive NHL were treated with 2 cycles of DHAP (Dexamethasone, Cisplatin and Cytarabine) and if responsive, randomly assigned to receive either DHAP for 4 additional cycles or high dose chemotherapy with BEAC (BCNU/Carmustine, Etoposide, Cytarabine and Cyclophosphamide) followed by ASCT, The results of this study revealed an overall survival (OS) benefit of 53 versus 32 percent (p= 0.038) in favor of the high dose chemotherapy arm. This approach has also been used in high risk patients who are in first remission (Haioun, C et al, 1997). Non-randomized trials of this high risk group have demonstrated high rates of progression free survival (FPS). Similarly, trials of HIV negative patients with Hodgkin Lymphoma have shown that ASCT can provide long term PFS for patients with relapsed disease (Linch, 1993). All these studies were done in the HIV negative population.

2.1. ASCT in HIV positive patients

ASCT in HIV positive patients was pioneered by the French in the pre-HAART era (Gabarre, J et al, 1996). The first patient was reported as a case study. He was a 40 year old male with HIV related NHL, receiving Zidovudine and Zalcitabine as antiretroviral treatment. He was treated with BEAM (BCNU, Etoposide, Cytarabine and Melphalan) chemotherapy for relapsed lymphoma followed by ASCT. His post-transplant course was complicated by several opportunistic infections including cytomegalovirus viremia, mycobacterium pneumonia and cryptosporidiosis. This report corroborated the fear that the immune impairment due to HIV augmented the infection risk. However, it also demonstrated that mobilizing stem cells and successful engraftment were feasible in this setting. In the post-HAART era, French investigators performed a study with fourteen patients with relapsed or refractory NHL. Eight patients died of which six deaths were from lymphoma. This study established that the mortality due to infection was substantially reduced, but that control of the underlying lymphoma remained the challenge (Gabarre et al, 2001). It set the stage for ASCT to be considered a feasible task in HIV patients, and revealed that infectious issues were manageable without apparent adverse consequences on the HIV infection.

Other centers have described similar findings. The larger City of Hope study had patients with less advanced lymphoma and disqualified chemotherapy refractory patients (Krishnan A, et al, 2005). The initial series consisted of 20 patients with HL or NHL. All patients were on HAART. The majority of patients underwent CBV (cyclophosphamide, BCNU, Etoposide) chemotherapy as conditioning. Engraftment times were comparable to HIV negative patients, median was 11 days. Despite efforts to continue HAART throughout the transplant period, only nine out of twenty were able to tolerate it. The remainder resumed it at a median of two months following ASCT. The poor tolerance of HAART was due to either nausea or mucositis. Transplant related mortality was low, as was the incidence of opportunistic infections. No patient died of an opportunistic infection. Although the CD4 count did nadir at 6 months, post-transplant follow up demonstrated that the underlying HIV disease did not deteriorate as a result of the transplant and the CD4 counts recovered to pre-transplant levels by one year in all patients. PFS and OS were 85%. The improved result compared to the French experience may be from selecting patients with less advanced disease and chemotherapy sensitive disease.

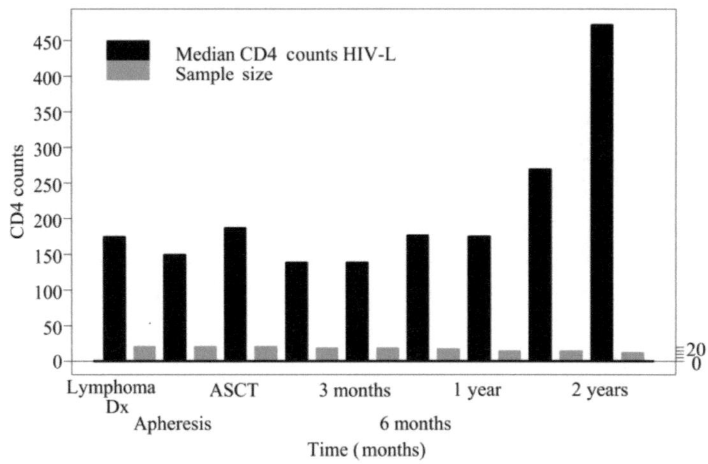

Figure 1. Median CD4 count trends during apheresis and after ASCT. Krishnan A et al. Blood 2005; 105:874-878 Blood: Journal of the American Society of Hematology by American Society of Hematology. Copyright 2009 Reproduced with permission of AMERICAN SOCIETY OF HEMATOLOGY (ASH) in the format Journal via Copyright Clearance Center.

The Italian cooperative group on AIDS and tumors (GIGAT) reported the long term results on 50 patients with HIV and relapsed or refractory lymphoma (Re A, et al, 2009). Similar to the City of Hope study, only patients with chemotherapy sensitive disease were selected to proceed with peripheral stem cell collection. Forty-six patients were already on HAART, two started at the time of study enrollment, and two at the time of stem cell mobilization. A minimum CD4 count of 100 cells/micro liter prior to initiating chemotherapy was a prerequisite. There were no eligibility criteria for viral load and therefore the viral loads at study entry ranged considerably. Thirteen patients withdrew before stem cell collection. Among these, two withdrawals were from early toxic deaths, one patient refusal, and the remaining ten patients had chemotherapy refractory disease. Eventually, twenty seven patients underwent ASCT. Of these, seven temporarily suspended HAART, some for similar reasons to the City of Hope experience with mucositis, and others for hepatotoxicity. All patients received BEAM (Carmustine/BCNU, Etoposide, Cytarabine and Melphalan) as the conditioning regimen. Three year progression free survival for the patients who proceeded to transplant was also similar to the City of Hope experience at 76.3%. Multivariate analysis of prognostic factors for survival showed that bone marrow involvement, performance status less than 2, and CD4 count below 100 cells/micro liter were significant. No significant HIV-associated infections were noted. In those patients on effective HAART therapy, the infectious risk was similar to patients without HIV who underwent ASCT. The high patient

http://dx.doi.org/10.5772/52686

withdrawal rate before transplantation displays the obstacles in treating these aggressive lymphomas.

The European Group for Blood and Marrow Transplantation conducted a retrospective, multicentre registry-based analysis of sixty eight patients from twenty institutions since 1999 (Balsalobre P et al, 2009). There were fifty patients with NHL and eighteen patients with HL. At the time of ASCT, sixteen patients were in first complete remission (CR1); forty four patients were in CR more than 1, partial remission, or chemotherapy-sensitive relapse; and eight patients had chemotherapy resistant disease. Most patients were treated with a chemotherapy based conditioning regimen (BEAM and variants). The median CD4 count at transplantation was 162 cells/micro litter, and eighty percent of patients had an HIV viral load under 200/mL. All patients engrafted at a median of eleven days, save one. The incidence of non relapse mortality (NRM) was 4.4% and 7.5% at 3 and 12 months, respectively. Three patients died from bacterial infection, two died of HIV related complications, and one patient died of an unknown cause while in CR. At a median follow-up of 32 months, progression free survival and overall survival were 56.5% and 61% at three years, respectively. On multivariate analysis, chemotherapy resistant disease and not attaining complete remission predicted poorer progression free survival and overall survival. This data indicates again similar to the HIV negative transplant setting, disease control with chemotherapy at the time of ASCT predicts a more favorable result.

Two case control studies also demonstrated that HIV status does not impact ASCT outcomes for lymphoma. The European Group for Blood and Marrow Transplantation undertook a retrospective study of 106 patients (Diez-Martin et al, 2009) which included 53 HIV-positive lymphoma patients who underwent transplant with controls matched for histology, non-age adjusted IPI (International Prognostic Index), and disease status at transplant. There were 66 percent NHL and 34 percent HL patients. Both groups were similar, other than the higher percentage of males, mixed cellularity Hodgkin lymphoma and patients receiving granulocyte colony stimulating factor before engraftment, and a smaller fraction receiving total body irradiation based conditioning within the HIV lymphoma cohort. With median follow-up of 30 months, progression free survival was 61 percent for the HIV-lymphoma group and 56 percent for the control lymphoma group. Overall survival was 61.5 percent for HIV-positive patients and 70 percent for controls (p = NS). There was a trend towards delay in platelet engraftment after transplant in the HIV group. It is uncertain whether this resulted from the more frequent granulocyte colony stimulating factor use in that cohort or to HAART therapy or to chronic HIV infection of the bone marrow. Incidence of relapse, overall survival and progression free survival were comparable in both groups. In the first year following ASCT, there was an elevated, but statistically insignificant non relapse mortality in the HIV lymphoma group, primarily from early bacterial infections. This data suggested that in the HAART era, HIV infection should not preclude lymphoma patients from undergoing ASCT. The authors recommended conscientious infection prophylaxis and vigilant immune recovery surveillance shortly following ASCT.

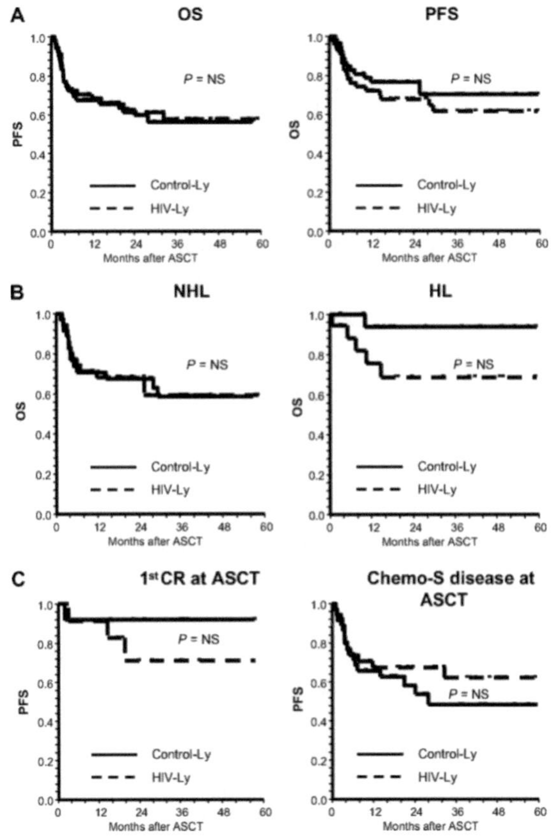

Figure 2. Survival according to HIV infection status: positive versus negative. Diez-Martin JL et al. Blood 2009; 113:6011-6014 Blood: Journal of the American Society of Hematology by American Society of Hematology. Copyright 2009 Reproduced with permission of AMERICAN SOCIETY OF HEMATOLOGY (ASH) in the format Journal via Copyright Clearance Center

City of Hope undertook a retrospective matched case-control study (Krishnan, et al, 2010) to study long-term outcome in HIV positive NHL patients (cases) and HIV negative NHL patients (controls). Twenty nine patients with HIV positive NHL were matched with HIV negative NHL controls with respect to sex, time to ASCT, year of transplant, histology, age, disease status, number of prior regimens, and conditioning regimen. A higher ratio of HIV positive NHL patients had high grade disease versus the HIV negative NHL controls. There were mostly male patients in both groups. The median CD4 count at study entry was 153.5, and the viral load was 6500. All patients in the HIV cohort were on HAART at the time of transplant; however thirteen patients had to interrupt treatment. The median follow-up for HIV-positive NHL patients was 62.4 months, and 48.4 months for the HIV-negative NHL controls. The median time to neutrophil engraftment was comparable for both groups. Non relapse mortality was also comparable for the two groups. Infectious complications did differ between the two groups, with more opportunistic infections occurring in the HIV-positive cohort, however this did not affect survival. There were more opportunistic viral infections in the HIV-positive group, with three cases of cytomegalovirus viremia, one case of adenovirus viremia, and one case of varicella infection. Disease free survival and overall survival were not significantly different between the two groups. The two year disease free survival for the HIV-positive NHL group was 76 percent and 56 percent for the HIV-negative group. The overall survival for both groups was also similar at 75 percent notwithstanding a higher proportion of poor risk HIV positive NHL patients.

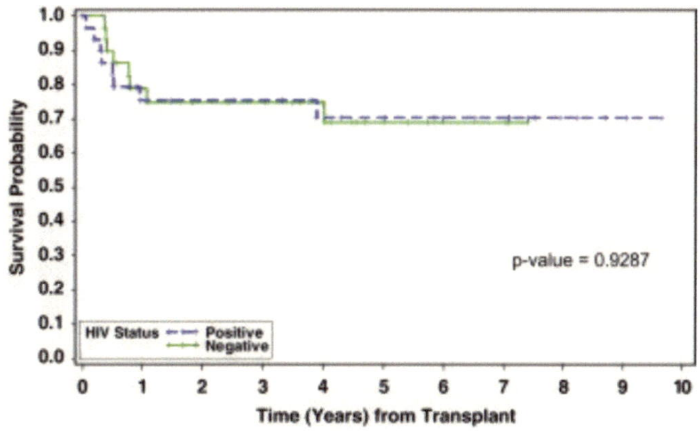

Figure 3. Probability of overall survival by HIV status. Krishnan A, Palmer J, Zaia J, et al. Vol. 16, (September 2010), pp. 1302-08. "Reprinted From: HIV Status Does Not Affect the Outcome of Autologous Stem Cell Transplantation (ASCT) for Non-Hodgkin Lymphoma (NHL) Biology of Blood and Marrow Transplantation 16:1302-1308 (2010), with permission from Elsevier"

Causes of death in the HIV-positive cohort were mostly from relapsed lymphoma, and not infection. Disease status at the time of transplant was the only clear predictor of outcome. This single-institution series corroborates the European data.

This data from the European Group for Blood and Marrow Transplantation (Balsalobre et al, 2009) and the City of Hope experience (Krishnan, et al, 2010) revealed better progression free survival rates in the HIV-positive lymphoma patients compared to their HIV-negative counterparts. This improved early outcome is interesting. Perhaps incorporating HAART in the regimen improves the result. Maybe transplant with high dose chemotherapy resets the clock on the immunologic effects of HIV, either by depleting the HIV reservoir or by its alterations on the T cell reconstitution. Inherent genetic variability may also play a part. Homozygosity for the 32-bp CCR5 allele CCR-Δ 32 has been shown to confer resistance to HIV infection (Liu R et al, 1996). This same deletion may also offer defense against lymphoma development in HIV patients (Dean M et al, 1999). A trial in the United States of ASCT for HIV lymphoma via the Bone Marrow Transplant Clinical Trials Network will prospectively analyze the genotypes and the CCR5 mutation to find its association with disease free survival. Correlative studies will also assess the pre and post-transplant HIV viral reservoir.

2.2. Immune recovery post transplant

An Italian study (Simonelli et al, 2010) prospectively evaluated 33 lymphoma patients of whom 24 were HIV positive and nine were HIV-negative. All patients had relapsed or refractory disease and both groups were given similar high dose chemotherapy and ASCT protocols. The study compared the immunological baseline features in the two groups. The study showed that front line chemotherapy resulted in immunodepression in the general population, which qualitatively differs from that observed in HIV-infected patients. HIV-positive patients had higher CD8+ T cell counts and inverted ratios of CD4+ cells to CD8+ cells than HIV-negative patients. There were no significant differences in the CD4+ cell compartment and thymic reservoir, between the groups. The authors attributed this finding to good control of HIV-RNA levels from ongoing HAART therapy. The initial differences in the dynamics of immune recovery between the populations also diminished with longer follow-up. Specifically, the CD8+ subpopulation, together with CD56+ NK cells quickly recovered in both groups of patients, leading, to a reversal of the ratio of CD4+ cells to CD8+ cells in the HIV-negative patients for up to two years following transplantation. In the HIV-infected population, high dose chemotherapy produced a different immune incompetence compared with conventional chemotherapy, which primarily impacted the CD4+ T cell subset without significantly affecting the CD4/CD8 ratio. In the first three months post ASCT, significantly more infectious episodes occurred in the HIV-positive group. The authors demonstrated that HIV-positive patients with early post-transplant infections had significantly lower CD4+ T cell counts during the third month post ASCT, compared with HIV-negative patients without infections. There was no difference in the frequency of infection or the dynamics of CD4+ T cell reconstitution beyond three months post ASCT. Overall, the study showed that high dose chemotherapy and ASCT in HIV-infected lymphoma patients does not worsen initial immune impairment or enhance viral replication or peripheral HIV reservoir in the long term. The temporary elevation in the incidence of early infectious events in the HIV-positive group may be related to an arrest in the CD4+ T cell count increment during the first three months post ASCT. There were no significant changes in the HIV DNA levels during the follow-up period, with values at 24 months significantly lower than those at baseline.

It is well-recognized that HIV persists at low levels in peripheral blood mononuclear cells, mostly in infected resting CD4+ T cells which constitute a stable reservoir for HIV, even when viral replication is well controlled with antiretroviral therapy. Analysis of HIV-1 DNA (HIV DNA) (Koelsch, KK et al, 2008) in peripheral blood mononuclear cells is therefore an accessible virological marker for estimating HIV infection. Bortolin's study of 22 patients with HIV associated relapsed or refractory lymphomas treated with salvage high dose chemotherapy followed by ASCT looked at the kinetics of the predictive value of HIV DNA. HIV DNA was measured by real-time PCR in the peripheral blood mononuclear cells. At baseline, HIV DNA was found to be associated with HIV-1 RNA (HIV RNA), but not with CD4 counts. HIV RNA load was under control throughout follow-up, while HIV DNA levels were nearly always detectable. The overall survival analysis demonstrated that patients with higher HIV DNA levels at baseline had a higher and nearly significant risk of death when compared with patients with lower levels (HR, 8.33, 95% CI 0.99 - 70.06, p=0.05). At the time of publication, of the 22 patients, 14 (63.6%) were still alive, of which 13 were in remission and one relapsed; 8 (36.5%) died, of which 6 deaths were from relapsed lymphoma and 2 were from opportunistic infections. Of note, baseline HIV DNA levels were significantly different between alive and deceased patients. Results from this study established HIV DNA as an valuable additional tool to optimize and tailor therapy, and also predict treatment outcome in these patients.

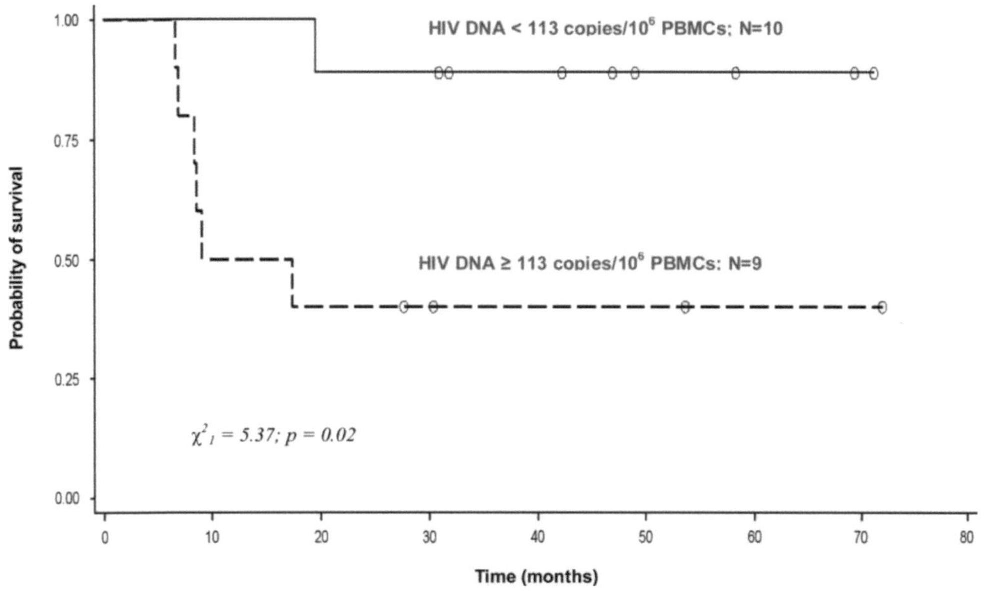

Figure 4. Kaplan–Meier curve showing survival according to baseline HIV DNA levels ($n = 19$) Bortolin MT, Zanussi S, Talamini R, et al. *AIDS Research and Human Retroviruses*. Vol. 26, No. 2, (2010), pp. 245-251. " The publisher for this copyrighted material is Mary Ann Liebert, Inc. publishers."

3. Allogeneic transplantation

Allogeneic transplantation refers to hematopoietic stem cells which come from an HLA matched donor. Allogeneic transplants typically have a higher morbidity and mortality than autologous transplants mostly due to infection or graft versus host disease. The 'graft' refers to the transplanted hematopoietic stem cells transplanted from the donor (sibling or matched unrelated donor) and the 'host' refers to the patient. In graft versus host disease, the donor's immune cells attack the recipient's organs. Virtually any organ can be affected, but frequently affected organs include the skin, liver and gut. Graft versus host disease (GVHD) is a major impediment to the success of bone marrow transplantation. Treatment and prevention of GVHD includes immunosuppressive medications and sometimes steroids. The incidence of chronic graft versus host disease (that occurring after 100 days post transplant) is up to 80% in recipients of allogeneic peripheral blood stem cells. On the other hand, allogeneic transplant has the advantage of lower rates of relapse due to the 'clean graft' as well as the immunologic effects of the donor graft, the so called graft versus tumor effect. These immunologic effects could be potentially even more beneficial in the treatment of HIV infection if the attendant risks of the procedure in the HIV infected patient could be overcome.

Allogeneic stem cell transplantation (alloSCT) is more difficult than ASCT in HIV infected individuals due to the need for chronic immunosuppression in an already immunosuppressed individual. Solid organ transplantation set the stage for allogeneic stem cell transplantation in that solid organ transplant patients also need chronic immunosuppression. There have been several published reports of solid-organ transplantation in HIV positive patients who are receiving HAART, which demonstrated that, in most cases, HIV infection does not affect the outcome of transplantation. Drug interactions were handled by requisite dose adjustments. The underlying HIV infection was controlled provided patients remained on antiretroviral therapy. (Ragni MV et al, 1999; Prachalias AA et al, 2001; Kuo PC, 2001; Gow PJ & Mutimer D, 2001 as cited in Halpern et al, 2002). Some solid organ transplant centers regard HIV patients akin to other high risk patients, for example, diabetics, or the elderly (Persad G et al, 2008).

The literature on allogeneic transplantation in HIV positive patients is considerably more limited than ASCT. Experience with ASCT in HIV-positive patients has shown that HIV infection did not impede engraftment provided myelosuppressive medications like azidothymidine were avoided. Therefore, in the allogeneic field, comparable engraftment times were expected. Allogeneic transplantation data indicates the rate of immune reconstitution after transplant is related to the type of conditioning regimen, HLA compatibility of the donor and host, and the occurrence of GVHD. In an allogeneic transplant with an HIV negative recipient, T lymphocyte recovery occurs by thirty days following transplant, although initially with primarily CD8+ T cells (Keever, CA et al, 1989). CD4+ cell recovery often takes up to six months.

Early reports of allogeneic transplant were in the pre-HAART period. Holland et al (1989) at Johns Hopkins published a case of a forty one year old male with HIV lymphoma who received a conditioning regimen consisting of total body irradiation and Cyclophosphamide followed by allogeneic bone marrow transplantation. Prior to the transplant, he was given high dose azidothymidine and following the transplant, he was given a lower dose. There was no significant regimen-related toxicity, and he engrafted at day seventeen, but thereafter died of lymphoma at day forty seven. At autopsy, no evidence of HIV, either by culture, or PCR was found in tissue specimens. Although the result was poor, this early report demonstrated the achievability of the procedure and raised the intriguing question, could allogeneic transplant be a route to treat HIV infection.

Woolfrey et al (2008) published a series of two HIV-positive patients who received nonmyeloablative transplants at the Fred Hutchinson Research Center. They received conditioning with Fludarabine and 200 cGy total body irradiation. They got HLA-matched peripheral blood stem cells, one from a sibling and the other from an unrelated donor. Post-transplantation cyclosporine and mycophenolatemofetil were given for graft versus host disease pro-

http://dx.doi.org/10.5772/52686

phylaxis. HAART was continued with adjustments to prevent drug interactions. The HIV RNA remained undetectable and no HIV associated infections were noted. The first patient died of GVHD. The second patient remained alive at the time of publication, more than 180 days following transplant. It is notable that both patients' donor cells expressed wild-type CCR5 co receptor, and not the CCRΔ32 allele which is linked with resistance to HIV infection. Reconstitution of CD4+ and CD8+ subsets was in accordance with other nonmyeloablative transplants. New HIV-1 specific CD8+ T cell responses were produced after transplant. The gradual loss of detectable proviral DNA in the patient who achieved full donor chimerism suggests that the reservoir of latently infected lymphocytes died out after transplantation. This study alluded to the dual benefits of allogeneic transplantation.

Larger studies are needed to determine if the benefits of allogeneic transplant can be preserved in the myeloablative setting with its accompanying elevated morbidity and mortality. The largest series was a retrospective study of thirty patients with various hematologic malignancies transplanted between 1987 and 2003 from the European Group for Blood and Marrow Transplantation (Gupta V, et al, 2007). Treatment related mortality at 100 days was 46 percent. There was a striking difference in survival in patients transplanted after 1996 after availability of HAART. Prior to 1996, only two out of twenty two patients survived, but after 1996, four out of eight patients survived. This study revealed that reduction of transplant related mortality and control of HIV infection together are imperative in carrying out successful allogeneic transplants in this population.

4. Allogeneic transplantation for HIV infection

Allogeneic hematopoietic stem cell transplantation has the exciting prospect of controlling the HIV infection. HIV-1 enters host cells by binding to a CD4 receptor and then interacting with either CCR5 or the CXC chemokine receptor (CXCR4). Homozygosity for a 32-bp deletion (delta 32) in the CCR5 allele confers natural resistance to infection with CCR5 tropic HIV strains (R5 HIV) because of the lack of CCR5 cell-surface expression. (Dean M et al, 1996 as cited in Allers et al, 2011)

A case report from Germany by Hutter et al (2009) published in the *New England Journal of Medicine* described a 40 year old patient with a ten year history of HIV who underwent allogeneic stem cell transplantation (SCT) in February 2007 for relapsed acute myelogenous leukemia from an HLA-matched unrelated donor who was homozygous for the CCR5 delta 32 allele. HAART was given until the day prior to transplantation. The patient relapsed at day 332 and was treated with a second transplant from the same donor after reinduction therapy with cytarabine and gemtuzumab along with single dose total body irradiation. There was no viral rebound twenty months after transplantation and discontinuation of antiretroviral therapy. Tissue sites, such as the intestines, serve as reservoirs, and were looked at to detect the HIV virus despite the absence of viremia. In this patient, the rectal biopsy performed at 159 days after transplant did reveal that CCR5-producing macrophages were still present in the intestinal mucosa, which demonstrated they had not yet been replaced by the new immune system. Although these long-lasting cells from the host can be viral reservoirs even after transplantation, HIV-1 DNA was not found in his rectal mucosa. Immunologic studies showed a loss of anti-HIV virus specific interferon gamma producing T cells. This indicated that HIV antigenic stimulation was not present post transplant. His viral load continued to be undetectable despite the presence of non-CCR5 tropic X4 virus variants. After nearly two years of follow-up, the patient's CD4 cell count normalized with all cells exhibiting the homozygous CCR5-deleted gene. This observation is notable because homozygosity for CCR5 delta 32 deletion is related to high but not complete resistance to HIV-1.

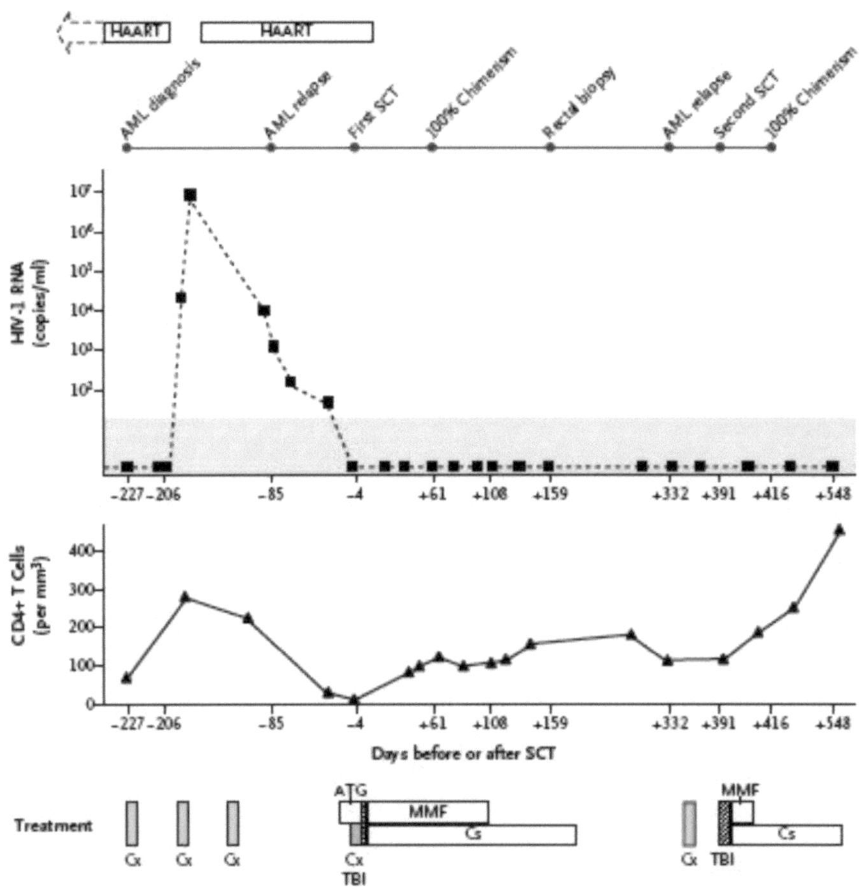

Figure 5. Clinical Course and HIV-1 Viremia. Hütter G, Nowak D, Mossner M, et al. Long-term control of HIV by CCR5 Delta32/Delta32 stem-cell transplantation. *The New England Journal of Medicine,* Vol. 360, No. 7, (February 2009) pp. 692-8. Permission granted. Copyright MMS

Allers et al (2011) published an article involving the same patient with extended follow-up, which reveals that he had remained off HAART and had no evidence of HIV disease for 45 months after the transplant. During his treatment course, he underwent multiple colonoscopies with biopsies to rule out GVHD, in addition to a liver biopsy and brain biopsy for evaluation of leukoencephalopathy. This study also looked at 10 HIV negative stem cell transplant controls and 15 HIV negative healthy controls, 5 of whom underwent colonoscopy as a cancer preventive examination. It was found that CD4+ T cell reconstitution increased continuously and, after two years reached levels within the normal range of age matched healthy patients. There was 100 percent donor chimerism, which was shown by absent CCR5 expression. Among the CD4+ T cells, there were more activated effector memory cells and less naïve cells when compared with healthy controls. CD4+ T cell reconstitution also occurred in the gut mucosa of the reported patient, similar to the stem cell transplant control patients, with cells exclusively derived from the donor hematopoietic system. There was more than a twofold increase in mucosal CD4+ T cells in the transplant patients compared to healthy controls, which demonstrates that conditioning and transplant elicits the enrichment of HIV target cells in the gut mucosal immune system.

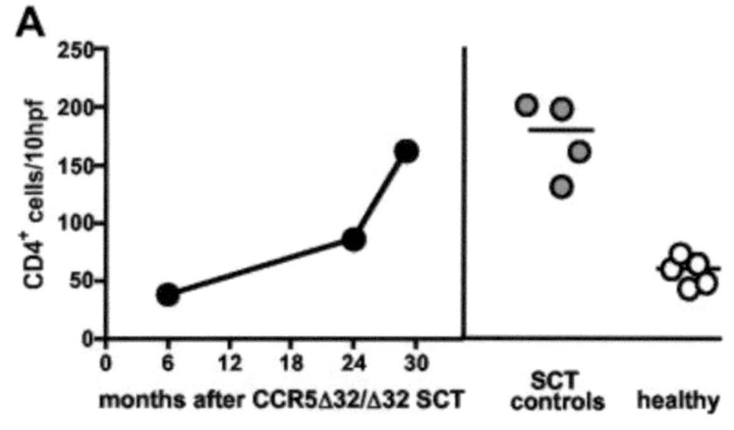

Figure 6. The mucosal immune system has been efficiently repopulated with donor-derived CD4+ T cells. (A) Immunohistochemical quantification of CD4+ T cells in colon tissue of the CR5Δ32/Δ32 SCT patient, SCT control patients (27 ± 9 months after transplantation), and healthy control patients. The horizontal lines denote the median values of each group. Allers K, Hütter G, Hofmann J, et al. *Blood.* Vol. 117, No. 10, (March 2011), pp. 2790-2799. Blood: journal of the American Society of Hematology by American Society of Hematology. Copyright 2009 Reproduced with permission of AMERICAN SOCIETY OF HEMATOLOGY (ASH) in the format Journal via Copyright Clearance Center

HIV RNA and DNA were not detected in the peripheral blood or biopsy specimens obtained from various tissues. These biopsies revealed that tissue macrophages were ultimately replaced by donor-derived macrophages without CCR5 expression (Parker and Sereti, 2011). The T cells of the reported patient do not express normal levels of CXCR4 and appear vulnerable to X4-tropic HIV. HIV specific antibodies declined over time, with only envelope antibodies being detectable at the time of publication.

The study suggests that CCR5Δ32/Δ32 SCT has probably led to a cure of HIV infection in this patient. However it remains difficult to conclusively demonstrate eradication of HIV and its latent reservoirs, and the chance of resurgence of lingering X4 strains which survived the chemotherapy and radiation, leading to X4 HIV rebound still exists. Host-originating

CD4+ T cells appear to be totally removed from the immune system; however tissue macrophages are practically resistant to conditioning and less susceptible to the cytopathic effects of HIV infection, making them resilient viral reservoirs (Swingler S et al, 2007). One of the most promising findings of this report was the demonstration that later in the course of immune reconstitution, host-originating macrophages became undetectable in the GI mucosa by both phenotypic and genotypic analysis. These findings suggest that the replacement of host tissue cells with donor derived cells has reduced the size of the viral reservoir during the course of the immune reconstitution, which consequently had reduced the risk of HIV rebound over time.

5. Gene therapy and the future

Gooley et al (2010) reported impressive decreases in allogeneic transplantation-related mortality. Nevertheless, the risk of allogeneic SCT is inappropriately high to recommend it in the absence of an underlying malignancy that requires it as therapy. It cannot be proposed as a treatment strategy for the bulk of HIV-infected patients who can live long healthy lives with the use of HAART. Homozygosity for the delta 32 mutation is only found in a minority of the population, so it is not feasible to find such HLA-matched donors for the majority of patients. Preferably, one would aspire to integrate the benefits of transplantation of cells with the CCR5 mutation without the hazards of allogeneic SCT. One potential way to achieve this would be to transplant autologous stem cells that were genetically modified to be CCR5 negative. We have performed two trials at the City of Hope using this approach. The most recent employed a lentivirus-based system to transduce stem cells with a combination of three forms of anti-HIV RNA. This incorporated RNA1 in the form of a short-hairpin RNA targeted to an exon in HIV-1 tat/rev, a decoy for the HIV tat reactive element and a ribozyme that targets the host cell CCR5 chemokine receptor. Krishnan et al (2008) reported four patients with AIDS-related lymphoma transplanted with autologous lentiviral-transduced modified stem cells and unmanipulated stem cells following high-dose chemotherapy. All patients engrafted and exhibited low levels of genetically modified cells. Future trials will address how to augment engraftment of the genetically modified stem cells. Further plans are for planned interruption of HAART which would further demonstrate the functionality of these genetically modified cells. It is likely that an amalgamation of approaches with an aim to limit CD4 T cell targets and target viral reservoirs may be necessary to achieve a cure.

6. Conclusion

In the HAART era, the barrier of HIV infection as an obstacle to transplant has been broken. The role of ASCT has been well established in the HIV negative population for the treatment of relapsed or high-risk lymphoma. Numerous studies have now shown that ASCT can be safely performed in HIV-positive patients, and that it may lead to durable remissions in patients with HIV-related lymphomas. Similar to well controlled diabetes, well controlled HIV infection does not significantly increase the risk of infections following ASCT if a program of adequate surveillance and prophylaxis is used. Allogeneic stem cell transplantation remains a more difficult task, is still in its infancy, and lacks larger studies. The Hutter and Allers experience of allogeneic SCT with a CCR5 negative donor has given a name and face to the cure of HIV. The task of finding more feasible options for the enormousglobal population living with HIV remains.

Author details

Nitya Nathwani

City of Hope National Medical Center, Duarte, USA

References

[1] Allers, K., Hütter, G., Hofmann, J., et al., & (2011, . (2011). Evidence for the cure of HIV infection by CCR5 (Delta) 32 (Delta) 32 stem cell transplantation.Blood. March 2011), , 117(10), 2790-2799.

[2] Balsalobre, P., Diez-Martin, J., Re, A., et al. (2009). Autologous stem-cell transplantation in patients with HIV-related lymphoma. Journal of Clinical OncologyMay 2009), , 27(13), 2192-2198.

[3] Biggar, R., Jaffe, E., Goedert, J., et al. (2006). Hodgkin Lymphoma and immunodeficiency in persons with HIV/AIDS. BloodDecember 2006, , 108(12), 3786-3791.

[4] Bortolin, M. T., Zanussi, S., Talamini, R., et al. (2010). Predictive value of HIV Type 1 DNA levels on overall survival in HIV-related lymphoma patients treated with high-dose chemotherapy (HDC) plus autologous stem cell transplantation (ASCT). *AIDS Research and Human Retroviruses*, 26(2), 245-251.

[5] Boue, F., Gabarre, J., Gisselbrecht, C., et al. (2006). Phase II trial of CHOP Plus Rituximab in Patients With HIV_Associated Non-Hodgkin's Lymphoma. Journal of Clinical Oncology.September 2006) , 24(25), 4123-4128.

[6] Dean, M., Jacobson, L. P., Mc Farlane, G., et al. (1999). Reduced risk of AIDS lymphoma in individuals heterozygous for the CCR5-DELTA32 mutation. Cancer Research-August 1999), , 3561-2564.

[7] Díez-Martín, J. L., Balsalobre, P., Re, A., et al. (2009). Comparable survival between HIV^+ and HIV^- non-Hodgkin and Hodgkin lymphoma patients undergoing autologous peripheral blood stem cell transplantation. *Blood*. 113. June 2009), (23), 6011-6014.

[8] Forman SJ, Blume KG, Thomas ED,(1994). Bone Marrow Transplantation.Blackwell Scientific Publications. 0-86542-253-2

[9] Gabarre, J., Choquet, S., Azar, N., et al. (2001). High Dose Chemotherapy with autologous stem cell transplantation for HIV associated lymphoma: A single center report on 14 patients. Blood 2001; 98: Abstract # 2092

[10] Gabarrre, J., Leblond, V., Sutton, L., et al. (1996). Autologous bone Marrow transplantation in relapsed HIV related Non-Hodgkin's lymphoma. Bone Marrow Transplantation 1996; 18: , 1195-1197.

[11] Gooley TA, Chien JW, Pergam SA, et al(2010). Reduced mortality after allogeneic hematopoietic-cell transplantation. The New England Journal of MedicineNovember 2010), , 363(22), 2091-2101.

[12] Grulich AE, Leeuwen MT, Falster MO, et al.(2007). Incidence of cancers in people with HIV/AIDS compared with immunosuppressed transplant recipients: a meta-analysis. Lancet. July 2007), , 370, 59-67.

[13] Gupta, V., Tomblyn, M., Pederson, T., et al. (2007). Allogeneic hematopoietic stem cell transplantation in HIV-positive patients with malignant and non-malignant disorders: a report from the center for international blood and marrow transplant research (CIBMTR). Biology of Blood and Marrow TransplantationSupplement, (February 2007) , 13(2), 5-6.

[14] Haioun, C., Lepage, E., Gisselbrecht, C., et al. (1997). Benefit of autologous bone marrow transplantation over sequential chemotherapy in poor risk aggressive non-Hodgkin's lymphoma: Updated results of the Prospective Study LNH87-2. Journal of Clinical OncologyMarch 1997), , 15(3), 1131-1137.

[15] Halpern SD, Ubel PA &Caplan AL(2002). Solid Organ Transplantation in HIV infected patients. The New England Journal of MedicineJuly 2002), , 347(4), 284-287.

[16] Holland, H. K., Saral, R., Rossi, J. J., et al. (1989). Allogeneic bone marrow transplantation, zidovudine and human immunodeficiency virus type 1 (HIV-1) infection. Annals of Internal Medicine.111(12) (December 1989), , 973-981.

[17] Hütter, G., Nowak, D., Mossner, M., et al. (2009). Long-term control of HIV by CCR5 Delta32/Delta32 stem-cell transplantation. The New England Journal of Medicine-February 2009) , 360(7), 692-698.

[18] Kaplan, LD, Strauss DJ, Testa, MA et al.(1997). Low-Dose Compared with Standard-Dose m-BACOD Chemotherapy for Non-Hodgkin's Lymphoma Associated with Human Immunodeficiency Virus Infection.The New England Journal of Medicine.June 1997) , 336, 1641-1648.

[19] Keever, Small. T. N., Flomenberg, N., et al. (1989). Immune Reconstitution following bone marrow transplantation: Comparison of recipients of T cell depleted marrow with recipients of conventional marrow grafts. BloodApril 1989) , 73(5), 1340-1350.

[20] Koelsch, K. K., Liu, L., Haubrich, R., et al. (2008). Dynamics of total, linear nonintegrated, and integrated HIV-1 DNA in vivo and in vitro. The Journal of Infectious Diseases. 197 (February 2008), , 411-419.

[21] Krishnan, A., Molina, A., Zaia, J., et al. (2005). Durable Remissions with autologous stem cell transplantation for high-risk HIV associated lymphomas. BloodJanuary 2005), , 105(2), 874-878.

[22] Krishnan, A., Palmer, J., Zaia, J., et al. (2010). HIV status does not affect the outcome of autologous stem cell transplantation (ASCT) for Non-Hodgkin Lymphoma (NHL). Biology of Blood and Marrow TransplantationSeptember 2010), , 16, 1302-1308.

[23] Krishnan, A., Zaia, J. A., Rossi, J., et al. (2008). First in Human Engraftment of Anti HIV lentiviral vector gene modified CD 34+ peripheral blood progenitor cells in the treatment of AIDS related lymphoma (ARL). Blood. 112: Abstract 2348

[24] Levine AM.(2000). Acquired immunodeficiency Syndrome-Related Lymphoma: Clinical Aspects. Seminars in OncologyAugust 2000), , 27(4), 442-453.

[25] Linch, D. C., Goldstone, A. H., Mc Millan, A., et al. (1993). Dose intensification with autologous bone marrow transplantation in relapsed and resistant Hodgkin's disease: results of a BNLI randomized trial. The Lancet. April 1993), , 341(8852), 1051-1054.

[26] Liu, R., Paxton, W., Choe, S., et al. (1996). Homozygous defect in HIV-1 coreceptor accounts for resistance of some multiply-exposed individuals to HIV-1 infection. CellAugust 1996), , 86, 367-377.

[27] Palella FJ, Delaney KM, Moorman AC, et al.(1998). Declining morbidity and mortality among patients with advanced human immunodeficiency virus infection. The New England Journal of MedicineMarch,1998), , 338(13), 853-860.

[28] Parker, R. ., Sereti, I., & (2011, . (2011). The power of 1 in HIV therapeutics.Blood. March 2011), , 117(10), 2745-2746.

[29] Persad, G. C., Little, R. F., & Grady, C. (2008). Including persons with HIV infection in cancer clinical trials. Journal of Clinical Onoclogy, March 2008), , 26(7), 1027-1032.

[30] Philip, T., Guglielmi, C., Hagenbeek, A., et al. (1995). Autologous bone marrow transplantation as compared with salvage chemotherapy in relapses of chemotherapy-sensitive non-Hodgkin's lymphoma. The New England Journal of Medicine. December 1995), , 333(23), 1540-1545.

[31] Re, A., Michieli, M., Casari, S., et al. (2009). High-dose therapy and autologous peripheral blood stem cell transplantation as salvage treatment for AIDS-related lymphoma: long-term results of the Italian Cooperative Group on AIDS and Tumors (GICAT) study with analysis of prognostic factors. BloodAugust 2009), , 114(7), 1306-1313.

[32] Simonelli, C., Zanussi, S., Pratesi, C., et al. (2010). Immune recovery after autologous stem cell transplantation is not different for HIV-infected versus HIV-uninfected pa-

tients with relapsed or refractory lymphoma. Clinical Infectious DiseasesJune 2010) , 1672-1679.

[33] Swingler, S., Mann, A. M., Zhou, J., et al. (2007). Apoptotic killing of HIV-1 infected macrophages is subverted by the viral envelope glycoprotein. PLoS PathogensSeptember 2007), , 3(9), 1281-1290.

[34] Woolfrey, A. E., Malhotra, U., Harrington, Rd., et al. (2008). Generation of HIV-1 specific CD8+ cell responses following allogeneic hematopoietic cell transplantation. Blood, October 2008), , 112(8), 3484-3487.

Section 2

HIV Screening

Chapter 4

Screening for HIV Infection in Pregnancy

Chi Dola, Maga Martinez, Olivia Chang and
Amanda Johnson

Additional information is available at the end of the chapter

http://dx.doi.org/10.5772/54551

1. Introduction

Approximately 100 to 200 infants annually in the United States are infected with HIV (CDC, 2007). Most were born to mothers who were unaware of their infected HIV status or who did not receive preventative services during their pregnancy to reduce transmission rates. Therefore, in 2006, the CDC updated its guidelines for screening of various populations for HIV, including pregnant women. Obstetricians and gynecologists are ideally suited to such screening of their patients during annual exams and prenatal visits.

1.1. Screening for HIV infection during prenatal care

Screening only patients who reported risk factors for the HIV infection will miss many infected women. Therefore, the current recommendation is for implementation of universal opt-out screening for HIV as early in pregnancy as possible (Branson et al., 2006). In this universal opt-out screening method, a patient is informed that HIV testing will be performed as a routine part of her prenatal care, unless she declines testing. She should be given written or oral information about HIV, including an explanation of the infection, the meaning of positive or negative test results, and measures that can be used to reduce perinatal transmission. She should also be given the opportunity to ask further questions. However, no informed consent is required. If a patient declines screening, this should be documented in the medical record, and screening should be offered at subsequent prenatal visits (Branson et al., 2006; ACOG, 2008). Retesting is recommended with each new pregnancy. Although these are the recommendations endorsed by the CDC and ACOG, healthcare providers must be aware of the laws regarding screening in their own states, which may differ from the above guidelines. Further information on state HIV testing laws can be obtained from state and local health departments.

Chou et al, estimated that the number needed to screen (NNS) in an area with 0.15% prevalence would be between 3,500 to 12,170 to prevent 1 case of perinatally-acquired HIV infection. In a high risk area with a prevalence of 5%, the NNS would be from 105 to 365 to prevent 1 case of perinatally-acquired infection (Chou et, 2005).

At this time, both conventional and rapid screening tests for HIV are available to the healthcare provider. Conventional testing consists of a screening test with an enzyme immunoassay (ELISA), followed by confirmatory testing of a positive result with Western blot or immunofluorescent antibody (IFA) testing. The sensitivity and specificity of this method of testing is greater than 99%. False positive results are rare even in the setting with low prevalence. Final results may not be available for several days to weeks. With rapid testing, a blood or saliva test for HIV antibodies is performed, and the results are often available within an hour. Confirmatory testing of a preliminary positive result is still required before a diagnosis of HIV can be made. A negative result with either the conventional or rapid screening test indicates a woman does not have HIV, and no further testing is needed, unless one suspects the patient was recently infected with HIV but has not produced an antibody response to the virus (ACOG, 2008; Rahangdale & Cohan, 2008). If the initial screening test is positive, but the confirmatory test is negative, the patient should be considered not infected, and no further testing is necessary.

1.2. Rescreening in the third trimester

Studies from several countries have demonstrated that pregnant women seem to be at increased risk for acquisition of HIV over their non-pregnant counterparts (Moodley et al., 2009; Gray et al., 2005; Sansom et al., 2003). Theories for this range from behavioral actions of the woman or her partner that put her at increased risk, to physiologic changes associated with pregnancy, including changes to the genital tract mucosa to changes in cellular immunity that may lead to increased susceptibility to HIV with pregnancy. Evidence has demonstrated that the rate of seroconversion during pregnancy may be as high as 2 to 3 percent in some areas (Moodley et al., 2009; Gray et al., 2005; Sansom et al., 2003). A study by Sansom, *et al* demonstrated that in a population with an HIV incidence of approximately 1 in 1000 person-years, the cost of repeat testing was offset by the savings in medical costs for prevention of an infected infant (Sansom et al., 2003). For the above reasons, repeat HIV testing is recommended in certain populations in the third trimester, preferably before 36 weeks gestation (Branson et al., 2006; ACOG, 2008). These populations include:

- Women living in areas with a high incidence of HIV/AIDs, including the 20 states with the highest incidence among women of child-bearing age
- Women who receive their healthcare in facilities where at least 1 in 1000 women screened for HIV are found to be infected
- Women who engage in high-risk behavior that puts them at risk for HIV acquisition (injection drug use, exchange of sex for drugs or money, diagnosis of another sexually transmitted infection in the past year, a sex partner who engages in injection drug use or high-

http://dx.doi.org/10.5772/54551

risk behaviors or is infected with HIV, or women who have had a new or more than one sexual partner during their pregnancy)

- Women with signs or symptoms of acute HIV infection

1.3. Screening of women with undocumented HIV status

Studies indicate that between 40 and 85 percent of infants infected with HIV are born to mothers whose HIV infection status is unknown prior to delivery (ACOG, 2008). If a woman without documentation of HIV status presents to labor and delivery, opt-out rapid HIV testing should be performed at time of her initial presentation. A positive result should prompt immediate treatment with antiretroviral prophylaxis without awaiting the result of confirmatory testing. If subsequent confirmatory testing shows the woman to be HIV negative, treatment may be discontinued. Similarly, if a woman has an unknown HIV status in the postpartum period, her infant should be tested by rapid screening. Antiretroviral treatment should be initiated with a positive result, as the benefits of such treatment are maximized when started within 48 hours of delivery (ACOG, 2008; Rahangdale & Cohan, 2008). Again, treatment may be stopped if confirmatory testing is negative.

The above recommendation for prenatal screening for HIV infection is summarized in table 1.

Timing	Screening test	Confirmatory Test
Initial prenatal care visit	Enzyme immunoassay (ELISA)	Western blot or immunofluorescent antibody (IFA) testing
Third trimester of pregnancy	Repeat ELISA in women at **high risk** for acquisition of HIV infection	Western blot or IFA testing
At time of labor and delivery for women with undocumented HIV status	Rapid HIV antibody screening test.	Western blot or IFA testing

Table 1. CDC and ACOG recommendation for screening for HIV infection during pregnancy.

2. Evidences supporting the effectiveness of current interventions to decrease mother-to-child transmission of HIV infection

Research in HIV infection reported several key factors in the transmission of the virus from the mother to the infant. The risk factors for transmission can be divided into: virologic/immunologic, maternal health status/behavior, and obstetrical factors (McGowan et al, 2000). High maternal plasma HIV-1 viral load, low maternal CD4 T-lymphocyte count, multidrug-resistant HIV genotype will increase the transmission rate. Certain maternal behavior (illicit drug use, cigarette smoking, breast feeding) or maternal health status (increased baseline weight or malnutrition or vitamin A deficiency) can increase the rate of mother-to-child transmission. Some obstetrical factors (vaginal delivery, prolonged rupture of membrane, fetal scalp electrode placement, chorioamnionitis, perineal lacerations, prematurity) can increase the vertical transmission rate (McGowan et al, 2000).

Other reports on perinatal transmission of HIV infection suggested that approximately 70% of the infections transmitted to the infant during the labor and delivery process; only 30% of the cases occurred during the antepartum period (Kourtis et al, 2006). Current interventions to prevent perinatal transmission of HIV infection included: prophylaxis therapy with antiretroviral medication, scheduled cesarean delivery and avoidance of breast feeding. These interventions resulted in decreasing transmission rate to 2% (Cooper et al, 2002). We will examine the evidence supporting these interventions.

2.1. Prophylaxis with antiretroviral agents

The Pediatric AIDS Clinical Trials Group (PACTG) 076 conducted a randomized controlled study and in 1994 published its landmark results demonstrating a reduction in perinatal HIV transmission by two-third with the antiretroviral medication Zidovudine (ZDV). HIV-infected mothers in the study group received a three-part regimen of antiretroviral medication. They received ZDV during pregnancy, intravenous ZDV during labor, and their infant received ZDV orally for 6 weeks (Conner et al, 1994). This trial reported a decrease in transmission rate from 26% in the placebo group to 8% in those patients who received ZDV. Later in the year of 1994, FDA approved the use of ZDV for reducing perinatal HIV transmission and the U.S. Public Health Service Task Force (USPHSTF) and CDC published their recommendations for the administration of this regimen in an effort to reduce mother-to-child transmission of the HIV infection (CDC, 2006).

In the late 1990s, additional antiretroviral medications were developed and the combined use of three or more of these drugs was found to greatly inhibit viral replication and allow improvement of the immune system. The combination of these medications was known as highly active antiretroviral therapy (HAART). In 1998, USPHSTF and CDC issued recommendation regarding HAART: pregnant women should receive HAART if they required the treatment for their disease status and all HIV-infected pregnant women should be offered HAART. USPHSTF and CDC at that time acknowledged that the benefits and risks to the fetus are uncertain (CDC, 1998). Four large U.S. and European cohort studies all concluded that regimens with two or more antiretroviral drugs were more effective than the one-drug regimen for reducing vertical transmission of the HIV infection (Cooper et al, 2002, Arch Pediatr Adolesc Med 2002, Clin Infect Dis *2005*, Mandelbrot et al, 2001).

For women diagnosed late in pregnancy and were not able to receive a full course of antiretroviral treatment, a short course of antenatal treatment, although less effective, also was proven to decrease perinatal transmission (Lallemant et al, 2000, Shaffer et al, 1999, Petra study 2002, Wiktor et al, 1999, Dabis et al, 1999, Chou et al, 2005). There was some reduction in the HIV infection transmission even when treatment was abbreviated to only antiretroviral regimen during labor (Moodley et al, 2003, Taha et al, 2003, Guay et al, 1999). However, neonatal prophylaxis alone in a mother who did not receive antiretroviral prophylaxis therapy was less effective in preventing HIV infection (Taha et al, 2003).

2.2. Scheduled cesarean delivery

A meta-analysis of 15 prospective cohort studies by the International Perinatal HIV Group (The International Perinatal HIV Group, 1999) included 8,533 mother-neonate pairs. Vertical HIV transmission was reduced by 50% when the mode of delivery was elective cesarean delivery. The effect of both antiretroviral therapy prophylaxis and cesarean delivery further reduced HIV transmission by 87 percent when compared with other modes of delivery (either vaginal delivery or non-elective cesarean delivery) and no antiretroviral therapy. However, in women who received HAART and achieved low HIV viral load levels (defined as less than 1,000 copies/ mL), current data is insufficient to determine whether elective cesarean delivery would offer further risk reduction. ACOG concluded that scheduled cesarean delivery should be discussed and recommended for HIV-infected women whose HIV-1 RNA viral load exceeds 1,000 copies/mL. Scheduled cesarean delivery was recommended as early as 38 weeks gestation to reduce the risk of labor or of prematurely ruptured membranes (ACOG, 1999).

2.3. Avoidance of breastfeeding

Breastfeeding was associated with an HIV transmission rate of 14% to 16% based on the results of two meta-analyses of observational studies (Dunn et al, 1992, John et al, 2001). A review of the literature did not reveal any randomized, controlled trials evaluating the HIV transmission rate associated with breastfeeding in the United States. A large, prospective cohort study in Italy included 3,770 babies and concluded that HIV infection rates were significantly higher in babies who were breastfed after the authors adjusted for other factors, including antiretroviral use (adjusted odds ratio, 10.20 [CI, 2.73 to 38.11]) (Arch Pediatr Adolesc Med., 2002, Chou et al, 2005).

In a study in Africa, women who breastfed and did not receive antiretroviral therapy had a probability of transmitting the HIV infection of 36.7% (CI, 29.4% to 44.0%) at 24 months and an infant mortality rate of 24.4% (CI, 18.2% to 30.7%). Those who formula fed their babies had a transmission probability of 20.5% (CI, 14.0% to 27.0%) and an infant mortality rate of 20.0% (CI, 14.4% to 25.6%) (Nduati et al, 2000).

As a result, in many countries, including the United States where formula feeding is readily available and inexpensive, breastfeeding is not recommended for infants of HIV-infected women (WHO, 2000).

3. Potential harms/risks as the result of prenatal HIV screening

We will next explore the potential risks as the results of prenatal HIV screening and the potential harms of the recommended interventions to reduce perinatal transmission of HIV infection (Table 2).

	Maternal risks	Fetal risks
Prenatal screening		
Screened positive	Discrimination from their partner Social ostracization from family and friends Anxiety and depression Abandonment and abuse from family and friend	
Screened falsely positive	Anxiety Social discrimination Relationship problems Unnecessary antiretroviral prophylaxis during labor	Potential risk for elective termination of pregnancy
Interventions to decrease perinatal transmission		
ART prophylaxis	Hepatic toxicity and hypersensitivity reaction (with Nevirapine) Development of drug resistance Gestational diabetes (with combination therapy including protease inhibitors)	Risks of neural tube defects with Sustive (Efavirenz) with first trimester exposure. ? Potential risk of mitochondrial toxicity and disorder Inconsistent data regarding increasing risk for preterm birth and low-birth weight
Scheduled cesarean delivery at 38 weeks	Post-operative morbidities, including: postpartum fever, hemorrhage, endometritis, urinary tract infection.	A trend toward higher risk of respiratory distress syndrome among neonates born by cesarean section (when compared to those born via vaginal delivery)

Table 2. Potential harms / risks from prenatal screening and strategic interventions to decrease perinatal transmission of HIV infection:

According to Katz, prenatal screening for HIV in pregnancy aims to test a presumably healthy population to discover asymptomatic women who are actually infected with HIV infection. These pregnant women might not have or perceive that they have risk factors for the HIV infection. This is different than the usual situation when a woman acknowledges her risk for the infection and requests the screening test. Most women would agree to be screened as they believe that they are doing everything they can for the health for their baby but they might not realize the full implication of a positive HIV test result on their lives. In some instances, they do not perceive that they are at risk for the infection and thus could be quite unprepared to receive the positive diagnosis. This could result in adverse effect on their emotional health, their pregnancy, and the family. Thus health care provider should

http://dx.doi.org/10.5772/54551

always be well prepared to provide the appropriate emotional support for a possibility of abnormal result (Katz, 2000).

Women tested positive for HIV infection can experience significant problems with discrimination from their partner, social ostracization from their family and members of the community (Provisional Committee on Pediatric AIDS, 1995, Samson et al, 1998). They were found to have higher anxiety and depression scores and many women fear abandonment or abuse, therefore, did not disclose their HIV status to their friend or families. (Lester, 1995) although no increased risk for intimate partner violence was noted according to one cohort study (Koenig et al, 2002, Chou et al, 2005)

Data on consequences of false-positive HIV infection diagnoses in pregnant women are mainly anecdotal as reported by Sheon et al. The potential risks from false-positive results included: elective termination of pregnancy, anxiety, social discrimination and relationship problems with their partner (Sheon et al, 1994, Chou et al, 2005).

False positive results from rapid HIV testing during labor result in 4 women receiving unnecessary antiretroviral prophylaxis out of 4,849 women tested (Bulterys et al, 2004).

4. Risks of Antiretroviral Therapy (ART) to fetus

4.1. Potential teratogenic effects of ART

Efforts continue to increase our knowledge of the potential teratogenic effects of the antiretroviral agents administered in pregnancy. The Antiretroviral Pregnancy Registry Steering Committee published their recent report of antiretroviral exposures during pregnancy from January 1989 through July 2007. They did not identify an increased risk of birth defects in those exposed to any of the antiretroviral therapy in the first trimester. The risk of birth defects among women exposed to antiretroviral therapy in first trimester was 2.8 per 100 live births, which is not different from the risk of birth defects in women exposed to these agents in the second or third trimester (2.6 per 100 live births), nor the CDC's reported background rate of birth defects of 2.72 per 100 live births (www.APRegistry.com, 2007, Bardeguez, 2009).

Four retrospective reports associated Sustiva (Efavirenz) with neural tube defects in infants born of mothers exposed to this medication in the first trimester (Bardeguez, 2009). There are discrepant results with regard to mitochondrial toxicity and disorders in children exposed in utero to antiretroviral therapy. Two deaths believed to be due to mitochondrial disorder were reported in children exposed in utero to nucleoside analogues (in specific, a combination of Zidovudine and Lamivudine regimen) (Blanche et al, 1999). However, European Collaborative report and systematic review of U.S. cohorts reports did not find evidence of clinical symptoms, or deaths due to mitochondrial dysfunction among HIV-negative infants exposed to antiretroviral agents in utero (Bardeguez, 2009).

Of infants exposed in utero to Zidovudine who were followed at 4 years to 6 years of life. The reports were reassuring. Normal growth, cognitive, and developmental function were noted in these infants at 4 years old. They did not sustain any tumors or deaths from cancer at 6 years old.

4.2. Association between ART and preterm birth and low-birth weight

Inconsistent results were noted among the reports studying the effects of combination antiretroviral therapy on two obsterics outcomes: preterm birth and low birth-weight. Lorenzi et al in 1998 first reported the association between combination antiretroviral therapy with preterm birth in a retrospective Swiss study of 30 women (Lorenzi et al, 1998). Subsequently, other European studies reported a similar association between combination antiretroviral therapy and preterm birth (The European Collaborative Study (ECS) andSwiss Mother + Child HIV Cohort Study (Mo-CHiV), 2000, Grosch-Woerner et al, 2008). However, this association was not found in U.S. studies until a recent study by Cotter et al. The authors prospectively collected the data from 1990 through 2002 on 999 women receiving antiretroviral regimen during pregnancy. They concluded that women who received combination therapy that included a protease inhibitor had an increased risk of preterm delivery (Cotter et al, 2006).

In a largest analysis to date, Tuomola et al did not find an increased rate of premature birth or low birth-weight infants among 2,123 HIV infected pregnant women from seven clinical studies who received combination ART and gave birth from 1990 through 1998.

5. Risks of ART to mothers

A large prospective study evaluating the rates of maternal toxicity, pregnancy complications, and peripartum morbidity among HIV-infected pregnant women receiving prenatal care and ART concluded that adverse events were rare. Gestational diabetes was noted to be highest among women who received combination therapy including protease inhibitors either before or during first trimester (Watts et al, 2004). Reports of potential risks of hepatic toxicity and hypersensitivity reaction were noted in pregnant women receiving the drug Nevirapine (Bardeguez, 2009).

Another valid concern is the potential development of drug resistance when ART was administered to the mother for a short period during pregnancy. Drug resistance was noted in 20 – 69% of women who received only intrapartum prophylaxis with single-dose nevirapine. This could decrease the choice of medications for these women should they later need treatment for their disease. Although, there are reports that this observed resistance dissolved over time. (Bardeguez, 2009). Limited exposure to zidovudine alone did not alter maternal disease progression, time until development of AIDS or death, or development of genotypic zidovudine resistance (Bardeguez et al, 2003).

6. Potential maternal risks from scheduled cesarean delivery

Cesarean deliveries could result in significant complications when compared to vaginal delivery even for HIV-negative women (Allen et al., 2003; Makoha et al., 2004). HIV-infected women with an immunodeficient state could potentially at risk for post-operative infectious morbidities. Most studies report that HIV-infected women are at higher risk for post-operative complications, mostly infectious, than the uninfected women (Coll et al., 2002; Grubert el al., 1999; Vimercati et al., 2000). The rate of complications is higher in those with severe immunodeficiency (Jamieson et al., 2007).

Read et al conducted a largest prospective observational study which included 1,186 HIV-infected women from The Women and Infants Transmission Study. The authors evaluated the postpartum morbidity among these infected women according to their mode of delivery. When compared to women who delivered vaginally, women who underwent scheduled cesarean delivery had an increased rate of postpartum fever (14.3%), hemorrhage (7.1%), endometritis (5.4%), urinary tract infection (5.4%), and any postpartum morbidity (26.7%) (Read et al, 2001).

7. Potential neonatal risks from scheduled cesarean delivery at 38 weeks gestation

In the absence of medical or obstetrical indications, ACOG recommends against scheduled cesarean delivery at less than 39 weeks of gestation, due to the increased risk of respiratory morbidity in the neonate born prior to this gestational age (ACOG, 2001). Neonatal morbidity is high even among those neonates born via cesarean delivery a few days younger than 39 weeks (Tita et al, 2011). However, both ACOG and U.S. Public Health Service recommend scheduled cesarean delivery at 38 weeks for HIV-infected women with viral load greater than 1,000 copies/ml (ACOG, 2001; Public Health Service Task Force, 2010). The scheduled cesarean delivery date is set at one week earlier than the usually required gestational age of 39 weeks to avoid onset of spontaneous labor and rupture of membranes which could increase perinatal transmission of HIV. Livingston et al and the IMPACT Protocol 1025 Study Group evaluated the risk of neonatal respiratory distress syndrome according to the mode of delivery and gestational age at delivery. They reported that the mode of delivery was not associated with respiratory distress syndrome. However, there was a trend toward a higher risk of respiratory distress syndrome among neonates delivered by either elective or non-elective cesarean section when compared to those delivered vaginally. Two out of 227 neonates born via scheduled cesarean delivery at 38 weeks gestation had respiratory distress syndrome (Livingston et al., 2010).

8. Conclusion

Current evidence supports prenatal HIV screening. The benefits from screening appear to outweight the small risks / harms to the fetus and mothers from the treatment interventions which significantly reduce perinatal-acquired HIV infection. We concluded the chapter by discussing the obstacles to the HIV prenatal screening and prevention interventions. Prenatal screening for HIV infection and implementation of Protocol 076 were lauded as a major public health success story and resulted in a significant decline in the number of children infected with HIV from their mother. However, in the United States, there are still about 100–200 infants born every year with perinatally acquired HIV infection (CDC, 2007). Lack of prenatal care remains one of the obstacles to prevention of perinatal transmission of HIV. In the United States about 5 to 10% of women do not pursue prenatal care or receive insufficient care (Kogan et al., 1998). HIV infected women, in particular, often do not receive prenatal care. In New York City, 50% of women infected with HIV who delivered in at a municipal hospital did not receive prenatal care (Minkoff et al., 1990). Of the HIV-infected women surveyed in Philadelphia, only one third reported adequate prenatal care, and 20% did not receive any care (Turner et al., 1996).

Even more worrisome, at the Medical Center of Louisiana in New Orleans, LA, 50% of the HIV-infected parturients who did not have prenatal care but presented to the hospital for labor and delivery did not disclose their HIV status to their physicians (CDC, 2004). Could it be because the HIV-infected women did not know of the available interventions that they put their infants at risk for the infection?

Several authors attempt to understand why HIV-infected women opted out of prenatal care and available interventions to decrease vertical transmission. Rothpletz-Puglia et al solicited opinions from a group of HIV-negative women about the process of prenatal HIV screening. The authors reported that fear was a big factor for declining testing. The women are afraid to find out they are HIV-infected. They are frightened to discover a partner's infidelity. They are fearful of being judged by their health care provider or of being denied medical care if they tested positive (Rothpletz-Puglia et al, 2001).

Lancioni et al. reported that HIV-infected women did not participate in prenatal care because they fear disclosing their status to their caretakers and being judged by them for continuing the pregnancy (Lancioni et al., 1999). In a recent report by Lindau et al, HIV-infected women who were interviewed were aware of the benefits of prophylaxis treatment yet most received insufficient or no prenatal care. They knew of their HIV infection diagnosis but most did not disclose their status to their caretaker when they presented for delivery at hospitals capable of providing prophylaxis treatment. They attributed health care providers' lack of sensitivity, violations of confidentiality, disdain for HIV infection and substance abuse as reasons for their non-participation in prenatal care, avoidance of treatment for HIV infection, and non-disclosure of their HIV status. Denial and fear were other barriers to HIV prophylaxis treatment (Lindau, 2006).

We agreed with Lindau et al that may be what is needed to further reduce perinatal transmission beyond the conventional models for prevention is to understand the HIV-infected women's point of view, their fears and concerns and to eliminate the disrespect treatment as perceived by them from the health care providers. It is hope that we can create a medical environment where these women will be confident of our compassion and care to disclose their status and to want to seek prenatal care and HIV prophylaxis treatment (Lindau, 2006).

http://dx.doi.org/10.5772/54551

Lastly, not only obstetricians and gynecologists need to follow the CDC and ACOG guidelines in providing opt-out prenatal screening for HIV they must receive appropriate training for pre and post screening counseling and must ensure patient confidentiality. More importantly, at every screening they must be prepared for positive results: they must be compassionate toward those tested positive and must have resources available for their emotional support beyond providing the standard medical interventions to decrease vertical transmission.

Author details

Chi Dola*, Maga Martinez, Olivia Chang and Amanda Johnson

*Address all correspondence to: cdola@tulane.edu

Department of Obstetrics and Gynecology, Tulane University School of Medicine, New Orleans, Louisiana, USA

References

[1] Allen, V. M, Connell, O, Liston, C. M, & Baskett, R. M. T.F. ((2003). Maternal morbidity associated with cesarean deliverywithout labor compared with spontaneous onset of labor at term. Obstet Gynecol 2003; , 102, 477-82.

[2] American College of Obstetricians and Gynecologists. ACOG Committee Opinion Routine Human Immunodeficiency Virus Screening. Obstetrics and Gynecology (2008). , 112: 401-403.(411)

[3] American College of Obstetricians and Gynecologists. ACOG Committee Opinion Prenatal and Perinatal Human Immunodeficiency Virus Testing: Expanded Recommendations. Obstetrics and Gynecology (2008). , 112: 739-742.(418)

[4] American College of Obstetricians and GynecologistsACOG committee opinion # 234. Scheduled cesarean delivery and the prevention of vertical transmission of HIV infection. May, (2000).

[5] Bardeguez, A. D, Shapiro, D. E, Mofenson, L. M, Coombs, R, Frenkel, L. M, Fowler, M. G, et al. Effect of cessation of zidovudine prophylaxis to reduce vertical transmission on maternal HIV disease progression and survival. J Acquir Immune Defic Syndr (2003). , 32, 170-81.

[6] Brabin, L. (2002). Interactions of the Female Hormonal Environment, Susceptibility to Viral Infections, and Disease Progression. *AIDS Patient Care and STDs*, 211 EOF-221 EOF.

[7] Branson, B. M, Handsfield, H. H, Lampe, M. A, Janssen, R. S, Taylor, A. W, Lyss, S. B, & Clark, J. E. Revised Recommendations for HIV Testing of Adults, Adolescents, and Pregnant Women in Health-Care Settings. MMWR Recommendations and Reports (2006).

[8] Bulterys, M, Jamieson, D. J, Sullivan, O, Cohen, M. J, Maupin, M. H, & Nesheim, R. S. et al. Rapid HIV-1 testing during labor: a multicenter study. JAMA. (2004). , 292219-23.

[9] Centers for Disease Control and PreventionDiagnoses of HIV infection and AIDS in the United States and dependent areas, (2010). HIV Surveillance Report. Atlanta (GA): CDC; 2012. Available at: http://www.cdc.gov/hiv/surveillance/resources/reports/2010report/pdf/2010_HIV_Surveillance_Report_pdf.Retrieved June 1, 2012.

[10] Centers for Disease Control and PreventionHIV/AIDS and women. Available at: http://www.cdc.gov/hiv/topics/women/overview_partner.htm.Retrieved June 29, (2012).

[11] Centers for Disease Control and PreventionHIV among women. Atlanta (GA): CDC; (2011). Available at: http://www.cdc.gov/hiv/topics/women/pdf/women.pdf.Retrieved June 1, 2012.

[12] Centers for Disease Control and PreventionHIV surveillance-United States, 1981-2008. MMWR. (2011). , 2011, 60-689.

[13] Centers for Disease Control and PreventionMother-to-Child (Perinatal) HIV Transmission and Prevention. CDC HIV/AIDS Fact Sheet (2007).

[14] Centers for Disease Control and PreventionPediatric HIV Surveillance. http://www.cdc.gov/hiv/topics/surveillance/resources/slides/pediatric.Accessed August 2, (2012).

[15] Centers for Disease Control and PreventionEstimated lifetime risk for diagnosis of HIV infection among Hispanics/Latinos-37 states and Puerto Rico, (2007). MMWR. , 59(40), 1297-1301.

[16] Centers for Disease Control and PreventionPublic Health Service Task Force recommendations for the use of antiretroviral drugs in pregnant women infected with HIV-1 for maternal health and for reducing perinatal HIV-1 transmission in the United States. MMWR (1998). (RR-2)

[17] Chou, R, Smits, A. K, Huffman, L. H, Fu, R, & Korthuis, P. T. US Preventive Services Task Force. Prenatal screening for HIV: A review of the evidence for the U.S. Preventive Services Task Force. Ann Intern Med. (2005). Jul 5;, 143(1), 38-54.

[18] Coll, O, Fiore, S, Floridia, M, et al. (2002). Pregnancy and HIV infection: a European consensus on management. AIDS, 2002; 16(suppl):S, 1-18.

[19] Connor, E. M, Sperling, R. S, Gelber, R, Kiselev, P, Scott, G, & Sullivan, O. MJ, et al. Reduction of maternal-infant transmission of human immunodeficiency virus type 1

with zidovudine treatment. Pediatric AIDS Clinical Trials Group Protocol 076 Study Group. N Engl J Med (1994). , 331, 1173-80.

[20] Cooper, E. R, Charurat, M, Mofenson, L, Hanson, I. C, Pitt, J, Diaz, C, et al. Combination antiretroviral strategies for the treatment of pregnant HIV-1-infected women and prevention of perinatal HIV-1 transmission. J Acquir Immune Defic Syndr (2002). , 29, 484-94.

[21] Dabis, F, Msellati, P, Meda, N, Welffens-ekra, C, You, B, Manigart, O, et al. month efficacy, tolerance, and acceptability of a short regimen of oral zidovudine to reduce vertical transmission of HIV in breastfed children in Cote d'Ivoire and Burkina Faso: a double-blind placebo-controlled multicentre trial. DITRAME Study Group. Diminution de la Transmission Mere-Enfant. Lancet (1999). , 353, 786-92.

[22] De Cock, K. M, Fowler, M. G, Mercier, E, et al. (2000). Prevention of Mother-to-child HIV transmission in resource-poor countries: translating research into policy and practice. JAMA. 283(9).

[23] Determinants of mother-to-infant human immunodeficiency virus 1 transmission before and after the introduction of zidovudine prophylaxisArch Pediatr Adolesc Med (2002). , 156, 915-21.

[24] Dunn, D. T, Newell, M. L, Ades, A. E, & Peckham, C. S. Risk of human immunodeficiency virus type 1 transmission through breastfeeding. Lancet. (1992). , 340585-8.

[25] Efficacy of three short-course regimens of zidovudine and lamivudine in preventing early and late transmission of HIV-1 from mother to child in TanzaniaSouth Africa, and Uganda (Petra study): a randomised, double-blind, placebo-controlled trial. Lancet (2002). , 359, 1178-86.

[26] European collaborative study and the Swiss Mother + Child HIV Cohort Study ((2000). Combination antiretroviral therapy andduration of pregnancy. AIDS. 2000;, 14, 2913-20.

[27] Gray, R. H, Li, X, Kigazi, G, Serwadda, D, Brahmbhatt, H, Wabwire-mangen, F, Nalugoda, F, Kiddugavu, M, Sweankambo, N, Quinn, T. C, Reynolds, S. J, & Wawer, M. J. Increased Risk of Incident HIV during Pregnancy in Rakai, Uganda: A Prospective Study. The Lancet (2005).

[28] Grubert, T. A, Reindell, D, Belohradsky, B. H, Gurtler, L, Stauber, M, & Dathe, O. Rates of postoperative complication among human immunodeficiency virus-infected women who have undergone obstetric and gynecologic surgical procedures. CID (2002). , 34, 822-30.

[29] Grosch-woerner, I, Puch, K, Maier, R. F, Niehues, T, Notheis, G, Patel, D, et al. Multicenter Interdisciplinary Study GroupGermany/Austria. Increased rate of prematurity associated with antenatal antiretroviral therapy in a German/Austrian cohort of-HIV-1-infected women. HIV Med. (2008). , 9, 6-13.

[30] Guay, L. A, Musoke, P, Fleming, T, Bagenda, D, Allen, M, Nakabiito, C, et al. Intrapartum and neonatal single-dose nevirapine compared with zidovudine for prevention of mother-to-child transmission of HIV-1 in Kampala, Uganda: HIVNET 012 randomised trial. Lancet (1999). , 354, 795-802.

[31] Hall, H. I, An, Q, Hutchinson, A. B, & Sansom, S. Estimating the lifetime risk of a diagnosis of the HIV infection in 33 states, (2004). J Acquir Immune Defic Syndr 2008;, 49, 294-7.

[32] Holtgrave, D. R, Hall, H. I, Rhodes, P. H, et al. (2009). Updated annual HIV transmission rates in the United States, 1977-2006. J Acquir Immune Defic Syndr , 50(2), 236-238.

[33] Grubert, T. A, Reindell, D, Kastner, R, Lutz-friedrich, R, Belohradsky, B. H, & Datha, O. Complications after caesarean section in HIV-1 infected women not taking antiretroviral treatment. Lancet, (1999). , 354, 1612-3.

[34] Jamieson, D. J, Read, J. S, Kourtis, A. P, Durant, T. M, Lampe, M. A, & Dominguez, K. L. Cesarean delivery for HIV-infected women: recommendations and controversies. Am J Obstet Gynecol. (2007). Sep;197(3 Suppl):S, 96-100.

[35] John, G. C, Richardson, B. A, Nduati, R. W, Mbori-ngacha, D, & Kreiss, J. K. Timing of breast milk HIV-1 transmission: a meta-analysis.. East Afr Med J. (2001). , 7875-9.

[36] Koenig, L. J, Whitaker, D. J, Royce, R. A, Wilson, T. E, Callahan, M. R, Fernandez, M. I, et al. Violence during pregnancy among women with or at risk for HIV infection.. Am J Public Health. (2002). , 92367-70.

[37] Kourtis, A. P, Lee, F. K, Abrams, E. J, et al. Mother-to-child transmission of HIV-1: timing and implications for prevention. Lancet Infect Dis. (2006). , 6, 726-732.

[38] Lancioni, C, Harwell, T, & Rutstein, R. M. (1999). Prenatal care and HIV infection. AIDS Patient Care STDS. 1999 Feb; 13 (2); , 97-102.

[39] Lallemant, M, & Jourdain, G. Le Coeur S, Kim S, Koetsawang S, Comeau AM, et al. A trial of shortened zidovudine regimens to prevent mother-to-child transmission of human immunodeficiency virus type 1. Perinatal HIV Prevention Trial (Thailand) Investigators. N Engl J Med (2000). , 343, 982-91.

[40] Lester, P, Partridge, J. C, Chesney, M. A, & Cooke, M. The consequences of a positive prenatal HIV antibody test for women. J Acquir Immune Defic Syndr Hum Retrovirol. (1995). , 10341-9.

[41] Lindau, S, Jerome, J, Miller, K, Monk, E, Garcia, P, & Cohen, M. (2006). Mothers on the margins: Implications for eradicating perinatal HIV. Social Science and Medicine, 62(1), 59-69.

[42] Livingston, E, Huo, Y, Patel, K, Brogly, S. B, Tuomala, R, Scott, G. B, Bardeguez, A, Stek, A, & Read, J. S. (2010). For the International Maternal Pediatric Adolescent AIDS Clinical Trials Group (IMPAACT) Protocol 1025 Study. Mode of Delivery and

Infant Respiratory Morbidity Among Infants Born to HIV-1 infected Women. Obstet Gynecol, 2010; 116(2 Pt 1): 335-343.

[43] Makoha, F. W, Felimban, H. M, Fathuddien, M. A, Roomi, F, & Ghabra, T. (2004). Multiple cesarean section morbidity. Int J Gynaecol Obstet 2004; , 87, 227-32.

[44] Mandelbrot, L, Landreau-mascaro, A, Rekacewicz, C, Berrebi, A, Benifla, J. L, Burgard, M, et al. Lamivudine-zidovudine combination for prevention of maternal-infant transmission of HIV-1. JAMA (2001). , 285, 2083-93.

[45] Marks, G, Crepaz, N, & Janssen, R. (2006). Estimating sexual transmission of HIV from persons aware and unaware that they are infected with the virus in the USA. Journal of Acquired Immune Deficiency Sydromes , 20(10), 1447-1450.

[46] Minkoff, H, Mccalla, S, & Feldman, J. (1990). The relationship of cocaine use to syphilis and HIV infection among inner city parturient women. Am J Obstet Gynecol. 1990;, 163, 521-526.

[47] Moodley, D, Moodley, J, Coovadia, H, Gray, G, Mcintyre, J, Hofmyer, J, et al. A multicenter randomized, controlled trial of nevirapine versus a combination of zidovudine and lamivudine to reduce intrapartum and early postpartum mother-to-child transmission of human immunodeficiency virus type 1. J Infect Dis (2003). , 187, 725-35.

[48] Moodley, D, Esterhuizen, T. M, Pather, T, Chetty, V, & Ngaleka, L. High HIV Incidence During Pregnancy: Compelling Reason for Repeat HIV Testing. AIDS (2009).

[49] Mother-to-child transmission of HIV infection in the era of highly active antiretroviral therapyClin Infect Dis (2005). , 40, 458-65.

[50] Nduati, R, John, G, Mbori-ngacha, D, Richardson, B, Overbaugh, J, Mwatha, A, et al. Effect of breastfeeding and formula feeding on transmission of HIV-1: a randomized clinical trial.. JAMA. (2000). , 2831167-74.

[51] Provisional Committee on Pediatric AIDSAmerican Academy of Pediatrics. Perinatal human immunodeficiency virus testing. Pediatrics. (1995). , 95303-7.

[52] Prejean, J, Song, R, Hernandez, A, Ziebell, R, Green, T, et al. Estimated HIV Incidence in the United States, (2011). PLoS ONE 2011 6(8): e17502. doi:10.1371/journal.pone.0017502., 2006-2009.

[53] Public Health Service Task Force(2010). Recommendations for use of antiretroviral drugs in pregnant HIV-infected women for maternal health and interventions to reduce perinatal HIV-1 transmission in the United States. 2010. Available at: http://aidsinfo.nih.gov/contentfiles/PerinatalGL.pdfRetrieved April 13, 2011., 1.

[54] Rahangdale, L, & Cohan, D. Rapid Human Immunodeficiency Virus Testing on Labor and Delivery. Obstetrics and Gynecology (2008).

[55] Read, J. S, Tuomala, R, Kpamegan, E, Zorrilla, C, Landesman, S, Brown, G, et al. Mode of delivery and postpartum morbidity among HIV-infected women: the women and infants transmission study. J Acquir Immune Defic Syndr (2001). , 26, 236-45.

[56] Rothpletz-puglia, P, Storm, D, Burr, C, & Samuels, D. Routine prenatal HIV testing: women's concern and their strategies for addressing concerns. Matern Child Health J (2012).

[57] Samson, L, & King, S. Evidence-based guidelines for universal counselling and offering of HIV testing in pregnancy in Canada.. CMAJ. (1998). , 1581449-57.

[58] Sansom, S. L, Jamieson, D. J, Farnham, P. G, Bulterys, M, & Fowler, M. G. Human Immunodeficiency Virus Retesting During Pregnancy: Costs and Effectiveness in Preventing Perinatal Transmission. Obstetrics and Gynecology (2003).

[59] Shaffer, N, Chuachoowong, R, Mock, P. A, Bhadrakom, C, Siriwasin, W, Young, N. L, et al. Short-course zidovudine for perinatal HIV-1 transmission in Bangkok, Thailand: a randomised controlled trial. Bangkok Collaborative Perinatal HIV Transmission Study Group. Lancet (1999). , 353, 773-80.

[60] Sheon, A. R, Fox, H. E, Alexander, G, Buck, A, Higgins, A, Mcdermott, S. M, et al. Misdiagnosed HIV infection in pregnant women: implications for clinical care.. Public Health Rep. (1994). , 109694-9.

[61] Shernoff, M, & Smith, R. HIV treatments: A history of scientific advance. Body Positive Magazine. July (2001).

[62] Sturt, A. S, Dokubo, E. K, & Sint, T. T. Antiretroviral therapy (ART) for treating HIV infection in ART-eligible pregnant women. Cochrane Database of Systematic Reviews (2010). Issue 3. Art. DOI:CD008440.(CD008440)

[63] Taha, T. E, Kumwenda, N. I, Gibbons, A, Broadhead, R. L, Fiscus, S, Lema, V, et al. Short postexposure prophylaxis in newborn babies to reduce mother-to-child transmission of HIV-1: NVAZ randomised clinical trial. Lancet (2003). , 362, 1171-7.

[64] Tita, A. T, Landon, M. B, Spong, C. Y, Lai, Y, Leveno, K. J, Varner, M. W, Moawad, A. H, Caritis, S. N, Meis, P. J, Wapner, R. J, Sorokin, Y, Miodovnik, M, Carpenter, M, Peaceman, A. M, Sullivan, O, Sibai, M. J, Langer, B. M, Thorp, O, Ramin, J. M, & Mercer, S. M. B.M.; Eunice Kennedy Shriver NICHD Maternal-Fetal Medicine Units Network. Timing of elective repeat cesarean delivery at term and neonatal outcomes. N Engl J Med, (2009). , 360(2), 111-20.

[65] The International Perinatal HIV GroupThe mode of delivery and the risk for vertical transmission of human immunodeficiency virus type a meta-analysis of 15 prospective cohort studies. N Engl J Med. (1999). , 1.

[66] Turner, B. J, Mckee, L. J, Siverman, N. S, et al. (1996). Prenatal care and birth outcomes of a cohort of HIV-infected women. J Acquir Immune Defic Syndr 1996; , 12, 259-67.

[67] UNFPA/UNICEF/WHO/UNAIDS Inter-Agency Task Team on Mother-to-Child Transmission of HIVNew data on the prevention of mother-to-child transmission of HIV and their policy implications: conclusions and recommendations. Geneva, Switzerland: World Health Organization; (2000).

[68] Vimercati, A, Greco, P, Loverro, G, Lopalco, P. L, Pansini, V, & Selvaggi, L. (2000). Maternal complications after caesarean section in HIV infected women. Eur J Obstet Gynecol Reprod Biol, 2000;, 90, 73-76.

[69] Watts, D. H, Lambert, J. S, Stiehm, E. R, Bethel, J, Whitehouse, J, Fowler, M. G, et al. Complications according to mode of delivery among human immunodeficiency virus-infected women with CD4 lymphocyte counts of < or = 500/microL. Am J Obstet Gynecol (2000). , 183, 100-7.

[70] Watts, D. H, & Balasubramanian, R. Maupin RT Jr, Delke I, Dorenbaum A, Fiore S, et al. Maternal toxicity and pregnancy complications in human immunodeficiency virus-infected women receiving antiretroviral therapy: PACTG 316. Am J Obstet Gynecol (2004). , 190, 506-16.

[71] Wiktor, S. Z, Ekpini, E, Karon, J. M, Nkengasong, J, Maurice, C, Severin, S. T, et al. Short-course oral zidovudine for prevention of mother-to-child transmission of HIV-1 in Abidjan, Cote d'Ivoire: a randomised trial. Lancet (1999). , 353, 781-5.

Chapter 5

Human Immunodeficiency Virus Testing Algorithm in Resource Limiting Settings

Teddy Charles Adias and Osaro Erhabor

Additional information is available at the end of the chapter

http://dx.doi.org/10.5772/53675

1. Introduction

Testing and counseling for human immunodeficiency virus (HIV) is now recognized as a priority in national HIV programs because it is the gateway to HIV/AIDS prevention, care, treatment, and support interventions. In order to ensure access to HIV testing for large populations and to facilitate access to antiretroviral treatment in the context of the World Health Organization's universal access strategy, radical scaling up of HIV testing and counseling services is being advocated globally.

The use of HIV rapid tests will facilitate this in many settings, particularly in services in which the people most likely to benefit from knowing their HIV status can be reached. These Settings include diagnostic and treatment services for tuberculosis and sexually transmitted infections; services linked to the prevention of mother-to-child transmission of HIV; the management of occupational and non-occupational exposures to HIV; at voluntary counseling and testing (VCT) sites; in remote areas where the creation and maintenance of a laboratory infrastructure is not possible; and where hard-to-reach populations have access to HIV testing (PAHO, 2008).

To date, HIV testing strategies has clear objective for diagnosis, surveillance and transfusion safety. The need for appropriate selection of testing platforms and protocol had also varied from setting to setting. In general, four criteria had underpinned the choice of most appropriate test or combination of tests for any given setting and depend on: General goal for testing, Diagnostic indices of sensitivity and specificity, Prevalence of HIV infection in the general population and Cost of testing (WHO, 2004).

HIV testing is the entry point for both care and prevention. In resource limiting settings, this declaration seems more valid than ever given the increase prevalence and incidence of HIV infection in these settings and current efforts at universal access for care and prevention. The aim of this chapter is to provide trend in HIV testing Algorithm- a combination and sequence of specific testing employed in given strategy for the confirmation of HIV status of an individual or sample.

In the evolving Chapter, we shall transit with set-out for HIV testing algorithms (with appropriate sub-themes) from HIV testing evolution and forms of testing to HIV testing strategies and algorithm platforms.

2. HIV testing

2.1. Evolution of HIV testing

HIV screening and diagnostic tests have been developed, and a variety of testing algorithms have come into use. HIV antibody tests have evolved from first generation HIV-1(clade B) viral lysate-based, indirect antibody enzyme immunoassays (EIAs) to third generation antigen-sandwich immunoassays that use synthetic peptide and recombinant DNA derived antigens that represent the immunodominant epitopes from diverse HIV-1 and HIV-2 strains. These third generation enzyme immunoassays have substantially enhanced sensitivity to divergent viral variants and have shortened the infection-to-seroconversion window period by more than 3 weeks compared with first generation tests. Assays have also been developed that detect and quantitate viral antigen (p24) and nucleic acids (HIV RNA or DNA) in blood, and in body fluids and tissues (Branson, 2010; WHO, 2009a).

These assays have seen increasing application in blood and organ donor screening, as well as in clinical diagnosis, prognosis, and therapeutic monitoring; and clinicians now have access to a broad and potentially confusing array of test options, each with its own advantages and limitations. Developing testing algorithms and interpretive criteria appropriate to a particular group of patients—high-risk adults; blood, plasma and organ donors; recently exposed healthcare workers; paediatric patients, and especially in resource limiting settings—poses a challenge, especially as new tests appear with tantalizing claims of enhanced performance (WHO, 2009a/b).

The laboratory diagnosis of the HIV infection is based on a two-stage strategy: a screening analysis followed by a confirmation analysis. A positive screening analysis must always be supplemented by a confirmation analysis on the same sample. An HIV infection can only be confirmed when the result of the confirmation analysis is positive and consistent results are obtained for two separate samples (PAHO, 2008).

Screening tests provide presumptive identification of specimens that contain antibody to HIV. These enzyme immunosorbent assays (EIAs) or simple/rapid immuno-diagnostics are selected for their high sensitivity of detecting antibodies to HIV. Supplemental or confirmatory tests, such as Western blot (WB), can be used to confirm infection in samples that are initially reactive on conventional EIAs. Alternatively, repetitive testing incorporating EIAs or rapid tests selected for their specificity may be used to confirm whether specimens found to be reactive for HIV antibodies with a particular screening test are specific to HIV. For practical purposes, resource-poor settings depend heavily on EIA and rapid tests for screening and confirmation (WHO, 2004).

2.2. Enzyme immunsorbent assays

EIAs are the most widely used screening tests because of their suitability for analyzing large numbers of specimens, particularly in blood screening centers. Since 1985, EIAs have progressed considerably from first to fourth generation assays: first generation assays were based on purified HIV whole viral lysates, however, sensitivity and specificity of these assays were poor; second generation assays used HIV-recombinant proteins and/or synthetic peptides, which enabled the production of assays capable of detecting HIV-1 and HIV-2. The assays had improved specificity, although their overall sensitivity was similar to that of first-generation assays. Third-generation assays used the solid phase coated with recombinant antigens and /or peptides and similar recombinant antigens and peptides conjugated to a detection enzyme or hapten that could detect HIV-specific antibodies bound to a solid phase. These assays could detect immunoglobulin M, early antibodies to HIV, in addition to IgG, thus resulting in a reduction of the seroconversion window. Fourth generation assays are very similar to third-generations tests but have the ability to detect simultaneously HIV antibodies and antigens. Typical fourth-generation EIAs incorporate cocktails of HIV-1 group M (HIV-1 p24, HIV-1 gp160), HIV-1 group O, and HIV-2 antigens (HIV-2 env peptide) (WHO, 2009a/b and 2004).

Furthermore, third and fourth-generation assays are able to detect IgM and IgG antibodies to both HIV-1 and HIV-2. These assays may reduce the 2-4 week time period, "window period" of detecting HIV antibodies (WHO, 2009b).

2.3. Rapid/simple assays

Simple, instrument-free assays are also available and are now widely used in Africa. They include agglutination, immunofiltration, and immunochromatographic assays. The appearance of a colored dot or line, or an agglutination pattern indicates a positive result. Most of these tests can be performed in less than 20 minutes, and are therefore called simple/rapid assays. Some simple tests, such as agglutination assays, are less rapid and may require about 30 minutes to 2 hours to be completed. In general, these rapid/simple tests are most suitable for use in settings that have limited facilities and process fewer than 100 samples per day (WHO, 2009b and 2004).

2.3.1. Importance of rapid/simple assays

Although EIA–based serodiagnostic algorithms are highly cost effective, their application in resource-poor settings is limited by several factors. They require well-trained personnel, need a consistent supply of electricity, and maintenance and cost of most equipment. Rapid assays have high sensitivity and specificity and perform as well as EIAs on specimens from persons seroconverting for non-B HIV-1 subtypes (Koblavi-Dème *et al*, 2001). Rapid enzyme assays circumvent the issue of low rates of return for serologic results associated with EIA-based testing algorithms because results can be delivered on the same day (Puro *et al*, 2004). In addition, their performance has improved considerably, and some do not require reconstitution of reagents or refrigeration; thus, making them very suitable for use in resource limited settings and hard to reach populations (Koblavi-Dème *et al*, 2001). Practical applications for the use of simple/rapid assays are in settings such as Voluntary Counseling and Testing (VCT) and Prevention of Mother to Child Transmission (PMTCT) programs. Studies have shown that using rapid assay testing algorithms result in remarkable increase in the number of HIV-positive women identified as eligible to receive the short-course therapy that reduces mother-to-child transmission of HIV (Sibailly *et al*, 2000).

3. HIV testing strategies and algorithm

3.1. Nature of algorithm/testing strategy

A testing algorithm for serologic diagnosis of HIV-infection is the sequence in which assays are performed to detect HIV antibody in a body fluid. The most common referenced testing algorithm employs an EIA to screen specimens with those found to be positive then confirmed by WB testing. This so-called conventional algorithm has several limitations (PAHO, 2008):

- WB is expensive and requires technical expertise.
- WB often yields indeterminate results with certain types of specimens with uncertain diagnostic significance, e.g., hyperimmunoglobulinemia specimens.
- Both ELISA and WB are time consuming and require a well-equipped laboratory infrastructure.

Various combinations of tests can be used: combinations of HIV EIAs; combinations of rapid tests; or an EIA in conjunction with rapid tests. The choice of strategy and of HIV tests should be determined by the quality of the tests and by the practicality of their implementation, logistics, and the cost-benefit analysis. Figure 1, depicts the WHO/UNAIDS testing strategies which can be adopted in diverse settings

In the WHO/UNAIDS testing strategies I – III, as applicable relative to testing objective (surveillance, blood screening, or diagnosis) or diagnostic indices (sero-prevalence in a given population and the duo of sensitivity and specificity of the test being used. The three HIV testing strategies recommended by WHO and UNAIDS are described below (Figure 1) (WHO, 2009a; UNAID/WHO, 1998).

http://dx.doi.org/10.5772/53675

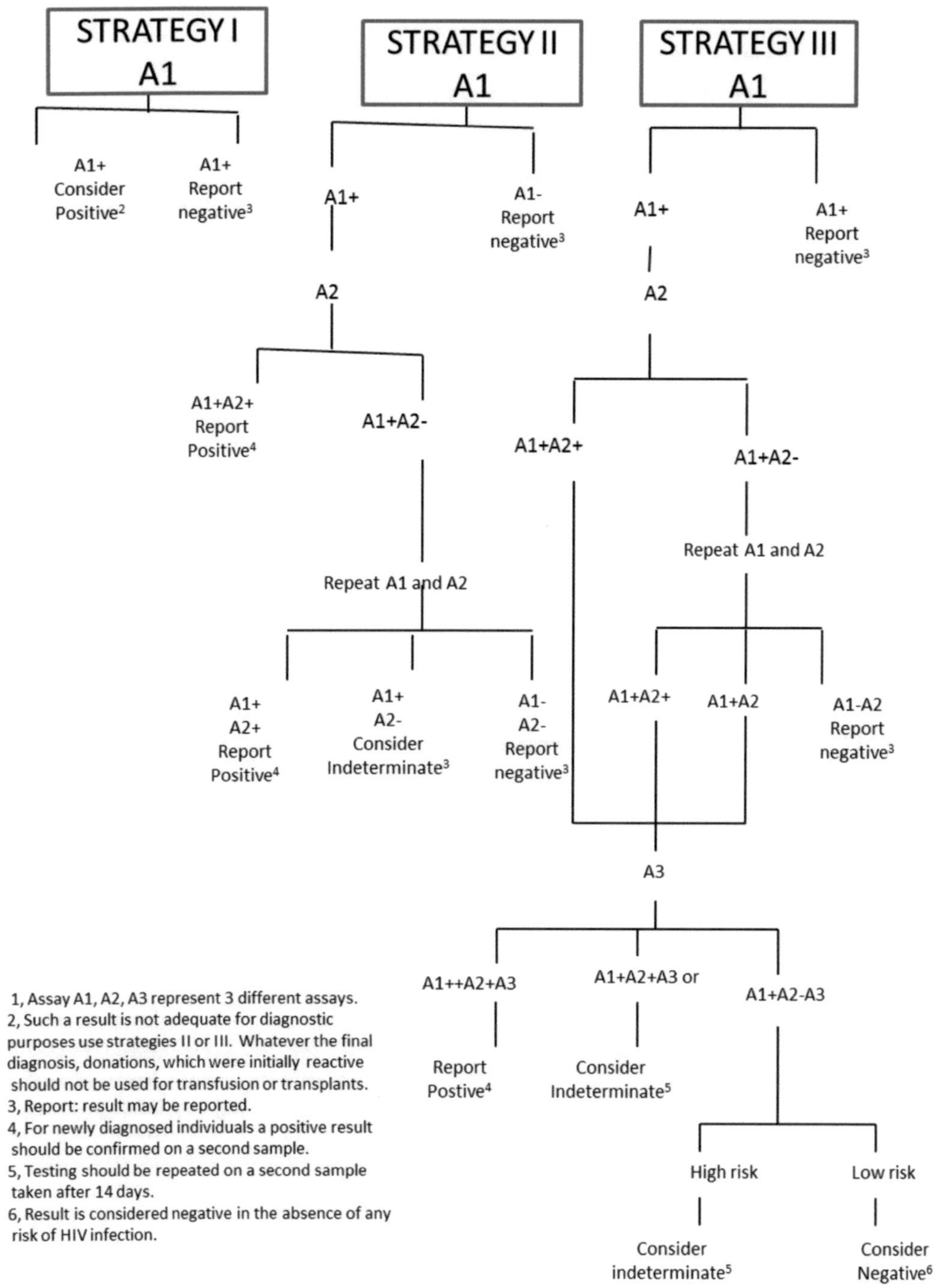

Figure 1. Schematic Representation of the WHO/UNAIDS HIV Testing Strategy(Adapted from WHO, 2009a/b and UN-AID/WHO,1998)

Strategy I:

- Requires one test.
- For use in diagnostic testing in populations with an HIV prevalence >30% among persons with clinical signs or symptoms of HIV infection.
- For use in blood screening, for all prevalence rates.
- For use in surveillance testing in populations with an HIV prevalence >10% (example: unlinked anonymous testing for surveillance among pregnant women at antenatal clinics). No results are provided.

Strategy II:

- Requires up to two tests.
- For use in diagnostic testing in populations with an HIV prevalence ≤30% among persons with clinical signs or symptoms of HIV infection or >10% among asymptomatic persons.
- For use in surveillance testing in populations with an HIV prevalence ≤10% (example: unlinked anonymous testing for surveillance among patients at antenatal clinics or sexually transmitted infection clinics). No results are provided.

Strategy III:

- Requires up to three tests.
- For use in diagnostic testing in populations with an HIV prevalence ≤10% among asymptomatic persons.

Sensitivity and specificity are two important factors that determine a test's accuracy in distinguishing between HIV-infected and uninfected individuals. It is crucial that the HIV tests used in the algorithms all have a sensitivity of at least 99% and a specificity of at least 98% (WHO, 2009a and 1997). There are commercially available HIV EIAs and HIV rapid tests that meet these criteria. When selecting HIV tests to be used in combination, it is important to select tests that do not share the same false positive and same false negative results. This information can be obtained from comparative evaluation studies of HIV test kits, such as those published in international scientific publications and in WHO reports (WHO, 2009a/b). It is recommended that such comparative evaluations of a select number of HIV test kits be conducted at the national and/or regional level prior to the establishment of the national HIV test algorithms. These principles apply to both conventional HIV EIA and HIV rapid tests. The national reference laboratory should validate a select number of test kits for use in the national HIV testing algorithms.

Specific implementation requirements must be considered when selecting tests kits and algorithms. For example, will testing be performed in a laboratory setting, or in a VCT or clinical setting without extensive laboratory facilities? In settings without extensive laboratory facilities or where clients do not return for follow-up visits, algorithms using only rapid tests are preferred. In situations in which patients return at regular intervals (e.g., TB clinics) or in prenatal clinics where blood specimens are taken for other testing purposes, the set-up may allow for HIV EIA-based algorithms or algorithms combining EIA and rapid tests (Owusu-Ofori et al, 2005; Routet et al, 2004).

Another factor determining the most cost-efficient approach is the volume of specimens to be processed daily or weekly. An EIA test is half the price of a rapid test, so if a particular setting processes 40 specimens a day and the laboratory has the required equipment, it is more cost effective to use EIAs than rapid tests. It is important that the HIV tests and algorithms be chosen carefully and with the aim of optimal integration into the existing health care facilities, minimizing the potential to disrupt their operations or unnecessarily overburden staff.

There are many strategies for HIV testing (Parekh *et al*, 2010; WHO, 2009a/b; P*aul et al, 2004*). WHO, CDC, and the Association of Public Health Laboratories have jointly developed one of the most useful references for HIV testing algorithms. These strategies can be divided into two approaches: serial (or sequential) testing and parallel testing.

3.2. Algorithm platforms

3.2.1. Serial/sequential testing strategy

In a Serial or sequential testing strategy, samples are initially tested with only one, highly sensitive assay. Samples that are reactive in the first assay are then re-tested using a second, highly specific assay. A third test may be performed, depending on the result of the second assay and the objective of the testing. Both the selection of and the order in which the assays are used are of the utmost importance for the final outcome of the tests. If test combinations are not carefully selected, individuals may be incorrectly diagnosed. WHO recommends sequential testing (Figure 2) in most settings because it is more economical, as the second test is required only when the initial test result is positive (Gershy=Damet *et al*, 2010; WHO, 2009a/b; Ferreira *et al*, 2005).

3.2.2. Parallel testing strategy

In a parallel testing strategy (Figure 3), samples are tested using two different assays simultaneously. This approach is rather expensive, as it virtually doubles the cost of testing in low- prevalence settings by requiring two tests at the outset. As with sequential testing, a third test may be performed preferably at the secondary level, where laboratory facilities and experienced staff are available, depending on the result of the assays and the objective of the testing (WHO, 2009a/b).

Therefore, the parallel testing strategy is recommended only in situations in which it can add value. Prenatal clinics provide one such example: A woman's first visit to the clinic may be to deliver her child, thus requiring a rapid decision whether an intervention to prevent mother-to-child transmission of HIV is needed. Other emergency situations, such as work accidents, sexual violence, and discordant couples also would benefit from this strategy. In these cases, two rapid tests using whole-blood finger-stick specimens in parallel will provide the answer in just 10–15 minutes. HIV rapid tests using wholeblood finger-stick specimens have great potential in situations where results need to be known quickly, or where taking a conventional venous sample is difficult (Gershy-Damet *et al*, 2010; WHO, 2009a/b; Ferreira *et al*, 2005).

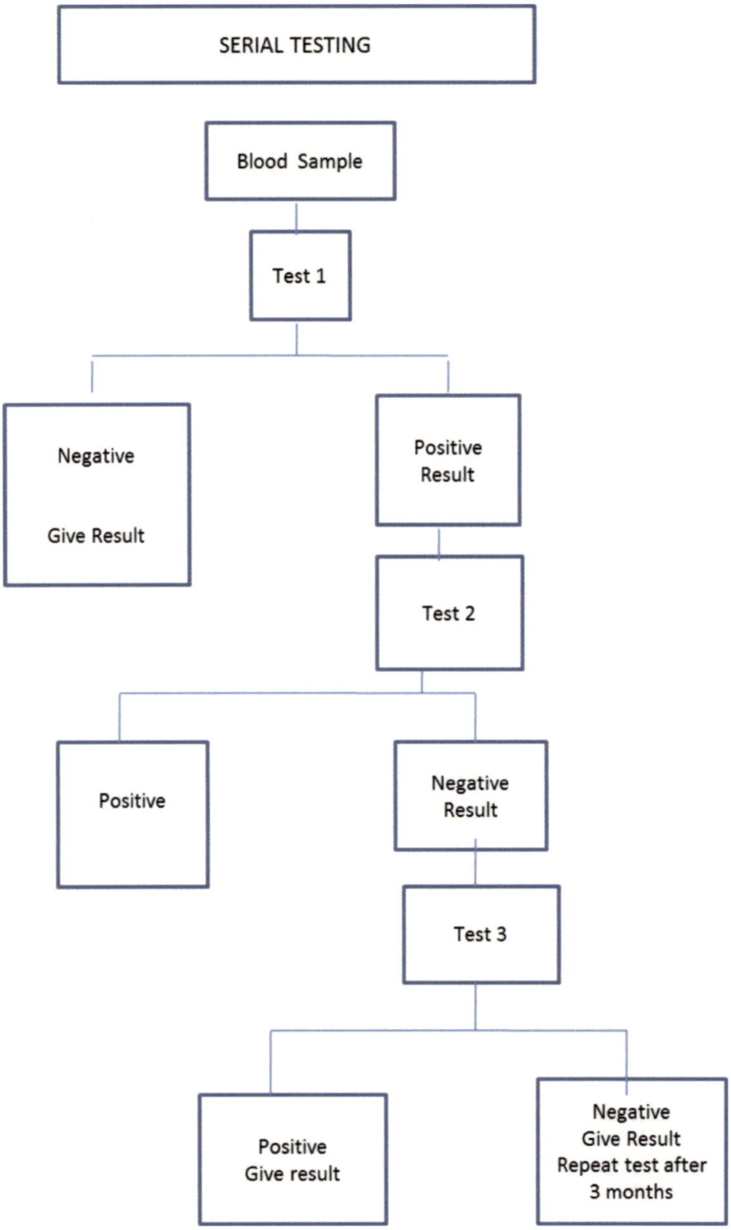

Figure 2. Serial/ Sequential Testing Algorithm (Adapted from WHO, 2009a/b)

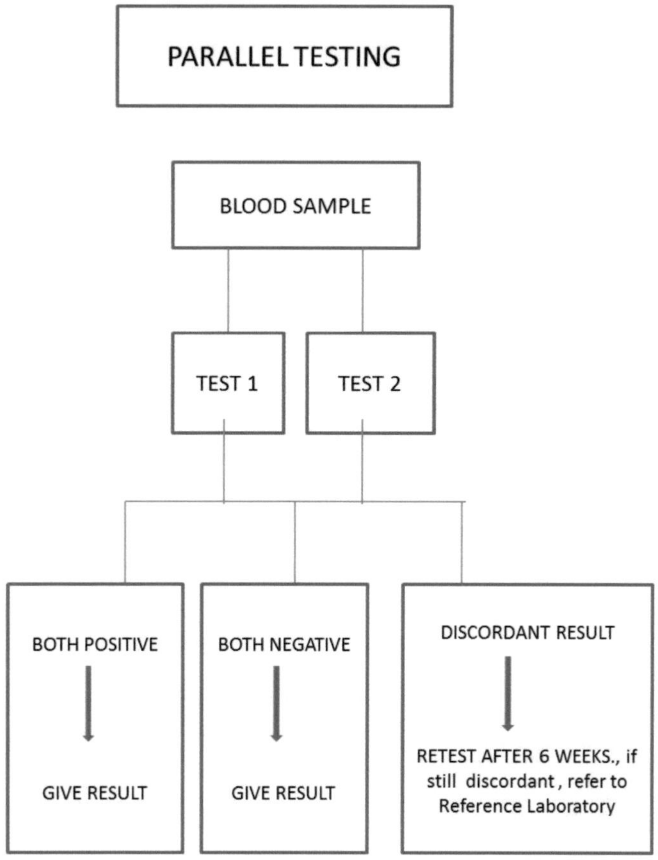

Figure 3. Parallel Testing Algorithm (Adapted from WHO, 2009a/b)

4. Conclusion

HIV testing is the essential entry point for both treatment and prevention. As in all societies, especially in Africa, high degree of genetic diversity exist. One implication for this is the need for each country to have an in-house evaluation of its country –specific testing strategy. The selection of a national algorithm is the responsibility of the country's Ministry of Health. The choice of sequential or parallel testing should be made after a thorough analysis of the scientific evidence, logistics, test performance requirements, and cost/affordability of the various algorithms.

Author details

Teddy Charles Adias[1*] and Osaro Erhabor[2]

*Address all correspondence to: teddyadias@yahoo.com

1 Bayelsa State College of Health Technology, Ogbia Town, Yenagoa, Nigeria

2 Department of Blood Sciences, Royal Bolton Hospital NHS Trust UK, Bolton, United Kingdom

References

[1] Branson BM (2010). The future of HIV testing. *JAIDS.* 55 (2): 102-105.

[2] Ferreira Junior OC, Ferreira C, Riedel M, Widolin MR, Barbosa-Júnior A (2005). HIV Rapid Test Study Group.Evaluation of rapid tests for anti-HIV detection in Brazil. *AIDS.*19(4):S70–75.

[3] Gershy-Damet G, Rotz P, Cross, D, *et al* (2010). The World Health Organization African region laboratory accreditation process: Improving the quality of laboratory systems in the African region. *Am J Clin Pathol. 134* : 393-400.

[4] Koblavi-Dème S, Maurice C, Yavo D, *et al* (2001). Sensitivity and specificity of HIV rapid serologic assays and testing algorithms in an antenatal clinic in Abidjan, Côte d'Ivoire. *J Clin Microbiol.* 39:1808-1812.

[5] Owusu-Ofori S, Temple J, Sarkodie F, Anokwa M, Candotti D, Allain JP (2005). Predonation screening of blood donors with rapid tests: Implementation and efficacy of a novel approach to blood safety in resource-poor settings. *Transfusion.* 45(2):133–140.

[6] Pan American Health Organisation (PAHO) (2008). Guidelines for the implementation of Reliable and Efficient Diagnostic HIV Testing, Region of the Americas.

[7] Parekh B, Kalou M, Alemnji G, Ou C, *et al* (2010). Scaling up HIV rapid testing in developing countries: comprehensive approach for implementing quality assurance. *Am J Clin Pathol. 134*: 573-84.

[8] Paul SM, Grimes-Dennis J, Burr CK, DiFerdinando GT (2003). Rapid diagnostic testing for HIV. Clinical implications. *N J Med* 100(9):11–14.

[9] Puro V, Francisci D, Sighinolfi L, Civljak R, Belfiori B, Deparis P, et al (2004) Benefits of a rapid HIV test for evaluation of the source patient after occupational exposure of healthcare workers. *J Hosp Infect.* 57(2):179–182.

[10] Rouet F, Ekouevi DK, Inwoley A, Chaix ML, Burgard M, Bequet L, et al (2004). Field evaluation of a rapid human immunodeficiency virus (HIV) serial serologic testing

algorithm for diagnosis and differentiation of HIV type 1 (HIV-1), HIV-2, and dual HIV-1–HIV-2 infections in West African pregnant women. *J Clin Microbiol.* 42(9): 4147–4153.

[11] Sibailly TS, Ekpini ER, Kamelan-Tanoh A, *et al* (2000). Impact of on-site HIV rapid testing with same-day post-test counseling on acceptance of short-course zidovudine for the prevention of mother-to-child transmission of HIV in Abidjan, Côte d'Ivoire. *The XIII International AIDS 2000 Conference.*

[12] UNAIDS/WHO (1998). UNAIDS/WHO Recommendations. The importance of simple/rapid assays in HIV testing. Weekly Epidemiological Record. 73:321-28.

[13] World Health Organisation (WHO) (2009a). *HIV assays. Operational characteristics.* Report 16. *Rapid assay*. Geneva.

[14] World Health Organisation (WHO) (2009b). Guidelines for using HIV testing technologies in surveillance: Selection, Evaluation and Implementation 2009 Update

[15] World Health Organisation (WHO) (2004). Rapid HIV tests: guidelines for use in HIV testing and counseling services in resource-constrained settings.

[16] WHO/UNAIDS (1997). Revised Recommendations for the selection and use of HIV antibody tests. WHO Weekly Epidemiol. *72:* 81-7.

Section 3

HIV and NeuroAIDS

Chapter 6

NeuroAIDS: Mechanisms, Causes, Prevalence, Diagnostics and Social Issues

Shailendra K. Saxena, Sneham Tiwari and
Madhavan P.N. Nair

Additional information is available at the end of the chapter

http://dx.doi.org/10.5772/55100

1. Introduction

Human immunodeficiency virus-1 (HIV-1) engulfs 33 millions of life as per the latest UN AIDS report [Saxena, Tiwari., *et al.*, 2012] and the effect worsens up when it causes dementia with alarming occurrence worldwide but the mechanism through which it happens is still not well understood, and is in the embryonic stages. The estimated overall prevalence of nervous system disorders among patients receiving highly active antiretroviral therapy but also requiring neurological care is over 25% (Singh *et al.*, 2011). According to WHO there are ~ 34 million people in the world infected with HIV. Out of that 95 percent of these cases as well as deaths from AIDS occur in the developing world. Dementia (HIV-associated dementia) is becoming common in HIV infected adults having prevalence up to 40% in western countries where clade B prevails (Sacktor *et al.*, 2007). Dementia cannot be considered as a disease by itself but it is the term used to describe a set of symptoms resulting from damages and disorders affecting the brain. These symptoms can be caused by a multitude of diseases and depend upon the specific brain regions affected. These symptoms appear as a variety of cognitive, behavioural, affective, motor, and psychiatric disorders. Dementia can be caused by a variety of diseases, known as neurodegenerative diseases resulting from protein aggregation in the brain. Many studies related to this area are been carried out in respect to this, to provide new insights (Saxena *et al.*, 2012). HIV-1 infects macrophages and microglia, and there is an indirect pathway to neuronal injury which happens due to release of macrophage, microglial and astrocytes toxins and viral proteins. The toxins which are released over stimulate neurons, form free radicals, finally leading to neurodegenerative diseases. The cognitive and motor dysfunction which is observed in HIV patients is termed as HIV associated dementia (HAD). The prevalence of the dementia is eventually increasing as AIDS patients are now surviving more. HIV-1 replicates in monocyte and macrophage but not as severe as in infected T cells and blood mononuclear cells (Sundaravaradan *et al.,* 2006). These cells differentiate and travel to several organs, henceforth acting as a source of infectious virus and secreted viral proteins to cause pathological issues and alternating several signalling pathways and distorting many cellular transcription factors, ultimately resulting in HIV-1 pathogenesis. Increased transcription leads to the upregulation of virus production, and hence increased production of viral proteins (gp120, Tat, Nef, and Vpr) (Gandhi et al., 2020; Samikkannu et al., 2010; Saiyed et al., 2011; Saxena et al., 2012; Saxena et al., 2012). The high concentration of these toxic proteins lead to distorted cellular functions, and increased production of toxic metabolites, finally leading to organ-specific like neuroAIDS, in case of viral entry inside the brain (Kilareski et al., 2009). Antiretroviral therapy has increased the lifespan of HIV patients, but CNS function often remains diminished sometimes developing into HIV-associated dementia and the severity and progression of dementia is studied to be increased with the effect of drug abuse [Reddy *et al.,* 2012; Ferris *et al.,* 2008].

2. Prevalence

The prevalence of HAD is estimated to be more than 30% of HIV infected patients, and it is still reported to be increasing (Dean *et al.*, 2012). Improvements in control of peripheral viral replication and the treatment of opportunistic infections, helps in extending life expectancy, resulting in an increase in neuropathogenesis. We are seeing a linear increase in prevalence in rich countries, but an exponential increase in low-income countries. Just under half of people with dementia live in high-income countries, 39% live in middle-income countries, and only 14% live in low-income countries. Increasing living standards, in low income countries such as India (Shankar *et al.*, 2005), may lead to increased life expectancy, which may increase the frequency of dementia cases. As biggest risk factor for dementia is age, a longer-living global population means there will be more people with dementia. The report predicts that the numbers of people with dementia will double every 20 years, to 65.7 million in 2030 and 115.4 million in 2050. Most of this increase will be in developing countries (Prince *et al.,* 2012). A more complete understanding of the pathogenesis of HAD will help in identifying therapeutic targets for its prevention and treatment. The global age standardized death rate for dementia is ~ 6.7 per 100,000 for males and 7.7 per 100,000 for females. According to the World Health Organization, dementia mortality rate for India is 13.5 per 100,000 males and 11.1 for 100,000 females, which is quite alarming (Prince *et al.,* 2012).

3. HIV- Mechanism of neuronal injury

Presently, neuropathogenesis is winning, because there is an incomplete knowledge about the mechanism of HIV infection causing neuronal injury and apoptosis in the host (Fig. 1). HIV enters the central nervous system through infected monocytes and leads to pathogenesis involving activation of macrophages and microglia and further toxin release, that activates several pathways leading to neuronal dysfunction. There are several extracellular and intracellular signalling pathways, which when activated lead to macrophage or microglial activation, and induction in neurons and astrocytes. These pathways are of potential therapeutic importance as targets for the prevention or treatment of neuropathogenesis.

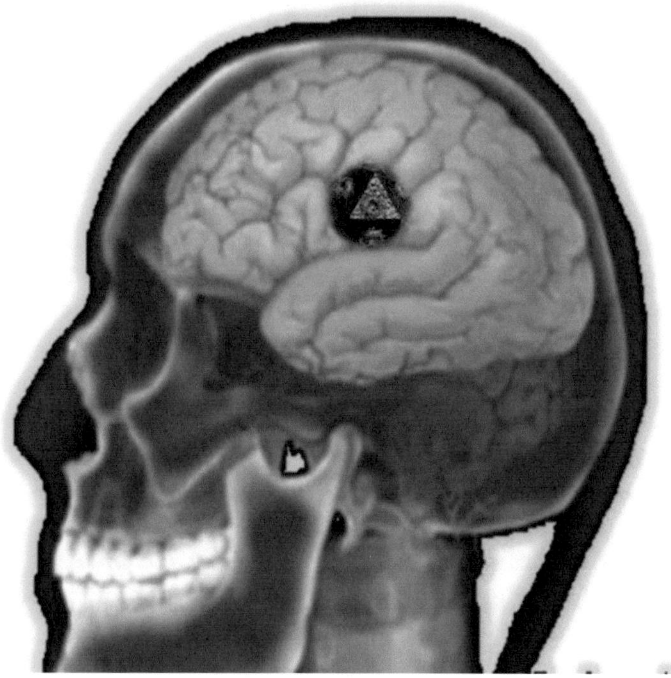

Figure 1. HIV virus can enter the CNS by altering the integrity of blood brain barrier.

4. Neuropathology of AIDS

HIV-1 is capable of causing a multi-system disorder including the CNS. HIV-1 enters the CNS at the early phase of infection, it persists and induces several motor and cognitive disorders leading to behavioural changes. Major clinical symptoms include impaired short term-memory, reduced mental concentration, weakness, slowness of hand and leg movement and depression accompanied by behavioural issues like personality disorders, lethargy and social withdrawal. These neurological and psychiatric symptoms caused by HIV-1 infection, constitute together as neuropathogenesis. A more subtle form of CNS dysfunction, known as minor cognitive motor disorder (MCMD), is also seen common in HIV patients. HAD cannot be controlled by HAART, HIV-1 infection becomes chronic and even rise in disease has been reported. The HIV-1 associated neuropathology is characterized by the infiltration of macrophages into the CNS, the formation of microglial nodules and multinucleated giant cells, astrocyte activation and damage; neuronal loss in ganglions and hippocampus, myelin damage, axonal damage and presence of HIV-1 in the CSF. MRI reports say that HIV infection is associated with progressive cortical atrophy which might be caused by neuronal loss and demyelination worsening in certain cognitive functions (Ghafouri *et al.*, 2006).

5. HIV entry into the brain and initiation of HAD

HIV-1 infects cells having major HIV-1 receptors, CD4 and CD8, and several chemokine receptors which are known to be as HIV-1 co-receptors which help in the attachment of the virus to the cell and membrane fusion leading to viral entry. Infected CD4+ T cells and monocytes circulating in the blood are the potential source of CNS infection. HIV-1 infected cells can be either highly active producers or low/non producers of viruses. Both types of infections occur in the CNS. Studies of different astrocytes cell lines, demonstrated the presence of large quantities of Rev in the cytoplasm. Changes in cell environment, like the elevation in the level of cytokines such as TNF-α and IL-1β, might reactivate virus production (Ghafouri *et al.*, 2006). During early infection, HIV enters the CNS (Bertin *et al.*, 2012) and attacks cells macrophages and microglial cells (Foley *et al.*, 2008). But along with this infection, periphery factors (non-CNS) are also important for initiating neurodegeneration and triggering dementia, which are like for example; increased number of circulating monocytes that express CD16 and CD69. The cells which get activated by viral entry, progressively adhere to the endothelium membrane of the brain microvasculature, and further transmigrate, triggering a spontaneous array of harmful processes which might finally lead to the loss of Blood Brain Barrier (BBB) integrity making it easy for virus to enter and replicate inside the brain. The BBB is crucial in HIV infection of the CNS. BBB is composed of specialized Human brain microvascular endothelial cells (HBMECs), which do not have any opening and are connected by intercellular junctions in an impermeable single layer. BBB plays a central role in neuropathogenesis as it serves as the channel through which free virus and infected immune cells enter the brain. The BBB loses its integrity and permeability due to progressive HIV infection and immune compromisation, which leads to easy entry of toxins, free virus, infected and activated monocytes into the brain. It has been reported that HIV-1 gp120 protein and also Tat protein are behind BBB disregulation. PKC signaling pathways and receptor-mediated Ca^{2+} release are the involved pathways resulting into cytotoxicity of the brain endothelial cells (Kanmogne *et al.*, 2005) leading to downregulation and rupture of tight junction proteins (TJPs) of HBMECs, by the induction of proteasome by HIV-1. It has been studied that circulating virus or envelope proteins may also cause BBB dysfunction during primary infection. CNS infection of HIV is detected by viral RNA load in CSF (Woods *et al.*, 2009; Morgan *et al.*, 2011). Chemokines like monocyte chemoattractant protein (MCP)-1 control PBMCs relocation through BBB. Cellular migration engages adhesion molecules and differential regulation of inflammatory cytokines, leading to BBB disintegration and finally immune

http://dx.doi.org/10.5772/55100

dysregulation by letting sufficient entry of infected or activated immune cells into the brain causing neuronal injury.

6. Types of CNS cells invaded by HIV-1

BBB is selectively permeable, made up of firmly concurrent brain microvascular endothelial cells, and its major role is to separate the CNS from the periphery. It manages the trafficking of cells and molecules across it into the brain parenchyma. For the purpose of brain entry, HIV-1 has to cross the BBB using several mechanisms which are still poorly understood and are unclear. Numerous *in vitro* experimentations have been done to understand the mechanisms of HIV-1 introduction into the CNS via BBB. It is reported that the severity of HIV-1 associated neuropathogenesis is dependent on amount of HIV DNA circulating in PBMCs (Shiramizu *et al.*, 2009). It is hypothesized that HIV-1 enters the CNS, in disguise as a commuter in cells trafficking till the brain (Verma *et al.*, 2010). CD4+ cells, like T cells and monocytes are infected by HIV-1, which circulate in blood and have the ability to cross the BBB and introduce the infection into CNS. Though presence of CD4 receptors in human brain microvascular endothelial cells is still a matter of debate whereas its presence is studied along with expression of HIV-1 co-receptors have also being reported on primary human brain's microvascular endothelial cells. Other proposed hypothesis for the entry of HIV-1 is the migration between/ transcytosis of endothelial cells. All types of the CNS cells like astrocytes (Wang *et al.*, 2009), oligodendrocytes, neurons, macrophage and microglia, are easily infected by HIV-1 as they have receptors and co-receptors for HIV-1 entry, but only macrophage and microglia get infected most commonly which are the resident immunocompetent cells of the brain (Gendleman *et al.*, 1985). Expression of CCL2/MCP-1 in astrocytes is enhanced by nef via calmodulin dependent pathway. Consequently, increased CCL2/MCP-1 functions as a chemoattractant for monocytes, thereby facilitating entry of monocytes into the brain (Lehmann *et al.*, 2006). Peripheral macrophage population is necessary to be refilled, which is compensated by the migration of monocytes into the CNS, resulting in major drawback of facilitating the entry of intracellular virus. Microglia and monocyte-derived macrophages are the main culprits of HIV-1 CNS infection. Immunostaining experiments have shown HIV-1 infection in parenchymal microglia, but it is still unclear that whether the HIV-1 immunopositive microglia receives influx of infected cells from blood or directly results from prolonged infection in the CNS. *In-vitro* experiments demonstrate that HIV-1 replication takes place in primary microglia isolated from adults and infants leading to cytopathology. Microglial cells are the major targets as they express CD4/CCR5 major receptors/co-receptors which is a necessity for HIV-1 infection. On the other hand astrocytes express CXCR4 and other HIV-1 coreceptors like CCR5, but do not express CD4 receptors and are still reported to be infected by HIV-1 mechanisms to which are still unclear. Also i*n vivo*, oligodendrocytes infection by HIV-1 remains unclear and less understood as they do not have CD4 receptors. Mostly there is absence of *in vivo* infection in neurons, however sometimes presence of HIV-1 DNA and proteins in neurons have been reported too, leading to need of further studies. Various pathways for the entry of virus into the brain have been studied like (i) direct entry, (ii) transcytosis, (iii) Trojan horse hypothesis for entry, which states that HIV enters the CNS via infected CD4 + AND T-cells which are capable of crossing BBB and they reach CNS and are also capable of transferring infection to other CNS cells too (Fig. 2).

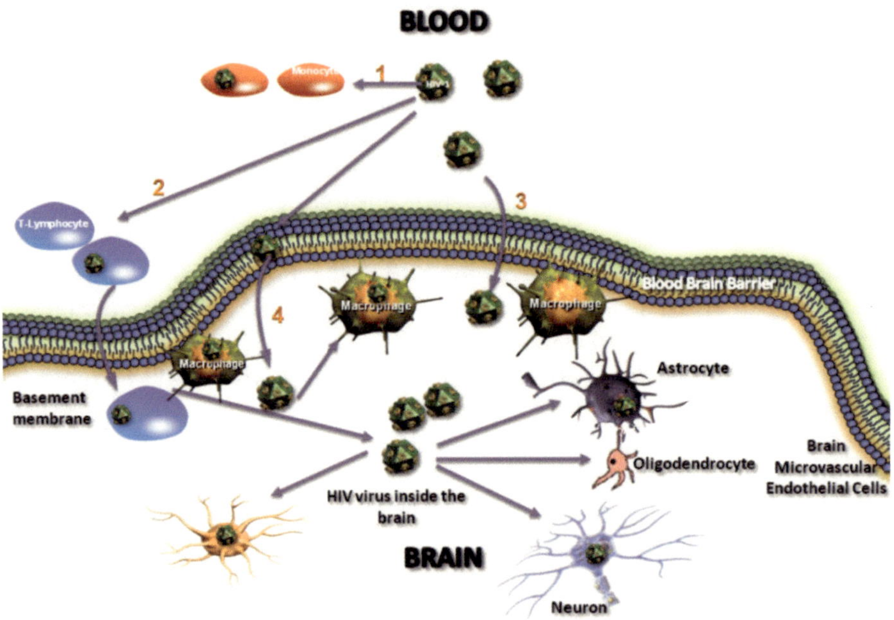

Figure 2. HIV-1 neuroinvasion. 1) "Trojan Horse hypothesis" for entry of HIV-1 into the brain via migration of infected monocytes which differentiate into perivascular macrophage. 2) The passage of infected CD4+ T cells into the brain. Other probable causes of CNS infection might be: 3) the direct entrance of the virus via tight junctions across the membrane and 4) entrance of HIV-1 by transcytosis phenomenon.

7. Crosstalk between the peripheral and CNS immunity

The way by which HIV-1-infected monocytes escape immune surveillance can be explained by "Trojan horse cell" model. The "support" needed for the viral entry is through CNS-produced chemokines like MCP-1 and IFN-γ-inducible peptide, CXCL10, whereas the "opposition" is through peripheral immune activation (Yadav *et al.*, 2009). Upon entry in the brain, HIV-1-infected blood-borne macrophages secrete proinflammatory cytokines like tumor necrosis factor alpha (TNF-α), interleukin-1 beta (IL-1β), and viral proteins which affect neuronal function (Brabers and Nottet, 2006). Within the brain, astrocytes serve as principal regulators for neural homeostasis. They bring out a neurotoxic secretory response in macrophages, resulting to upregulation of certain acids and metabolites, chemokines, and cytokine secretions. They can also alter macrophage phenotype, which may help in neuroprotection. But on the contrary astrocytes can also influence autocrine and paracrine inflammatory cascades, which may lead to immune activation, increased viral infection, and allowance of cellular entry via BBB (Kraft-Terry *et al.,* 2010). Also CD16+ monocytes are linked to infection of the brain as they can be easily infected by the virus, they carry virus into the brain and help in viral dissemination and serve as viral reservoirs as they are apoptosis resistant. HIV proteins like nef require adaptive selection in brain for efficient replication in macrophages or when it is exposed to brain specific immune selection (Olivieri *et al.,* 2010). Neuropsychiatric disorders associated with HIV infection result in substantial morbidity and fatality. HIV injures the CNS and PNS, leading to neuropsychiatric disorders, which together constitute for neuroAIDS (McCombe *et al.*,2009), which includes neurocognitive disorders like HAD, minor neurocognitive disorder (HAND), mania, anxiety, depression, seizures, myelopathy and neuropathy, and also involves display of several symptoms like neurocognitive impairment, mood disorders, neuropathic pain, epilepsy, addiction, physical disability, loss of memory, mood swings etc (Fig.3).

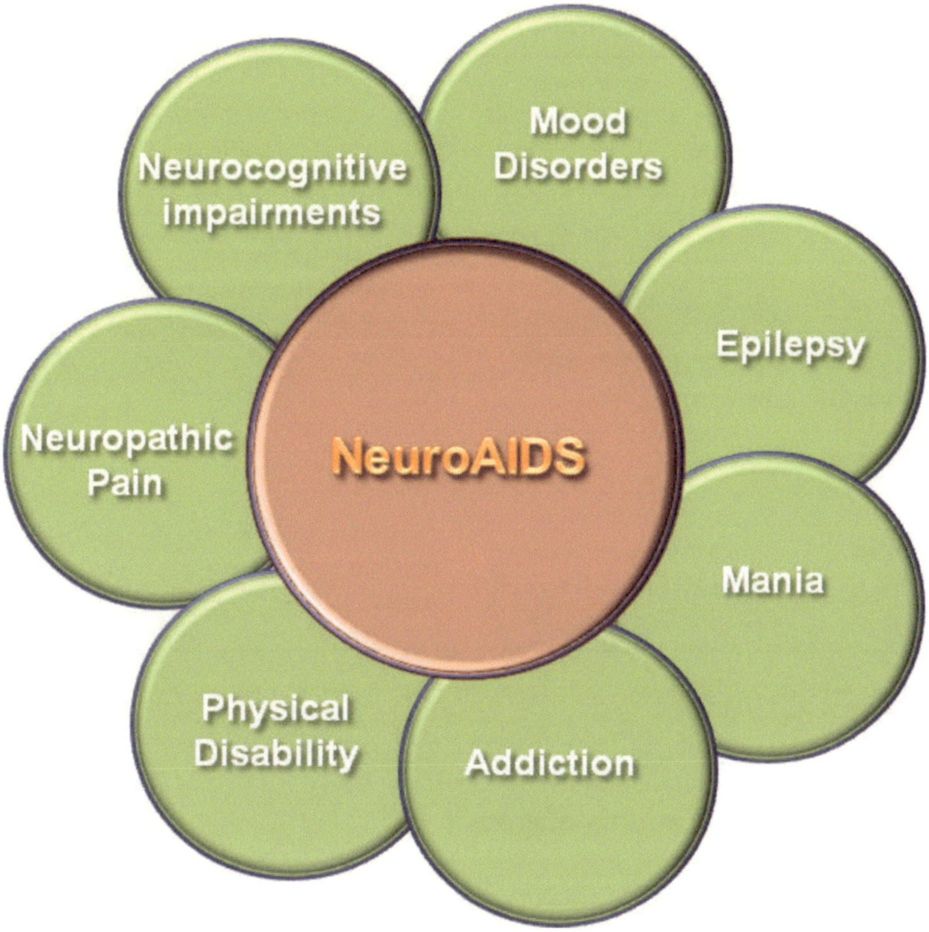

Figure 3. Associated disorders and symptoms which are commonly seen in patients suffering from neuroAIDS.

8. Forms of dementia

One form of dementia is Alzheimer's disease caused by amyloid pathology, during which peptides of amyloid-β generate and clump together into plaques which release toxic fragments of amyloid-β leading to neuropathogenesis. Another form of dementia is caused by vascular pathology in which blood vessels leak and hence deprives small areas of the brain of blood and oxygen, which damage brain tissue resulting in cognitive defects. Both forms exist equally, even though Alzheimer pathology is more common, but it coexists with vascular pathology. (Abott *et al.*, 2011).

TYPES OF DEMENTIA

Dementia type	Symptoms	Neuropathological findings	Percentage of total dementia cases
Alzheimer's	Weakened memory power, leading to confusion, disinterest depression and bad judgement skills.	Formation of amyloid plaques and also neurofibrillary tangles.	50–80%
Vascular dementia	Memory is weakened, but not as intense as in the case of Alzheimer's patients.	Causing microstrokes due to reduced blood flow to brain	20–30%
Frontotemporal dementia	Personality disorders, mood swings and difficulty in understanding different languages.	Damage limited to frontal and temporal lobes	5–10%
Dementia with Lewy bodies	Weakened memory power, leading to confusion, disinterest depression and bad judgement skills, hallucinations and tremors.	Cortical Lewy bodies (of the protein a-synuclein) inside neurons.	<5%

Table 1. Displaying the types of dementia and their prevelance. (Source: Abbott A. Dementia: a problem for our age. *Nature*. 2011; 475(7355): S2-4)

9. Knowing dementia and its diagnosis

Dementia is considered as loss of memory and other cognitive abilities which reduces the lifespan of patients. Dementia is often associated with physical, mental and financial burden. 37% of the dementic population in developing countries have vulnerable living environment and they require specialised care. Diagnosis of dementia involves investigations for

http://dx.doi.org/10.5772/55100

decline in memory and disturbance in several cognitive abilities like coherent speech, understanding spoken or written language, recognizing objects, executing motor activities, sensory function, thinking abstractly, making sound judgments, planning and carrying out complex tasks. Dementia reduces the lifespan of affected people. In the developed countries life span after dementia diagnosis can be expected to be ~7 years, but in low and middle income countries survival may be shorter. Dementia symptoms and linked issues can be understood in three stages of early stage (1-2 years) which is often overlooked because the onset of dementia is gradual, making it difficult to predict when it begins, leading to problems in talking, memory loss. Secondly, the middle stage (2-5 years) which makes patients life more difficult and restricted, giving them difficulty in day-to-day living and forgetting recent events and people's names, etc. Thirdly, the late stage (>5 years) leading to total dependence and inactivity, serious memory disturbances difficulty in physical works like walking, eating, incapability of communicating, not recognizing familiar objects, displaying inappropriate behavior in public etc.

HIV associated dementia, referred as the syndrome of cognitive and motor dysfunction resulting in progressive neurodegeneration observed after infection with human HIV-1, also known as HIV encephalopathy (HIV-E) and AIDS dementia complex (ADC) (Kaul *et al.*, 2001). In the last stage of HIV, HAD a severe neurological complication affects 15–20% of the patients (Van de Bovenkamp *et al.*, 2002). The relationship between spreading of HIV in brain tissue and pathology has not been thoroughly assessed in HAART era (Lamers *et al.*, 2010). Inspite of preventing former end stage complications of AIDS by HAART however, with increased survival times, the prevalence of minor HIV-1 associated cognitive impairment appears to be rising among AIDS patients. Further, HIV-1 associated dementia (HAD) is still prevalent in treated patients as well as attenuated forms of HAD and CNS opportunistic disorders (Ghafouri *et al.*, 2006). Infected macrophages with HIV have an ability to cross BBB infect inhabitant brain macrophages initiating the development of HAD. Cytokines are released from infected resident brain macrophages which further attract more macrophages to sites of infection and a series of self-inflammatory process emerges (Williams *et al.*, 2002). Studies have suggested that the process of entering in the CNS causing HAD mostly depends on the HIV variants as some HIV variants have capability of entering in the CNS and develops HAD but in contrast other variants don't have capability to develop HAD even after entering in the CNS (Fischer-Smith *et al.*, 2008; Fischer-Smith *et al.*, 2005).

10. Underlying mechanisms and issues

Some studies suggest that neurological involvement of infected patients occurs at different frequencies, depending on the HIV subtype involved in the infection (Liner 2nd *et al.*, 2007). HIV-1 Subtype D has more prominent chance for developing dementia (89%) than subtype A (24%) in the patients localized in a region of Uganda, Africa suggesting genetic determinants exist within HIV that influence the ability of the virus to replicate in the central nervous system. HIV-1 proteins have been shown to be released from HIV infected cell and/ or they have found to be present in the extracellular milieu in the HIV-1-

infected brain. In vitro, neurotoxic and/or neuromodulatory effects have been shown by HIV proteins: nef, env, tat, rev, vpr and vpu that might play a role in the development of HIV-1-associated dementia in vivo (Sactor *et al.*, 2009).

11. Fight against dementia

Dementia is engulfing bigger proportion of HIV patients and is expected to worsen more. It is expected that a significant proportion of dementia is driven by amyloid-β. But so far none of the amyloid-based strategies has been successful, but still drug developers are strategising on the concept which can combat against it. More reliable biomarkers are being developed potentially making it possible to carry out trials on patients before symptoms. Some scientists are also wondering to target vascular pathology as well, which is equally responsible for causing dementia. So cholesterol level lowering drugs and blood pressure reducing drugs are also given long term to patients, who are at higher risk of heart attack which may also help protect from dementias as well (Abott *et al.*, 2011). There are several extracellular and intracellular signalling pathways, which when activated lead to macrophage or microglial activation, and induction in neurons and astrocytes. These pathways may act as a potential therapeutic importance as drug targets against neuropathogenesis. NeuroAIDS is challenge to patients, their families, society and our country, thus development of preclinical models appropriate for new compounds testing with neurotrophic and neuroprotective potential is necessary (Crews *et al.*, 2008; Williams *et al.*, 2008).

12. Therapeutic developments

The biggest issue which comes in front of drug developers is the incapability of the drugs to cross the BBB, which leads to low bioavailability of the drugs into the CNS. HIV-1 protease inhibitors are totally incapable in entering the CNS, while other HIV-1 therapies such as zidovudine (AZT) are reported to have efficient BBB penetration. Recently, a broad range of nanomedicines are being developed to improve drug delivery across BBB, development of nanoparticulate– antiretroviral therapy (nanoART), against CNS disorders as the structure of the BBB, efflux pumps and the expression of metabolic enzymes make it difficult for the regular drug to reach brain. Nanoformulations can evade the BBB and can boost CNS-directed drug delivery (Fig. 4) (Saxena *et al.*, 2012; Nowacek *et al.*, 2010; Nowacek *et al.*, 2009). Efforts are been done in finding long-lasting injectable antiretrovirals to avoid the challenges of therapy adherence (Baert *et al.*, 2009). To specifically target the CNS, NPs are synthesized with various combinations of ART therapies to be taken up by monocytes and carried into the CNS for release at sites of HIV-1 infection, for example Indinavir nanoART and p24 loaded and coated NP, which are providing new avenues for treating or even preventing the spread of HIV-1 in the brain. Adjunctive therapeutics ART is engaged in making combinatory drugs against virus mutation. Efforts are being made to improve penetrability of ART across the BBB, but importance of considering drug toxicity and elicited cellular response for various ART regiments is always a necessity. Adjunctive therapy like platelet-activating factor (PAF) antagonist, PMS-601, are demonstrated to reduce HAND symptoms and even combination of ART and PAF antagonists, are also studied to have role in reducing neurodegeneration. All of these are also being developed as therapies for neurodegenerative disorders which may prove to be a boon in the combat against NeuroAIDS. Need of the hour is to device an exact combination of CNS-penetrating nanoART and adjunctive therapies, which might be able to help us against neurocognitive symptoms (Kraft-Terry *et al.*, 2010).

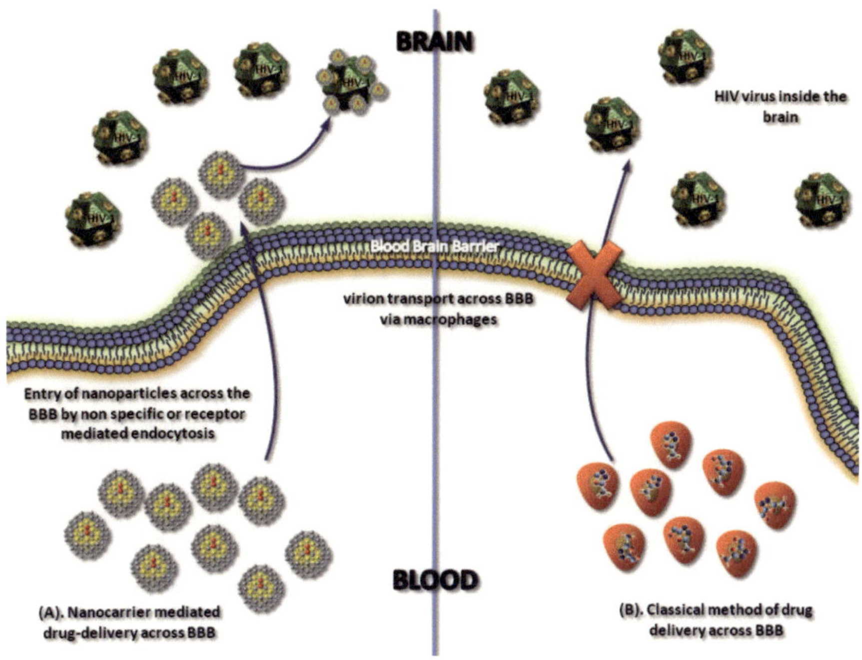

Figure 4. Comparative display of nanocarrier mediated method of drug delivery (A) versus the classical method of drug delivery across the Blood Brain Barrier (BBB), which is less efficient than the former in the process of drug delivery.

13. Future implications and need of the hour

Since dementia is quite prevalent in HIV patients, in developed countries and has also been reported to extend its grip towards developing countries as well due to increase in patient survival rates and life expectancy due to HAART treatment and increased living standards. Low prevalence of HAD in underdeveloped and developing countries have been attributed to under diagnosis, short life expectancy and short survival following HIV infection associated with opportunistic infections and also low prevalence of HIV related neuroinfections and pathology is not available due to inadequate medical facilities, social stigma and ignorance that lead to under diagnosis (Vivithanaporn *et al.*, 2010). So a need of collaboratory studies is there which can be used, for learning the cause, prevalence and diagnosis of neuropathogenesis. A synchronised effort is needed by researchers, drug makers, physicians, policy makers, government bodies nationally as well as globally. A proper and deep understanding about the entry of the virus into the CNS and the various mechanisms it employs to undertake the host machinery would be of great help in understanding the issue and combating against the virus.

Author details

Shailendra K. Saxena[1], Sneham Tiwari[1] and Madhavan P.N. Nair[2]

1 Centre for Cellular and Molecular Biology (CCMB-CSIR), Hyderabad, India

2 College of Medicine, Florida International University, Miami, USA

References

[1] Abbott, A. (2011). Dementia: a problem for our age." *Nature*. 475(7355): S, 2-4.

[2] Baert, L, Klooster, t, Dries, G, François, W, Wouters, M, Basstanie, A, Iterbeke, E, Stappers, K, Stevens, F, Schueller, P, Van Remoortere, L, Kraus, P, Wigerinck, G, & Rosier, P. J. ((2009). Development of a long-acting injectable formulation with nanoparticles of rilpivirine (TMC278) for HIV treatment." *Eur J Pharm Biopharm. 72*(3), 502-508.

[3] Bertin, J, Barat, C, Méthot, S, & Tremblay, M. J. (2012). Interactions between prostaglandins, leukotrienes and HIV-1: possible implications for the central nervous system." *Retrovirology*. 9:4.

[4] Brabers, N. A, & Nottet, H. S. (2006). Role of the pro-inflammatory cytokines TNF-alpha and IL-1beta in HIV-associated dementia." *Eur J Clin Invest.* , 36(7), 447-458.

[5] Crews, L, Lentz, M. R, Gonzalez, R. G, Fox, H. S, & Masliah, E. (2008). Neuronal injury in simian immunodeficiency virus and other animal models of neuroAIDS." *J Neurovirol.* , 14(4), 327-339.

[6] Dean, D, & Berger, J. R. (2012). Neuro-AIDS in the developing world." *Neurology.* , 78(7), 499-500.

[7] Ferris, M. J, Mactutus, C. F, & Booze, R. M. (2008). Neurotoxic profiles of HIV, psychostimulant drugs of abuse, and their concerted effect on the brain: current status of dopamine system vulnerability in NeuroAIDS." *Neurosci Biobehav Rev.* , 32(5), 883-909.

[8] Fischer-smith, T, & Rappaport, J. (2005). Evolving paradigms in the pathogenesis of HIV-1-associated dementia." *Expert Rev Mol Med.* , 7(27), 1-26.

[9] Fischer-smith, T, Bell, C, Croul, S, Lewis, M, & Rappaport, J. (2008). Monocyte/macrophage trafficking in acquired immunodeficiency syndrome encephalitis: lessons from human and nonhuman primate studies." *J Neurovirol.*, 14(4), 318-326.

[10] Foley, J, Ettenhofer, M, Wright, M, & Hinkin, C. H. (2008). Emerging issues in the neuropsychology of HIV infection." *Curr HIV/AIDS Rep.*, 5(4), 204-211.

[11] Gandhi, N, Saiyed, Z. M, Napuri, J, Samikkannu, T, Reddy, P. V, Agudelo, M, Khatavkar, P, Saxena, S. K, & Nair, M. P. (2010). Interactive role of human immunodeficiency virus type 1 (HIV-1) clade-specific Tat protein and cocaine in blood-brain barrier dysfunction: implications for HIV-1-associated neurocognitive disorder." *J Neurovirol.*, 16(4), 294-305.

[12] Gendelman, H. E, Narayan, O, Molineaux, S, Clements, J. E, & Ghotbi, Z. (1985). Slow, persistent replication of lentiviruses: role of tissue macrophages and macrophage precursors in bone marrow." *Proc Natl Acad Sci U S A.*, 82(20), 7086-7090.

[13] Ghafouri, M, Amini, S, Khalili, K, & Sawaya, B. E. (2006). HIV-1 associated dementia: symptoms and causes." *Retrovirology.* 19;3: 28.

[14] Kanmogne, G. D, Primeaux, C, & Grammas, P. (2005). HIV-1 gp120 proteins alter tight junction protein expression and brain endothelial cell permeability: implications for the pathogenesis of HIV-associated dementia." *J Neuropathol Exp Neurol.*, 64(6), 498-505.

[15] Kaul, M, Garden, G. A, & Lipton, S. A. (2001). Pathways to neuronal injury and apoptosis in HIV-associated dementia." *Nature.*, 410(6831), 988-994.

[16] Kilareski, E. M, Shah, S, Nonnemacher, M. R, & Wigdahl, B. (2009). Regulation of HIV-1 transcription in cells of the monocyte-macrophage lineage." *Retrovirology.* 6:118.

[17] Kraft-terry, S. D, Stothert, A. R, Buch, S, & Gendelman, H. E. (2010). HIV-1 neuroimmunity in the era of antiretroviral therapy." Neurobiol Dis., 37(3), 542-548.

[18] Lamers, S. L, Poon, A. F, & Mcgrath, M. S. (2011). HIV-1 nef protein structures associated with brain infection and dementia pathogenesis." *PLoS One.* 6(2): e16659.

[19] Lamers, S. L, Salemi, M, Galligan, D. C, Morris, A, Gray, R, Fogel, G, Zhao, L, & Mcgrath, M. S. (2010). Human immunodeficiency virus-1 evolutionary patterns associated with pathogenic processes in the brain." *J Neurovirol.*, 16(3), 230-241.

[20] Lehmann, M. H, Masanetz, S, Kramer, S, & Erfle, V. (2006). HIV-1 Nef upregulates CCL2/MCP-1 expression in astrocytes in a myristoylation- and calmodulin-dependent manner." *J Cell Sci.* 119(Pt 21): 4520-4530.

[21] Liner, K. J. nd, Hall, C.D. and Robertson, K.R. ((2007). Impact of human immunodeficiency virus (HIV) subtypes on HIV-associated neurological disease." *J Neurovirol.*, 13(4), 291-304.

[22] Mccombe, J. A, Noorbakhsh, F, Buchholz, C, Trew, M, & Power, C. (2009). NeuroAIDS: a watershed for mental health and nervous system disorders." *J Psychiatry Neurosci.*, 34(2), 83-85.

[23] Morgan, E. E, Woods, S. P, Delano-wood, L, & Bondi, M. W. Grant I; HIV Neurobehavioral Research Program (HNRP) Group. ((2011). Intraindividual variability in HIV infection: evidence for greater neurocognitive dispersion in older HIV seropositive adults." *Neuropsychology.*, 25(5), 645-654.

[24] Nowacek, A, & Gendelman, H. E. (2009). NanoART, neuroAIDS and CNS drug delivery." *Nanomedicine* (Lond)., 4(5), 557-574.

[25] Nowacek, A. S, Mcmillan, J, Miller, R, Anderson, A, Rabinow, B, & Gendelman, H. E. (2010). Nanoformulated antiretroviral drug combinations extend drug release and antiretroviral responses in HIV-1-infected macrophages: implications for neuroAIDS therapeutics." *J Neuroimmune Pharmacol.* Epub, 5(4), 592-601.

[26] Olivieri, K. C, Agopian, K. A, Mukerji, J, & Gabuzda, D. (2010). Evidence for adaptive evolution at the divergence between lymphoid and brain HIV-1 nef genes." *AIDS Res Hum Retroviruses.*, 26(4), 495-500.

[27] Prince, M, Acosta, D, Ferri, C. P, Guerra, M, & Huang, Y. Llibre Rodriguez, J.J.,Salas, A., Sosa, A.L., Williams, J.D., Dewey, M.E., Acosta, I., Jotheeswaran, A.T. and Liu, Z. ((2012). Dementia incidence and mortality in middle-income countries, and associations with indicators of cognitive reserve: a 10/66 Dementia Research Group population-based cohort study." *Lancet. 380*(9836), 50-58.

[28] Prince, M, Brodaty, H, Uwakwe, R, Acosta, D, Ferri, C. P, Guerra, M, Huang, Y, & Jacob, K. S. Llibre Rodriguez, J.J., Salas, A., Sosa, A.L., Williams, J.D., Jotheeswaran, A.T. and Liu, Z. ((2012). Strain and its correlates among carers of people with dementia in low-income and middle-income countries. A 10/66 Dementia Research Group population-based survey." *Int J Geriatr Psychiatry.*, 27(7), 670-82.

[29] Reddy, P. V, Pilakka-kanthikee, S, Saxena, S. K, Saiyed, Z, & Nair, M. P. (2012). Interactive Effects of Morphine on HIV Infection: Role in HIV-Associated Neurocognitive Disorder." *AIDS Res Treat.* 2012: 953678.

[30] Sacktor, N, Nakasujja, N, Robertson, K, & Clifford, D. B. (2007). HIV-associated cognitive impairment in sub-Saharan Africa--the potential effect of clade diversity." *Nat Clin Pract Neurol.*, 3(8), 436-443.

[31] Sacktor, N, Nakasujja, N, Skolasky, R. L, Rezapour, M, Robertson, K, Musisi, S, & Quinn, T. C. (2009). HIV subtype D is associated with dementia, compared with subtype A, in immunosuppressed individuals at risk of cognitive impairment in Kampala, Uganda." *Clin Infect Dis.*, 49(5), 780-786.

[32] Saiyed, Z. M, Gandhi, N, Agudelo, M, Napuri, J, Samikkannu, T, Reddy, P. V, Khatavkar, P, Yndart, A, Saxena, S. K, & Nair, M. P. (2011). HIV-1 Tat upregulates ex-

pression of histone deacetylase-2 (HDAC2) in human neurons: implication for HIV-associated neurocognitive disorder (HAND)." *Neurochem Int.* , 58(6), 656-64.

[33] Samikkannu, T, Rao, K. V, Gandhi, N, Saxena, S. K, & Nair, M. P. (2010). Human immunodeficiency virus type 1 clade B and C Tat differentially induce indoleamine 2,3-dioxygenase and serotonin in immature dendritic cells: Implications for neuroAIDS." *J Neurovirol.* , 16(4), 255-263.

[34] Saxena, S. K, Gupta, A, Bhagyashree, K, Saxena, R, Arora, N, Banerjee, A. K, Tripathi, A. K, Chandrasekar, M. J, Gandhi, N, & Nair, M. P. (2012). Targeting strategies for Human immunodeficiency virus: a combinatorial approach." *Mini Rev Med Chem.* , 12(3), 236-254.

[35] Saxena, S. K, Shrivastava, G, Tiwari, S, & Nair, M. P. N. (2012). HIV-1 Nef: hacker of the host cell." *Future Virol.* 7(2), 117-120

[36] Saxena, S. K, Shrivastava, G, Tiwari, S, Swamy, M. A, & Nair, M. P. (2012). Modulation of HIV pathogenesis and T-cell signaling by HIV-1 Nef." *Future Virol.* , 7(6), 609-620.

[37] Saxena, S. K, Tiwari, S, & Nair, M. P. (2012). Nanotherapeutics: emerging competent technology in neuroAIDS and CNS drug delivery." *Nanomedicine (Lond).* , 7(7), 941-944.

[38] Saxena, S. K, Tiwari, S, & Nair, M. P. (2012). A global perspective on HIV/AIDS." *Science.* 337(6096): 798.

[39] Shankar, S. K, Mahadevan, A, Satishchandra, P, Kumar, R. U, Yasha, T. C, Santosh, V, Chandramuki, A, Ravi, V, & Nath, A. (2005). Neuropathology of HIV/AIDS with an overview of the Indian scene." *Indian J Med Res. 121*(4), 468-488.

[40] Shiramizu, B, Williams, A. E, Shikuma, C, & Valcour, V. (2009). Amount of HIV DNA in peripheral blood mononuclear cells is proportional to the severity of HIV-1-associated neurocognitive disorders." *J Neuropsychiatry Clin Neurosci.* , 21(1), 68-74.

[41] Singh, R, Kaur, M, & Arora, D. (2011). Neurological complications in late-stage hospitalized patients with HIV disease." *Ann Indian Acad Neurol.* , 14(3), 172-177.

[42] Sundaravaradan, V, Saxena, S. K, Ramakrishnan, R, Yedavalli, V. R, Harris, D. T, & Ahmad, N. (2006). Differential HIV-1 replication in neonatal and adult blood mononuclear cells is influenced at the level of HIV-1 gene expression." *Proc Natl Acad Sci U S A.* , 103(31), 11701-11706.

[43] Van de BovenkampM., Nottet, H.S. and Pereira, C.F. ((2002). Interactions of human immunodeficiency virus-1 proteins with neurons: possible role in the development of human immunodeficiency virus-1-associated dementia." *Eur J Clin Invest.* , 32(8), 619-627.

[44] Verma, A. S, Singh, U. P, Dwivedi, P. D, & Singh, A. (2010). Contribution of CNS cells in NeuroAIDS." *J Pharm Bioallied Sci.* , 2(4), 300-306.

[45] Vivithanaporn, P, Heo, G, Gamble, J, Krentz, H. B, Hoke, A, Gill, M. J, & Power, C. (2010). Neurologic disease burden in treated HIV/AIDS predicts survival: a population-based study." *Neurology.* , 75(13), 1150-1158.

[46] Wang, T, Gong, N, Liu, J, Kadiu, I, Kraft-terry, S. D, Schlautman, J. D, Ciborowski, P, Volsky, D. J, & Gendelman, H. E. (2008). HIV-1-infected astrocytes and the microglial proteome." *J Neuroimmune Pharmacol.* , 3(3), 173-186.

[47] Williams, K. C, & Hickey, W. F. (2002). Central nervous system damage, monocytes and macrophages, and neurological disorders in AIDS." *Annu Rev Neurosci.* , 25, 537-562.

[48] Williams, R, Bokhari, S, Silverstein, P, Pinson, D, Kumar, A, & Buch, S. (2008). Nonhuman primate models of NeuroAIDS." *J Neurovirol. 14*(4), 292-300.

[49] Woods, S. P, Moore, D. J, Weber, E, & Grant, I. (2009). Cognitive neuropsychology of HIV-associated neurocognitive disorders." *Neuropsychol Rev.* , 19(2), 152-168.

[50] Yadav, A, & Collman, R. G. (2009). CNS inflammation and macrophage/microglial biology associated with HIV-1 infection." *J Neuroimmune Pharmacol.* , 4(4), 430-447.

Chapter 7

Human Immunodeficiency Virus Infection and Co-Morbid Mental Distress

Peter J. Chipimo and Knut Fylkesnes

Additional information is available at the end of the chapter

http://dx.doi.org/10.5772/53696

1. Introduction

HIV/AIDS is probably the most challenging and pressing health issue of our time. Current estimates show that over 40million people are now living with HIV. Despite the availability of antiretroviral therapy, the provision of this treatment continues to pose a big challenge for various reasons. Globally, of the 6 million people requiring treatment, only 8% receive it – with considerable geographical inequity ie. High income countries vs. low income countries. Despite understanding the risk factors for HIV infection, the incidence of new HIV cases has not reduced at an acceptable rate. An unprecedented number of people still have no access to treatment and continue to die from HIV related problems. This has brought about devastating social and economic consequences at country level, family level and at personal level. A considerable number of individuals suffer from mental disorders resulting from being HIV infected. Independently, mental disorders make a substantial independent contribution to the burden of disease worldwide. The recognition of mental disorders as a major contributor to the global burden of disease has led to an increase in the demand for the inclusion of mental health services in primary health care as well as in community-based health surveys in order to improve screening, diagnosis and treatment of mental distress. It is estimated that, neuropsychiatric conditions account for up to 15% of all disability-adjusted life-years, and up to 30% of those attributable to non-communicable diseases. Neuropsychiatric disorders also account for 1.2 million deaths every year. These figures are most likely underestimated as official statistics especially in low and middle income countries are scanty and unreliable. In sub-Saharan Africa, it has been reported that 20–30% of primary health care centre attendees present with depressive symptoms as the first or secondary reason for seeking medical care. A study conducted in Tanzania revealed a 41.6% prevalence of depressive symptoms among primary health care patients while a similar study in Uganda reported a 20–30% prevalence of psychological disorders and depression among health care seekers. These research findings have also shown heightened risk for common mental disorders among the women i.e. a female to male ratio of 1.5–2.0. Other determinants have been found to include low socioeconomic position indicated by poor access to resources, unemployment and low educational attainment. It has also been shown to be higher among those with poor socio-support networks such as the unmarried, widowed and divorced. Mental disorders interact with many other health conditions, communicable and non-communicable. They commonly affect individuals with medical conditions and have been associated with adverse impacts on several measures of morbidity and mortality. Depressed patients have been shown to have worse physical, social and overall health than other patients. Of particular interest to this chapter is the interaction between HIV and mental distress

2. HIV and mental distress

Early stages of HIV epidemic

In the early stages of the HIV epidemic, the individuals who were affected did not know that their behaviour predisposed them to a potentially fatal disease. The epidemic also mushroomed at the time of a liberal and tolerant culture and dis-inhibited sexual restraint. Hence multiple sexual partners spread the epidemic in communities where these behaviours were more rampant. Intravenous drug use also contributed to the early spread of the epidemic. In the low and middle income countries, factors surrounding poor socio-economic position (poor education and low income) and inability to negotiate for condom use due to the disparity between the male and female gender have emerged as stronger predictors. Several early and recent epidemiologic studies elucidated these risk factors and more concerted effort was placed on public education directed at prevention. Other more recent innovations directed at rolling-back HIV infection have included massive male circumcision campaigns, innovation directed at the girl child to reduce early teenage pregnancies and early marriages and the introduction of Highly Active Anti-Retroviral Therapy (HAART). Recently efforts have been directed at the role mental distress plays in determining acquisition of HIV infection, initial individual's reaction and post-infection adaptation. Further poor mental health has been associated with subsequent development of AIDS.

Mental distress

Mental distress in the context of this book chapter refers to a term used by users of mental health services as well as some mental health practitioners in describing a wide array of experiences of a patient's life that commonly manifest as somatic symptoms and held to be out of the ordinary, distressing, troubling or confusing for the patient, without actually being ill in the medical sense. Chipimo and Fylkesnes identified some of the common causes of mental distress in a study conducted among primary health care centers in Zambia. (Table 1)

http://dx.doi.org/10.5772/53696

Category of factor	Frequency	Symptoms/comments
Worries about money	51	Concerns about rent, day-to-day living, school fees
Problems of the mind	47	Recurrent headaches, sleeplessness, unhappiness, trouble thinking, loss of appetite, night mares
Unknown cause of symptoms	32	Most common among informants not acknowledging symptoms as an illness or as mental distress, suggested witchcraft
Relationship with spouse and family members	26	Commonest among women, included crying more than usual, unhappiness, headaches, sleeplessness.
Ill health	24	Sleeplessness, daily life suffering, inability to play useful role in life, tiredness
Low self-esteem	16	Worthlessness, loss of interest, unhappiness, crying more than usual, difficulty enjoying daily activities, experience of stigma
Recent life events	6	Bereavement, divorces, newly diagnosed with chronic disease including HIV. Included symptoms of restlessness, sleeplessness, trouble thinking, headache, unhappiness

Table 1. Factors associated with Mental Distress as identified by the informants (Chipimo & Fylkesnes, 2011)

The term mental distress is seen by users of mental health services as less stigmatizing as it fits better with the social model of disability, since everyone experiences mental distress at one time or the other. The other synonym is psychological distress. The term is also often preferred as they feel it better captures the uniqueness and personal nature of their experiences. Mental distress is often thought of as being a concept with a wider scope than the regularly used traditional term, mental illness. The later being a specific set of symptoms medically defined in psychiatry, for example: Mania, schizophrenia, anxiety disorders, depression etc. Difficult life situations such as: poor social-support structures, bereavement, stress, poor sleep, drug and alcohol abuse can induce mental distress. These inducers could be temporary and resolve without further medical intervention. However individuals who have protracted episodes and endure such symptoms longer are more likely to be diagnosed with mental illness. This definition is not without controversy and often these terms are used interchangeably.

Double tragedy

Mental distress has been recognised as a crucial factor to some individual's ability to modify their behaviour to prevent HIV infection. With effective treatment options now available, care for HIV has become more dynamic and has transformed the HIV squeal from terminal care to chronic care. This further complicates the scenario as mental disorders have further been recognised as severely complicating treatment. These factors work in tandem with HIV causing direct damage on the brain, creating turmoil in the lives of the infected and further exacerbates mental disorders. Further the mental disorders reduce the individual's ability to effectively change behaviour thus increasing the risk of infection and morbidity. Published literature showing that individuals with pre-existing mental disorders are at increased risk for contracting HIV/AIDS has been largely indirect. However consistent reports from several countries have suggested that individuals with mental disorders have a higher sero-prevalence for HIV/AIDS and that mental distress generally precedes HIV infection. This is valid given that significant risk of HIV transmission exists within an individual's network. Frequencies of 30-60% behavioural risk factors that have been identified among individuals with mental distress include: high rates of unprotected sexual contact, poor adherence to condom use and injection-drug abuse. In a study conducted among gay men with depressive symptoms, use of alcohol and drugs before sex were identified as independent predictors for sero-conversion. In a systematic review comparing an HIV sero-positive group and HIV sero-negative control group, the prevalence of depression in the sero-positive group was two times higher than in the sero-negative (OR 2.0, 95% CI 1.3-3.0).

3. Aetiology of HIV related mental distress

HIV related mental distress can occur in multiple phases in which premorbid psychological and social adjustment issues play a vital role. Additionally other social factors such as household income, culture, religion and family circumstances also influence and can alter an individual's reaction to a diagnosis of HIV and subsequent adaptation to living with the diagnosis. The same factors have also been shown to influence and pose high risk of being infected With HIV. Put together all these factors singly or severally affect the clinical presentation and management of HIV patients. It is as such imperative that these factors are addressed and assessed in both the Voluntary-Counselling-and-Testing (VCT) and in the pre-HAART assessment. A self-perpetuating cycle (figure 1) of increasing morbidity appears to occur between HIV and mental distress; HIV infection leads to development of mental distress and/or pre-existing mental distress predispose to HIV infection. In their study, Chipimo and Fylkesnes (2009) showed that HIV infection has both a direct and indirect effects on genesis of mental distress.

Direct effect

HIV infection has been known to affect all other organ systems in the human body and is said to have replaced syphilis as the "great imitator" in the central nervous system (CNS) and almost any psychiatric or neurological presentation is possible. The CNS is the second most commonly affected organ in patients with AIDS. HIV can cause direct organic brain tissue damage thus leading to the development of mental disorders (Psychotic and non-psychotic). Virtually any mental disorder is possible. Among the most notable are depression and anxiety, personality disorders and dementia. The mechanisms explaining the development of these mental disorders are largely poorly understood but the presence of HIV-1-binding sites in the brain (chemokine receptors) allows HIV-1 to infect macrophages and microglia. It is however thought that it does not affect neurons, although neurons are injured and die by apoptosis. The pathway to neuronal injury is thought to be through release of macrophage, microglial and astrocyte toxins alongside the contribution of direct injury on the neurons by viral proteins. These toxins overstimulate neurons, resulting in the formation of free radicals and excitotoxicity, similar to other neurodegenerative diseases.

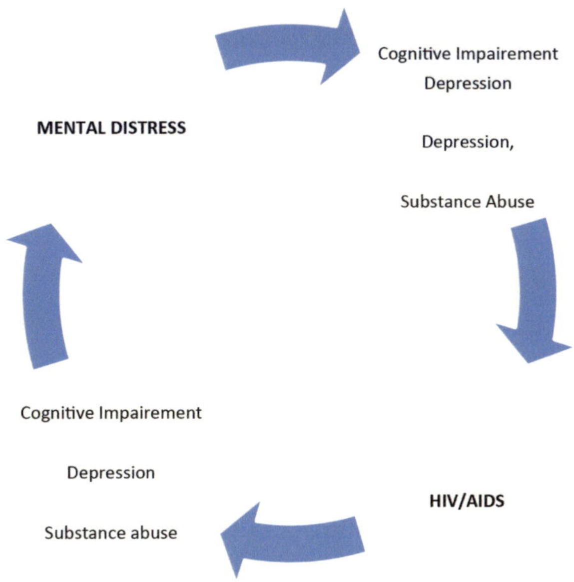

Figure 1. Self-perpetuating cycle of increasing morbidity: HIV/AIDS and Mental Distress (Chipimo, 2011)

Many HIV related opportunistic infections may involve the brain and lead to mental disorders. The four most frequent conditions are toxoplasmosis, progressive multifocal leukoencephalopathy (PML), cryptococcosis and cytomegalovirus infection. Although the incidence of these infections among patients with AIDS has decreased in the past years as a consequence of the introduction of highly active antiretroviral therapy (HAART), they remain a major cause of morbidity and mortality in this patient group. However, highly active antiretroviral drugs themselves such as, Zidovudine, Didanosine and Effervirenz have been associated with development of manic episodes

Indirect effect

Chipimo and Fylkesnes (2009) studied the relationship between HIV and mental distress in a population with high prevalence of HIV infection and low awareness of own HIV sero-status. In this study structural equation modeling (SEM) was used to establish the relationship between HIV infection and mental distress using maximum likelihood ratio as the method of estimation. The model indicated that underlying factors such as residence (rural or urban), level of education, marital status and age were inter-correlated as determinants for mental distress. Further Mental distress was found to be directly related to self-perceived risk and worry about being HIV infected, HIVsero-status and self-rated health. Further indirect inter-relationships were also found between self-rated health, self-perceived risk and worry about being HIV infected, and the underlying factors, namely age, residence, socio-economic position and education. Therefore self-rated health and self-perceived risk and worry about being HIV infected appear to be important mediators between underlying factors and mental distress. They are also important mediators between HIV status and mental distress. The results suggest that HIV infection has a substantial effect on mental distress both directly and indirectly. This effect was mediated through self-perceptions of health status, found to capture changes in health perceptions related to HIV, and self-perceived risk and worry of actually being HIV infected.

4. Prevalence of HIV related mental distress

Prevalence studies conducted world over have shown that when compared to the general population, mental disorders where considerably higher among the HIV infected individuals. However most of these studies have been conducted in the high income countries were the disease burden is relatively low and confined to selected groups for example Injection drug users and Homosexuals. Similar data in sub-Saharan Africa, where the HIV epidemic has its worse impact is limited. Therefore, given that mental disorders manifest in the majority of HIV infected individuals over the course of the illness, a simple assumption would then be that the prevalence reported in published studies represent an underestimate of the actual prevalence. A meta-analytic study identified 13 studies on mental disorders and HIV infection in low and middle income countries. The prevalence of mental disorders varied widely among these studies. Most of the studies done in Africa with HIV positive participants have shown differing but high percentages of mental distress, for example, Orange free state, South Africa 40%, rural Ethiopia 14% and Botswana 28%. In a study done in Zambia, Chipimo and Fylkesnes (2009) found a 13% prevalence of mental distress within the general population with a 2.0 higher odds ratio among the HIV infected. In Uganda, Musisi et. al. (2006) showed a 42% prevalence of depression among HIV infected individuals while in another study, Musisi & Kinyanda reported a prevalence of 41% among HIV infected adolenscents.

5. Presentation of HIV related mental distress

Diagnosis of mental disorders in HIV infection is a relatively rarely made diagnosis in sub-Saharan Africa. Studies have reported that physicians tend to be oblivious to psychological problems in HIV in the presence of a physical ailment. Further, the clinical presentation of mental distress in HIV infection presents a diagnostic challenge. This is often because the clinical Indictors of mental disorders are often masked by the symptoms of HIV infection. It is also a challenge for health care providers to distinguish between mental distress and grief. This calls for careful history taking that probes for previous history of mental disorders in the patient, suicide attempts, family history of mental illness, poor social support structures and a history of recent adverse events (deaths in family, physical violence, divorce, stigma).

Symptoms

Several studies have shown that mental distress often presents as somatisation. In a population based survey, Chipimo and Fylkesnes (2009) reported that the most frequently reported symptoms among the HIV infected were:

1. difficulty enjoying life,
2. feeling that their daily life was suffering,
3. poor sleep
4. low energy levels.

Among patients attending Primary Health Care, the most commonly reported symptoms observed by Chipimo and Fylkesnes (2010) were:

1. feelings of unhappiness,
2. loss of interest,
3. inability to enjoy daily life,
4. poor sleep
5. frequent headaches

Women reported these symptoms more than men in both studies. Musisi and Akena (2009) reported similar battery of symptoms and further added that, an otherwise asymptomatic HIV infected individual presenting with symptoms of fatigue and insomnia should be assessed for severe depression. These and other more pathognomonic symptoms put together allow clinicians to make a diagnosis of a full blown psychiatric disorder. The recognised HIV related psychiatric disorders are:

1. Anxiety disorders and depression
2. Psychotic disorder (Primary or secondary)
3. HIV-related Mania
4. HIV-related Dementia
5. HIV-related Delirium
6. Drug abuse ie. Substance and Alcohol abuse

6. Impact of HIV related mental distress on course and prognosis

There is a general lack of reported/ published follow-up studies on HIV related mental distress. However left untreated mental distress has an effect on the cell mediated immunity, where it causes impairments in T-cell mediated functions, reduced natural-killer cell counts and cytotoxicity. Depression in particular, has reproducibly been associated with decreased numbers and altered functioning of natural killer lymphocytes. It can also lead to an increase in activated CD8 T lymphocytes and viral load. By so doing mental distress can predict the onset and progression of both physical and social disability in HIV infection. Further, Co-morbid mental distress can delay health seeking hence reducing the likelihood of diagnosis and so can affect treatment and outcome in HIV infection. They may also adversely affect adherence to medication and activities to prevent disease and promote health.

7. Management

Mental disorders episodes are known to cluster around specific times in the course of the illness, such as, the period of diagnosis of HIV, period when the infected individual starts declining in health or the period in the early stages of HIV dementia. However, an episode of mental distress can occur at any point in the course of the illness. In the early stages social support alone can suffice alongside psychotherapy. However, in the later stages anti-depressants such as Imipramine or Amitriptyline can be used. Selective serotonin re-uptake inhibitors such as Fluoxetine may also be prescribed.

However the mainstay of management should fall around the time of diagnosis with adequate pre and post testing counseling surrounding the HIV test. The HIV counseling process should also be optimized to conditions that allow for higher acceptability of the counseling process. A Clinical trial study conducted in Zambia showed higher acceptability for Home-based-Voluntary-Counseling and testing as opposed to facility based counseling. Such innovative means of facilitating the counseling process will by induction lead to better acceptance of the HIV sero-status thus preventing subsequent maladjustment disorders. This has been shown in literature to reduce the risk of suicide at the initial diagnosis. Additionally follow-up counseling at every stage in the disease process emphasizing safer sex should be promoted alongside care giver support. This support should especially be extended to the most vulnerable; the women, children, orphans and those of low socio-economic position in society.

8. Conclusion

Mental disorders are common place in HIV infection and potentiate the course, progression and prognosis of the HIV disease process. The direct and indirect impact of HIV on the infected individual has conversely also been associated with mental distress episodes. Mental disorder and HIV/AIDS also have a lot of socio-demographic factors in common that have been attributed to each of their development. Therefore, a combination of these two disease entities leads to devastating morbidity and mortality, especially in the most affected communities. This thus emphasizes the need for prompt screening, diagnosis and treatment of mental distress in HIV infection.

Author details

Peter J. Chipimo[1,2] and Knut Fylkesnes[1]

1 University of Bergen, Faculty of Medicine, Centre for International Health, Norway

2 University of Zambia, School of Medicine, Department of Public Health, Zambia

References

[1] Bock PJ, Markovitz D. Infection with HIV-2. AIDS. 2001;15(Suppl 5):S35-45.

[2] Chipimo P.J. Fylkesnes K, Mental distress in the general population in Zambia: Impact of HIV and social factors: BMC Public Health. 2009; 9: 298. http://www.ncbi.nlm.nih.gov/pmc/articles/PMC2744699/

[3] Chipimo Peter J, Mental health in the era of HIV. Investigating mental distress, its determinants, conceptual models and the impact of HIV in Zambia. BORA-UiB 2011 http://hdl.handle.net/1956/4882

[4] Chipimo PJ, Fylkesnes K. Comparative validity of screening instruments for Mental Distress in Zambia. Clinical practice & Epidemiology in Mental Health. 2010;6:4-15.

[5] Chipimo PJ, Tuba M, Fylkesnes K, Conceptual models for Mental Distress among HIV infected and uninfected: A contribution to clinical practice and research in primary health-care centers in Zambia. BMC Health Services Research 2011; 11:7 1-12

[6] Chipimo, Peter Jay: Mental Distress and the Impact of HIV: Data from a Population-Based Survey in Zambia, Master thesis (2007) http://www.uib.no/cih/en/research/cih-master-theses

[7] Department of Health and Human Services (Ed). A Pocket Guide to Adult HIV/AIDS Treament January edition 2005

[8] DeVellis RF. Scale Development: Theory and Application. London: SAGE Publications; 2003.

[9] Escobar JI, Waitzkin H, Silver RC, Gara M, Holman A. A bridged somatization: a study in primary care. Psychosom Med. 1998;60:466-72.

[10] Gottlinger HG. The HIV-1 assembly machine. AIDS. 2001;15(Suppl 5):S13-20.

[11] Jenkins R. Sex differences in minor psychiatric morbidity: a survey of a homogeneous population. Social Science and Medicine. 1985;20(9):887-99.

[12] Kigozi FN, Flisher AJ, Lund C, Funk M, Banda M, Bhana A, et al. Mental health policy development and implementation in four African Conutries. Journal of health psychology. 2007;12(3):505-16.

[13] Kitahata MM, Gange SJ, Abraham AG, et al. Effect of early verses defered anti-retroviral therapy for HIV on survival. N Engl Med. 2009;360(18):1815-26.

[14] Kroenke K, Spitzer RL, Williams JB, et al. Physical symptoms in primary care: Predictors of psychiatric disorders and functional impairement. Arch Fam Med. 1994;3:774-9.

[15] Kuehner C. Gender diffferences in unipolar depression: an update of epidemiological findings and possible explanations. Acta Psychiatr Scand. 2003;108:163-74.

[16] Maier W, Gansicke M, Gater R, Rezaki M, Tiemens B, Urzua RF. Gender differences in the prevalence of depression: A survey in primary care. J Affect Disord. 1999;53:241-52.

[17] Mathers CD, Loncar D. Projections of global mortality and burden of disease from 2002 to 2030. Plos Med. 2006;3(e442).

[18] McCaffery JM, Frasure-Smith N, Dude MP, et al. Common genetic vulnerability to depressive symptoms and coronary artery disease: a review and development of candidate genes related to inflamation and serotonin. Psychosom Med. 2006;68:187-200.

[19] Murray CJL, Lopez AD, et al. The global burden of disease and injuries series: A comprehensive assessment of Mortality and disability, Injuries and Risk factors 1990 and projected to 2020. Volume 1: Cambridge, MA; 1996.

[20] Ngoma MC, Prince M, Mann A. Common mental disorders among those attending primary health clinics and traditional healers in urban Tanzania. Br J Psychiatry. 2003;183:349-55.

[21] Ovuga EBL, Boardman A, Oluka GAO. Traditional healers and mental illness in Uganda. Psychiatric Bull. 1999;23:276-9.

[22] Palella FJ, Delaney KM, Moorman AC, Loveless MO, Fuhrer J, Satten GA, et al. Declining morbidity and mortality among patients with advanced human immunodeficiency virus infection. N Engl Med. 1998;338(13):853-60.

[23] Patel V, Abas M, Broadhead J, Todd CH, Reeler AP. Depression in developing countries: Lessons from Zimbabwe. BMJ. 2001;322(482).

[24] Rachlis AR, Zarowny DP. Guidelines for anti-retroviral therapy for HIV infection. Canadian HIV trials Network Antiretroviral Working Group. CMAJ. 1998;158(4): 496-505.

[25] Sax PE, Baden LR. When to start anti-retroviral therapy- ready when you are? N Engl Med. 2009;360(18):1897-9.

[26] Saz P, Dewey ME. Depression symptoms and mortality in persons aged 65 and over living in the community: a systematic review of the literature. Int J Geriatric Psychiatry. 2001;16:622-30.

[27] Strong K, Mather C, Leeder S, Beaglehole R. Preventing Chronic diseases: How many lives can we save? Lancet. 2005;366:1578-82.

[28] Tatt ID, Barlow KL, Nicoll A. The public health significance of HIV-1 subtypes. AIDS. 2001;15(Suppl 5):S59-71.

[29] Vieweg WV, Julius DA, Fernandez A, et al. Treatmeant of depression in patients with coronary heart disease. Am J Med. 2006;119:567-73.

[30] Wilson D, Naidoo S, Bekker L, Cotton M, Maartens G. Handbook of HIV medicine. Cape Town: Oxford University press; 2002.

[31] Young TN, Arens FJ, Kennedy GE, Laurie JW, Rutherford G. Antiretroviral post-exposure prophylaxis (PEP) for occupational HIV exposure. Cochrane Database Syst Rev. 2007;1(CD002835).

Chapter 8

Neurological Manifestations of HIV-1 Infection and Markers for HIV Progression

Rehana Basri and Wan Mohamad Wan Majdiah

Additional information is available at the end of the chapter

http://dx.doi.org/10.5772/54026

1. Introduction

Human immunodeficiency virus, or HIV, is the virus that causes acquired immune deficiency syndrome (AIDS). The acquired immunodeficiency syndrome (AIDS) was first described in 1981 in USA. In 1983, human immunodeficiency virus type-1 (HIV-1) was isolated, and in the following year it was demonstrated clearly that it was the causative agent of AIDS. The disease is a major health problem in many parts of the world. The high prevalence and striking diversity of neurological disorders complicating AIDS were recognized in 1983 (Snider et al., 1983). AIDS was associated with distinct neurological syndromes, such as dementia, myelopathy and painful neuropathy that appeared to result from the HIV itself. Over the last 30 years, there has been increasing recognition of the role that auto antibodies play in neurological disorders. During the past decade, AIDS has become a global health problem with 182,000 000 cases reported from 152 countries. It is estimated that nearly five to ten million people are infected worldwide with HIV-1. With a mean incubation period from time of infection to the development of AIDS of eight to 10 years, it is projected that nearly all HIV-1-infected individual will develop AIDS within the next 15 years (Quinn, 1990). It has become increasingly evident that the vast majority of HIV-1 infected people will eventually develop AIDS or an AIDS-related condition (De Wolf and Lange, 1991) with a median time of progression to AIDS of 7-10 years from infection in adults (Lui *et al.*, 1988; Bacchetti and Moss, 1989) and shorter periods in infants and elderly patients (Medley et al., 1987; Auger et al., 1988; Lagakos & DeGruttola, 1989). In the United States alone, 104, 210 cases of AIDS and more than 61,000 deaths have been reported. Sexual, parenteral as well as perinatal transmission routes have remained the major modes of transmission, although the proportion of cases within each risk behaviour category has changed. Recently, there has been a dramatic increase in the proportion of AIDS patients who have acknowledged as IV drug user or have heterosexual contact with other individuals at high risk for HIV infection (Quinn, 1990).

In Sub-Saharan Africa, 22.5 million people living with HIV (68% of the global infections) and 1.6 million AIDS death in 2007 (76% of the AIDS deaths worldwide). In recent years, global efforts have increased substantially. The most encouraging improvements have been in Sub-Saharan Africa where the number of people being treated with anti-retrovirals has increased tenfold from 2003 to 2006 (Peters et al., 2008). The decline of HIV infection in some regions was partially offset by a rise in new infections in other parts of the globe, particularly in Asia and Eastern Europe (Delpech & Gahagan, 2009). It was estimated that over 5 million people in South Asia living with HIV/AIDS. Almost 90% of those infected live in India. Other countries in the region such as Bangladesh, Pakistan and Nepal have a low HIV prevalence in general population (Abeysena & De Silva, 2005).

2. Back ground of immune defence mechanisms

Humoral immunity and complement system: immunity that is mediated by secreted antibodies produced in the cells of the B lymphocyte. Cell mediated immunity : is an immune response that does not involve antibodies but rather involves the activation of macrophages, natural (NK), antigen-specific cytotoxic T-lymphocytes.

2.1. Causes of immunosuppression primary: Antibody deficiency, combined antibody

Antibody deficiency, combined antibody and cellular deficiency, Complement deficiency. Acquired: Extremes of age, Diabetes, Chronic alcoholism, HIV infection, Connective tissue diseases, Organ failure (renal, hepatic), Malignancy, Iatrogenic (chemotherapy, radiotherapy, Transplantation). HIV is a retrovirus that primarily infects vital organs of the human immune system such as CD4+ T cells (a subset of T cells), macrophages and dendritic cells. It directly and indirectly destroys CD4+ T cells (Alimonti et al 2003).

2.2. Cells affected

The virus entering through which ever route and acts primarily on the following cells: Lymphoreticular system: CD_4+ T-Helper cells, Macrophages, Monocytes, B-lymphocytes, Certain endothelial cells and Central nervous system: Microglia, Astrocytes, Oligodendrocytes, and Neurones.

2.3. Relation of CD4 T cell count

Neurologic Complications increase with decline in CD_4 T cell count. CD_4 T cell count > 500/μl – Earlystage – Demyelinating Neuropathies, CD_4 T cell count 200 to 500 – Mid stage – Dementia - VZV radiculities and CD_4 T cell count <200 –advance stage → Dementia, Myelopathy, Painful-neuropathy.

2.4. Immune deficiency & clinical disease

Clinical manifestations, Susceptibility to infections, Lymphoreticular malignancies, autoimmune disease.

http://dx.doi.org/10.5772/54026

3. Neurological menifestations of HIV-1 infections

HIV is neuroinvasive, it does not directly infect neurons. The major brain reservoirs for HIV infection and replication are microglia and macrophages. Astrocytes can be infected but are not a site of active HIV replication. HIV-associated neurologic complications are indirect effects of viral neurotoxins (viral proteins gp120 and tat) and neurotoxins released by infected or activated microglia, macrophages and astrocytes. Neurologic manifestations occur over the entire spectrum of HIV disease. Fifty to 70% of patients experienced acute clinical syndrome 1 to 6 wks after infection, Neuro Manifestations occur in 10% involves Multiple Parts of nervous system. Some Monophonic illness Meningitis, Meningioencephalitis, Seizures, Myelopathy, Cranial and Peripheral Neuropathy linked to primary HIV and recover within 1 week. Neurological opportunistic infections and malignancies predominated in early reports, but it became also clear that AIDS was associated with distinct neurological syndromes, such as Acute/subacute diffuse encephalopathy Progressive dementia, Focal mass lesions, Acute stroke like presentation, Meningitis, Multiple cranial neuropathies and Acute/subacute myelopathy.

3.1. HIV encephalopathy

(AIDS Dementia Complex or HIV associated Dementia) is a late complication of HIV infection and progresses slowly over months seen in pts with CD_{4T} cell Count >350cells/μl. Dementia is a major feature but aphasia, apraxia and afnofia uncommon, motor abnormality like unsteady gait, poor balance, tremor and in late stage develop apathy & lack of initiative – leads to vegetative state mania (table 1). Neuro imaging: MRI & CT demonstrate cerebral atrophy, Basal ganglia calcification in children. CSF: MonoNucleatz cells increase, Protein increase, RNA can be detected and HIV can be cultured. Infective: CMV ventriculoencephalitis, Varicella encephalitis, Herpes encephalitis, Toxoplasma encephalitis (rare).

[redacted]

Table 1. Clinical staging of HIV Encephalopathy

Treatment:

Combination anti retro viral therapy is beneficial and rapid improvement in cognitive function.

3.2. HIV-associated dementia

The major direct effect of HIV infection on the immune system is the profound and progressive loss of CD4 lymphocytes. This leads to impaired cellular immunity, and a dysregulation of macrophages, with the overproduction of a variety of proinflammatory cytokines and chemokines (Griffin, 1997). HIV can enter the nervous system early after infection, but productive infection is rarely detectable before immunosuppression has developed. Based upon phylogenetic analysis of HIV gp160, the route of central nervous system (CNS) infection appears to primarily involve infected monocytes (Liu et al., 2000) as well as free viral particles and HIV proteins crossing a disrupted blood–brain barrier. The presentation of HIV-D includes cognitive, behavioral, and motor dysfunction, and suggests a predominant subcortical involvement (Navia et al., 1986). In the early stages, memory loss, mental slowing, reading and comprehension difficulties, and apathy are frequent com plaints (Fig. 1) (Mc Arthur et al., 2003).

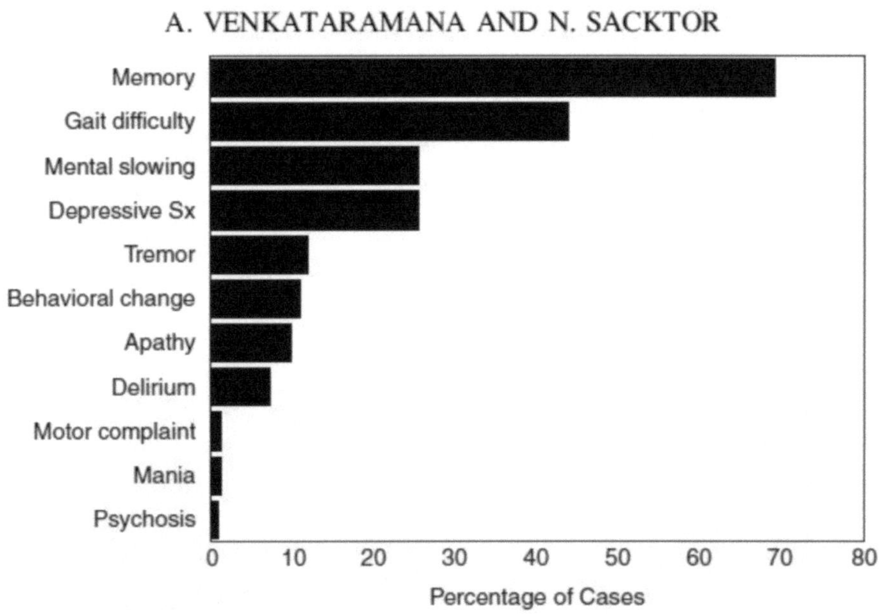

Figure 1. Frequency of symptoms in HIV dementia among 300 subjects personally examined at JHU HIV Neurology program (McArthur et al., 2003).

The cognitive deficits of HIV- D are characterized primarily by (1) memory loss that is selective for impaired retrieval; (2) impaired ability to manipulate acquired knowledge; (3) personality changes including apathy, inertia, and irritability; and (4) general slowing of all thought processes. Gait disturbance and impairment of fine manual dexterity are common early manifestations. Examination findings include impaired rapid movements of eyes and limbs,

http://dx.doi.org/10.5772/54026

diffuse hyperreflexia, frontal release signs, and sometimes Parkinsonism (Mirsattari et al., 1998). A recent study suggests that antiretroviral drug combinations with drugs that have better CSF penetration are associated with greater CSF viral load suppression and may be associated with greater improvement in neuropsychological test deficits compared to antiretroviral drug combinations with drugs that have poor CSF penetration (Letendre et al., 2004). Antiretroviral drugs with the highest CSF:plasma ratios or with profound effects on viral replication in the periphery with a resulting decrease in virus entry into the CNS (e.g., zidovudine, stavudine, abacavir, nevirapine, efavirenz, and indinavir) are likely to be the most efficacious for the treatment of HIV-D. Affective: Apathy (depression-like features), Irritability, Mania, new onset psychosis. Behavioral: Psychomotor retardation (slowed speech or response time), Personality changes, Social withdrawal. Cognitive: Lack of visuospatial memory (misplacing things), Lack of vasomotor coordination, Difficulty with complex sequencing (difficulty in performing previously learned complex tasks), Impaired concentration and attention-Impaired verbal memory (word-finding ability), Mental slowing. Motor: Unsteady gait, loss of balance, Leg weakness, dropping things, Tremors, poor handwriting and decline in fine motor skills.

3.3. HIV associated neuropathy

Symptomatic neuropathies occur in approximately 10% to 15%. Pathologic evidence of peripheral nerve involvement is present in virtually all end-stage AIDS patients. The most common complaints are numbness, parethesias and painful dysestesias. Zanetti et al., (2004) reported mild distal dysestesia that neither interfered with the activities of daily living nor required specific therapy. The main neurological sign was distal symmetric sensory alteration (in 97.1% of the patients) in the four limbs but mainly in the feet. The etiology and pathogenesis of peripheral neuropathy associated with HIV infection is uncertain. It can be caused by the direct or indirect action of HIV and antibody production, or secondary to infections (CMV, MAC), toxic effects of certain drugs (isoniazid, vincristine, d4T, ddi, ddC), or nutritional deficiencies (vitamin B12) (Rizzuto et al., 1995; Dalakas et al., 1988; Figg, 1991; Browne et al., 1993; Pike, 1993; Abrams et al., 1994; Kieburtz et al., 1991; Norton et al., 1996; Gill et al., 1990; Simpson et al.,1995). Almost all patients with HIV that had diagnosis of peripheral neuropathy were taking drugs probably neurotoxic (ddi, d4t,ddC isoniazid) (Zanetti et al., 2004) to determine the effect of 5 weeks of individualized acupuncture treatment, delivered in a group setting, on pain and symptoms of peripheral neuropathy associated with HIV infection. In addition, the acupuncture regimen reduced pain/aching/burning and pins/needles/numbness in the upper and lower limbs (Phillips et al., 2004).

3.4. HIV related to myelopathy with polyradiculopathy

The most common cause of spinal cord disease in AIDS patients is AIDS-associated myelopathy, with a reported prevalence of 20% to 55% in different series (Gray et al., 1990; Henin et al., 1992; Petito et al., 1985; Goldstick, 1985; Dal et al., 1994; Artigas et al., 1990). Clinical symptoms and signs of myelopathy included spastic paraparesis, gait disturbance, urinary problems, and impotence in males, hyperreflexia, and a variable degree of sensory loss. A clinical rating of the severity of the myelopathy was established by a neurologist blinded to the MR findings. The myelopathy was rated as mild, moderate, or severe: mild if there were only subjective complaints of leg stiffness, heaviness, cramps, or subjective bladder dysfunction (not incontinence), together with objective findings of increased tone, hyperreflexia, or extensor plantar responses; moderate if there was objectively demonstrable weakness of the lower extremities or incontinence; and severe if the patient was not independently ambulatory. The MR findings of the spinal cord were subsequently correlated with the clinical rating of the severity of the myelopathy. June et al, 1999, reported spinal cord MR features were abnormal in 18 (86%) of the 21 patients (table 2). The most common finding was spinal cord atrophy, seen in 15 patients (71%) (Fig 2).

MR Findings in the Spinal Cord	No. of Patients	Clinical Rating of Severity of Myelopathy, No. (%)		
		Mild	Moderate	Severe
Normal MR findings	3	2 (66.7)	0	1 (33.3)
Cord atrophy	15	3 (20.0)	9 (60.0)	3 (20.0)
Intrinsic cord signal abnormality	6	1 (16.7)	2 (33.3)	3 (50.0)
Atrophy plus cord signal abnormality	3	1 (33.3)	0	2 (66.7)

Table 2. American Journal of Neuroradiology 20:1412-1416 (9 1999)

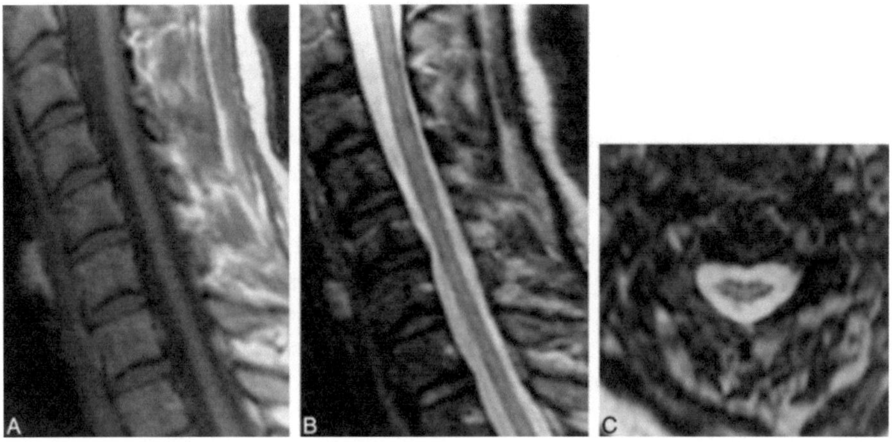

Figure 2. American Journal of Neuroradiology 20:1412-1416 (9 1999)

AIDS-associated myelopathy is characterized pathologically by discrete or coalescent intramyelin and periaxonal vacuolation, with cellular debris and lipid-laden macrophages, in the white matter of the spinal cord. The axons are usually intact, but in severe vacuolization, they may become disrupted. It typically involves the lateral and posterior columns of the cervical and thoracic cord (Henin et al., 1992; Petito et al., 1985; Dal et al., 1994; Tan et al., 1995). The effect of HAART on improving the symptoms or slowing the progression of HIV-associated myelopathy is not known. A pilot study using high doses of oral L-methionine led to improvement in clinical and electrophysiologic features of the disease in an open-label clinical trial (Dorfman et al., 1997). Uncontrolled clinical experience no benefit from corticosteroids and intravenous immunoglobulin (IVIG).

3.5. HIV-Associated Neuromuscular Weakness Syndrome (HANWS)

Toxic events secondary to use of HAART can be observed globally. Recently, Simpson et al. 2004, reported a heterogeneous syndrome termed the HIV-associated neuromuscular weakness syndrome (HANWS) which seems to be related to hyperlactatemia and stavudine and/or didanosine exposure. Rapidly ascending neuromuscular weakness syndrome," associated with lactic acidosis syndrome in HIV-infected patients. Majority dramatic motor weakness developed over days to weeks (resembling GBS ▪ respiratory failure and death in several patients. Systemic symptoms included nausea, vomiting, weight loss, abdominal distention, hepatomegaly, and lipoatrophy. Stavudine, Lamivudine and Efavirenz are most commonly used ARV agent. Muscle weakness worsened even after discontinuation of ARV therapy. Rapidly progressive sensorimotor polyneuropathy and myopathy observed. In recent years, a spectrum of metabolic and morphologic alterations has emerged among HIV-infected patients receiving HAART. Additionally, neurological syndromes, such as antiretroviral toxic neuropathy, have been clinically well characterized (Höke & Cornblath, 2004; Keswani et al., 2002). Diagnostic information find out by severe axonal neuropathy, increase Serum lactate level twice times than normal, decrease Serum bicarbonate and arterial pH level, increase serum CPK level. Electrophysiology; EMG-NCV: severe axonal neuropathy in most of the cases, demyelinating features may be seen admixed or in isolation and myopathic features may be noted. Nerve and Muscle Biopsy: Important in evaluating patients with HANWS. Mitochondrial studies with morphology assessment and mitochondrial DNA (mtDNA) quantification may be needed to further elucidate the role of mitochondrial toxicity in this syndrome Treatment: As was observed in this report, the antiretroviral most often associated with HANWS was stavudine. Avoiding stavudine or didanosine, the nucleosides with the highest association with mitochondrial toxicity, may be a satisfactory alternative in the long run. The treatment of HANWS is controversial and important since this is potentially a fatal syndrome. Our experience reinforces the recommendation that early interruption of HAART and clinical support is beneficial. Initiate systemic treatment for lactic acidosis syndrome and supportive treatment for the neurologic component in a monitored setting. Neuromuscular weakness - corticosteroids, intravenous immunoglobulins, vitamins (B1, B12), and plasmapheresis have been used (Luciano et al., 2003).

3.6. Toxoplasmosis

Toxoplasmosis is the leading cause of focal central nervous system (CNS) disease in AIDS. CNS toxoplasmosis in HIV-infected patients is usually a complication of the late phase of the disease. Toxoplasmosis has been an indicator disease for AIDS since the early days of the human immunodeficiency virus (HIV) epidemic (Horowitz et al., 1983; Luft et al., 1984). CNS toxoplasmosis begins with constitutional symptoms and headache. Later, confusion and drowsiness, seizures, focal weakness, and language disturbance develop. Without treatment, patients progress to coma in days to weeks. On physical examination, personality and mental status changes may be observed. Seizures, hemiparesis, hemianopia, aphasia, ataxia, and cranial nerve palsies may be evident. Occasionally, symptoms and signs of a radiculomyelopathy predominate. Serologic studies in patients with CNS toxoplasmosis may demonstrate rising titers of anti-toxoplasma immunoglobulin G (IgG) antibodies, CD4 counts < 100 cells mm^{-3} and CSF findings are non-specific. Detection of T.gondii DNA by PCR has only moderate sensitivity. MRI typically reveals multiple enhancing lesions with perifocal oedema and mass effect in the basal ganglia and gray white matter interface of the cerebral hemispheres. Any part of the brain can be affected, mostly solitary in appearance. Standard therapy consists of pyrimethamine, sulfadiazine, and folinic acid in combination. Trimethoprim-sulfamethoxazole (TMP-SMZ) can be used as an alternative regimen (Dedicoat et al., 2006). A Cochrane data base review failed to find a significant difference between standard therapy and TMP-SMZ. Clindamycin can be used in patients allergic to sulfa drugs. Effective antiretroviral therapy is equally important (Dedicoat et al., 2006; Fung et al., 1996; Bertschy et al., 2006; Behbahani et al., 1995). Most common cause of cerebral mass lesion, Sub acute course with fever, headache, confusion or cognitive disturbances with focal deficits, Seizures 24 – 29 %, rarely psychotic features. Imaging – Multiple mass lesions at grey – white junction & basal ganglia, CSF – Non specific, Antibody to T. Gondi, PCR recently developed.

3.7. AIDS related primary CNS lymphoma

A relationship between congenital or acquired immune deficiency (AIDS) and lymphoma was first recognised more than 30 years ago. An association between non-Hodgkin's lymphoma (NHL) and the acquired immune deficiency syndrome became evident in the early 1980s. Lymphoma occurring in the HIV-infected individual may be systemic, may primarily involve the central nervous system, or may be localised in the body cavities. Systemic lymphoma is the most common presentation, accounting for approximately 80% of all cases. The histology usually is diffuse large cell, immunoblastic, or small non-cleaved cell lymphoma. Primary CNS lymphoma accounts for approximately 20% of all cases. Most patients are profoundly immunosuppressed and typically have a CD4 lymphocyte count below 50/ml. Approximately two-thirds or more of them have AIDS-defining conditions prior to the development of primary CNS lymphoma (Gill et al., 1985; Goldstein, 1991). The lesions are typically few in number (1–3), large (2–4 cm), and contrast enhances approximately 50% of the time (Fine & Mayer 1993). Lesions are most common in the cerebrum, but also occur frequently in the cerebellum, basal ganglia and brain stem, and are nearly always found to be multifocal at autopsy (Loureiro et al., 1988; MacMahon et al., 1991). The lymphoma cells tend to be distributed along vascular channels as perivascular cuffs, are of B cell origin, display large cell and immunoblastic histologies. Subacute presentation with headache, impaired cognition, focal cerebral dysfunction. D/D – Toxoplasmosis, PML. Imaging – Multiple enhancing periventricular or subependymal lesions, CSF – EBV nucleic acid in CSF being studied. NHL are of higher grade and advanced stage. Response and tolerance to chemotherapy is poor. Systemic lymphoma in patients with HIV infection is a potentially curable disease, although the potential for cure is less than in immunocompetent individuals. Appropriate use of supportive care is an important component of therapy (Table 3) (Sparano, 2001).

Indication	Drug(s)
Primary infection prophylaxis	
Pneumocystis carinii, Toxoplasma	TMP-SMZ 1 DS QD
Oral and/or oesophageal candidiasis	Fluconazole 100 mg QD
MAI Complex (CD4 <50/ul)	Azithromycin 1200 mg weekly
Secondary infection prophylaxis	
Herpes simplex infections	Acyclovir 400 mg BID or 200 mg TID
Cytomegalovirus infection	Ganciclovir 1 g TID
Mycobacterium–avium complex	Clarithromycin 500 mg BID plus ethambutol 15 mg/kg QD, with or without rifabutin 300 mg QD
Toxoplasma gondii	Sulphadiazine 1–1.5 gm q6h, pyrimethamine 25–75 mg QD, Leucovorin 10–25 mg QD — QID
Cryptococcus neoformans	Fluconazole 200 mg QD
Salmonella bacteraemia	Ciprofloxacin 500 mg BID
Haematopoietic growth factors	
For selected patients in whom the risk of febrile neutropenia ⩾40%	G-CSF 5 mcg/kg or GM-CSF 250 mcg/M^2 s.c. daily beginning after completion of chemotherapy and continue until neutrophil recovery
Antiretroviral agents	
Selecting patients for therapy	Follow NIH guidelines (http://www.hivatis.org)
Role of therapy in controlling malignancy	
Kaposi's sarcoma	Essential
Lymphoma	Unknown
Other tumours	Unknown
Factors influencing selection of agents	
May be used with myelosuppressive drugs	Didanosine, zalcitabine
Avoid with myelosuppressive drugs/regimens	Zidovudine
Avoid with neurotoxic drugs/regimens	Didanosine, zalcitabine, stavudine
May alter the metabolism of cytotoxic drugs metabolised by cytochrome p450 enzymes	All protease inhibitors and non-nucleoside RTIs

QD. Daily; TID, three times daily; BID, two times daily; QID, four times daily; s.c., subcutaneous; G CSF, granulocyte colony stimulating factor; GM,CSF, granulocyte-macrophage colony stimulating factor, NIH, national institute of health; RTIs, reserve transcript inhibitors.

Table 3. Suggested supportive care for the patient with HIV infection and lymphoma or other malignancies. European Journal of Cancer 37 (2001) 1296–1305

Appropriate supportive care and CNS prophylaxis might improve outcome. In patients with HIV infection, the differential diagnosis of a patient with focal brain lesions includes PCNSL, cerebral toxoplasmosis, and other infections. Focal brain lesions have also been described in conjunction with relapsed systemic lymphoma (Desai et al., 1999). A proposed algorithm for the diagnostic approach to a patient with HIV infection and focal brain lesions is shown in Fig. 3.

3.8. HIV related progressive multifocal leukoencephalopathy

Progressive Multifocal Leukoencephalopathy (PML) is a rare demyelinating disease (focal neurological disease & cognitive impairment) of the CNS caused by reactivation of JC virus (JCV) 1. Radiographic evidence of white matter disease with subcortical involvement – 'scalloped' appearance. CSF – Non specific. Primary infection occurs in childhood and the virus remains latent in the kidney or lymphoid organs thereafter. In the setting of cellular immunosuppression, the virus may spread to the central nervous system, leading to a lytic infection of oligodendrocytes and subsequent demyelination. Classically, PML was observed in patients with advanced HIV infection, lymphoproliferative disorders and transplant recipients. There is no specific treatment for PML, but the survival in HIV-infected PML patients has increased substantially during the last decade. Before the introduction of highly active antiretroviral therapy (HAART), only 10% patients with PML lived for more than a year. In contrast, recent studies have shown at least 50% one-year survival of HIV- infected PML patients (Falco et al., 2008; De Luca et al., 2008). However, the prognosis of PML associated with other immunosuppressive conditions remains poor. Immune recovery associated with HAART has resulted in a better prognosis for HIV-infected PML patients. The prompt institution of HAART in HIV infected PML patients is the most effective therapeutic approach in increasing survival in this group. Several studies have shown that PML survival increased from 10 to 50% in the last decade (Falco et al., 2008; De Luca et al., 2008; Cinque et al., 2003; Bamford et al., 1989; Du Pasquier et al., 2004; Koralnik et al., 2004; Gasnault et al., 2003; Antinori et al., 2003). In a recent study, JCV-peptide loaded dendritic cells from PML patients, HIV-infected individuals and healthy control subjects could elicit a strong cellular immune response mediated by CD8+ cytotoxic T lymphocytes cell response *in vitro* (Marzocchetti et al, 2009), which suggests that autologous dendritic cell-based immunotherapy could be a potential therapeutic option for PML.

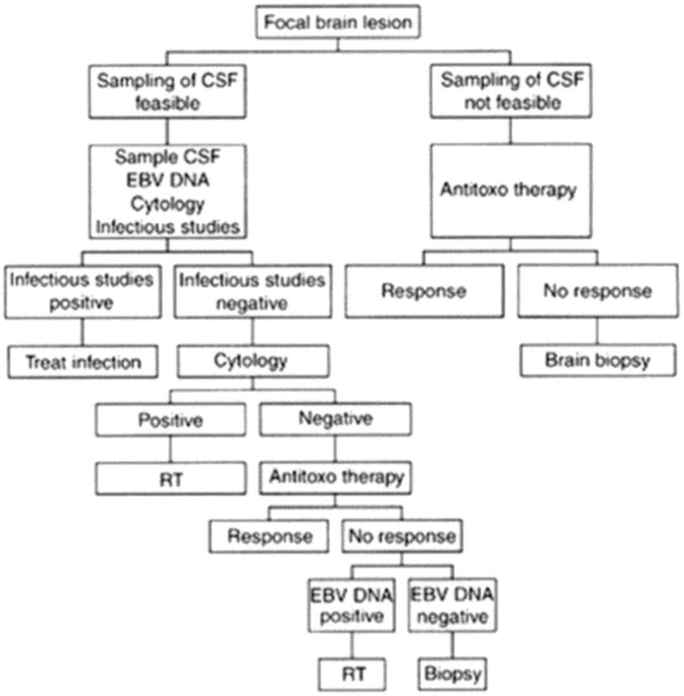

CSF, cerebrospinal fluid
Antitoxo, antitoxoplasmosis
RT, radiotherapy

Figure 3. Algorithm for management of HIV – infected individuals with focal brain lesions European Journal of Cancer 37 (2001) 1296–1305

http://dx.doi.org/10.5772/54026

3.9. Neurological approach to immunocompromized patients due to HIV-1

Central nervous system pathogens in specific immunocompromised-host (HIV-1) categories based upon presentation like Meningitis, Meningoencephalitis, and Encephalitis. Cryptococcal meningitis is seen in populations but cryptococcomas are much more frequent in the latter. Encephalitis and cerebral abscesses usually do not produce cerebrospinal fluid (CSF) changes unless the lesion communicates with the ventricular or subarachnoid spaces. Discrete white matter lesions have a narrower differential including calcineurin-induced demyelination usually in the posterior territory and progressive multifocal leukoencephalopathy (JC papova virus) which is characteristically nonenhancing and without mass effect. Meningoencephalitis due to Toxoplasma gondii continues to be the predominant pathogen in HIV-1 disease even with highly active antiretroviral therapy (HAART) exposure (Peter K. Linden, 2009).

3.10. Neurogenic manifestation of HIV infection in children

Twenty percent of children present with severe symptoms or die in infancy, Prognosis is related to: a) Greater inoculation of HIV b) Earlier infection with immature immune system c) Immune escape from mother. Asceptic Meningitis or Meningoencephalitis does not occur in infants. Acquired Microcephali, cerebral vasculopathy and basal ganglia, Calcification are unique in children. OIS are rare in children, here absolute CD_4T cell count less helpful. HIV-DNA PCR on peripheral blood lymphocytes can help to diagnosis. Avoid vaginal delivery, plan caesarean section and avoid breast feeding.

4. Markers for HIV progression

A combination of different markers is required to predict plasma human immunodeficiency virus type 1 (HIV-1) disease progression (Fahey et al., 1990; Saves et al., 2001). Levels of plasma HIV-1 RNA and CD4 + cell count are highly predictive of progression to AIDS or death (Hughes et al., 1997; Mellors et al., 1997; Saves et al., 2001). However, variations of these markers do not explain all variations of disease progression and the relative prognostic value of laboratory markers of HIV disease are not the same at different stages of the disease. Therefore the use of markers of immune activation has been suggested (Graham, 1996; Saves et al., 2001). CD4+ cell count (CD4) and RNA viral loads (RNA) are the two most commonly used prognostic markers of the clinical progression of HIV infection for HIV infection (Hammer et al., 2006; Gilks et al., 2006). Besides, there are various additional markers for HIV progression such as CD8+ cell count, anti-HIV antibodies, p24 antigen, hemoglobin concentration, platelet concentration as well as erythrocyte sedimentation rate (ESR). Various predictors for progression to AIDS among HIV-positive homosexual men have beed identified. These include low absolute number and/or percentage of CD4+ lymphocytes, low CD8+ cell count, low concentration of anti-HIV antibodies, p24 antigenaemia, decreased concentration of haemoglobin, increased titre of IgG antibody to cytomegalovirus, raised serum IgA and IgM values, raised concentrations in the serum of interleukin-2 receptor, neopterin and beta2-microglobulin (Gafa et al., 1993). Among these markers, the percentage of CD4+ cells was found to be the best predictor of HIV progression (Fahey et al., 1990), followed by serum concentrations of neopterin and beta2-microglobulin, IgA, interleukin-2 receptors and p24 antigen. Only a few studies have the predictive values of these serological markers which have been evaluated in cohorts of IVDUs (Gafa et al., 1993). De Wolf & Lange, (1993) observed that several laboratory markers become most noticeably established as predictors of progression from asymptomatic HIV-1 infection to AIDS: (1) Decline in antibody reactivity to HIV core proteins p24 and p17; (2) Appearance of persistent HIV-1 p24 antigenemia; (3) Declining numbers and percentages of peripheral blood CD4-positive lymphocytes; (4) Elevated serum beta2-microglobulin concentration and (4) Elevated serum and urine neopterin concentrations.

4.1. Immunological and virological markers

Based upon scientific literature, immunological and virological markers have been proven as prognostic indicators for progression of HIV disease. The most widely studied marker, the CD4 + lymphocyte count was found to be the best single indicator of the stage of the illness (Zeller et al., 1996). HIV infects CD4+ T lymphocytes selectively and causes the destruction of CD4+ T cells directly as well as indirectly leading to gradual loss of the CD4 T cell numbers in peripheral circulation. Hence, the CD4+ T cell counts are being used to monitor the disease progression in HIV infection, to decide the threshold for initiation of anti-retro viral therapy, to monitor the efficacy of Anti Retrroviral treatment and to initiate prophylactic treatment for opportunistic infections (OIs) (Atlh Nicholson, 1997; Pattanapanyasat & Thakat, 2005). Measuring the CD4+ lymphocytes count remains the most effective means of evaluating of the clinical prognosis of patients infected with Human Immunodeficiency Virus (HIV) (Stein et al., 1992). This measurement has been universally accepted as a uniform means for the clinical staging of patients infected with HIV and those progressing to AIDS (Levine et al., 2000) and for the determination of the commencement of antiretroviral therapy and for monitoring the response to antiretroviral therapy (Evans-Gilbert et al., 2004).

4.2. CD4+ cell count

CD4+ T lymphocyte play a central regulatory role in the immune response. The decrease in CD4+ T cell numbers can compromise the normal immune functions of the body. Hence, the number of CD4+ T cells in the circulation provides important information regarding the immune competence of an individual (Thakar et al., 2011). HIV primarily targets CD4 cells. As HIV disease progresses, CD4 cell counts decline, typically by about 30-100 cells/µl per year (depending on viral load), leaving a person increasingly vulnerable to infections and cancers. People with CD4 cell counts above 500 cells/µl generally have relatively normal immune function and are at low risk for opportunistic infections (Hammer et al., 2006). The clinical staging of HIV disease and the relative risk of developing opportunistic infections have historically relied on the CD4 cell count as the principle laboratory marker of immune status (Kleinman et al., 1998; Patton et al., 2003). HIV disease is commonly categorized on the basis of three levels of immunodeficiency: relative immune competence (CD4 cell count > 500/µl; ≥ 29%), early immune suppression (CD4 cell count between 200/µl and 500/ µl); 4%-28%) and severe immune suppression (CD4 cell count <200/µl and 500/ µl); <14%) (CDC, 1993).

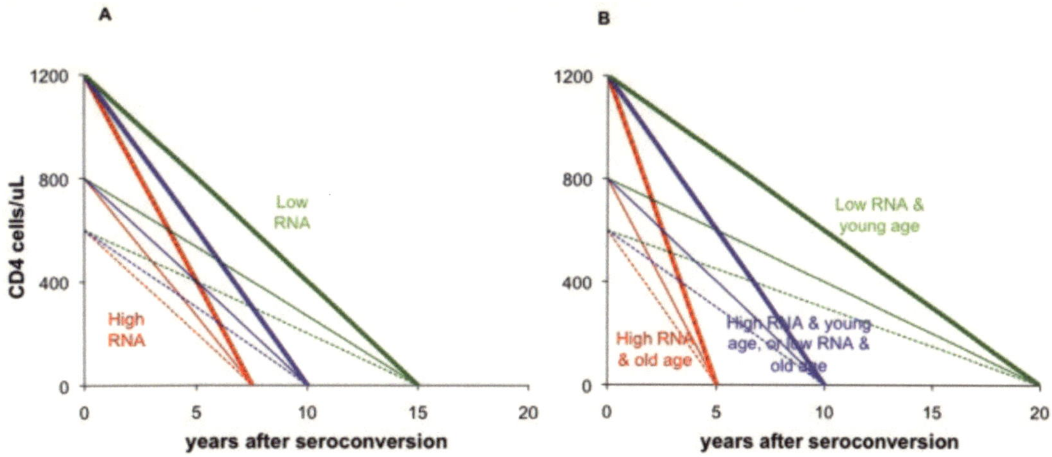

Figure 4. Schematic natural history model of HIV-1 replication driving rates of CD4 decline and clinical progression (Korenromp et al., 2009)

4.3. CD8+ cell count

There are two types of T cells carry the CD8 surface molecule: T-suppressor cells, which inhibit immune responses, and killer T cells (also known as cytotoxic T lymphocytes, or CTLs), which target and kill infected or cancerous cells. As with CD4 cells, a variety of factors can cause CD8 cell counts to fluctuate. CD8 cell counts typically rise over time in people with HIV, but (unlike CD4 cells) CD8 cell numbers do not independently predict disease progression, and their relation to immune status is not well understood (Vajpayee & Mohan 2011).

4.4. CD4 and CD8 cell percentage

Because absolute CD4 and CD8 cell counts are so variable, some physicians prefer to look at CD4 or CD8 cell percentages, the proportion of all lymphocytes that are CD4 or CD8 cells. Percentages are usually more stable over time than absolute counts. A normal CD4 cell percentage in a healthy person is about 30-60 per cent, while a normal CD8 cell percentage is 15-40 per cent (Taylor et al., 1989).

4.5. CD4/CD8 cell ratio

The CD4/CD8 cell ratio is calculated by dividing the CD4 cell count by the CD8 cell count. A normal CD4/CD8 cell ratio is about 0.9-3.0 or higher, there are at least 1-3 CD4 cells for every CD8 cell. In people with HIV this ratio may be much lower, with many more CD8 cells than CD4 cells (Giorgi, 1993).

4.6. HIV viral load

Viral load tests measure the amount of HIV RNA in the blood. The presence of RNA indicates that the virus is actively replicating or multiplying. Along with the CD4 cell count, viral load is one of the most valuable measures for predicting HIV disease progression and gauging when anti-HIV treatment is indicated and how well it is working. Viral load is expressed either as copies of RNA per milliliter of blood (copies/ml) or in terms of logs. A log change is an exponential or 10-fold change. For example, a change from 100 to 1,000 is a 1 log (10-fold) increase, while a change from 1,000,000 to 10,000 is a 2 log (100-fold) decrease. If the level of HIV is too low to be measured, viral load is said to be undetectable, or below the limit of quantification. However, undetectable viral load does not mean that HIV has been eradicated; people with undetectable viral load maintain a very low level of virus. Even when HIV is not detectable in the blood, it may be detectable in the semen, female genital secretions, cerebrospinal fluid, tissues, and lymph nodes (Calmy et al., 2004; Petti et al., 2006; WHO, 2006). In primary HIV infection, patients may present with flu-like symptoms which usually occur during the first weeks of HIV-1 infection. It is associated with peak levels of HIV-1 RNA viremia, which subsequently declines until reaching a set point, where levels remain for months to years. Initial studies suggested that those with more symptomatic acute infection and longer duration of illness have faster rates of progression to AIDS (Koenig et al., 2006). A viral load of 100,000 copies/ml or more is considered high, while levels below 10,000 copies/ml are considered low. Research has consistently shown that higher viral loads are associated with more rapid HIV disease progression and an increased risk of death. Current U.S. HIV treatment guidelines (Koenig et al., 2006) recommend that people should consider starting treatment if their viral load is above 55,000 copies/ml (revised upward from 10,000 copies/ml in the previous guidelines). Importantly, most studies that have correlated viral load and HIV disease progression have been done in men; more recent research indicates that women may progress to AIDS at lower viral load levels, suggesting that the treatment threshold should perhaps be revised downward for women (Monica et al., 2002).

4.7. Beta2-microglobulin (β2-microglobulin)

β2-microglobulin is a low molecular weight protein that forms light chain of the class I major histocompatibility complex (MHC) which present on the surface of most somatic cells including T and B lymphocytes as well as macrophages (Cresswell et al., 1974; Lawlor et al., 1990; De Wolf and Lange 1991). It exhibits amino acid homology with the constant region of immunoglobins (Dar & Singh, 1999; Fauci & Lane, 1998; Quin & Benson, 1994). Circulating β_2-MG is generated during normal MHC I turnover (Lawlor et al., 1990) and thus is not specific to HIV-related cell death. Stimulation of lymphoid cells increases β2-microglobulinproduction. Elevated serum concentration are seen in renal failure, hepatitis, rheumatoid arthritis, myeloproliferative disorders, lymphoproliferative disorders, infectious mononucleosis, influenza A and cytomegalovirus infection (De wolf and Lange, 1991). Free β2-microglobin can be measured in both serum and urine and levels of urine β2-microglobin correlate with the degree of progression of HIV disease. It spikes in acute infection, declines and then rises during the infection. Levels of β2-microglobin are elevated in a variety of conditions characterized by lymphocyte activation and/ or lymphocyte destruction; *e.g.* lymphoproliferative syndromes, autoimmune diseases, viral infection and in patients with renal diseases. It can be measured in serum or plasma by using radio immunoassay radio immunoassay (RIA) or competivive ELISA based tests. B2-microglobin measurement has several advantages as a laboratory assay to help determine prognosis. By contrast with CD4 cell count which requires special procedures for specimen handling and processing, β2-microglobin can be measured with a serological assay and equipment available in many laboratories (Vajpayee & Mohan, 2011). Increased concentrations of this molecule are predictive of progression of HIV infection to AIDS (Moss et al., 1988).

4.8. Neopterin

Neopterin (6-D- erythrohydroxy-propylpterin) is a low molecular weight compound derived from an intermediate product of the *de novo* biosynthesis of tetrahydrobiopterin from guanosine triphosphate (GTP) (Dar & Singh, 1999; Fauci & Lane, 1998; Quin & Benson, 1994). It is an early marker of HIV infection. The levels rise further on progression from pre AIDS to clinical AIDS (Vajpayee & Mohan 2011). It is produced by macrophages after stimulation with gamma interferon. The levels have also been found to be associated with progression of HIV-1-related disease (Fuchs et al., 1988; Melmed et al., 1989; Kramer et al., 1989; De Wolf and Lange 1991) but the predictive value is slightly inferior to that of β2-microglobulin levels. Since neopterin levels are stimulated by HIV infection, measurement of neopterin levels can be useful in monitoring progression and evaluating antiviral therapy (Vajpayee & Mohan 2011).

4.9. Additional markers

Haematological manifestations of HIV infection are common and more frequently occur with progression of the disease. Therefore the complete blood count (CBC) is one of the important haematological parameters which need to checked for HIV patients. They may have low blood cell counts (cytopenias) due to chronic HIV infection or as a side effect of medications, particularly drugs that damage the bone marrow, where all blood cells are produced. Blood cell counts are typically reported as the number of cells per μl of blood (cells/μl) or as a percentage of all blood cells. HIV patients should be checked for CBC for every six months, and more often if they are experiencing symptoms or taking drugs associated with low blood cell counts (De Santis et al., 2011; Olayemi et al, 2008).

4.9.1. Red and white blood cells

Anemia is common in HIV positives. HIV itself and various OIs such as *Mycobacterium avium* complex (MAC) can affect red blood cells and their oxygen-carrying capacity (Volberding et al., 2003; Owiredu et al., 2011). People with HIV infection should be especially concerned with neutrophil and lymphocyte levels, in particular CD4 and CD8 cell counts. Neutrophils normally make up about 50-70 per cent of all white blood cells. Various anti-HIV drugs, OI medications [including ganciclovir (Cytovene), used to treat cytomegalovirus, or CMV], and cancer chemotherapies that suppress the bone marrow may lead to neutropenia (Firnhaber, 2010).

4.9.2. Platelets

Platelets are necessary for blood clotting. A normal platelet count is about 130,000-440,000 cells/μl. Low platelet counts (thrombocytopenia) - which can lead to easy bruising and excessive bleeding may be caused by certain drugs, autoimmune reactions, accelerated destruction by the spleen, or HIV disease itself (Torre & Pugliese, 2008). In 2012, Parinitha & Kulkarni study the haematological changes in HIV infection with correlation to CD4+ cell count. In their study, they found that among 250 patients studied, anaemia was seen in 210 (84%) of cases. Thrombocytopenia occurs in 45 (18%) cases. Majority of cases (70%) had CD4+ cell counts below 200 cells/mm3. Fifty-four cases (21.6%) had CD4 cell counts between 200 to 499 cells/mm3 and 21 (8.4%) cases had CD4 count more than 500 cells/mm3. In patients with CD4 counts less than 200 cells/mm3, anaemia was seen in 91.4% cases, leucopenia in 26.8% cases, lymphopenia in 80% cases and thrombocytopenia in 21.7% cases.

5. Summary

The prevalence of neurological associated with HIV-1 is estimated at 15 to 50% of patients (Dalakas et al., 1988; Cornblath et al., 1988; So et al., 1988; Monte et al., 1988; Gabbai et al., 1990). But it may be almost 100% when a pathological study is performed (Rizzuto et al., 1995; Gabbai et al., 1990). The etiology and pathogenesis of neurological disease associated with HIV infection is uncertain. It can be caused by the direct or indirect action of HIV and antibody production, or secondary to infections (CMV, MAC), toxic effects of certain drugs (isoniazid, vincristine, d4T, ddi, ddC), or nutritional deficiencies (vitamin B12) (Rizzuto et al., 1995; Dalakas et al., 1988; Figg et al., 1991; Browone et al., 1993; Pike et al., 1993; Abram et al., 1994; Kieburtz et al., 1991). HIV seropositive patients may be overlooked or misdiagnosed. A discerning clinical analysis may be helpful in the diagnosis of this common disease and several laboratory markers become most noticeably established as predictors of HIV-1 infection.

Author details

Rehana Basri* and Wan Mohamad Wan Majdiah

*Address all correspondence to: rehana@kk.usm.my

Neurology Craniofacial Sciences & Oral Biology, School of Dental Science, Universiti Sains, Malaysia

References

[1] Abeysena C. & De Silva HJ (2005). HIV in South Asia. Medicine, 33, 42-43

[2] Abrams DI, Goldman AI, Launer C, Korvick JA, Neaton JD, Crane LR, Grodesky M, Wakefield S, Muth K, Kornegay S (1994). A comparative trial of didano-sine or zalcitabine after treatment with zidovudine in patients with human immunodeficiency virus infection. *N Engl J Med* 330: 657-662.

[3] Alimonti JB., Ball T.B.& Fowke K.R. (2003). "Mechanisms of CD4+ T lymphocyte cell death in human immunodeficiency virus infection and AIDS". *J Gen Virol* 84: 1649–1661

[4] Antinori A, Cingolani A, Lorenzini P, Giancola ML, Uccella I, Bossolasco S, Grisetti S, Moretti F, Vigo B, Bongiovanni M, Del Grosso B, Arcidiacono MI, Fibbia GC,Mena M, Finazzi MG, Guaraldi G, Ammassari A, d'Arminio Monforte A, Cinque P, De Luca A. (2003). Clinical epidemiology and survival of progressive multifocal leukoencephalopathy in the era of highly active antiretroviral therapy: data from the Italian Registry Investigative Neuro AIDS (IRINA). *J Neurovirol* 9, Suppl 1:47–53.

[5] Artigas J., Grosse G. & Niedobitek F. (1990). Vacuolar myelopathy in AIDS: a morphologic analysis. *Pathol Res Pract* 186:228– 237

[6] Atlh Nicholson J.A. (1997). Revised guidelines for the performance of CD4+ T cell determinations in persons with human immunodeficiency virus infection. *Morb Mortal Wkly Rep* 46:41–29.

[7] Auger I, Thomas P, De Gruttola V, Morse D, Moore D, Williams R, Truman B, Lawrence CE. (1988). Incubation periods for paediatric AIDS patients. *Nature* 336: 575-77

[8] Bacchetti P. & Moss A.R. (1989). Incubation time of AIDS in San Francisco. *Nature* 338: 251-53

[9] Bamford J.M., Sandercock P.A., Warlow C.P. & Slattery J. (1989). Interobserver agreement for the assessment of handicap in stroke patients. *Stroke* 20(6): 828

[10] Behbahani R., Moshfeghi M. & Baxter J.D. (1995). Therapeutic approaches for AIDS-related toxoplasmosis. *Ann Pharmacother* 29 (7-8): 760-8.

[11] Browne MJ, Mayer KH, Chafee SB, Dudley MN, Posner MR, Steinberg SM, Graham KK, Geletko SM, Zinner SH, Denman SL. (1993). 2',3'-didehydro-3'- deoxythymidine (d4T) in patients with AIDS and AIDS-related complex: a phase I trial. *J Infect Dis* 167: 21-29

[12] Calmy A., Klement E., Teck R., Berman D., Pecoul B. & Ferradini L. (2004). Simplifying and adapting antiretroviral treatment in resource-poor settings: a necessary step to scaling-up. *AIDS* 18: 2353–60

[13] Center for Disease Control and Prevention. (1993). Revised classification system for HIV infection and expanded surveillance case definition for AIDS among adolescents and adults. *MMWR Morb Mortal Wkly Rep* 1992; 41 (RR-17): 1-9.

[14] Cinque P., Koralnik I.J. & Clifford D.B. (2003). The evolving face of human immunodeficiency virus-related progressive multifocal leukoencephalopathy: defining a consensus terminology. *J Neurovirol* 9 Suppl 1:88–92

[15] Cornblath D.R. & McArthur J.C. (1988). Predominantly sensory neuropathy in patients with AIDS and AIDS-related complex. *Neurology* 38: 794-796

[16] Cresswell P, Springer T, Strominger JL, Turner MJ, Grey HM, Kubo RT. (1974). Immunological identity of the small subunit of HLA-A antigens and β2-microglobulin and its turnover on the cell membrane. *Proc Natl Acad Sci USA* 71: 2123-27

[17] Dalakas M.C. & Pezeshkpour G.H. (1988). Neuromuscular diseases associated with human immunodeficiency virus infection. *Ann Neurol* 23: 38-48

[18] Dal Pan, G.J., Glass J.D. & McArthur J.C. (1994). Clinicopathologic correlations of HIV-1-associated vacuolar myelopathy: an autopsybased case-control study. *Neurology* 44: 2159–64

[19] Dar L. & Singh Y.G.K. (1999). Laboratory tests for monitoring stage and progression of HIV infection. In HIV testing manual by NICD and NACO. New Delhi: CBS Publishers. 114–25

[20] Dedicoat M. & Livesley N. (2006). Management of toxoplasmic encephalitis in HIV-infected adults (with an emphasis on resource-poor settings). *Cochrane Database Syst Rev* 3:CD005420

[21] De la Monte SM, Gabuzda DH, Ho DD, Brown RH Jr, Hedley-Whyte ET, Schooley RT, Hirsch MS, Bhan AK. (1988). Peripheral neuropathy in the acquired immunodeficiency syndrome. *Ann Neurol* 23: 485-492

[22] Delpech V. & Gahagan J. (2009). The global epidemiology of HIV. *Medicine* 37: 317-20

[23] De Luca A, Ammassari A, Pezzotti P, Cinque P, Gasnault J, Berenguer J, Di Giambenedetto S, Cingolani A, Taoufik Y, Miralles P, Marra CM, Antinori A; Gesida. (2008).Cidofovir in addition to antiretroviral treatment is not effective for AIDS-associated progressive multifocal leukoencephalopathy: a multicohort analysis. *AIDS* 22(14): 1759–1767

[24] De Santis GC, Brunetta DM, Vilar FC, Brandão RA, de Albernaz Muniz RZ, de Lima GM, Amorelli-Chacel ME, Covas DT, Machado AA. (2011). Hematological abnormalities in HIV-infected patients. *Int J Infect* Dis.15: e808–11.

[25] Desai J., Mitnick R.J., Henry D.H., Llena J., Sparano J.A. (1999). Patterns of central nervous system recurrence in patients with systemic human immunodeficiency virus-associated non-Hodgkin's lymphoma. *Cancer* 86: 1840–1847

[26] Dorfman D., DiRocco A., Simpson D., Tagliati M., Tanners L. & Moise J. (1997). Oral methionine may improve neuropsychological function in patients with AIDS myelopathy: results of an open-label trial. *AIDS* 11(8): 1066-7

[27] Du Pasquier R.A., Kuroda M.J., Zheng Y., Jean-Jacques J., Letvin N.L., Koralnik I.J. (2004). A prospective study demonstrates an association between JC virus-specific cytotoxic T lymphocytes and the early control of progressive multifocal leukoencephalopathy. *Brain* 127(Pt 9): 1970–1978

[28] De Wolf F. & Lange J.M.A. (1991). Serologic and Immunologic Markers in the Course of HIV-1 Infection. Clinics in Dermatology: 1-11

[29] Evans-Gilbert T., Pierre R., Steel-Duncan J.C., Rodriguez B., Whorms S., Hambleton IR., Figueroa JP. & Christie CD. (2004). Antiretroviral drug therapy in HIV-infected Jamaican children. *West Indian Med J* 53(5):322–326

[30] Fahey JL, Taylor JM, Detels R, Hofmann B, Melmed R, Nishanian P, Giorgi JV. (1990). The prognostic value of cellular and serologic markers in infection with human immunodeficiency virus type I. *N Engl J Med* 322: 166-72

[31] Falcó V, Olmo M, del Saz SV, Guelar A, Santos JR, Gutiérrez M, Colomer D, Deig E, Mateo G, Montero M, Pedrol E, Podzamczer D, Domingo P, Llibre JM. (2008). Influence of HAART on the clinical course of HIV-1-infected patients with progressive multifocal leukoencephalopathy: results of an observational multicenter study. *J Acquir Immune Defic Syndr* 49(1):26–31.

[32] Fauci A.S. & Lane H.C. (1998). HIV disease: AIDS and related disorders. Chapter 308. In: Fauci AS, Braunwald E, Wilson JD, Martin JB, Kaspar DL, Hauser SL, Longo DL, editors. *Harrison's principles of internal medicine.* 14th ed. New York: Mc Graw Hill: 1816–8

[33] Figg W.D. (1991). Peripheral neuropathy in HIV patients after isoniazid therapy. *Drug Intell Clin Pharm* 25: 100-101

[34] Fine H.A. & Mayer R.J. (1993). Primary central nervous system lymphoma. *Ann Intern Med* 119: 1093–1104

[35] Firnhaber C., Smeaton L., Saukila N., Flanigan T., Gangakhedkar R. & Kumwenda J. et al. (2010). Comparisons of anemia, thrombocytopenia, and neutropenia at initiation of HIV antiretroviral therapy in Africa, Asia, and the Americas. *Int J Infect Dis* 14:e1088–92

[36] Fung H.B. & Kirschenbaum H.L (1996). Treatment regimens for patients with toxoplasmic encephalitis. *Clin Ther* 18(6): 1037-56; discussion 1036

[37] Fuchs D., Hansen A. & Reibnegger G. et al. (1988). Neopterin as a marker for activated cell-mediated immunity: Application in HIV infection. *Immunol Today* 9: 150-55

[38] Gabbai A.A, Schmidt B., Castelo A., Oliveira A.S.B, Lima J.G.C. (1990). Muscle biopsy in AIDS and ARC: analysis of 50 patients. *Muscle Nerve* 13,541-4

[39] Gafa S., Giudici M.G., Pezzotti P. & Rezza G. (1993). IgA as a marker of clinical progression among HIV-seropositive intravenous drug users. *Journal of Infection* 26: 33-38

[40] Gasnault J., Kahraman M., de Goer de Herve M.G., Durali D., Delfraissy J.F. & Taoufik Y. (2003). Critical role of JC virus-specific CD4 T-cell responses in preventing progressive multifocal leukoencephalopathy. *AIDS* 17(10):1443–49

[41] Gill P, Rarick M, Bernstein-Singer M, Harb M, Espina BM, Shaw V, Levine A. (1990). Treatment of advanced Kaposi's sarcoma using combination of bleomycin and vincristine. *Am J Clin Oncol* 13 : 315-319

[42] Gill P.S., Levine A.M., Meyer P.R. (1985). Primary central nervous system lymphoma in homosexual men: clinical, immunologic, and pathologic features. *Am J Med* 78 : 742–748

[43] Gilks CF, Crowley S, Ekpini R, Gove S, Perriens J, Souteyrand Y, Sutherland D, Vitoria M, Guerma T, De Cock K. (2006). The WHO public-health approach to antiretroviral treatment against HIV in resource-limited settings. *Lancet* 368: 505–10

[44] Giorgi J.V. (1993). Characterization of T lymphocyte subset alterations by flow cytometry in HIV disease. *Ann NY Acad Sci* 677:126–37.

[45] Goldstein J.D, Dickson D.W. & Moser F.G. (1991). Primary central nervous system lymphoma in acquired immunodeficiency syndrome: a clinical and pathologic study with results of treatment with radiation. *Cancer* 67: 2756–65

[46] Goldstick L., Mangybur T.I. & Bode R. (1985). Spinal cord degeneration in AIDS. *Neurology* 35: 103–6

[47] Griffin D.E. (1997). Cytokines in the brain during viral infection: clues to HIV-associated dementia. *J Clin Invest* 100: 2948–51

[48] Gray F., Gherardi R., Trotot P., Fenelon G. & Poirier J. (1990). Spinal cord lesions in the acquired immune deficiency syndrome (AIDS). *Neurosurg Rev* 13: 189–194

[49] Graham N.M.H. (1996). The role of immunologic and viral markers in predicting clinical outcome in HIV infection. *AIDS 10*: S21-S25

[50] Hammer SM, Saag MS, Schechter M, Montaner JS, Schooley RT, Jacobsen DM, Thompson MA, Carpenter CC, Fischl MA, Gazzard BG, Gatell JM, Hirsch MS,Katzenstein DA, Richman DD, Vella S, Yeni PG, Volberding PA; International AIDS Society-USA panel. (2006). Treatment for adult HIV infection: 2006 Recommendations of the International AIDS Society-USA panel. *JAMA* 296: 827–43

[51] Henin D., Smith T.W., De Girolami U, Sughayer M, Hauw J.J. (1992). Neuropathology of the spinal cord in the acquired immunodeficiency syndrome. *Hum Pathol* 23: 1106–14

[52] Höke A. & Cornblath. D.R. (2004). Peripheral neuropathies in human immunodeficiency virus infection. *Clin Neurophysiol* 57(Suppl): S195-S210

[53] Horowitz S.L , Bentson J.R., Benson F., Davos I., Pressman B. & Gottlieb M.S. (1983). CNS toxoplasmosis in acquired immunodeficiency syndrome. *Arch Neurol* 40: 649–52

[54] Hughes MD, Johnson VA, Hirsch MS, Bremer JW, Elbeik T, Erice A, Kuritzkes DR, Scott WA, Spector SA, Basgoz N, Fischl MA, D'Aquila RT. (1997). Monitoring plasma HIV-1 RNA levels in addition to CD4+ lymphocyte count improves assessment of antiretroviral therapeutic response: ACTG Protocol Virology Substudy Team. *Ann Int Med* 126: 929-938

[55] J.A. Sparano (2001). Clinical aspects and management of AIDS-related lymphoma. *European Journal of Cancer* 37, 1296–1305

[56] Phillips KD, Skelton WD, Hand GA (2004). Effect of acupuncture administered in a group setting on pain and subjective peripheral neuropathy in persons with human immunodeficiency virus disease. The journal of alternative and complementary medicine 10:3, 449–455.

[57] Keswani S.C., Pardo C.A., Cherry C.L., Höke A. & McArthur J.C. (2002). HIV-associated sensory neuropathies. *AIDS* 16: 2105-2117

[58] Kieburtz K.D., Giang D.W., Shiffer R.B., Vakil N. (1991). Abnormal vitamin B12 metabolism in human immunodeficiency virus infection: association with neurological dysfunction. *Arch Neurol* 48: 312-314

[59] Kleinman S, Busch MP, Hall L, Thomson R, Glynn S, Gallahan D, Ownby HE, Williams AE. (1998). False positive HIV-1 test results in a low-risk screening setting of voluntary blood donation. *JAMA* 280 (12): 1080-5

[60] Koralnik I.J. (2006). Progressive multifocal leukoencephalopathy revisited: Has the disease outgrown its name? *Ann Neurol* 60(2): 162–173

[61] Koralnik I.J , Schellingerhout D , Frosch M.P. (2004). Case records of the Massachusetts General Hospital. Weekly clinicopathological exercises. Case 14-2004. A 66-year-old man with progressive neurologic deficits. *N Engl J Med* 350 (18): 1882–1893

[62] Koenig S.P., Kuritzkes D.R., Hirsch M.S., Leandre F., Mukherjee J.S. & Farmer P.E. et al. (2006). Monitoring HIV treatment in developing countries. *BMJ* 332: 602–4

[63] Krämer A, Wiktor SZ, Fuchs D, Milstien S, Gail MH, Yellin FJ, Biggar RJ, Wachter H, Kaufman S, Blattner WA. (1989). Neopterin: A predictive marker of acquired immune deficiency syndrome in human immunodeficiency virus infection. *J Acquir Immune Defic Syndr* 2: 291-96

[64] Lawlor D.A., Zemmour J., Ennis P.D. & Parham P. (1990). Evolution of class-I MHC genes and proteins: from natural selection to thymic selection. *Annu Rev Immunol* 8: 23–63

[65] Lagakos S.W. & DeGruttola V. (1989). The conditional latency distribution of AIDS for persons infected by blood transfusions. *J Acquir Immune Defic Syndr* 2: 84-87

[66] Letendre SL, McCutchan JA, Childers ME, Woods SP, Lazzaretto D, Heaton RK, Grant I, Ellis RJ; HNRC Group. (2004). Enhancing antiretroviral therapy for human immunodeficiency virus cognitive disorders. *Ann Neurol* 56: 416–423

[67] Levine A.M., Seneviratne L., Espina B.M., Wohl A.R., Tulpule A., Nathwani B.N. &Gill PS. (2000). Evolving characteristics of AIDS-related lymphoma. *Blood* 96(13): 4084–90

[68] Liu Y, Tang XP, McArthur JC, Scott J, Gartner S. (2000). Analysis of human immunodeficiency virus type 1 gp160 sequences from a patient with HIV dementia: evidence for monocyte trafficking into brain. *J Neurovirol* 6: S70–S81

[69] Lui K.J, Lawrence D.N & Morgan W.M. (1988). A model-based estimate of the mean incubation period for AIDS in homosexual men. *Science* 240: 1333-35

[70] Loureiro C, Gill P.S., Meyer P.R., Rhodes R., Rarick M.U. & Levine A.M. (1988). Autopsy findings in AIDS-related lymphoma. *Cancer* 62: 735–739

[71] Luciano C.A., Pardo C.A. & McArthur J.C. (2003). Recent developments in the HIV neuropathies. *Curr Opin Neurol* 16: 403-9

[72] Luft B.J., Brooks R.G., Conley F.K., McCabe R.E., Remington J.S. (1984). Toxoplasmic encephalitis in patients with acquired immune deficiency syndrome, *JAMA* 252: 913–7

[73] Lui KJ, Darrow WW, Rutherford GW 3rd. (1988). A model-based estimate of the mean incubation period for AIDS in homosexual men. *Science* 240: 1333-35

[74] Mac Mahon, E.M, Glass, J.D, Hayward, S.D, Mann, R.B, Becker, P.S, Charache, P, McArthur, J.C, & Ambinder, R.F. (1991). Epstein Barr virus in AIDS-related primary central nervous system lymphoma. *Lancet* 338: 969–973

[75] Marzocchetti A, Lima M, Tompkins T, Kavanagh DG, Gandhi RT, O'Neill DW, Bhardwaj N, Koralnik IJ. (2009). Efficient in vitro expansion of JC virus-specific CD8(+) T-cell responses by JCV peptide-stimulated dendritic cells from patients with progressive multifocal leukoencephalopathy. *Virology* 383(2): 173–177

[76] McArthur JC, Haughey N, Gartner S, Conant K, Pardo C, Nath A, Sacktor N. (2003). Human immunodeficiency virus-associated dementia: an evolving disease. *J Neurovirol* 9: 205–221

[77] Medley G.F., Anderson R.M., Cox D.R. & Billard L. (1987). Incubation period of AIDS in patients infected via blood transfusion. *Nature* 328: 719-21

[78] Mellors JW, Muñoz A, Giorgi JV, Margolick JB, Tassoni CJ, Gupta P, Kingsley LA, Todd JA, Saah AJ, Detels R, Phair JP, Rinaldo CR Jr. (1997). Plasma viral load and CD4+ lymphocyte as prognostic markers of HIV-1 infection. *Ann Int Med* 126: 946-954

[79] Melmed RN, Taylor JM, Detels R, Bozorgmehri M, Fahey JL.Melmed. (1989). Serum neopterin changes in HIV-infected subjects: indicator of significant pathology CD4 T cell changes and the development of AIDS. *J Acquire Immune Defic Syndr* 2: 70-76

[80] Mirsattari S.M., Power C. & Nath A. (1998). Parkinsonism with HIV infection. *Mov Disord* 13: 684–9

[81] Monica G., Peter B., Paolo M., Thomas C.Q., Fulvia V. & Ruth M.G. (2002). Does patient sex affect human immunodeficiency virus levels? *Clin Infect Dis* 35:313–22

[82] Moss AR, Bacchetti P, Osmond D, Krampf W, Chaisson RE, Stites D, Wilber J, Allain JP, Carlson J. (1988). Seropositivity for HIV and the development of AIDS or AIDS related condition: three year follow up of the San Francisco General Hospital cohort. *Br Med J* 296: 745–50

[83] Navia B.A., Cho E.S., Petito C.K, Price RW. (1986). The AIDS dementia complex: II. Neuropathology. *Ann Neurol* 19: 525–35

[84] Norton G.R., Sweeney J., Marriott D., Law M.G., Brew B.J. (1996). Association between HIV distal symmetric polyneuropathy and *Mycobacterium avium* complex infection. J Neurol Neurosurg

[85] Olayemi E., Awodu O.A. & Bazuaye G.N. (2008). Autoimmune hemolytic anemia in HIV-infected patients: a hospital based study. *Ann Afr Med*

[86] Owiredu W.K., Quaye L., Amidu N. & Addai-Mensah O. (2011). Prevalence of anaemia and immunological markers among ghanaian HAART-naïve HIV-patients and those on HAART. *Afr Health Sci* 11: 2–15

[87] Petito C.K, Navia B.A, Cho E.S, Jordan BD, George DC, Price RW (1985). Vacuolar myelopathy pathologically resembling subacute combined degeneration in patients with the acquired immunodeficiency syndrome. *N Engl J Med* 312: 874–879

[88] Peter K.L. (2009). Approach to the Immunocompromised Host with Infection in the Intensive Care Unit. *Infect Dis Clin N Am* 23 535–556.

[89] Pike I.M. & Nicaise C. (1993). The didanosine expanded access program: safety analysis. *Clin Infect Dis* 16, S63-S68

[90] Parinithas S. & Kulkarni M. (2012). Haematological changes in HIV infection with correlation to CD4 cell count. *Australas Med J* 5(3): 157-62

[91] Patton LL. (2003). HIV disease. *Dent Clin N Am* 47: 467-492

[92] Pattanapanyasat K. & Thakar MR. (2005). CD4+ T cell count as a tool to monitor HIV progression & anti-retroviral therapy. *Indian J Med Res* 121: 539–49

[93] Peters P.J., Kilmarx P.H.& Mastro T.D. (2008). AIDS: Global Epidemiology. Encyclopedia of Virology (3rd Edition): 56-68

[94] Petti C.A., Polage C.R., Quinn T.C., Ronald A.R. & Sande M.A. (2006). Laboratory medicine in Africa: a barrier to effective health care. *Clin Infect Dis* 42:377–82

[95] Quinn T.C. (1990). The Epidemiology of the human immunodeficiency virus. *Annals of Emergency Medicine* 19: 225-32

[96] Quin J.W. & Benson E.M. (1994). It is HIV: Immediate and long term plans. Chapter 24. In: Stewart G, editor. Could it be HIV? 2nd ed. Sydney, Australia: Australasian medical publishing company Ltd; 66–9

[97] Rizzuto N, Cavallaro T, Monaco S, Morbin M, Bonetti B, Ferrari S, Galiazzo-Rizzuto S, Zanette G, Bertolasi L. (1995). Role of HIV in the pathogenesis of distal symmetrical peripheral neuropathy. *Acta Neuropathol* (Berl) 90: 244-50

[98] Simpson D.M. & Tagliati M. (1995). Nucleoside analogue-associated peripheral neuropathy in human immunodeficiency virus infections. *J Acquir Immune Def Syndr Hum Retrovirol* 9, 153-161

[99] Snider WD., Simpson DM., Nielsen S., Gold JW., Metroka CE., Posner JB. (1983). Neurological complications of acquired immune deficiency syndrome: analysis of 50 patients," *Ann Neurol* 14: 403-418.

[100] So Y.T., Holtzman D.M., Abrams D.I. & Olney R.K. (1988). Peripheral neuropathy associated with acquired immunodeficiency syndrome: prevalence and clinical features from a population-based survey. *Arch Neurol* 45: 945-48

[101] Saves M., Morlat P., Chene G., Peuchant E., Pellegrin I, Bonnet SF., Bernard N., Lacoste D., Salamon R. & Beylot J. (2001). Prognostic value of plasma markers of immune activation in patients with advanced HIV disease treated by combination antiretroviral therapy. *Clinical Immunology* Vol 99. (3): 347-352.

[102] Sparano J.A (2001). Clinical aspects and management of AIDS-related lymphoma European Journal of Cancer 37: 1296–1305

[103] Stein D.S., Korvick J.K. & Vermund SH. (1992). CD4+ Lymphocyte cell enumeration for prediction of clinical course of human immunodeficiency virus disease: a review. *J Infect Dis* 165: 352–363

[104] Tan S.V., Guiloff R.J. & Scaravilli F. (1995). AIDS-associated vacuolar myelopathy: a morphometric study. *Brain* 118: 1247–61

[105] Taylor J.M.G., Fahey J.L., Detels R. & Giorgi J.V. (1989). CD4 percentage, CD4 number, and CD4:CD8 ratio in HIV infection: Which to choose and how to use. *J Acquir Immune Defic Syndr* 2:114–24

[106] Thakar MR, Abraham PR, Arora S, Balakrishnan P, Bandyopadhyay B, Joshi AA, Devi KR, Vasanthapuram R, Vajpayee M, Desai A, Mohanakrishnan J, Narain K, Ray K, Patil SS, Singh R, Singla A, Paranjape RS. (2011). Establishment of reference CD4+ T cell values for adult Indian population. *AIDS Res Ther* 8: 35.

[107] Torre D. & Pugliese A. (2008). Platelets and HIV-1 infection: old and new aspects. *Curr HIV Res* 6: 411–8

[108] Vajpayee M. & Mohan T. (2011). Current practices in laboratory monitoring of HIV infection. *Indian J Med Res* 134 (6): 801-22

[109] Volberding P.A., Baker K.R. & Levine A.M. (2003). Human immunodeficiency virus hematology. *Haematol Am Soc Hematol Educ Program*: 294–313

[110] World Health Organization : Geneva. (2006). Antiretroviral therapy for HIV infection in adults and adolescents in resource-limited settings: towards universal access.

[111] Zeller J.M., McCain N.L. & Swanson B. (1996). *Journal of the Association of Nurses in AIDS care* Vol 7. Issue 1: 15-17

[112] Zanetti C, Manzano GM, Gabbai AA (2004). The frequency of peripheral neuropathy in a group of HIV positive patients in brazil. *Arq Neuropsiquiatr* 62(2-A): 253-256

Chapter 9

Persistence of HIV-Associated Neurocognitive Disorders in the Era of Antiretroviral Therapy

Jennifer M. King, Brigid K. Jensen,
Patrick J. Gannon and Cagla Akay

Additional information is available at the end of the chapter

http://dx.doi.org/10.5772/52683

1. Introduction

HIV-Associated Neurocognitive Disorders (HAND) is a serious menifestation of HIV infection in the central nervous system (CNS), and encompassess a wide spectrum of cognitive, behavioral, and motor deficits [1-3]. While the implementation of combination antiretroviral therapy (ART) has dramatically increased the life expectancy and led to significant improvements in the clinical presentation and progression of HAND, an estimated 50% of HIV-infected patientscontinue to suffer from implications of HAND in the ART era, with as much as 20% of these exhibiting symptoms of HIV-associated dementia (HAD), the most severe form of HAND [3-6]. The brain regions affected in patients with HAND has changed in the ART era in parallel to the changes observed in the clinical picture; a more subtle and insidious cortical damage mainly in the hippocampus and the temporal cortex is observed, in contrast to the overt subcortical damage seen before ART [7-10]. The underlying causes of these changes are not fully elucidated; however, examination of the post-mortem tissue reveals the persistence of synaptic and dendritic damage in the affected brain regions [3, 11]. Emerging evidence suggests that controlling viral replication in the periphery or in the CNS may not be sufficient to control the underlying neuropathological processes that culminate in the development of HAND. The impact of HAND on the quality of life, adherence to drug regimens, and co-morbidities especially in an aging HIV population with decreased cognitive reserves, is of major concern. In this chapter, we will examine the major factors that continue to impact the CNS of HIV-infected individuals, and introduce new challenges in the successful treatment of HAND.

2. Clinical presentation and neuropathology of HAND

According to the diagnostic criteria established for the assessment of neurocognitive impairment in HIV-infected individuals, the neurological deficits in HAND patients are divided into three diagnostic groups. This classification is based on the neuropsychological evaluation of multiple cognitive domains, including simple motor skills or sensory perceptual ability, complex perceptual motor skills, attention and working memory, learning and memory recall, verbal and language, abstraction and executive function. Asymptomatic neurocognitive impairment (ANI) is defined as acquired impairment in at least two cognitive domains without a decline in activities of daily living (ADL), while mild to moderate neurocognitive impairment that affects ADL is termed minor neurocognitive disorder (MND). Moderate to severe impairment in two or more domains with marked impact on ADL is defined as HAD. Additionally, behavioral and emotional problems such as depression, psychosis and anxiety are commonly observed in HAND patients. Since the multi-drug regimens that form the basis of ART have become the mainstay of HIV, the clinical presentation and the course of HAND have become more unpredictable. The severity of deficits appears to fluctuate over time during the course of infection: some patients may experience continuing decline in cognitive abilities, while others may recover from HAD and exhibit only minor deficits for the remainder of the disease. While clinical studies clearly establish that suppression of viral replication below the level of detection is paramount to a more favorable outcome, the clinical course of HAND, once diagnosed, cannot be predicted successfully in most patients.

While microglial nodules, multinucleated giant cells and astrogliosis, all of which are associated with HIV-induced inflammatory changes, are not as frequently found in post-mortem HAND brain tissue after ART, dendritic and synaptic damage still persist [12-16]. For example, several studies have reported the presence of deoxynucleotidyltransferase-mediated dUTP nick-end labeling (TUNEL)-positive cells, DNA laddering and structural changes with electron microscopy [17, 18]. Importantly, these markers of neuronal death correlate with activation of immune cell populations suggesting that the inflammatory mediators secreted by these cells may play a role in initiating the death cascades [1, 19]. Given the chronic nature of the HIV infection in the ART era, co-existing conditions which can activate immune responses and precipitate a neuroinflammatory environment independent of infection are likely to contribute to the development of persistent neuropathology, and need to be addressed for a more efficient clinical approach and more favorable outcomes. Foremost, it is necessary to examine the mechanisms of neuronal injury in order to successfully expound on the contribution of confounding factors on the persistence of HAND.

The two major cell types targeted by HIV are $CD4^+$ T cells and the cells of monocyte/macrophage lineage. HIV infection of the $CD4^+$ T cells ends in the selective loss of this cell population, leading to severe immunodeficiency [20]. More relevant to HAND, HIV also targets monocytes early during infection [20]. In the healthy brain, the BBB and the blood-cerebrospinal fluid barriers are the first lines of defense against invading pathogens; however, HIV can circumvent these barriers and enter the CNS within infected monocytes [21, 22]. According to this model, supported by a multitude of *in vitro* and *in vivo* studies, the infected monocytes differentiate into macrophages, and constitute the viral reservoirs in the CNS [23-26]. Moreover, these cells release a variety of molecules, some of them known neurotoxins, leading to the eventual neuronal damage and dysfunction observed in HAND. Importantly, unlike other cell types that readily undergo replication, neurons in their post-mitotic state are more vulnerable to immune cell damage which can disrupt critical neuronal functions. Additionally, recent focus in efforts towards a cure in HIV is purging the virus from its reservoirs, by reactivating pro-viral DNA [27-31]. Thus, it is crucial to examine the impact of HIV infection on immune cells for a better understanding of the neuropathology of HAND, and for the development of successful paradigms for HIV reactivation and purging.

3. The immunology of HAND

3.1. Initiation of immune response in the CNS

HIV initially enters helper T lymphocytes and monocytes in the periphery via viral glycoproteins, gp120 and gp41, which are part of the HIV envelope [32]. These glycoproteins engage with the CD4 on the host cell membrane; however, this fusion step requires the presence of a chemokine co-receptor, C-X-C chemokine receptor type 4 (CXCR4) in lymphocytes,orC-C chemokine type 5 (CCR5) / C-C chemokine type 3 (CCR3) in macrophages [32, 33]. Of all the cell types in the brain, only macrophages and microglia express CD4 antigen, are commonly infected by HIV, and are capable of productive infection. There is very limited evidence for HIV infection of the glial cells, which if present, has not been conclusively shown as being productive [34]. More importantly, HIV cannot infect neurons as these cells lack CD4 co-receptors.

The CNS of a healthy adult human has a relatively low presence of cellular components of the immune system [35, 36]. The CNS presents the immune system with unique problems with trafficking of immune cells and the recognition of foreign antigen when present. First, the BBB constitutes a physical barrier for the entry of cells and macromolecules from the periphery into the CNS. Additionally, there is minimal expression of major histocompatibility class II (MHC class II) molecules and an absence of professional antigen presenting cells such as dendritic cells, all of which are required for antigen presentation and adaptive immune response activation. However, it has been extensively shown that brain derived factors act to suppress or counter-regulate the actions of pro-inflammatory mediators in the CNS where immune surveillance is not sufficient. For example, transforming growth factor-β (TGF-β) has the ability to inhibit the activation of macrophages, T lymphocytes, and natural killer (NK) cells, and has been shown to possess neuroprotective capabilities [37-41]. Interestingly, increased TGF-β protein levels are reported in the frontal cortex of HAD patients, and elevated TGF-βimmunoreactivity has been detected in reactive astrocytes and mononuclear cells of the white matter in HIV-infected CNS [42, 43]. Similar roles have been proposed for BDNF, NT-3, and NGF, among others, during HIV infection in the CNS [44, 45].

In the initial stages of HIV infection, the number of $CD4^+$T cells decreases as a consequence of uncontrolled viral replication. While the impact of primary HIV infection on specific $CD8^+$ T cell subpopulations is not clear, there is an overall expansion of this cell population [46]. In this environment, infected monocytes can enter the CNS, establish and maintain productive infection, and HAND becomes clinically manifest. Perivascular macrophages are replenished throughout life by the migration of circulating monocytes to the brain, a process enhanced in an inflammatory environment [47]. Several studies have shown that the number of activated macrophages, rather than the viral load,correlates best with the axonal damage and synaptic loss observed in the HAND brain [11, 14, 48, 49]. In addition, indirect markers of macrophage activation, such as neopterin and β2-microglobulin, are elevated in the CSF of HAND patients [50-52]. Further, soluble factors that are known to be released by macrophages and glia, such as quinolinic acid, tumor necrosis factor-α (TNF-α), reactive oxygen species (ROS), and cytokines such as CXCL12 (stromal cell-derived factor-1, SDF-1), CCL2 (monocyte chemotactic protein-1, MCP-1), and interleukin-6 (IL-6), are also elevated in the CSF of HAND patients [53-57]. These findings reinforce the model which proposes monocyte-derived macrophages and microglia as major instigators of the neuropathological processes in the course of disease development in HAND.

It should be noted that viral proteins such as gp120 and transactivator of transcription (Tat) can directly activate uninfected macrophages [58-62]. Additionally, one mechanism of injury that is proposed to account for neuronal damage in the absence of neuronal infection by HIV involves direct neurotoxicity by these viral proteins. Several *in vitro* studies have shown that these viral proteins that are released and/or shed by the infected macrophages/microglia can induce direct synaptic and neuronal damage [63-65]. However, the indicators of neuroinflammation continue to persist despite successful suppression of replication in the CSF to levels below the limit of detection with ART, suggesting that other, less direct mechanisms of injury might be major contributors to the underlying neuropathology.

3.2. The role of cytokines and chemokines in HAND neuropathology

A number of indirect mechanisms for the pathogenesis of HAND have been proposed [1, 25, 66]. These mechanisms are not mutually exclusive, and may be synergistic based on the common background of macrophage activation and release of cytokines and chemokines.As a protective measure to suppress viral production, macrophages are responsible for the production of inflammatory mediators including TNF-α, IL (interleukin)-1, interferon-α (IFN-α) and nitric oxide synthase (NOS) [33, 59]. However, the release of these pro-inflammatory cytokines can activate the uninfected macrophages, and can induce the migration of leukocytes into the CNS [62]. For example, in HIV-1 transgenic (Tg) rats, elevated levels of IL-1β and TNF-α and increased expression of arachidonic acid cascade enzymes have been implicated in neuronal damage and cognitive and behavioral impairment [67]. A recent study indicates that similar changes could contribute to cognitive impairment in HIV-infected patients despite an effective ART [68]. *In vivo* studies suggest that the progression of HAND may be predicted by high concentrations of TNF-α in plasma, and polymorphisms in the TNF-α promoter are associated with HAND to a degree [69, 70]. Interestingly, functional *ex-*

vivo studies have shown that the macrophages and B-lymphocytes isolated from HIV-infected patients are activated despite viral suppression by ART [71]. Further, *in vitro* experiments show that HIV reactivation can be achieved by cytokine and chemokine stimulation [30, 33]. These findings are especially important in light of recent concerns regarding viral latency and its contribution to the persistence of HAND [29].

In the CNS,chemoattractant cytokines, or chemokines have been demonstrated as essential factors in neuroinflammation and related neuronal injury and loss through their regulation of inflammatory responses. Post-mortem studies have revealed up-regulation of chemokines and chemokine receptors in the brains of patients with HAND [25, 26, 56, 72-75]. The best-characterized chemokines up-regulated in HAND are the β-chemokines CCL2, CCL5, and CX3CL1, and the alpha chemokine CXCL12. For example, the levels of one of the more potent chemokines, CCL2 correlate with the likelihood and severity of HAND [76, 77]. In addition, an intriguing regulatory role for the chemokine CCR5 was demonstrated that its activation led to cell death via caspase-3 mediated apoptosis in a neuroblastoma cell line [78]. Further, induction of apoptosis has also been reported with CXCL12 in primary neuroglial cultures in the absence of the HIV viral protein gp120. However, results from several recent studies suggest that the changes in the expression of these chemokines may indicate neuroprotective efforts in response to the neuroinflammatory environment [79]. Further studies are needed to dissect the roles of chemokines in HAND pathogenesis, as they take part in a crucial phase in immune responses, and provide attractive targets for modulation in resolving HAND persistence.

The mechanisms by which the neuroinflammatory environment eventually ends in damage to the neurons are not precisely known; however, several mechanisms are likely candidates. Studies suggest that the neuronal damageis a result of indirect effects of viral proteins as well as inflammatory mediators [1, 66]. Gp120 and Tat are reported to induce neuronal apoptosis by activating death-associated proteases, caspases, specifically caspase-3 in *in vitro* and *in vivo* disease models [80]. Another mechanism proposes a role for excitotoxicity secondary to impaired glutamate reuptake by astrocytes which are overwhelmed by pro-inflammatory factors [81]. The well-defined cascade of excitotoxic injury includes excess Ca^{2+} influx into the neuronal cytoplasm. Several downstream events secondary to such increases in Ca^{2+} such as excess free radical production and oxidative stress, and the activation of Ca^{2+}-dependent death proteases, calpains and caspases, will be detrimental to neurons, especially in an environment with inadequate glial support and ongoing inflammation due to immune cell activation [1, 66].

3.3. Neuroinflammation in HAND

The persistence of immune activation in the CNS and the peripheral nervous system (PNS) of HIV-infected individuals in the ART era is supported by several lines of evidence. The relatively low levels of HIV RNA in the presence of widespread neuropathological changes in the CNS and PNS of HAND patients, and the lack of evidence of HIV infection of neuronal cells *in vivo and in vitro* hint at the possibility of chronic immune activation as a factor in the persistence of HAND. Recent clinical evidence shows that ART reduces intrathecal immunoactivation in treated patients; however, a significant percentage of patients continue to exhibit signs of ongoing inflammation [49, 50, 82, 83]. Further, even after successful reduction of HIV RNA levels below the limit of detection for several years, patients present with increased levels of inflammatory markers such as CSF neopterin and intrathecal IgG [52]. It is thus apparent that ART is not sufficient to prevent or control HAND. One major factor to consider in addressing this failure is that ART may not be efficient and/or sufficient in controlling the inflammatory cascade triggered by HIV infection.

Once HIV replication is established in the CNS, the initial chemotactic and inflammatory factor production leads to further recruitment and activation of monocytes/macrophages, creating a perpetual neuroinflammatory environment. The phenomenon of monocyte/ macrophage recruitment can be explained by a "push and pull" mechanism [47]. Two key chemokines that play a role in the recruitment, or "pull", of monocytes are CCL2 and fractalkine (CXCL1).CCL2 is considered to be the more critical factor involved in the infiltration of monocytes and lymphocytes across the BBB in the HAND brain [79]. Multiple cell types of the CNS have been shown to produce CCL2 in models of inflammation, in which CCL2 is a part of a signaling mechanism for recruitment of monocytes/macrophages from the periphery. For example, leukocyte infiltration into the brain parenchyma has been demonstrated upon pertussis toxin challenge in CCL2 transgenic mice [84]. More importantly, HIV-infected leukocyte transmigration across BBB is dependent on CCL2 in an *in vitro* model of disease [85]. Further, CCL2 has been shown to directly damage the endothelial cell junctions of the BBB [86]. These findings clearly indicate a significant role for CCL2 in the "pull" of monocyte/macrophages across the BBB in HAND. Interestingly, CCL2 levels remain elevated in the CSF of HAND patients on ART, implicating that ongoing trafficking might be occurring despite viral suppression, and warrants further investigations into the persistence of HAND in the era of ART [83].

The "push" aspect of the monocyte/macrophage recruitment involves the expansion in peripheral blood neuroinvasive monocyte population. It has been shown that individuals with HAND exhibit an expanded population of $CD14^+$ peripheral blood monocytes that co-express CD16, which is considered a more mature population [21]. These $CD14^+/CD16^+$ monocytes are preferentially susceptible to infection, and can serve as a reservoir harboring proviral DNA. The entry of monocytes into the brain plays a key role in initiating the series of events that lead to HAND, and although antiretrovirals hinder viral replication, they may have minimal effects on the continued transmigration of monocytes into the brain. One study showed that a single exposure of the CNS to the neurotoxic viral protein Tat led to the infiltration of peripheral blood monocytes and resulted in prolonged disruption of CNS function [87]. Thus, continuous and efficient viral suppression in the periphery is critical in achieving suppressed inflammation in the CNS, and is of prime importance in the fight against HAND.

While macrophages and microglia play primary roles in HIV infection in the CNS, other glial cells also contribute to the neuroinflammation and neurotoxicity in the HAND brain. One important cell type that needs to be mentioned in the neuroinflamatory processes in HAND is the astrocytic cell population. As the most abundant cells in the CNS, astrocytes

http://dx.doi.org/10.5772/52683

provide neurotrophic support, and are involved in repair processes for neurons. Further, astrocytes are physiological regulators of microglial and macrophage inflammatory responses, and indirectly modulate neuronal survival through reduction of the macrophage inflammatory response. However, their dysfunction, as a result of HIV infection, will lead to the dysregulation of the local cytokine/chemokine balance. Evidence has shown that astrocytes are key mediators in the regulation of microglial function and its influence on the onset and the progression of HAND [55, 88]. Viral proteins gp120, and Tat both activate astrocytes to produce pro-inflammatory cytokines TNF-α, IL-6, and IL-1β as well as the pro-inflammatory chemokines CCL2 and CXCL10 [34, 55, 89-91]. The contribution of these pro-inflammatory mediators by astrocytes as well as the release of pro-inflammatory cytokines IL-1β and TNF-α by microglia and macrophage will only exacerbate the inflammatory environment in the HIV-infected CNS.

Although the pathogenic mechanisms of HAND are likely to be multifactorial (Table 1), cellular activation with the initiation and persistence of the immune system in the CNS play a pivotal role in this disease progression. Continued CNS inflammation is an essential factor in many neurodegenerative diseases and HIV infection induces a cascade of inappropriate immune responses in the CNS. The initial immunological response has protective intentions through macrophage activation, but with persistent infection, the inflammatory response becomes toxic to the neurons through the production of pro-inflammatory cytokines and chemokines. Further, the decreased viral load in the CNS is accompanied by persistent microglial activation and inflammation. Ineffective drug penetrance into the CNS, which continues to be a challenge, can initiate the development of resistance to ART via permitting mutations to the virus which allows the CNS to become a reservoir for the infection. As HIV-infected macrophages are shown to be resistant to apoptosis,this will end in exacerbating the virus reservoir in the CNS.

Inflammatory Responses During HIV-1 Brain Infection
Macrophage Activation (M1 phenotype)
Micogial nodules
Multinucleated Giant Cells in Central White Matter and Deep Gray Matter
Astrogliosis
Cytokines
Transforming Growth Factor-beta (TGF-β)
Tumor Necrosis Factor-alpha(TNF-α)
Interleukin-6 (IL-6)
Interleukin-1 (IL-1)
Chemokines
Monocyte Chemotactic Protein-1 (MCP-1)
Interferon Gamma Induced Protein-10 (IP-10)
MHC class II presentation

Table 1. Pathological and laboratory evidence for immune activation in the CNS after HIV infection.

It should also be noted that the impact of HIV infection in the peripheral tissue will ultimately impact the immune responses in the CNS. Thus, co-morbidities such as co-infections, substance abuse, malignancies and antiretroviral drug toxicities, as well as general inflammatory processes in the periphery, such as oxidative stress should be taken into account when assessing the relationships between immune responses and the neuropathological processes occurring in the HAND brain. This approach will provide more efficient tools, and will have a greater impact on resolving the persistence of HAND.

4. Oxidative stress in neurodegenerative diseases

Oxidative stress is a shared pathological finding in a myriad of neurodegenerative diseases including Alzheimer Disease, Parkinson Disease, Multiple Sclerosis (MS), Amyotrophic Lateral Sclerosis (ALS), and HAND [92, 93]. While it is clear that chronic oxidative stress which will overwhelm the protective capacities of the cellular endogenous antioxidant responses may be responsible in part for the neuronal death occurring in these conditions, in many neurodegenerative diseases it is difficult to ascertain whether oxidative stress is the causative factor for disease pathology and progression, or rather a resultant downstream event of other cellular dysfunctions [92-95]. Nonetheless, in HAND, several lines of evidence suggest that both HIV and antiretroviral compounds may result in oxidative and nitrosative stress in the periphery and in the CNS [96-102]. Deficits in total antioxidant levels and increases in the markers for oxidative stress are still observed in individuals on stable ART regimens with undetectable viral titers, necessitating the need for adjunctive therapies to ameliorate this imbalance [103, 104]. As has been suggested in a variety of neurodegenerative conditions, antioxidant supplementation or upregulation of the endogenous antioxidant response in cells of the CNS may ameliorate the neuronal damage and death in HAND [1, 93, 94, 105].

4.1. Oxidative stress in the era of ART

The evidence of disrupted antioxidant balance and oxidative stress represent a continued concern for HIV-infected individuals even when virus is successfully controlled by ART [102]. To understand the magnitude and implications of this problem, it is important to understand the initial disruptions to the antioxidant system that were observed in infected individuals, and determine whether ART contributed to the resolution or the exacerbation of these problems.

Oxidative stress prior to ART:As early as 1988, while researchers were just beginning to understand the HIV virus, Sönnerborg and colleagues determined that plasma levels of malondialdehyde in adults with HIV infection were elevated up to 30% when compared with controls [106]. Malondialdehyde is the breakdown product of polyunsaturated lipids by reactive oxygen species, and is a mainstay in terms of a biological marker for measuring the relative levels of lipid peroxidation and oxidative stress in individuals [107]. A multitude of studies followed, showing significant increases in the levels of free radicals, hydroperoxides, hydroxynoneal, and oxidation of thiols in infected individuals, and confirming that malondialdehyde is increased significantly in infected adults, as well as children [108-118]. The metabolic synthesis of lipids is closely tied to the oxidative state of the cell and the lipids residing in the cell membrane, as certain enzymes such as sphingomyelinase, are sensitive to the oxidative status of the cell and regulate their activity based on cellular need [119]. Studies looking into the production of sphingolipids illustrated an overproduction of both sphingomyelin and ceramides with HIV-infection, suggesting a lipid imbalance caused by the virus [115, 116, 119]. Additionally, studies showed remarkable deficiencies in antioxidant micronutrients including zinc, selenium, Vitamin C, Vitamin D, Vitamin E and beta-carotene (Vitamin A) [109, 110, 118, 120-126]. Conflicting reports exist on perturbation of total antioxidant status prior to ART, with severalclinical studies reporting decreased total antioxidant capacity [108, 113, 118], while Repetto *et al.* described an increase in the overall antioxidant capacity as individuals progressed to AIDS [114]. The discrepancies between these findings are likely based on the assays utilized to determine "total antioxidant capacity", as different enzymatic approaches target different portions of the antioxidant system.

Activity levels of superoxide dismutase (SOD), which catalyzes the detoxification of the oxidant superoxide into hydrogen peroxide and water, were assessed by a variety of laboratories. Elevated SOD activity was observed in all evaluated HIV-infected individuals, with further increases occuringwith disease progression to AIDS. In addition, increases in SOD mRNA levels were reported in individuals with HAD, as compared to those who were neurocognitively normal [114, 127, 128]. These changes in SOD were observed in microglial cells, as well as in HIV-infected macrophages, suggesting a virus-triggered induction [128]. An essential antioxidant found in the brain which buffers many reactive oxygen species is glutathione. In HIV-infected patients, overall glutathione levels were found to be reduced, and the remaining glutathione was greatly skewed to the oxidized versus reduced form. [114, 127, 129, 130]. The enzyme glutathione peroxidase, which promotes the conversion of hydrogen peroxide to water through the use of glutathione, was also decreased, illustrating a severe imbalance in this system whose goal is to maintain cellular redox homeostasis [121]. Another deleterioius consequence of rampant pro-oxidants within cells is oxidative modification of DNA bases. Increased levels of 5-hydroxyuracil, 5-hydroxycytosine, 8-hydroxyadenine and 8-hydroxyguanine were found when comparing DNA isolated from lymphocytes of HIV-infected individuals versus uninfected controls [131]. One other common product of an imbalanced oxidative state which is beginning to gain more interest and research focus is peroxynitrite. This compound, which is formed when superoxide reacts with nitric oxide, is detectable through its nitrotyrosine moiety, and is found at higher levels and with more frequency in the brains of patients with HAD, compared with those who are neurocognitively normal [128]. In addition to the generation of superoxide as a direct result of HIV infection, the virus also increases mRNA expression of inducible nitric oxide synthase (iNOS), which enables a precipitous accumulation of this deleterious oxidation product [128].Further research in the Nath laboratory has illustrated that thirteen proteins with nitrotyrosine modifications are present in the CSF of individuals with HIV-infection. Individuals with dementia had the highest levels of these nitrites and nitrates. Importantly, three of these proteins were significantly elevated in individuals who showed declines in neurocognitive assessment over a period of 6 months [101].

While it appears that there is not an all-or-nothing increase or decrease in antioxidant capacity, the evidence is clear that the components of the antioxidant defense system prior to ART were greatly affected by HIV-infection, and that the capabilities of endogenous antioxidant response were not able to alleviate damaging oxidative alterations to proteins and DNA.

Persistence of oxidative stress in the era of ART: In the ART era, oxidative stress is still pervasive in individuals living with well controlled HIV-infection [102]. In 2007, a group at the University of Pennsylvania sought to ascertain whether ART had an effect on inflammation and oxidative stress in the brains of HIV-infected individuals through utilization of chemical-shift magnetic resonance spectroscopy. Through careful analysis of lipid, lactate, and creatine levels, they determined that the inflammation and oxidative stress initiated by the HIV infection was not ameliorated in ART-treated individuals, compared to seronegative controls [132]. While these effects were observed in all HAND patients, the levels of oxidative stress markers were higher in those with more severe cognitive deficits [132].

Lipid peroxidation is still rampant despite effective viral control. While a couple of studies report decreased levels in markers of lipid peroxidation in ART-medicated patients, as compared with those not receiving ART, multiple studies have shown persistent statistically significant increases in hydroperoxides, isoprostanes, and malondialdehyde in ART-treated HIV-infected individuals, compared to seronegative controls [103, 113, 133-139]. Interestingly, two independent groups have determined in patient blood samples that the levels of peroxide species and oxidative stress are higher in patients on protease inhibitor (PI) based regimens, as compared with those in individuals on non-nucleoside reverse transcriptase inhibitor (NNRTI) based regimens, implicating a role for the protease inhibitor class in induction or exacerbation of oxidative stress [138, 140].

Micronutrient deficiencies are still problematic with ART, and while most patients have adequate plasma concentrations of vitamins C, D, and E, reported levels are still considered sub-optimal and lower than seronegative patients [123, 141]. While subsequent reports have indicated that zinc and selenium deficits are no longer observed in individuals on ART, further definitive confirmation of these findings is necessary [142, 143]. Additionally, in studies which evaluated the serum of adults and the saliva of children, the total antioxidant status was found to be decreased in ART treated HIV-patients when compared to HIV-negative controls, mirroring findings in studies conducted in the pre-ART era [104, 144].

While several studies have indicated that introduction of ART has been accompanied by an improvement in overall glutathione status, this effect is not totally rectified and imbalances still occur [129]. In particular, numerous groups have shown that circulating glutathione levels are still markedly reduced in HIV-infected individuals, when compared with age-matched controls, with the ratio of oxidized to reduced glutathione remaining out of balance [112, 133-135, 145]. Unfortunately, studies investigating nitrosative stress and nitrosylated proteins in HIV-infected individuals on ART are still lacking; however, the Nath, Hammond, and Sutliff laboratories have been investigating nitrosative stress in HIV, and it is likely that such reports are forthcoming.

It has been reported that HIV-positive individuals do not have altered levels of 8-hydroxy-2'-deoxyguanosine [8-oxoG) in their urine regardless of ART or lipodystrophy status [146]. While these findings appear to be promising, in a very recent study, autopsy tissue from frontal cortex was stained for both nuclear and mitochondrial 8-oxoG. The levels of this oxidized DNA product were significantly increased in cases of HAND, suggesting that ART, or ART in combination with ongoing infection may promote DNA oxidative modification, cellular dysfunction damage and death [147]. Additionally, the presence of clastogenic factors, which cause chromosomal breaks and DNA damage and which may be released from cells under conditions of oxidative stress, was observed in the plasma of all HIV-patients tested by Edeas *et al*. [148]. This was true ofpatients that were both asymptomatic and symptomatic for AIDS-defining pathologies, and was independent of ART status [148]. The effects of these clastogenic factors appear to persist in multiple cell populations implicated in HAND pathogenesis. For example, in leukocytes obtained from HIV-infected individuals, the percentage of cells exhibiting DNA fragmentation was increased in individuals on ART, as compared with those who were ART- naïve [135]. However, the results of this study have not addressed the possible contribution of latent or low level of infection to the findings. Due to pervasive oxidative damage and antioxidant imbalance despite effective long-term viral control in patients, it is now imperative to recognize the direct effect that viral enclaves and antiretroviral drugs themselves may have on perpetuating these effects. Further studies are needed to investigate the independent effects of ART and the virus on oxidative damage in the CNS, as well as in the periphery in order to better determine therapeutic interventions to resolve these dysfunctions.

4.2. Oxidative stress induction by HIV

Exhaustive research has been conducted in order to determine the effects of the HIV on infected cells and the cytotoxic factors released from these cells. As addressed earlier, it is now clear that HIV-infected macrophages secrete a variety of neurotoxic substances including glutamate, nitric oxide, and superoxide [96]. Within actively infected human myeloid-monocytic cell lines or monocyte-derived macrophages, HIV induces an increase in superoxide anions, with a concomitant increase in superoxide to combat these factors [128, 149]. Mollace and colleagues have demonstrated that the supernatants from HIV-infected human primary macrophages induced oxidative stress in astrocytes, as indicated by increases in malondialdeyde levels [150]. They further showed that these supernatants, which contained excess superoxide, induced astrocytic apoptosis, confirming HIV-mediated toxicity of this secreted product [150]. In a similar fashion, in HIV-infected monocytes, an induction of nitric oxide synthase and subsequent increase nitric oxide was observed [151]. It is also interesting to note that elevated oxidative stress in the form of intracellular singlet oxygen is capable of reactivating latent HIV through long terminal repeat (LTR) transactivation in infected monocytes or lymphocytes, suggesting that the virus may rely on oxidative stress signaling cascades for continuation of long-term infection or viral rebound [152].

The amino acid and neurotransmitter glutamate is normally secreted from neurons into the synaptic cleft, and is quickly removed and recycled through the actions of astrocytes. This molecule normally activates the N-methyl D-aspartate (NMDA) receptor on neurons, and allows for Ca^{2+} entry into the cell. However, it has been clearly demonstrated that excessive extracellular levels of glutamate resulting from overstimulation of neurons, impaired reuptake by astrocytes, or release from other cell populations within the brain can lead to hyperactivation of NMDA channels, subsequent increases in Ca^{2+} levels in the neuronal cytoplasm, resulting in excitotoxic neuronal death [153]. In 2001, Jiang *et al.* demonstrated through a series of elegant experiments that the molecule responsible for the neurotoxicity observed on neuronal cultures was a molecule of less than 3,000 kilodaltons, was not sensitive to trypsin digestion, and that its neurotoxic effect was blocked by a selective NMDA receptor antagonist, MK-801. It was through this study, as well as a subsequent study by O'Donnell *et al.* that the increased levels of extracellular glutamate secreted by HIV-infected macrophages may be a major factor in HIV-infected macrophage mediated indirect neuronal death [154]. The increases in extracellular glutamate appears to be an effect of dysregulation of the glutamate synthesis pathway, as inhibition of the mitochondrial glutaminase enzyme blocks the production and the secretion of glutamate from HIV-infected macrophages [155-157]. As was distinctly noted in human patient samples, a marked deficiency of glutathione and an imbalance between the oxidized and the reduced glutathione was observed. Within cells, glutaminase is the enzyme which converts glutamine to glutamate. It is tempting to consider that the oxidative stress resulting from the lack of the antioxidant properties of glutamine may be very tightly coupled to a depletion of glutamine from cells by hyperactivation of glutaminase enzymes, precipitating an overproduction of glutamate and triggering an excitotoxic neuronal death pathway.

Similar to effects of whole virus *in vivo*, when gp120 and Tat were injected into the brains of rats, both of these viral proteins induced lipid peroxidation and glutathione depletion [158]. Additionally, both of these proteins significantly reduced intracellular glutathione, and increased malondialdehyde in immortalized brain endothelial cells, showing that the oxidative status of these cells would also be directly affected by the presence of virus. This is of particular importance as the altered oxidative status of these endothelial cells comprising the BBB will have potential impact on not only the integrity of the BBB, but also on the monocyte/macrophage transmigration to the CNS, an important factor in the persistence of HAND [159]. Further, when applied to neurons in culture, gp120 and Tat induce disruptions in the lipid metabolism, leading to increased levels of sphingomyelin, ceramide, and hydroxynoneal,paralleling disruptions in these pathways observed in the neurons of HAND patients [116].

Studies that investigated gp120 separately have revealed that it is capable of inducing ROS formation, and activating the antioxidant response in astrocytes [91, 160]. Studies looking into the production of oxidant species by gp120 have shown that superoxide ions as well as nitric oxide are involved in neuronal toxicity [100, 161]. Mechanistically, gp120-induced nitric oxide formation is dependent on a mannose-specific endocytic lectin in macrophages, while gp120-induced expression and upregulation of iNOS selectively occurs in astrocytes in human fetal neuroglial cultures [100, 162]. Multiple studies have shown that in neurons undergoing gp120-induced toxicity, a significant increase in intracellular Ca^{2+}, likely released from intracellular stores,preceeded death, suggesting at a mechanism of activation of calpains or other pro-death cellular machinery [63, 160].

Studies investigating Tat-induced neuronal death have revealed that this viral protein triggered the accumulation of ROS when exogenously applied to a variety of cell types, including lymphocytes, microglia, brain microvascular endothelial cells (BMECs) and neurons, as well as in HeLa cells expressing Tat [163-166]. When directly injected into striatum of rats, Tat produced dramatic increases in protein oxidative modifications and protein carbonyls [167]. Protein carbonyls were also markedly increased in HeLa cells expressing Tat, supporting *in vivo* data [166]. In addition, decreased levels of glutathione were observed in cardiac myocytes and BMECs exposed to recombinant Tat protein, Tat-expressing transgenic mice, and in Tat-expressing HeLa cells [164, 168-170]. Two studies pinpointed the involvement of manganese-dependent superoxide dismutase (Mn-SOD) as a key player in Tat- induced cellular changes. By expressing Tat in HeLa cells, the laboratories of Lehman and McCord convincingly showed that Tat suppressed the RNA, protein, and activity levels of Mn-SOD, while inducing no changes in the Cu,Zn SOD enzyme levels [166, 170]. In HIV-infected individuals, plasma levels of SOD were increased in plasma, and these changes were in parallel with disease progression to AIDS. If the results from these HeLa cell studies can be expanded to other cell populations, it is tempting to speculate that perhaps this overall increase in SOD activity is a compensatory mechanism resulting from the Tat-induced alterations in Mn-SOD activity and the subsequent increases in superoxide ions that cannot be eliminated. The overexpression of Tat in HeLa cells also led to decreases in overall glutathione levels, with a lower ratio of reduced to oxidized glutathione in the remaining supply, mimicking the effect seen in HIV-infected individuals *in vivo* and in HIV-infected macrophages *in vitro* [166, 170].

Finally, studies focusing on microglia have shown that the expression of HIV viral protein R (Vpr) can induce oxidative stress pathways, and can activate HIV latent gene expression [171]. When exogenously applied to human fetal astrocytes, the oxidative stress caused by Vpr causes decreases in intracellular ATP and glutathione, and skews remaining glutathione in favor of the oxidized versus reduced form [172].

In summary, exhaustive *in vivo* and *in vitro* studies indicate that HIV viral proteins themselves can induce, precipitate and augment oxidative stress in multiple cell types, of both peripheral and CNS tissue. These findings further emphasize the importance of complete inhibition of viral replication in alleviating oxidative stress via antiretroviral therapy. However, emerging evidence suggests that antiretroviral drugs themselves might inadvertently lead to oxidative stress.

4.3. Oxidative stress and ART

Due to the requirement for lifelong adherence to antiretroviral regimens to prevent viremia and immune system compromise, it is necessary to investigate the effects of these compounds in a cellular context. Many of these drugs are associated with negative side effects, and have been linked to the metabolic syndrome, atherosclerosis, lipodystrophy, proteasome inhibition and the unfolded protein response [173-175]. Additionally, it has become apparent that these compounds themselves produce oxidative stress, even in the absence of virus, and may in fact be contributing to the persistence of oxidative stress in patients with well controlled viral load [97, 102].

HIV is highly susceptible to mutations, mostly due to the error-prone reverse transcription step during replication, and underlies the emergence of drug resistant mutations over time in patients treated with single antiretroviral drugs in the early 1990s. Additionally, the development of more sensitive methods for HIV RNA detection revealed the presence of viral reservoirs in multiple tissues, including the CNS. These findings led to the revision of antiretroviral therapy, which, until that time included mostly single antiretroviral drug regimens. A multiple drug treatment approach, termed ART, was implemented to aim at different steps in the HIV replication. Currently recommended ART regimens include a cocktail of nucleoside/nucleotide reverse-transcriptaseinhibitors (NRTIs/NtRTIs), non-nucleoside reverse-transcriptase inhibitors (nNRTIs), protease inhibitors (PIs), and to a lesser extent, entry inhibitors and integrase inhibitors(Panel on Antiretroviral Guidelines for Adults and Adolescents. Guidelines for the use of antiretroviral agents in HIV-1-infected adults and adolescents.Department of Health and Human Services.Available at http://aidsinfo.nih.gov/contentfiles/lvguidelines/AdultandAdolescentGL.pdf). This approach has led to improved immune function, long-term viral suppression; and underlies the reductions in HIV-associated morbidity and mortality in the era of ART. The recently updated guidelines recommend ART initiation to all HIV- infected, ART-naive individuals irrespective of CD4$^+$ counts and the impact of early initiation of ART on HIV-associated neurological complications remain to be seen. While a concensus has been reached regarding the time to initiate ART based on CD4 cell counts, AIDS-defining illnesses, and certain co-morbidity factors; the panel did not clearly outline strategies to best eradicate the viral reservoirs in the CNS, and to decrease the risk of developing HAND among infected patients.

In the meantime, one major approach to better control HAND has been to implement therapies that include drugs which achieve therapeutic concentrations in the CNS. While HIV can circumvent the BBB barrier, complex drug transport and efflux mechanisms at this junction hampers effective antiretroviral concentrations in the brain parenchyma. Recent efforts to address this hurdle have led to the establishment of CNS penetrance effectiveness (CPE) score, an algorithm based on the chemical structure, pharmacodynamic and pharmacokinetic data of antiretroviral drugs [176-178]. In summary, an antiretroviral drug with high CPE score is small in size (molecular mass below 400-500 kDa), has high lipid solubility and low protein binding, and it is not a substrate for drug transport or efflux proteins. Unfortunately, results of several clinical studies which incorporated CPE into the design and the analysis of outcomes are not conclusive [176, 178-183]. While a positive correlation between CPE scores and neurological outcomes are observed in several studies, one study revealed that ART regimens with higher CPE scores might be associated with worse neurocognitive performance [184].

These studies investigating the effect of CPE scores on neurological outcomes have inherent caveats. First, due to the limited methodologies, the clinical studies cannot assess the drug concentrations in the brain parenchyma, and instead depend on the CSF levels, which are usually based on measurements after a single-dose administration of the drug. Several factors, such as poor drug adherence and the impact of co-prescribed drugs on the pharmacokinetics of antiretroviral drugs can impact the CNS concentrations and can confound the measured outcomes.Additionally, the escape of drug-resistant viral species into the CNS and their establishment in viral reservoirs early during infection can lead to the rise of drug-resistant HIV species in the CNS, and can hinder the efforts to assess the impact of CPE scores on neurological outcomes. Further, co-morbidity factors impacting the integrity of the BBB should also be considered in assessing drug availability in the CNS. Among these factors are cancer, infections, and drug and alcohol abuse, all of which are shown to alter BBB integrity independent of HIV infection, and should be considered when CPE scores are established and evaluated [185-187]. One final factor to consider in evaluating the long-term effectiveness of ART is the potential direct toxicities of antiretroviral drugs in the CNS, especially given the interest in implementation of ART regimens with better CNS penetrance and possibly developing nanoART as part of treatment plans. Antiretroviral drugs have known side-effects in the periphery, including dyslipidemia, and lipohypertrophy. Further, antiretroviral drug-associated toxicity is well documented in the peripheral nervous system, and potential CNS toxicities secondary to ART exist. Oxidative damage elicited by antiretroviral drugs is of particular interest, given ample evidence of ongoing oxidative stress in the HAND brain, as described above.

In several cavalier studies, researchers eloquently demonstrated in several cell populations (human adipocytes, monocytes, myeloid cell lines, and human aortic endothelial cells) that a variety of drugs from the PI and NRTI families, alone or in combinations, induced the production of ROS, hydrogen peroxide, and factors promoting monocyte recruitment. The compounds reported to induce these changes included PIs: indinavir, nelfinavir, lopinavir, ritonavir, saquinavir, atazanavir and NRTIs: stavudine (d4T), zidovudine (AZT), and didanosine [97-99, 188-191]. The compounds amprenavir (PI) and abacavir (NRTI) were consistently reported as lacking these effects, making these drugs good candidates for inclusion in regimens to be prescribed to patients with HAND [98].

As the first available antiretroviral drug, AZT has been extensively studied. While AZT may not be a mainstay drug of choice for customized optimal regimens, as the primary ART compound available in resource-limited developing countries, it is still of importance to understand its cellular effects. AZT was approved for treatment in 1987, and as early as 1992 the Papoian laboratory reported deficits in mitochondrial enzymes and uncoupling of the electron transport chain (ETC) [192]. The disruption of the ETC is a primary cause of mitochondrial based intracellular ROS accumulation and mitochondrial DNA oxidation, an effect since expounded upon in multiple laboratories after acute AZT exposure in isolated heart mitochondria and primary human cardiomyocytes, and after chronic gestational AZT exposure in mouse liver and kidney and in the lung and brain of fetal patas monkeys [193-196]. This compound has also been shown to increase mitochondrial lipid peroxidation, deplete intracellular glutathione, and lead to oxidation of remaining glutathione, ultimately inducing a caspase-3- and caspase-7- dependent apoptotic death [193, 195, 197]. When another NRTI, d4T was investigated, it also was shown to produce ROS, mitochondrial oxidative stress, oxidized mitochondrial DNA, and altered activity of mitochondrial oxidative phosphorylation enzymes [198, 199]. Similarly, NRTI zalcitabine (ddC) also induces oxidative stress, as evidenced by the accumulation of protein carbonyls and nitrotyrosine modifications. Interestingly, this study also reported that the better-tolerated cytidine analog lamivudine (3TC) did not produce these effects, suggesting that 3TC may be considered as an alternative to reduce oxidative stress, and that future compounds generated from this structural base may behave similarly [200]. Interestingly, in contrast to studies in human lymphoid cells, Brandmann and collegues have recently reported that in astrocytes AZT, lamivudine, efavirenz, and nevirapine do not appear to reduce intracellular levels of glutathione [190]. Whether or not these compounds behave similarly in neurons and other cell populations in the CNS remains to be elucidated.

In the non-nucleoside reverse transcriptase inhibitor (nNRTI) drug class, efavirenz applied to a human hepatoblastoma cell line resulted in superoxide generation, depletion of intracellular glutathione, and decrease in mitochondrial function and membrane potential that was independent of mitochondrial DNA replication [201]. In addition, efavirenz has also been linked to neuropsychological side effects in HIV-infected patients, and it is probable that the specific oxidative stress effects on mitochondria and glutathione may play a role in the neurotoxicity of this compound, as neurons are particularly sensitive to perturbations in the antioxidant system [201, 202].

Within the protease inhibitor class, both ritonavir and amprenavir have been associated with increased superoxide anion production, while ritonavir has been shown to cause increases in nitrotyrosine levels in porcine coronary arteries [203]. On the other hand, both indinavir and nelfinavir have been shown to induce a time and concentration dependent depletion of intracellular glutathione in astrocytes as well as in pancreatic beta cells [99, 190]. Nelfinavir is of particular interest, as it suppresses cytosolic, rather than mitochondrial superoxide dismutase levels, and induces a necrotic rather than apoptotic cell death cascade in an adipocyte cell line [99, 204]. Future studies of this compound will undoubtedly prove interesting and may have important implications in patients with regard to their neurocognitive outcomes associated with this compund. Finally, it is interesting to note that multiple studies investigating the oxidative effects of the thymidine analogs in the NRTI class have reported increased ROS, hydrogen peroxide, and nitric oxide intermediates but no superoxide anions [188, 205].

Currently, there is no information on possible oxidative effects of the entry inhibitor, integrase inhibitor, and mutation inhibitor drug classes. Similarly, the lack of published studies for the neuroglial cell populations in the brains of HAND patients is surprising. Several posters at national and international meetings over recent years have addressed this important issue, and hopefully these reports will be forthcoming [206, 207]. In order to design custom drug regimens which will not precipitate, or can ameloirate oxidative stress, cellular dysfunction and death, it is critical to have an understanding of the cellular effects of each currently approved antiretroviral compound, and to design future compounds with minimal oxidative effects. Further, it is possible that the continued dysfunction in superoxide production and superoxide dismutase levels in patients may be due to the effects of more than one drug in a multi-drug regimen. Thus, designing future combinations which do not precipiateoxidative stressis of utmost importance in efforts to resolve the persistence of HAND observed in the ART era.

4.4. Potential therapeutic avenues for oxidative stress in ART era

Since the manifestations of oxidative stress induced by HIV and ART have emerged, it has also become evident to scientists that boosting the endogenous antioxidant response may be a valid and encouraging adjunctive therapeutic option. Within the cell, the antioxidant response is mediated through the activation of transcription factor NF-E2 (nuclear factor (erythroid-derived 2)-related factor-2 (Nrf2)and its myriad of effector phase II and III detoxifying enzymes. Relevant to the previously discussed aberrations in oxidant detoxification, this pathway upregulates superoxide dismutase, peroxiredoxins, thioredoxins, and multiple glutathione biosynthesis enzymes [208, 209].

In vitro, multiple compounds which act upon the Nrf2 pathway have proven effective in ameliorating the oxidative effects of viral infection, viral proteins or antiretroviral drugs. Among these compounds are resveratrol, dimethyl fumarate, N-acetylcysteine, and curcurmin [189, 191, 193, 203, 210]. Antioxidants which have not yet been shown to act through the Nrf2 pathway, but which have similar effects *in vitro* include dihydroxybenzyl alcohol, water soluble vitamin E (trolox), glutathione mimetic tricyclodecan-9-yl-xanthogenat, and acetyl-l-carnitine [188, 200, 201, 211]. An alternative approach to specifically inhibit the actions of NADPH oxidase through the compound diphenyleneiodonium, was able to specifically prevent the effects of PIs, but not NRTIs in human adipocytes [98]. This interesting finding suggests that the different antiretroviral classes may lead to ROS production through different mechanisms, and that specific therapeutics targeting individual oxidant-producing enzymes or pathways may need to be considered for specific ART regimens.

An alternative approach to activating Nrf2 pathway is supplementation with the antioxidant vitamin C (ascorbate), which is capable of directly scavenging reactive oxygen and nitrogen species. This method has been shown to be effective in counteracting the deleterious effects of gp120, as well as nelfinavir *in vitro*, and has been shown to have beneficial outcomes in patients, when supplemented to ART regimens [100, 195, 204]. Along these same lines, supplementation with a variety of other antioxidants and micronutrients including minocycline, glutathione replenishing peptide alpha-lipoic acid, selenium, vitamin A, Vitamin E, and a multivitamin regimen including vitamins A, C, E selenium and coenzyme Q10 have demonstrated partial protection from the deleterious oxidative effects of HIV/SIV and ART *in vivo*, with particular emphasis on restoration of the total blood glutathione levels [127, 195, 212-214]. Finally, the NMDA-receptor blocker memantine, and monoamide oxidase type B inhibitor selegiline, approved for treatment in Alzheimer and Parkinson Diseases, respectively, have also been proposed as potential therapeutics for HAND [1, 214]. Memantine might exert therapeutic effects through reduction of residual virus-mediated glutamate excitotoxicity, and selegiline has been reported to be capable of reducing oxygen-based free radicals [215, 216]. The use of these compounds and their efficacy in reducing oxidative damage in HAND are still in early stages. Initial studies were confounded by the fact that much damage was already present in late stage HAD patients and a protective effect at this stage was not evident [217]. Further work with these compounds will require identifying patients with ANI or MND to enroll in longitudinal studies to determine whether these compounds will have long-term benefit.

Going forward, it is imperative that the oxidative stress imposed by HIV and ART are targeted by adjunctive therapies. As research progresses with the quest for eliminating viral reservoirs and designing more effective, less toxic antiretroviral compounds, it is important to keep in mind that oxidative stress is and will continue to be a persistent burden, especially in a patient population with a significantly enhanced life expectancy.

5. The impact of co-morbidities on HAND

HIV, once an acute and catastrophic infection, has now become a chronic and manageable disease, with advances made in diagnosis and treatment. These changes are reflected in the increases in life expectancy from 5 years to up to the projected 50 years from the time of diagnosis. However, with the increased lifespan, co-morbidities, such as chronic co-infections, substance abuse, and aging have become major contributors to HAND persistence, and need to be addressed for successful evaluation and treatment of HAND.

The compromised immune system in an HIV-infected individual increases the risk of opportunistic infections in the CNS, much like that observed in the peripheral tissue. Most commonly observed infections, CNS toxoplasmosis, cryptococcosis, CNS tuberculosis, and cytomegalovirus encephalitis can be treated successfully by a combination of antimicrobials, antiviral and antiretroviral drugs. However, there are several other viral agents that can either directly target or indirectly compromise CNS, and cannot be readily managed by antiretroviral drugs or chemotherapeutics. One important virus with serious complications in HAND patients is JC virus, the causative agent of progressive multifocal leukoencephelopathy (PML). While approximately 60-80% of adults globally are seropositive for JC virus, it leads to the development of PML mostly in individuals who are immuno-compromised, either due to an underlying cancer or immunosuppressive treatment, or who are HIV-positive. The current incidence of PML in HIV patients is 3%. Studies have shown that JC virus can traffic across the BBB within the B cells, can enter the CNS as a free virus, or can infect brain vascular endothelial cells. Once in the CNS, JC virus causes the lytic infection of oligodendrocytes, and results in multifocal demyelination in multiple regions of the white matter. Thus, PML may exacerbate white matter loss that may already be occurring in HAND patients. Further, the most efficient, however limited, treatment for PML, which is immune restoration with aggressive antiretroviral therapy, can potentiate immune reconstitution inflammatory syndrome (IRIS). IRIS, a T-cell mediated encephalitis, can precipitate further injury and worsening of neurological symptoms. While fatality due to PML in HIV-infected individuals can be as high as 50%, the number of cases with non-lethal PML is increasing and PML may be contributing to the persistence of HIV-associated neurological complications.

Hepatitis B and C (HBV and HCV) are also commonly found in HIV-infected individuals due to the shared risk factors of contracting the virus. While these viruses are not thought to target the primary cells of the CNS, a recent study has reported the presence of HCV antigens in astrocytes and the cells of the macrophage/microglial lineage in the human brain. Additionally, there is limited evidence suggesting that HCV core protein might be detrimental to neurons *in vitro* and *in vivo*. Further, several studies have suggested that HCV and HIV can potentiate each other's replication. Currently, there is no conclusive data regarding a possible correlation between HCV presence in the CNS and the neurocognitive deficits in HAND patients. However, the potential implications of HCV infection in the CNS are at least three-fold. First, HCV co-infection can hinder the efforts to suppress HIV replication in the CNS. Second, weakened immune system function secondary to HCV will negatively impact subsequent alleviation of neurocognitive functions. Finally, compromised functioning of CNS support cells, mainly astrocytes, secondary to concomitant HCV infection will augment the neuroinflammatory environment with a negative impact on neuronal health. These implications may underlie the evidence that suggests that viral suppression and $CD4^+$ cell recovery is not as successful in the presence of HCV, and might partially explain the sporadic data suggesting that worse neurocognitive impairment is observed in HIV-HCV co-infected patients [184].

Illicit drug use, as well as alcohol abuse, put HIV-positive patients at a greater risk for HAND [6, 218-224]. The prevalence of HIV infection is 11-17% among illicit drug users, and methamphetamine (METH) is among the most frequently abused drug with well-known toxic effects on the BBB and in the CNS [220]. HIV-infected patients using METH exhibit more neurocognitive deficits, compared to those not using METH. These findings are likely due to the effects of METH on several fronts in the CNS. First, extensive studies have conclusively shown that METH alters the BBB permeability through direct damage to the BMECs, which in turn can augment HIV access to the CNS. Additionally, METH can exert neurotoxic effects in the CNS through oxidative stress and mitochondrial dysfunction [184], and precipitate further synaptic and neuronal damage. METH may also interfere with the expected benefits of ART in several ways. Most importantly, studies have shown that altered patient behavior due to METH use can interfere with drug adherence. Secondly, altered BBB function in a patient using METH can potentially alter antiretroviral access to the CNS, hindering efforts to establish an efficient regimen with limited side effects.

6. Aging and HAND

The widespread use of ART has drastically decreased the incidence of AIDS-related complications and improved the long-term prognosis of HIV-positive individuals. Currently, 30% of the HIV-positive population in the United States is over the age of 50,and by 2015 it is estimated that more than 50% will be over the age of 50 [225, 226]. Despite this remarkable development, the life expectancy for ART-treated HIV-positive individuals remains 10-30 years less than that of uninfected individuals [227]. Given the rapid global expansion of this population, it has become increasingly important to understand the risk factors that lie at the intersection of HIV, ART, and aging.

Older HIV-positive patients, including those treated with ART, are at increased risk for systemic diseases including atherosclerosis, liver and kidney failure, cancer, and osteoporosis [227, 228]. The aging brain may also be more vulnerable to the effects of HIV as older adults display an increased susceptibility to HAND, and emerging evidence suggests an increased prevalence of neurodegenerative diseases, including Alzheimer and Parkinson, in this patient population [229, 230]. It remains unclear if the increased prevalence of HAND is a result of HIV and related comorbidities, including hypertension, insulin resistance, and lipodystrophy, or other confounding factors such as immunosenescence and ART toxicities, all of which are likely to impact CNS disease progression in older HIV-positive individuals [231, 232].

Antiretroviral therapy effectively limits HIV disease progression, maintains patients in a state of partial immune competence, and arrests subjects in a pre-symptomatic state [233]. However, despite the ability of ART to reduce plasma HIV RNA to undetectable levels, HIV-positive individuals remain at higher risk for opportunistic illnesses and premature death [234, 235]. Thus, ART may reduce, but does not appear to eliminate, premature and/or accelerated aging in HIV-infected individuals. This may be attributed to many factors including drug toxicity and slower immune recovery following ART initiation in older patients, compared to younger adults [236]. Furthermore, advanced age has been linked to decreased production of T cells, B cells, and cytokines as well as to chronic immune activation, the latter of which may be linked to the breakdown of gut-associated lymphoid tissue (GALT) and to the elevated levels of systemic lipopolysaccharide (LPS) [237, 238].

Older patients also display a dampened recovery of CD4 cells following treatment with ART, which may increase their risk for systemic diseases ranging from heart disease to cancer [238]. Thus, it is not surprising that advanced age at seroconversion and/or onset of ART treatment is considered a major risk factor for severe HIV disease [239, 240]. Goetz, *et al.* performed a retrospective study on HIV-positive patients receiving ART treatment at the Veteran's Administration Greater Los Angeles Medical center between 1996 and 1999, and found that for every 10 years of additional age at the onset of ART treatment, the rate of CD4 cell replenishment decreased by 35 cells per microliter of blood [241]. Yet, despite the obvious benefits of beginning ART treatment in asymptomatic HIV-positive individuals, there remain significant concerns for initiating drug therapy sooner than necessary and how this may negatively impact drug toxicity, long-term patient outcome, and the evolution of drug resistant strains of HIV [240, 242]. Based on the updated recommendations for treatment initiation, as mentioned previously, all HIV-infected individuals will be put on ART regimen upon diagnosis, and the impact of this approach on older patients will be revealing.

Lower CD4 count, in addition to advanced age, also places older patients at a nearly fourfold higher risk for liver-related mortality compared to younger patients [243]. This risk is exacerbated by other factors commonly afflicting ART-treated, HIV-positive individuals including diabetes, alcohol abuse, as well as antiretroviral and cholesterol drug toxicity [243]. Among all non-AIDS-related complications, liver disease is the primary cause of death in

http://dx.doi.org/10.5772/52683

HIV-positive patients [243]. In addition, older HIV-positive individuals are at increased risk for frailty, bone loss and non-AIDS related cancers [244, 245]. It remains unclear if HIV itself places older individuals at higher risk for heart disease compared to older, HIV-negative individuals, though specific classes of antiretrovirals, especially protease inhibitors, have been linked to atherosclerosis [237, 246, 247].

The CNS is particularly susceptible to the synergistic neurodegenerative effects of HIV and aging. Several studies have demonstrated that, compared to younger (age 20 to 39 years) cohorts, older HIV-positive individuals (age > 50 years) display decreased neurocognitive functioning in several areas including memory, psychomotor speed, and executive functions [225, 248, 249]. The persistence of HAND in individuals with an undetectable viral load and CD4 cell counts greater than 200/μL is not well understood and may be a result of aging-associated processes rendering the cells of the CNS more vulnerable.

Several recent neuroimaging studies have begun to address the structural, physiological, and functional changes in the CNS in the context of HIV and aging. Six MRI investigations that assessed the structural changes in the brains of older HIV-positive individuals between 1998 and 2012 found evidence of premature or accelerated aging characterized by significant brain atrophy in the basal ganglia, cerebellum, and frontal and temporal brain regions, when compared to seronegative controls [231]. However, several diffusion tensor imaging (DTI) studies found only normal, age-dependent changes in mean diffusion and fractional anisotropy, which reflects the directionality of water diffusion in the brain, and is greater along organized white matter tracts but decreased in pathologically damaged, disorganized tracts [231, 250-252].

Other studies have employed proton magnetic resonance spectroscopy (MRS) to assess the changes in brain metabolite levels that are indicative of neuronal damage and death or glial activation. Ernst and Chang demonstrated a five-fold acceleration of aging effects in a relatively young (mean age 36 years) ART-naïve, HIV-positive cohort, as compared to HIV-negative controls, as reflected by increased levels of glial activation markers, myoinositol (MI) and choline compounds (CHO), and a decrease in the neuronal marker, N-acetylaspartate (NAA) [253]. A recent multicenter MRS study of slightly older (ages 30-70], ART-treated HIV-positive individuals demonstrated elevated MI and CHO in all brain regions of patients with asymptomatic or mild neurocognitive impairment, but decreased levels of MI in those with dementia, which the authors interpreted as premature microglial senescence [231, 254]. In addition, this study found an age-dependent decrease in NAA in frontal white matter, but only in patients with HAD [254]. Thus, while ART-naïve HIV-positive patients show evidence of increased, age-dependent glial activation and neuronal damage leading to accelerated aging, ART-treated individuals show only signs of premature aging [231].

As mentioned previously, the clinical and pathological hallmarks of post-ART HAND differ from those in the pre-ART era. While HAD presented as a subcortical dementia afflicting the basal ganglia and white matter, some post-ART studies suggest the focus of neuroinflammation has shifted primarily to the hippocampus, even in effectively treated patients [255-257]. Furthermore, there is emerging evidence that pathologic similarities exist between HAND and some common neurodegenerative disorders such as Alzheimer Disease, which is characterized by the presence of extracellular beta amyloid (Aβ) plaque deposits, and intracellular neurofibrillary tangles composed of hyperphosphorylated Tau [228, 233, 258, 259]. *In vitro* work involving the viral protein Tat has demonstrated the ability of this viral protein to inhibit the activity of the Aβ-degrading enzyme, Neprilysin, and the ability to bind to the receptor for advanced glycation end products, all of which may promote Aβ accumulation in the CNS. Indeed, some individuals with HAND display CSF levels of Aβ42 comparable to those observed in AD patients [228, 260, 261]. However, a recent report utilizing the amyloid-binding, carbon 11-labeled Pittsburgh compound B (11C-PiB) and PET imaging found that irrespective of neurocognitive impairment, HIV-positive individuals showed no increase in 11C-PiB levels, highlighting a potential key difference between Aβ metabolism in HAND vs. AD despite some overlapping pathological features [258].

Among the studies underlining the similarities between HAND and AD, Esiri *et al.* were the first to report a predisposition to plaque formation in the brains of pre-ART HIV-positive individuals [262]. Such pathological changes have been observed in HIV-positive patients despite successful virologic control with ART, suggesting that antiretrovirals either cannot achieve therapeutic concentrations within the brain parenchyma, allowing for ongoing viral replication and neuroinflammation, or may have toxic effects that could facilitate neurodegeneration [263, 264]. To address the latter concern, several reports investigated differences in either phospho-tau or beta amyloid levels in ART-naïve vs. ART-treated individuals. Two groups independently reported elevated Aβ deposition in the hippocampus of ART-treated individuals compared to pre-ART patients, yet Anthony *et al.* reported only increased hyperphosphorylated tau, but no Aβ deposition in the hippocampus and entorhinal cortex of HIV-positive individuals [257, 259, 265]. To date, no group has reported concomitant phospho-tau and Aβ plaque depositions in the same brain samples from HIV-positive cohorts. Differences in patient age and ART-regimens, as well as the antibodies used to detect Aβ may account for the varied outcomes of these reports.

Importantly, the aforementioned studies highlight the potentially under-appreciated concern of antiretroviral-associated toxicity and its effect on neuropsychological outcomes in long-term ART-treated patients. As described earlier, ART drugs have been linked to wide-ranging, peripheral metabolic and neural disturbances that could themselves influence the progression of HAND and foretell potential mechanisms of toxicity in the CNS [246, 266-276]. While CNS effects of ART are poorly understood, Schweinsburg et al. demonstrated an association between NRTIs and decreased levels of frontal white matter NAA, which they attributed to NRTI-mediated mitochondrial dysfunction and depletion of cellular respiration [268]. Confounding the issue of direct CNS toxicity of antiretroviral medications is the variability in BBB permeability amongst different drug classes as determined by various physicochemical properties such as plasma protein binding, lipophilicity, and molecular size.

Although it is a widely held that ART regimens with higher CNS penetrance generally confer greater neuropsychological outcomes in HIV-positive individuals, numerous clinical studies have suggested these regimens may negatively impact cognition. In a prospective study, Marra et al. found a significant association between highly CNS-penetrant ART regimens and worse neurocognitive and motor performance, despite decreased CSF HIV RNA in a small HIV-positive cohort [181]. In addition, Robertson et al. reported an improvement in neuropsychological outcome in a cohort of patients with interrupted drug treatment [277]. Studies using SCID mice, which display neuropathological hallmarks similar to those associated with HIV, showed reduced viral load and astrogliosis following administration of ART, but no improvement in cognitive dysfunction [278]. Altogether, these studies reinforce an emerging hypothesis that antiretroviral drugs may be contributing to the rising prevalence of HAND in the aging HIV-positive population.

However, many clinical studies have demonstrated beneficial effects on neurocognitive functioning by ART regimens with high CPE scores [279, 280]. A cross-sectional study of 2636 adults from the AIDS Clinical Trials Group Longitudinal Linked Randomized Trials (ALLRT cohort), on effective ART for at least 6 weeks showed better neurocognitive performance in individuals receiving ART medications with higher CPE scores [281]. In some cases, participants required more than 3 antiretrovirals to treat HIV in the CNS. Letendre et al. demonstrated improvements in cognition over a 15-week period in patients beginning ART with higher CPE ART regimens [282]. Another recent investigation utilized MRS imaging to investigate the effect of different CPE ART regimens with different CPE scores on changes in brain NAA metabolite levels. Over 48 weeks, HIV-positive, ART-naïve individuals receiving the regimens with highest CPE scores displayed the highest increases in NAA levels, and showed the greatest improvement in a battery of neuropsychological tests [283]. These studies suggest that ART medications with higher CNS penetrance may have a neuroprotective effect in successfully treated HIV-positive adults. However, given the well-characterized toxicities of ART medications in the periphery, and the potential impact of related co-morbidities on CNS pathology, it may be necessary to consider adjunctive therapies to minimize the synergistic effects of ART and aging in HIV-positive individuals.

7. Summary

The advent of ART has profoundly changed the landscape of disease; however, neurocognitive impairments continue to be debilitating to patients with the expected life expectancy closer to that of the uninfected population. A better understanding and appreciation of the confounding factors has become more acute as the recent focus in the race to cure AIDS has shifted towards the eradication of latent viral reservoirs, including those in the CNS. It is imperative to anticipate and control the immune responses due to viral reactivation, the potential neurotoxicities of viral proteins in the brain parenchyma when latent viral progeny is activated, and the oxidative damage that may be precipitated by viral particles and the activated immune cells. These factors will be even more crucial to control in the aging brain with limited cognitive reserves.

Author details

Jennifer M. King, Brigid K. Jensen, Patrick J. Gannon and Cagla Akay*

*Address all correspondence to: akayc@upenn.edu

Department of Pathology, School of Dental Medicine, University of Pennsylvania, Philadelphia, USA

References

[1] Lindl KA, Marks DR, Kolson DL, Jordan-Sciutto KL. HIV-associated neurocognitive disorder: pathogenesis and therapeutic opportunities. J Neuroimmune Pharmacol. (Review). 2010 Sep;5 (3):294-309.

[2] Antinori A, Arendt G, Becker JT, Brew BJ, Byrd DA, Cherner M, et al. Updated research nosology for HIV-associated neurocognitive disorders. Neurology. 2007 Oct 30;69 (18):1789-99.

[3] Heaton RK, Clifford DB, Franklin DR, Jr., Woods SP, Ake C, Vaida F, et al. HIV-associated neurocognitive disorders persist in the era of potent antiretroviral therapy: CHARTER Study. Neurology. 2010 Dec 7;75 (23):2087-96.

[4] Dore GJ, Correll PK, Li Y, Kaldor JM, Cooper DA, Brew BJ. Changes to AIDS dementia complex in the era of highly active antiretroviral therapy. AIDS (London, England). 1999 Jul 9;13 (10):1249-53.

[5] Dore GJ, Li Y, McDonald A, Ree H, Kaldor JM. Impact of highly active antiretroviral therapy on individual AIDS-defining illness incidence and survival in Australia. Journal of acquired immune deficiency syndromes (1999). 2002 Apr 1;29 (4):388-95.

[6] Power C, Boisse L, Rourke S, Gill MJ. NeuroAIDS: an evolving epidemic. Can J Neurol Sci. 2009 May;36 (3):285-95.

[7] Price RW, Brew B, Sidtis J, Rosenblum M, Scheck AC, Cleary P. The brain in AIDS: central nervous system HIV-1 infection and AIDS dementia complex. Science. 1988;239:586-92.

[8] Gongvatana A, Schweinsburg BC, Taylor MJ, Theilmann RJ, Letendre SL, Alhassoon OM, et al. White matter tract injury and cognitive impairment in human immunodeficiency virus-infected individuals. J Neurovirol. 2009 Apr;15 (2):187-95.

[9] Thompson PM, Dutton RA, Hayashi KM, Toga AW, Lopez OL, Aizenstein HJ, et al. Thinning of the cerebral cortex visualized in HIV/AIDS reflects CD4+ T lymphocyte decline. Proc Natl Acad Sci U S A. 2005 Oct 25;102 (43):15647-52.

[10] Cohen RA, Harezlak J, Schifitto G, Hana G, Clark U, Gongvatana A, et al. Effects of nadir CD4 count and duration of human immunodeficiency virus infection on brain

volumes in the highly active antiretroviral therapy era. J Neurovirol. 2010 Feb;16 (1): 25-32.

[11] Ellis R. HIV and antiretroviral therapy: impact on the central nervous system. Prog Neurobiol. 2010 Jun;91 (2):185-7.

[12] Everall I, Vaida F, Khanlou N, Lazzaretto D, Achim C, Letendre S, et al. Cliniconeuropathologic correlates of human immunodeficiency virus in the era of antiretroviral therapy. J Neurovirol. 2009 Sep;15 (5-6):360-70.

[13] Everall IP, Heaton RK, Marcotte TD, Ellis RJ, McCutchan JA, Atkinson JH, et al. Cortical synaptic density is reduced in mild to moderate human immunodeficiency virus neurocognitive disorder. HNRC Group. HIV Neurobehavioral Research Center. Brain Pathol. 1999 Apr;9 (2):209-17.

[14] Masliah E, Heaton RK, Marcotte TD, Ellis RJ, Wiley CA, Mallory M, et al. Dendritic injury is a pathological substrate for human immunodeficiency virus-related cognitive disorders. HNRC Group. The HIV Neurobehavioral Research Center. Ann Neurol. 1997 Dec;42 (6):963-72.

[15] Zheng J, Thylin MR, Cotter RL, Lopez AL, Ghorpade A, Persidsky Y, et al. HIV-1 infected and immune competent mononuclear phagocytes induce quantitative alterations in neuronal dendritic arbor: relevance for HIV-1-associated dementia. Neurotox Res. 2001 Oct;3 (5):443-59.

[16] Gelman BB, Schuenke K. Brain aging in acquired immunodeficiency syndrome: increased ubiquitin-protein conjugate is correlated with decreased synaptic protein but not amyloid plaque accumulation. J Neurovirol. 2004 Apr;10 (2):98-108.

[17] Kolson DL, Sabnekar P, Baybis M, Crino PB. Gene expression in TUNEL-positive neurons in human immunodeficiency virus-infected brain. J Neurovirol. 2004;10 Suppl 1:102-7.

[18] Wiley CA, Achim CL, Hammond R, Love S, Masliah E, Radhakrishnan L, et al. Damage and repair of DNA in HIV encephalitis. J Neuropathol Exp Neurol. 2000 Nov;59 (11):955-65.

[19] Gonzalez-Scarano F, Martin-Garcia J. The neuropathogenesis of AIDS. Nat Rev Immunol. 2005 Jan;5 (1):69-81.

[20] Fauci AS. The human immunodeficiency virus: infectivity and mechanisms of pathogenesis. Science. 1988 Feb 5;239 (4840):617-22.

[21] Williams DW, Eugenin EA, Calderon TM, Berman JW. Monocyte maturation, HIV susceptibility, and transmigration across the blood brain barrier are critical in HIV neuropathogenesis. J Leukoc Biol. 2012 Mar;91 (3):401-15.

[22] Roberts TK, Buckner CM, Berman JW. Leukocyte transmigration across the blood-brain barrier: perspectives on neuroAIDS. Front Biosci. 2010;15:478-536.

[23] Liu NQ, Lossinsky AS, Popik W, Li X, Gujuluva C, Kriederman B, et al. Human immunodeficiency virus type 1 enters brain microvascular endothelia by macropinocytosis dependent on lipid rafts and the mitogen-activated protein kinase signaling pathway. J Virol. 2002 Jul;76 (13):6689-700.

[24] Gendelman HE, Lipton SA, Tardieu M, Bukrinsky MI, Nottet HS. The neuropathogenesis of HIV-1 infection. (see comment). (Review) (107 refs). 1994 Sep.

[25] Gonzalez-Scarano F, Martin-Garcia J. The neuropathogenesis of AIDS. (Review) (173 refs). 2005 Jan.

[26] Kaul M, Zheng J, Okamoto S, Gendelman HE, Lipton SA. HIV-1 infection and AIDS: consequences for the central nervous system. (Review) (199 refs). 2005 Aug.

[27] Carter CC, Onafuwa-Nuga A, McNamara LA, Riddell Jt, Bixby D, Savona MR, et al. HIV-1 infects multipotent progenitor cells causing cell death and establishing latent cellular reservoirs. Nat Med. 2010 Apr;16 (4):446-51.

[28] Hakre S, Chavez L, Shirakawa K, Verdin E. HIV latency: experimental systems and molecular models. FEMS Microbiol Rev. 2012 May;36 (3):706-16.

[29] Lafeuillade A. Eliminating the HIV reservoir. Curr HIV/AIDS Rep. 2012 Jun;9 (2): 121-31.

[30] Saleh S, Wightman F, Ramanayake S, Alexander M, Kumar N, Khoury G, et al. Expression and reactivation of HIV in a chemokine induced model of HIV latency in primary resting CD4+ T cells. Retrovirology. 2011;8:80.

[31] Vandergeeten C, Fromentin R, Chomont N. The role of cytokines in the establishment, persistence and eradication of the HIV reservoir. Cytokine Growth Factor Rev. 2012 Aug;23 (4-5):143-9.

[32] Wilen CB, Tilton JC, Doms RW. Molecular mechanisms of HIV entry. Adv Exp Med Biol. 2012;726:223-42.

[33] Devadas K, Hardegen NJ, Wahl LM, Hewlett IK, Clouse KA, Yamada KM, et al. Mechanisms for macrophage-mediated HIV-1 induction. J Immunol. 2004 Dec 1;173 (11):6735-44.

[34] Gorry PR, Ong C, Thorpe J, Bannwarth S, Thompson KA, Gatignol A, et al. Astrocyte infection by HIV-1: mechanisms of restricted virus replication, and role in the pathogenesis of HIV-1-associated dementia. Curr HIV Res. 2003 Oct;1 (4):463-73.

[35] Wraith DC, Nicholson LB. The adaptive immune system in diseases of the central nervous system. J Clin Invest. 2012 Apr 2;122 (4):1172-9.

[36] Ransohoff RM, Brown MA. Innate immunity in the central nervous system. J Clin Invest. 2012 Apr 2;122 (4):1164-71.

[37] Fairweather D, Cihakova D. Alternatively activated macrophages in infection and autoimmunity. J Autoimmun. 2009 Nov-Dec;33 (3-4):222-30.

[38] Fujiwara N, Kobayashi K. Macrophages in inflammation. Curr Drug Targets Inflamm Allergy. 2005 Jun;4 (3):281-6.

[39] Tesseur I, Wyss-Coray T. A role for TGF-beta signaling in neurodegeneration: evidence from genetically engineered models. Curr Alzheimer Res. 2006 Dec;3 (5): 505-13.

[40] Wahl SM, Allen JB, McCartney-Francis N, Morganti-Kossmann MC, Kossmann T, Ellingsworth L, et al. Macrophage- and astrocyte-derived transforming growth factor beta as a mediator of central nervous system dysfunction in acquired immune deficiency syndrome. J Exp Med. 1991 Apr 1;173 (4):981-91.

[41] Wahl SM. The role of transforming growth factor-beta in inflammatory processes. Immunol Res. 1991;10 (3-4):249-54.

[42] Johnson MD, Gold LI. Distribution of transforming growth factor-beta isoforms in human immunodeficiency virus-1 encephalitis. Hum Pathol. 1996 Jul;27 (7):643-9.

[43] Dhar A, Gardner J, Borgmann K, Wu L, Ghorpade A. Novel role of TGF-beta in differential astrocyte-TIMP-1 regulation: implications for HIV-1-dementia and neuroinflammation. J Neurosci Res. 2006 May 15;83 (7):1271-80.

[44] Samah B, Porcheray F, Dereuddre-Bosquet N, Gras G. Nerve growth factor stimulation promotes CXCL-12 attraction of monocytes but decreases human immunodeficiency virus replication in attracted population. J Neurovirol. 2009 Jan;15 (1):71-80.

[45] Meeker RB, Poulton W, Markovic-Plese S, Hall C, Robertson K. Protein changes in CSF of HIV-infected patients: evidence for loss of neuroprotection. J Neurovirol. (Research Support, N.I.H., Extramural). 2011 Jun;17 (3):258-73.

[46] Heath SL, Sabbaj S, Bansal A, Kilby JM, Goepfert PA. CD8 T-cell proliferative capacity is compromised in primary HIV-1 infection. Journal of acquired immune deficiency syndromes (1999). 2011 Mar;56 (3):213-21.

[47] Yadav A, Collman RG. CNS inflammation and macrophage/microglial biology associated with HIV-1 infection. J Neuroimmune Pharmacol. 2009 Dec;4 (4):430-47.

[48] Tozzi V, Balestra P, Bellagamba R, Corpolongo A, Salvatori MF, Visco-Comandini U, et al. Persistence of neuropsychologic deficits despite long-term highly active antiretroviral therapy in patients with HIV-related neurocognitive impairment: prevalence and risk factors. Journal of acquired immune deficiency syndromes (1999). 2007 Jun 1;45 (2):174-82.

[49] Yilmaz A, Price RW, Spudich S, Fuchs D, Hagberg L, Gisslen M. Persistent intrathecal immune activation in HIV-1-infected individuals on antiretroviral therapy. Journal of acquired immune deficiency syndromes (1999). 2008 Feb 1;47 (2):168-73.

[50] Yilmaz A, Fuchs D, Hagberg L, Nillroth U, Stahle L, Svensson J-O, et al. Cerebrospinal fluid HIV-1 RNA, intrathecal immunoactivation, and drug concentrations after

treatment with a combination of saquinavir, nelfinavir, and two nucleoside analogues: the M61022 study. BMC Infectious Diseases. 2006;6 (1):63.

[51] Edén A, Fuchs D, Hagberg L, Nilsson S, Spudich S, Svennerholm B, et al. HIV-1 Viral Escape in Cerebrospinal Fluid of Subjects on Suppressive Antiretroviral Treatment. Journal of Infectious Diseases. 2010 December 15, 2010;202 (12):1819-25.

[52] Hagberg L, Cinque P, Gisslen M, Brew B, Spudich S, Bestetti A, et al. Cerebrospinal fluid neopterin: an informative biomarker of central nervous system immune activation in HIV-1 infection. AIDS Research and Therapy. 2010;7 (1):15.

[53] Achim CL, Masliah E, Heyes MP, Sarnacki P, Hilty C, Baldwin M, et al. Macrophage Activation Factors
in the Brains of AIDS Patients. Journal of neuro-AIDS. 1996;1 (2):1-16.

[54] Achim CL, Wiley CA. Inflammation in AIDS and the role of the macrophage in brain pathology. Curr Opin Neurobiol. 1996;9 (3):221-5.

[55] Conant K, Garzino-Demo A, Nath A, McArthur JC, Halliday W, Power C, et al. Induction of monocyte chemoattractant protein-1 in HIV-1 Tat-stimulated astrocytes and elevation in AIDS dementia. Proc Natl Acad Sci U S A. 1998 Mar 17;95 (6): 3117-21.

[56] Gisolf EH, van Praag RM, Jurriaans S, Portegies P, Goudsmit J, Danner SA, et al. Increasing cerebrospinal fluid chemokine concentrations despite undetectable cerebrospinal fluid HIV RNA in HIV-1-infected patients receiving antiretroviral therapy. Journal of acquired immune deficiency syndromes (1999). 2000 Dec 15;25 (5):426-33.

[57] Sippy BD, Hofman FM, Wallach D, Hinton DR. Increased expression of tumor necrosis factor-alpha receptors in the brains of patients with AIDS. J Acquir Immune Defic Syndr Hum Retrovirol. 1995 Dec 15;10 (5):511-21.

[58] Tomkowicz B, Lee C, Ravyn V, Cheung R, Ptasznik A, Collman RG. The Src kinase Lyn is required for CCR5 signaling in response to MIP-1beta and R5 HIV-1 gp120 in human macrophages. Blood. 2006 Aug 15;108 (4):1145-50.

[59] Lee C, Tomkowicz B, Freedman BD, Collman RG. HIV-1 gp120-induced TNF-{alpha} production by primary human macrophages is mediated by phosphatidylinositol-3 (PI-3) kinase and mitogen-activated protein (MAP) kinase pathways. J Leukoc Biol. 2005 Oct;78 (4):1016-23.

[60] Chihara T, Hashimoto M, Osman A, Hiyoshi-Yoshidomi Y, Suzu I, Chutiwitoonchai N, et al. HIV-1 proteins preferentially activate anti-inflammatory M2-type macrophages. J Immunol. 2012 Apr 15;188 (8):3620-7.

[61] Turchan-Cholewo J, Dimayuga VM, Gupta S, Gorospe RM, Keller JN, Bruce-Keller AJ. NADPH oxidase drives cytokine and neurotoxin release from microglia and macrophages in response to HIV-Tat. Antioxid Redox Signal. 2009 Feb;11 (2):193-204.

[62] Pu H, Tian J, Flora G, Lee YW, Nath A, Hennig B, et al. HIV-1 Tat protein upregulates inflammatory mediators and induces monocyte invasion into the brain. Mol Cell Neurosci. 2003 Sep;24 (1):224-37.

[63] Agrawal L, Louboutin JP, Marusich E, Reyes BA, Van Bockstaele EJ, Strayer DS. Dopaminergic neurotoxicity of HIV-1 gp120: reactive oxygen species as signaling intermediates. Brain Res. 2010 Jan 8;1306:116-30.

[64] Louboutin JP, Agrawal L, Reyes BA, Van Bockstaele EJ, Strayer DS. Protecting neurons from HIV-1 gp120-induced oxidant stress using both localized intracerebral and generalized intraventricular administration of antioxidant enzymes delivered by SV40-derived vectors. Gene Ther. 2007 Dec;14 (23):1650-61.

[65] Agrawal L, Louboutin JP, Reyes BA, Van Bockstaele EJ, Strayer DS. HIV-1 Tat neurotoxicity: a model of acute and chronic exposure, and neuroprotection by gene delivery of antioxidant enzymes. Neurobiol Dis. 2012 Feb;45 (2):657-70.

[66] Gannon P, Khan MZ, Kolson DL. Current understanding of HIV-associated neurocognitive disorders pathogenesis. Curr Opin Neurol. (Research Support, N.I.H., ExtramuralReview). 2011 Jun;24 (3):275-83.

[67] Rao JS, Kim HW, Kellom M, Greenstein D, Chen M, Kraft AD, et al. Increased neuroinflammatory and arachidonic acid cascade markers, and reduced synaptic proteins, in brain of HIV-1 transgenic rats. J Neuroinflammation. 2011;8:101.

[68] Kusao I, Shiramizu B, Liang CY, Grove J, Agsalda M, Troelstrup D, et al. Cognitive performance related to HIV-1-infected monocytes. J Neuropsychiatry Clin Neurosci. 2012 Dec 1;24 (1):71-80.

[69] Rostasy K, Monti L, Yiannoutsos C, Wu J, Bell J, Hedreen J, et al. NFkappaB activation, TNF-alpha expression, and apoptosis in the AIDS-Dementia-Complex. J Neurovirol. 2000 Dec;6 (6):537-43.

[70] Pemberton LA, Stone E, Price P, van Bockxmeer F, Brew BJ. The relationship between ApoE, TNFA, IL1a, IL1b and IL12b genes and HIV-1-associated dementia. HIV Med. 2008 Oct;9 (8):677-80.

[71] Lichtfuss GF, Cheng WJ, Farsakoglu Y, Paukovics G, Rajasuriar R, Velayudham P, et al. Virologically Suppressed HIV Patients Show Activation of NK Cells and Persistent Innate Immune Activation. J Immunol. 2012 Aug 1;189 (3):1491-9.

[72] Goldberg SH, van der Meer P, Hesselgesser J, Jaffer S, Kolson DL, Albright AV, et al. CXCR3 expression in human central nervous system diseases. Neuropathol Appl Neurobiol. 2001 Apr;27 (2):127-38.

[73] Letendre S, Zheng J, Kaul M, Yiannoutsos C, Ellis R, Taylor M, et al. Chemokines in cerebrospinal fluid correlate with cerebral metabolite patterns in HIV-infected individuals. Journal of NeuroVirology. 2011;17 (1):63-9.

[74] Martin-Garcia J, Kolson DL, Gonzalez-Scarano F. Chemokine receptors in the brain: their role in HIV infection and pathogenesis. AIDS (London, England). 2002 Sep 6;16 (13):1709-30.

[75] van der Meer P, Ulrich AM, Gonzalez-Scarano F, Lavi E. Immunohistochemical analysis of CCR2, CCR3, CCR5, and CXCR4 in the human brain: potential mechanisms for HIV dementia. Exp Mol Pathol. 2000 Dec;69 (3):192-201.

[76] Dhillon NK, Williams R, Callen S, Zien C, Narayan O, Buch S. Roles of MCP-1 in development of HIV-dementia. Front Biosci. 2008;13:3913-8.

[77] Monteiro de Almeida S, Letendre S, Zimmerman J, Lazzaretto D, McCutchan A, Ellis R. Dynamics of monocyte chemoattractant protein type one (MCP-1) and HIV viral load in human cerebrospinal fluid and plasma. Journal of neuroimmunology. 2005 Dec;169 (1-2):144-52.

[78] Cartier L, Dubois-Dauphin M, Hartley O, Irminger-Finger I, Krause KH. Chemokine-induced cell death in CCR5-expressing neuroblastoma cells. Journal of neuroimmunology. 2003 Dec;145 (1-2):27-39.

[79] Kraft-Terry SD, Stothert AR, Buch S, Gendelman HE. HIV-1 neuroimmunity in the era of antiretroviral therapy. Neurobiol Dis. 2010 Mar;37 (3):542-8.

[80] Alirezaei M, Watry DD, Flynn CF, Kiosses WB, Masliah E, Williams BR, et al. Human immunodeficiency virus-1/surface glycoprotein 120 induces apoptosis through RNA-activated protein kinase signaling in neurons. J Neurosci. 2007 Oct 10;27 (41): 11047-55.

[81] O'Donnell LA, Agrawal A, Jordan-Sciutto KL, Dichter MA, Lynch DR, Kolson DL. Human immunodeficiency virus (HIV)-induced neurotoxicity: roles for the NMDA receptor subtypes. J Neurosci. 2006 Jan 18;26 (3):981-90.

[82] Abdulle S, Hagberg L, Gisslen M. Effects of antiretroviral treatment on blood-brain barrier integrity and intrathecal immunoglobulin production in neuroasymptomatic HIV-1-infected patients. HIV Med. 2005 May;6 (3):164-9.

[83] Kamat A, Lyons JL, Misra V, Uno H, Morgello S, Singer EJ, et al. Monocyte Activation Markers in Cerebrospinal Fluid Associated With Impaired Neurocognitive Testing in Advanced HIV Infection. Journal of acquired immune deficiency syndromes (1999). 2012 Jul 1;60 (3):234-43.

[84] Schellenberg AE, Buist R, Del Bigio MR, Khorooshi R, Toft-Hansen H, Owens T, et al. Blood-brain barrier disruption in CCL2 transgenic mice during pertussis toxin-induced brain inflammation. Fluids and barriers of the CNS. 2012 Apr 30;9 (1):10.

[85] Eugenin EA, Osiecki K, Lopez L, Goldstein H, Calderon TM, Berman JW. CCL2/monocyte chemoattractant protein-1 mediates enhanced transmigration of human immunodeficiency virus (HIV)-infected leukocytes across the blood-brain barrier: a potential mechanism of HIV-CNS invasion and NeuroAIDS. J Neurosci. (Compara-

tive StudyResearch Support, N.I.H., ExtramuralResearch Support, Non-U.S. Gov't). 2006 Jan 25;26 (4):1098-106.

[86] Roberts TK, Eugenin EA, Lopez L, Romero IA, Weksler BB, Couraud PO, et al. CCL2 disrupts the adherens junction: implications for neuroinflammation. Lab Invest. 2012 Aug;92 (8):1213-33.

[87] Lu SM, Tremblay ME, King IL, Qi J, Reynolds HM, Marker DF, et al. HIV-1 Tat-induced microgliosis and synaptic damage via interactions between peripheral and central myeloid cells. PLoS One. 2011;6 (9):e23915.

[88] Markowitz AJ, White MG, Kolson DL, Jordan-Sciutto KL. Cellular interplay between neurons and glia: toward a comprehensive mechanism for excitotoxic neuronal loss in neurodegeneration. Cellscience. 2007 Jul 27;4 (1):111-46.

[89] Benos DJ, Hahn BH, Bubien JK, Ghosh SK, Mashburn NA, Chaikin MA, et al. Envelope glycoprotein gp120 of human immunodeficiency virus type 1 alters ion transport in astrocytes: implications for AIDS dementia complex. Proc Natl Acad Sci U S A. 1994 Jan 18;91 (2):494-8.

[90] Kolson DL, Buchhalter J, Collman R, Hellmig B, Farrell CF, Debouck C, et al. HIV-1 Tat alters normal organization of neurons and astrocytes in primary rodent brain cell cultures: RGD sequence dependence. AIDS Res Hum Retroviruses. 1993 Jul;9 (7): 677-85.

[91] Reddy PV, Gandhi N, Samikkannu T, Saiyed Z, Agudelo M, Yndart A, et al. HIV-1 gp120 induces antioxidant response element-mediated expression in primary astrocytes: Role in HIV associated neurocognitive disorder. Neurochem Int. 2011 Jul 3.

[92] Shukla V, Mishra SK, Pant HC. Oxidative stress in neurodegeneration. Adv Pharmacol Sci. 2011;2011:572634.

[93] Reynolds A, Laurie C, Mosley RL, Gendelman HE. Oxidative stress and the pathogenesis of neurodegenerative disorders. Int Rev Neurobiol. 2007;82:297-325.

[94] Melo A, Monteiro L, Lima RM, Oliveira DM, Cerqueira MD, El-Bacha RS. Oxidative stress in neurodegenerative diseases: mechanisms and therapeutic perspectives. Oxid Med Cell Longev. 2011;2011:467180.

[95] Ramsey C, Glass CA, Montgomery MB, Lindl KA, Ritson GP, Chia LA, Hamilton RL, Chu CT, Jordan-Sciutto KL. Expression of Nrf2 in Neurodegenerative Diseases. J Neuropathol Exp Neurol. 2007;66 (1):75-85.

[96] Lipton S. Update on current models of HIV-related neuronal injury: platelet-activating factor, arachidonic acid, and nitric oxide. Adv Neuroimmunol. 1994;4 (3):181-8.

[97] Mondal D, Pradhan L, Ali M, Agrawal KC. HAART drugs induce oxidative stress in human endothelial cells and increase endothelial recruitment of mononuclear cells: exacerbation by inflammatory cytokines and amelioration by antioxidants. Cardiovasc Toxicol. 2004;4 (3):287-302.

[98] Lagathu C, Eustace B, Prot M, Frantz D, Gu Y, Bastard JP, et al. Some HIV antiretrovirals increase oxidative stress and alter chemokine, cytokine or adiponectin production in human adipocytes and macrophages. Antivir Ther. 2007;12 (4):489-500.

[99] Chandra S, Mondal D, Agrawal KC. HIV-1 protease inhibitor induced oxidative stress suppresses glucose stimulated insulin release: protection with thymoquinone. Exp Biol Med (Maywood). 2009 Apr;234 (4):442-53.

[100] Walsh KA, Megyesi JF, Wilson JX, Crukley J, Laubach VE, Hammond RR. Antioxidant protection from HIV-1 gp120-induced neuroglial toxicity. J Neuroinflammation. 2004 May 27;1 (1):8.

[101] Cherry CL, Duncan AJ, Mackie KF, Wesselingh SL, Brew BJ. A Report on the Effect of Commencing Enfuvirtide on Peripheral Neuropathy. AIDS Research and Human Retroviruses. 2008;24 (8):1027-30.

[102] Blas-Garcia A, Apostolova N, Esplugues JV. Oxidative stress and mitochondrial impairment after treatment with anti-HIV drugs: clinical implications. Curr Pharm Des. 2011 Dec 1;17 (36):4076-86.

[103] Hulgan T, Morrow J, D'Aquila RT, Raffanti S, Morgan M, Rebeiro P, et al. Oxidant stress is increased during treatment of human immunodeficiency virus infection. Clin Infect Dis. 2003 Dec 15;37 (12):1711-7.

[104] Mandas A, Iorio EL, Congiu MG, Balestrieri C, Mereu A, Cau D, et al. Oxidative imbalance in HIV-1 infected patients treated with antiretroviral therapy. Journal of biomedicine & biotechnology. 2009;2009:749575.

[105] Calkins M, Johnson DA, Townsend JA, Vargas MR, Dowell JA, Williamson TP, Kraft AD, Lee JM, Li J, Johnson JA. The Nrf2/ARE Pathway as a Potential Therapeutic Target in Neurodegenerative Disease. Antiox Redox Sig. 2009;11 (3):497-508.

[106] Sonnerborg A, Carlin G, Akerlund B, Jarstrand C. Increased production of malondialdehyde in patients with HIV infection. Scand J Infect Dis. 1988;20 (3):287-90.

[107] Moore K, Roberts LJ, 2nd. Measurement of lipid peroxidation. Free radical research. 1998 Jun;28 (6):659-71.

[108] McLemore JL, Beeley P, Thorton K, Morrisroe K, Blackwell W, Dasgupta A. Rapid automated determination of lipid hydroperoxide concentrations and total antioxidant status of serum samples from patients infected with HIV: elevated lipid hydroperoxide concentrations and depleted total antioxidant capacity of serum samples. Am J Clin Pathol. 1998 Mar;109 (3):268-73.

[109] Favier A, Sappey C, Leclerc P, Faure P, Micoud M. Antioxidant status and lipid peroxidation in patients infected with HIV. Chem Biol Interact. 1994 Jun;91 (2-3):165-80.

[110] Allard JP, Aghdassi E, Chau J, Salit I, Walmsley S. Oxidative stress and plasma antioxidant micronutrients in humans with HIV infection. Am J Clin Nutr. 1998 Jan;67 (1):143-7.

[111] Malvy DJ, Richard MJ, Arnaud J, Favier A, Amedee-Manesme O. Relationship of plasma malondialdehyde, vitamin E and antioxidant micronutrients to human immunodeficiency virus-1 seropositivity. Clin Chim Acta. 1994 Jan 14;224 (1):89-94.

[112] Walmsley SL, Winn LM, Harrison ML, Uetrecht JP, Wells PG. Oxidative stress and thiol depletion in plasma and peripheral blood lymphocytes from HIV-infected patients: toxicological and pathological implications. AIDS (London, England). 1997 Nov 15;11 (14):1689-97.

[113] Jareno EJ, Bosch-Morell F, Fernandez-Delgado R, Donat J, Romero FJ. Serum malondialdehyde in HIV seropositive children. Free Radic Biol Med. 1998 Feb;24 (3):503-6.

[114] Repetto M, Reides C, Gomez Carretero ML, Costa M, Griemberg G, Llesuy S. Oxidative stress in blood of HIV infected patients. Clin Chim Acta. 1996 Nov 29;255 (2): 107-17.

[115] Sacktor N, Haughey N, Cutler R, Tamara A, Turchan J, Pardo C, Vargas D, Nath A. Novel markers of oxidative stress in actively progressive HIV dementia. Journal of neuroimmunology. 2004;157:176-84.

[116] Haughey NJ, Cutler RG, Tamara A, McArthur JC, Vargas DL, Pardo CA, et al. Perturbation of sphingolipid metabolism and ceramide production in HIV-dementia. Ann Neurol. 2004 Feb;55 (2):257-67.

[117] Turchan J, Pocernich CB, Gairola C, Chauhan A, Schifitto G, Butterfield DA, Buch S, Narayan O, Sinai A, Geiger J, Berger JR, Elford H, Nath A. Oxidative stress in HIV demented patients and protection ex vivo with novel antioxidants. Neurology. 2003;60:307-14.

[118] Suresh DR, Annam V, Pratibha K, Prasad BV. Total antioxidant capacity--a novel early bio-chemical marker of oxidative stress in HIV infected individuals. J Biomed Sci. 2009;16:61.

[119] Haughey NJ, Steiner J, Nath A, McArthur JC, Sacktor N, Pardo C, et al. Converging roles for sphingolipids and cell stress in the progression of neuro-AIDS. Front Biosci. 2008;13:5120-30.

[120] Droge W, Eck HP, Mihm S. Oxidant-antioxidant status in human immunodeficiency virus infection. Methods Enzymol. 1994;233:594-601.

[121] Ogunro PS, Ogungbamigbe TO, Elemie PO, Egbewale BE, Adewole TA. Plasma selenium concentration and glutathione peroxidase activity in HIV-1/AIDS infected patients: a correlation with the disease progression. Niger Postgrad Med J. 2006 Mar;13 (1):1-5.

[122] Dworkin BM, Rosenthal WS, Wormser GP, Weiss L. Selenium deficiency in the acquired immunodeficiency syndrome. JPEN J Parenter Enteral Nutr. 1986 Jul-Aug;10 (4):405-7.

[123] Sudfeld CR, Wang M, Aboud S, Giovannucci EL, Mugusi FM, Fawzi WW. Vitamin D and HIV Progression among Tanzanian Adults Initiating Antiretroviral Therapy. PLoS ONE. 2012;7 (6):e40036.

[124] Srinivas A, Dias BF. Antioxidants in HIV positive children. Indian J Pediatr. 2008 Apr;75 (4):347-50.

[125] Bilbis LS, Idowu DB, Saidu Y, Lawal M, Njoku CH. Serum levels of antioxidant vitamins and mineral elements of human immunodeficiency virus positive subjects in Sokoto, Nigeria. Ann Afr Med. 2010 Oct-Dec;9 (4):235-9.

[126] Oliveira KF, Cunha DF, Weffort VR. Analysis of serum and supplemented vitamin C and oxidative stress in HIV-infected children and adolescents. J Pediatr (Rio J). 2011 Nov-Dec;87 (6):517-22.

[127] Delmas-Beauvieux MC, Peuchant E, Couchouron A, Constans J, Sergeant C, Simonoff M, et al. The enzymatic antioxidant system in blood and glutathione status in human immunodeficiency virus (HIV)-infected patients: effects of supplementation with selenium or beta-carotene. Am J Clin Nutr. 1996 Jul;64 (1):101-7.

[128] Boven LA, Gomes L, Hery C, Gray F, Verhoef J, Portegies P, et al. Increased peroxynitrite activity in AIDS dementia complex: implications for the neuropathogenesis of HIV-1 infection. J Immunol. (Research Support, Non-U.S. Gov't). 1999 Apr 1;162 (7): 4319-27.

[129] Aukrust P, Svardal AM, Muller F, Lunden B, Berge RK, Ueland PM, et al. Increased levels of oxidized glutathione in CD4+ lymphocytes associated with disturbed intracellular redox balance in human immunodeficiency virus type 1 infection. Blood. 1995 Jul 1;86 (1):258-67.

[130] Buhl R, Jaffe HA, Holroyd KJ, Wells FB, Mastrangeli A, Saltini C, et al. Systemic glutathione deficiency in symptom-free HIV-seropositive individuals. Lancet. 1989 Dec 2;2 (8675):1294-8.

[131] Jaruga P, Jaruga B, Olczak A, Halota W, Olinski R. Oxidative DNA base damage in lymphocytes of HIV-infected drug users. Free radical research. 1999 Sep;31 (3): 197-200.

[132] Roc AC, Ances BM, Chawla S, Korczykowski M, Wolf RL, Kolson DL, et al. Detection of Human Immunodeficiency Virus Induced Inflammation and Oxidative Stress in Lenticular Nuclei With Magnetic Resonance Spectroscopy Despite Antiretroviral Therapy. 2007. p. 1249-57.

[133] Wanchu A, Rana SV, Pallikkuth S, Sachdeva RK. Short communication: oxidative stress in HIV-infected individuals: a cross-sectional study. AIDS Res Hum Retroviruses. 2009 Dec;25 (12):1307-11.

[134] Flourie F, Arab K, Gagnieu MC, Tardy JC, Jeanblanc F, Livrozet JM, et al. (Redox status in HIV+ patients under HAART). Ann Biol Clin (Paris). 2004 Nov-Dec;62 (6): 713-5.

[135] Gil L, Tarinas A, Hernandez D, Riveron BV, Perez D, Tapanes R, et al. Altered oxidative stress indexes related to disease progression marker in human immunodeficiency virus infected patients with antiretroviral therapy. Biomed Pharmacother. 2010 Sep 25.

[136] Ibeh BO, Obidoa O, Nwuke C. Lipid Peroxidation Correlates with HIVmRNA in Serodiscordant Heterosexual HIVpartners of Nigerian Origin. Indian J Clin Biochem. 2011 Jul;26 (3):249-56.

[137] Ibeh BO, Emeka-Nwabunnia IK. Increased oxidative stress condition found in different stages of HIV disease in patients undergoing antiretroviral therapy in Umuahia (Nigeria). Immunopharmacol Immunotoxicol. 2012 Apr 28.

[138] Masia M, Padilla S, Bernal E, Almenar MV, Molina J, Hernandez I, et al. Influence of antiretroviral therapy on oxidative stress and cardiovascular risk: a prospective cross-sectional study in HIV-infected patients. Clin Ther. 2007 Jul;29 (7):1448-55.

[139] Ngondi JL, Oben J, Forkah DM, Etame LH, Mbanya D. The effect of different combination therapies on oxidative stress markers in HIV infected patients in Cameroon. AIDS Res Ther. 2006;3:19.

[140] Hurwitz BE, Klimas NG, Llabre MM, Maher KJ, Skyler JS, Bilsker MS, et al. HIV, metabolic syndrome X, inflammation, oxidative stress, and coronary heart disease risk : role of protease inhibitor exposure. Cardiovasc Toxicol. 2004;4 (3):303-16.

[141] Stephensen CB, Marquis GS, Jacob RA, Kruzich LA, Douglas SD, Wilson CM. Vitamins C and E in adolescents and young adults with HIV infection. Am J Clin Nutr. 2006 Apr;83 (4):870-9.

[142] Stephensen CB, Marquis GS, Douglas SD, Kruzich LA, Wilson CM. Glutathione, glutathione peroxidase, and selenium status in HIV-positive and HIV-negative adolescents and young adults. Am J Clin Nutr. 2007 Jan;85 (1):173-81.

[143] Sundaram M, Saghayam S, Priya B, Venkatesh KK, Balakrishnan P, Shankar EM, et al. Changes in antioxidant profile among HIV-infected individuals on generic highly active antiretroviral therapy in southern India. Int J Infect Dis. 2008 Nov;12 (6):e61-6.

[144] Padmanabhan V, Rai K, Hegde AM, Shetty S. Total antioxidant capacity of saliva in children with HIV. J Clin Pediatr Dent. 2010 Summer;34 (4):347-50.

[145] Awodele O, Olayemi SO, Nwite JA, Adeyemo TA. Investigation of the levels of oxidative stress parameters in HIV and HIV-TB co-infected patients. J Infect Dev Ctries. 2012 Jan;6 (1):79-85.

[146] Paul S, Bogdanov MB, Matson WR, Metakis L, Jacobs J, Beal MF. Urinary 8-hydroxy-2'-deoxyguanosine, a metabolite of oxidized DNA, is not elevated in HIV patients on combination antiretroviral therapy. Free radical research. 2003 May;37 (5): 499-502.

[147] Zhang Y, Wang M, Li H, Zhang H, Shi Y, Wei F, et al. Accumulation of nuclear and mitochondrial DNA damage in the frontal cortex cells of patients with HIV-associated neurocognitive disorders. Brain Res. 2012 Jun 6;1458:1-11.

[148] Edeas MA, Emerit I, Khalfoun Y, Lazizi Y, Cernjavski L, Levy A, et al. Clastogenic factors in plasma of HIV-1 infected patients activate HIV-1 replication in vitro: inhibition by superoxide dismutase. Free Radic Biol Med. 1997;23 (4):571-8.

[149] Kimura T, Kameoka M, Ikuta K. Amplification of superoxide anion generation in phagocytic cells by HIV-1 infection. FEBS letters. 1993 Jul 12;326 (1-3):232-6.

[150] Mollace V, Salvemini D, Riley DP, Muscoli C, Iannone M, Granato T, et al. The contribution of oxidative stress in apoptosis of human-cultured astroglial cells induced by supernatants of HIV-1-infected macrophages. J Leukoc Biol. 2002 Jan;71 (1):65-72.

[151] Bukrinsky MI, Nottet HS, Schmidtmayerova H, Dubrovsky L, Flanagan CR, Mullins ME, et al. Regulation of nitric oxide synthase activity in human immunodeficiency virus type 1 (HIV-1)-infected monocytes: implications for HIV-associated neurological disease. J Exp Med. 1995 Feb 1;181 (2):735-45.

[152] Piette J, Legrand-Poels S. HIV-1 reactivation after an oxidative stress mediated by different reactive oxygen species. Chem Biol Interact. 1994 Jun;91 (2-3):79-89.

[153] Szydlowska K, Tymianski M. Calcium, ischemia and excitotoxicity. Cell Calcium. 2010 Feb;47 (2):122-9.

[154] Jiang ZG, Piggee C, Heyes MP, Murphy C, Quearry B, Bauer M, et al. Glutamate is a mediator of neurotoxicity in secretions of activated HIV-1-infected macrophages. Journal of neuroimmunology. 2001 Jul 2;117 (1-2):97-107.

[155] Erdmann N, Zhao J, Lopez AL, Herek S, Curthoys N, Hexum TD, et al. Glutamate production by HIV-1 infected human macrophage is blocked by the inhibition of glutaminase. J Neurochem. 2007 Jul;102 (2):539-49.

[156] Zhao J, Lopez AL, Erichsen D, Herek S, Cotter RL, Curthoys NP, et al. Mitochondrial glutaminase enhances extracellular glutamate production in HIV-1-infected macrophages: linkage to HIV-1 associated dementia. J Neurochem. 2004 Jan;88 (1):169-80.

[157] Huang Y, Zhao L, Jia B, Wu L, Li Y, Curthoys N, et al. Glutaminase dysregulation in HIV-1-infected human microglia mediates neurotoxicity: relevant to HIV-1-associated neurocognitive disorders. J Neurosci. 2011 Oct 19;31 (42):15195-204.

[158] Banerjee A, Zhang X, Manda KR, Banks WA, Ercal N. HIV proteins (gp120 and Tat) and methamphetamine in oxidative stress-induced damage in the brain: potential role of the thiol antioxidant N-acetylcysteine amide. Free Radic Biol Med. 2010 May 15;48 (10):1388-98.

[159] Price TO, Ercal N, Nakaoke R, Banks WA. HIV-1 viral proteins gp120 and Tat induce oxidative stress in brain endothelial cells. Brain Res. 2005 May 31;1045 (1-2):57-63.

[160] Viviani B, Corsini E, Binaglia M, Galli CL, Marinovich M. Reactive oxygen species generated by glia are responsible for neuron death induced by human immunodeficiency virus-glycoprotein 120 in vitro. Neuroscience. 2001;107 (1):51-8.

[161] Dawson VL, Dawson TM, Uhl GR, Snyder SH. Human immunodeficiency virus type 1 coat protein neurotoxicity mediated by nitric oxide in primary cortical cultures. Proc Natl Acad Sci U S A. 1993 Apr 15;90 (8):3256-9.

[162] Pietraforte D, Tritarelli E, Testa U, Minetti M. gp120 HIV envelope glycoprotein increases the production of nitric oxide in human monocyte-derived macrophages. J Leukoc Biol. 1994 Feb;55 (2):175-82.

[163] Kruman, II, Nath A, Mattson MP. HIV-1 protein Tat induces apoptosis of hippocampal neurons by a mechanism involving caspase activation, calcium overload, and oxidative stress. Exp Neurol. 1998 Dec;154 (2):276-88.

[164] Toborek M, Lee YW, Pu H, Malecki A, Flora G, Garrido R, et al. HIV-Tat protein induces oxidative and inflammatory pathways in brain endothelium. J Neurochem. 2003 Jan;84 (1):169-79.

[165] Israel N, Gougerot-Pocidalo MA. Oxidative stress in human immunodeficiency virus infection. Cell Mol Life Sci. 1997 Dec;53 (11-12):864-70.

[166] Flores SC, Marecki JC, Harper KP, Bose SK, Nelson SK, McCord JM. Tat protein of human immunodeficiency virus type 1 represses expression of manganese superoxide dismutase in HeLa cells. Proc Natl Acad Sci U S A. 1993 Aug 15;90 (16):7632-6.

[167] Aksenov MY, Hasselrot U, Bansal AK, Wu G, Nath A, Anderson C, et al. Oxidative damage induced by the injection of HIV-1 Tat protein in the rat striatum. Neurosci Lett. 2001 Jun 1;305 (1):5-8.

[168] Raidel SM, Haase C, Jansen NR, Russ RB, Sutliff RL, Velsor LW, et al. Targeted myocardial transgenic expression of HIV Tat causes cardiomyopathy and mitochondrial damage. Am J Physiol Heart Circ Physiol. 2002 May;282 (5):H1672-8.

[169] Choi J, Liu RM, Kundu RK, Sangiorgi F, Wu W, Maxson R, et al. Molecular mechanism of decreased glutathione content in human immunodeficiency virus type 1 Tat-transgenic mice. J Biol Chem. 2000 Feb 4;275 (5):3693-8.

[170] Westendorp MO, Shatrov VA, Schulze-Osthoff K, Frank R, Kraft M, Los M, et al. HIV-1 Tat potentiates TNF-induced NF-kappa B activation and cytotoxicity by altering the cellular redox state. The EMBO journal. 1995 Feb 1;14 (3):546-54.

[171] Deshmane SL, Mukerjee R, Fan S, Del Valle L, Michiels C, Sweet T, et al. Activation of the oxidative stress pathway by HIV-1 Vpr leads to induction of hypoxia-inducible factor 1alpha expression. J Biol Chem. 2009 Apr 24;284 (17):11364-73.

[172] Ferrucci A, Nonnemacher MR, Cohen EA, Wigdahl B. Extracellular human immunodeficiency virus type 1 viral protein R causes reductions in astrocytic ATP and glutathione levels compromising the antioxidant reservoir. Virus Res. 2012 Jun 9.

[173] Vidal F, Gutierrez F, Gutierrez M, Olona M, Sanchez V, Mateo G, et al. Pharmacogenetics of adverse effects due to antiretroviral drugs. AIDS reviews. (Research Support, Non-U.S. Gov'tReview). 2010 Jan-Mar;12 (1):15-30.

[174] Zhou H, Gurley EC, Jarujaron S, Ding H, Fang Y, Xu Z, Pandak WM, Hylemon PB. HIV protease inhibitors activate the unfolded protein response and disrupt lipid metabolism in primary hepatocytes. Am J Physiol Gastrointest Liver Physiol. 2006;291:G1071-G80.

[175] Zhou H, Pandak WM, Lyall V, Natarajan R, Hylemon PB. HIV Protease Inhibitors Activate the Unfolded Protein Response in Macrophages: Implication for Atherosclerosis and Cardiovascular Disease. Mol Pharmacol. 2005;68:690-700.

[176] Letendre S, Marquie-Beck J, Capparelli E, Best B, Clifford D, Collier AC, et al. Validation of the CNS Penetration-Effectiveness rank for quantifying antiretroviral penetration into the central nervous system. Arch Neurol. 2008 Jan;65 (1):65-70.

[177] Letendre SL, Ellis RJ, Ances BM, McCutchan JA. Neurologic complications of HIV disease and their treatment. Top HIV Med. 2010 Apr-May;18 (2):45-55.

[178] Tozzi V, Balestra P, Salvatori MF, Vlassi C, Liuzzi G, Giancola ML, et al. Changes in Cognition During Antiretroviral Therapy: Comparison of 2 Different Ranking Systems to Measure Antiretroviral Drug Efficacy on HIV-Associated Neurocognitive Disorders. JAIDS Journal of Acquired Immune Deficiency Syndromes. 2009;52 (1): 56-63 10.1097/QAI.0b013e3181af83d6.

[179] Garvey L, Winston A, Walsh J, Post F, Porter K, Gazzard B, et al. Antiretroviral therapy CNS penetration and HIV-1-associated CNS disease. Neurology. 2011 Feb 22;76 (8):693-700.

[180] Lanoy E, Guiguet M, Bentata M, Rouveix E, Dhiver C, Poizot-Martin I, et al. Survival after neuroAIDS. Neurology. 2011 February 15, 2011;76 (7):644-51.

[181] Marra CM, Zhao Y, Clifford DB, Letendre S, Evans S, Henry K, et al. Impact of combination antiretroviral therapy on cerebrospinal fluid HIV RNA and neurocognitive performance. AIDS (London, England). 2009 Jul 17;23 (11):1359-66.

[182] Smurzynski M, Wu K, Letendre S, Robertson K, Bosch RJ, Clifford DB, et al. Effects of central nervous system antiretroviral penetration on cognitive functioning in the ALLRT cohort. AIDS (London, England). 2011;25 (3):357-65 10.1097/QAD.0b013e32834171f8.

[183] Cysique LA, Vaida F, Letendre S, Gibson S, Cherner M, Woods SP, et al. Dynamics of cognitive change in impaired HIV-positive patients initiating antiretroviral therapy. Neurology. 2009 August 4, 2009;73 (5):342-8.

[184] Marra CM, Zhao Y, Clifford DB, Letendre S, Evans S, Henry K, et al. Impact of combination antiretroviral therapy on cerebrospinal fluid HIV RNA and neurocognitive performance. AIDS. 2009 Jul 17;23(11):1359-66.

[185] Ramirez SH, Potula R, Fan S, Eidem T, Papugani A, Reichenbach N, et al. Methamphetamine disrupts blood-brain barrier function by induction of oxidative stress in brain endothelial cells. J Cereb Blood Flow Metab. 2009 Dec;29 (12):1933-45.

[186] Shiu C, Barbier E, Di Cello F, Choi HJ, Stins M. HIV-1 gp120 as well as alcohol affect blood-brain barrier permeability and stress fiber formation: involvement of reactive oxygen species. Alcohol Clin Exp Res. 2007 Jan;31 (1):130-7.

[187] Qin L, He J, Hanes RN, Pluzarev O, Hong JS, Crews FT. Increased systemic and brain cytokine production and neuroinflammation by endotoxin following ethanol treatment. J Neuroinflammation. 2008;5:10.

[188] Ferraresi R, Troiano L, Roat E, Nemes E, Lugli E, Nasi M, et al. Protective effect of acetyl-L-carnitine against oxidative stress induced by antiretroviral drugs. FEBS letters. 2006 Dec 11;580 (28-29):6612-6.

[189] Manda K, Banerjee A, Banks WA, Ercal N. Highly active antiretroviral therapy drug combination induces oxidative stress and mitochondrial dysfunction in immortalized human blood-brain barrier endothelial cells. Free Rad Biol and Med. 2011;50:801-10.

[190] Brandmann M, Tulpule K, Schmidt MM, Dringen R. The antiretroviral protease inhibitors indinavir and nelfinavir stimulate Mrp1-mediated GSH export from cultured brain astrocytes. J Neurochem. 2012 Jan;120 (1):78-92.

[191] Touzet O, Philips A. Resveratrol protects against protease inhibitor-induced reactive oxygen species production, reticulum stress and lipid raft perturbation. AIDS (London, England). 2010 Jun 19, 2010;24 (10):1437-47.

[192] Lewis W, Gonzalez B, Chomyn A, Papoian T. Zidovudine induces molecular, biochemical, and ultrastructural changes in rat skeletal muscle mitochondria. J Clin Invest. 1992 Apr;89 (4):1354-60.

[193] Gao RY, Mukhopadhyay P, Mohanraj R, Wang H, Horvath B, Yin S, et al. Resveratrol attenuates azidothymidine-induced cardiotoxicity by decreasing mitochondrial reactive oxygen species generation in human cardiomyocytes. Mol Med Report. 2011 Jan-Feb;4 (1):151-5.

[194] de la Asuncion JG, del Olmo ML, Sastre J, Pallardo FV, Vina J. Zidovudine (AZT) causes an oxidation of mitochondrial DNA in mouse liver. Hepatology. 1999 Mar;29 (3):985-7.

[195] de la Asuncion JG, Del Olmo ML, Gomez-Cambronero LG, Sastre J, Pallardo FV, Vina J. AZT induces oxidative damage to cardiac mitochondria: protective effect of vitamins C and E. Life Sci. 2004 Nov 19;76 (1):47-56.

[196] Bialkowska A, Bialkowski K, Gerschenson M, Diwan BA, Jones AB, Olivero OA, et al. Oxidative DNA damage in fetal tissues after transplacental exposure to 3'-azido-3'-deoxythymidine (AZT). Carcinogenesis. 2000 May;21 (5):1059-62.

[197] Yamaguchi T, Katoh I, Kurata S. Azidothymidine causes functional and structural destruction of mitochondria, glutathione deficiency and HIV-1 promoter sensitization. Eur J Biochem. 2002 Jun;269 (11):2782-8.

[198] Velsor LW, Kovacevic M, Goldstein M, Leitner HM, Lewis W, Day BJ. Mitochondrial oxidative stress in human hepatoma cells exposed to stavudine. Toxicol Appl Pharmacol. 2004 Aug 15;199 (1):10-9.

[199] Gerschenson M, Nguyen VT, St Claire MC, Harbaugh SW, Harbaugh JW, Proia LA, et al. Chronic stavudine exposure induces hepatic mitochondrial toxicity in adult Erythrocebus patas monkeys. J Hum Virol. 2001 Nov-Dec;4 (6):335-42.

[200] Opii WO, Sultana R, Abdul HM, Ansari MA, Nath A, Butterfield DA. Oxidative stress and toxicity induced by the nucleoside reverse transcriptase inhibitor (NRTI)--2',3'-dideoxycytidine (ddC): relevance to HIV-dementia. Exp Neurol. 2007 Mar;204 (1):29-38.

[201] Apostolova N, Gomez-Sucerquia LJ, Moran A, Alvarez A, Blas-Garcia A, Esplugues JV. Enhanced oxidative stress and increased mitochondrial mass during efavirenz-induced apoptosis in human hepatic cells. Br J Pharmacol. 2010 Aug;160 (8):2069-84.

[202] Ciccarelli N, Fabbiani M, Di Giambenedetto S, Fanti I, Baldonero E, Bracciale L, et al. Efavirenz associated with cognitive disorders in otherwise asymptomatic HIV-infected patients. Neurology. 2011 Apr 19;76 (16):1403-9.

[203] Chai H, Yan S, Lin P, Lumsden AB, Yao Q, Chen C. Curcumin blocks HIV protease inhibitor ritonavir-induced vascular dysfunction in porcine coronary arteries. J Am Coll Surg. 2005 Jun;200 (6):820-30.

[204] Vincent S, Tourniaire F, El Yazidi CM, Compe E, Manches O, Plannels R, et al. Nelfinavir induces necrosis of 3T3F44-2A adipocytes by oxidative stress. Journal of acquired immune deficiency syndromes (1999). 2004 Dec 15;37 (5):1556-62.

[205] Amatore C, Arbault S, Jaouen G, Koh AC, Leong WK, Top S, et al. Pro-oxidant properties of AZT and other thymidine analogues in macrophages: implication of the azido moiety in oxidative stress. ChemMedChem. 2010 Feb 1;5 (2):296-301.

[206] Jensen BK, Akay C, Lindl KA, Jordan-Sciutto K. Involvement of the Antioxidant response pathway in neuroglial, neuronal, and astrocytic cultures exposed to antiretroviral compounds.. The International Symposium on NeuroVirology; New York, NY, USA. Journal of NeuroVirology2012. p. S51.

[207] Akay C, Cooper M, Odeleye A, Jensen BK, White M, Vassoler F, et al. Antiretroviral Drugs Induce Oxidative Stress and Neuronal Damage in the Central Nervous System. The International Symposium on NeuroVirology; 2012; New York, N.Y., USA: Journal of NeuroVirology; 2012. p. S5.

[208] Li W, Kong A. Molecular Mechanisms of Nrf2-Mediated Antioxidant Response. Molecular Carcinogenesis. 2009;48:91-104.

[209] Shih A, Johnson DA, Wong G, Kraft AD, Jiang L, Erb H, Johnson JA, Murphy TH. Coordinate Regulation of Glutathione Biosynthesis and Release by Nrf2-Expressing Glia Potently Protects Neurons from Oxidative Stress. J Neurosci. 2003;23 (8): 3394-406.

[210] Cross SA, Cook DR, Chi AW, Vance PJ, Kolson LL, Wong BJ, et al. Dimethyl fumarate, an immune modulator and inducer of the antioxidant response, suppresses HIV replication and macrophage-mediated neurotoxicity: a novel candidate for HIV neuroprotection. J Immunol. (Research Support, N.I.H., Extramural). 2011 Nov 15;187 (10):5015-25.

[211] Weakley SM, Jiang J, Lu J, Wang X, Lin PH, Yao Q, et al. Natural antioxidant dihydroxybenzyl alcohol blocks ritonavir-induced endothelial dysfunction in porcine pulmonary arteries and human endothelial cells. Med Sci Monit. 2011 Sep;17 (9):BR235-41.

[212] Meulendyke KA, Pletnikov MV, Engle EL, Tarwater PM, Graham DR, Zink MC. Early minocycline treatment prevents a decrease in striatal dopamine in an SIV model of HIV-associated neurological disease. J Neuroimmune Pharmacol. 2012 Jun;7 (2): 454-64.

[213] Jariwalla RJ, Lalezari J, Cenko D, Mansour SE, Kumar A, Gangapurkar B, et al. Restoration of blood total glutathione status and lymphocyte function following alpha-lipoic acid supplementation in patients with HIV infection. J Altern Complement Med. 2008 Mar;14 (2):139-46.

[214] Batterham M, Gold J, Naidoo D, Lux O, Sadler S, Bridle S, et al. A preliminary open label dose comparison using an antioxidant regimen to determine the effect on viral load and oxidative stress in men with HIV/AIDS. Eur J Clin Nutr. 2001 Feb;55 (2): 107-14.

[215] Kutzing MK, Luo V, Firestein BL. Protection from glutamate-induced excitotoxicity by memantine. Ann Biomed Eng. 2012 May;40 (5):1170-81.

[216] Nagatsu T, Sawada M. Molecular mechanism of the relation of monoamine oxidase B and its inhibitors to Parkinson's disease: possible implications of glial cells. J Neural Transm Suppl. 2006 (71):53-65.

[217] Schifitto G, Yiannoutsos CT, Ernst T, Navia BA, Nath A, Sacktor N, et al. Selegiline and oxidative stress in HIV-associated cognitive impairment. Neurology. 2009 Dec 8;73 (23):1975-81.

[218] Bhaskaran K, Mussini C, Antinori A, Walker AS, Dorrucci M, Sabin C, et al. Changes in the incidence and predictors of human immunodeficiency virus-associated dementia in the era of highly active antiretroviral therapy. Ann Neurol. 2008 Feb;63 (2): 213-21.

[219] Nath A. Human immunodeficiency virus-associated neurocognitive disorder: pathophysiology in relation to drug addiction. Ann N Y Acad Sci. 2010 Feb;1187:122-8.

[220] Cadet J, Krasnova I. Interactions of HIV and methamphetamine: Cellular and molecular mechanisms of toxicity potentiation. Neurotoxicity Research. 2007;12 (3):181-204.

[221] Durazzo TC, Rothlind JC, Cardenas VA, Studholme C, Weiner MW, Meyerhoff DJ. Chronic cigarette smoking and heavy drinking in human immunodeficiency virus: consequences for neurocognition and brain morphology. Alcohol. 2007 Nov;41 (7): 489-501.

[222] Miguez-Burbano MJ, Lewis JE, Moreno J, Fishman J. Cognitive performance and the thymus among HIV-infected subjects receiving HAART. Biologics. 2008 Jun;2 (2): 321-7.

[223] Miguez-Burbano MJ, Nair M, Lewis JE, Fishman J. The role of alcohol on platelets, thymus and cognitive performance among HIV-infected subjects: are they related? Platelets. 2009 Jun;20 (4):260-7.

[224] Winston A, Garvey L, Scotney E, Yerrakalva D, Allsop JM, Thomson EC, et al. Does acute hepatitis C infection affect the central nervous system in HIV-1 infected individuals? J Viral Hepat. 2010 Jun;17 (6):419-26.

[225] Malaspina L, Woods SP, Moore DJ, Depp C, Letendre SL, Jeste D, et al. Successful cognitive aging in persons living with HIV infection. J Neurovirol. Feb;17 (1):110-9.

[226] Mateen FJ, Mills EJ. Aging and HIV-related cognitive loss. Jama. Jul 25;308 (4):349-50.

[227] Deeks SG. Immune dysfunction, inflammation, and accelerated aging in patients on antiretroviral therapy. Top HIV Med. 2009 Sep-Oct;17 (4):118-23.

[228] Xu J, Ikezu T. The comorbidity of HIV-associated neurocognitive disorders and Alzheimer's disease: a foreseeable medical challenge in post-HAART era. J Neuroimmune Pharmacol. 2009 Jun;4 (2):200-12.

[229] Tisch S, Brew B. Parkinsonism in hiv-infected patients on highly active antiretroviral therapy. Neurology. 2009 Aug 4;73 (5):401-3.

[230] Alisky JM. The coming problem of HIV-associated Alzheimer's disease. Medical hypotheses. 2007;69 (5):1140-3.

[231] Holt JL, Kraft-Terry SD, Chang L. Neuroimaging studies of the aging HIV-1-infected brain. J Neurovirol. Aug;18 (4):291-302.

[232] Gannon P, Khan MZ, Kolson DL. Current understanding of HIV-associated neurocognitive disorders pathogenesis. Curr Opin Neurol. Jun;24 (3):275-83.

[233] Anthony ICB, J.E. Neuropathological Findings Associated with Long-Term HAART. In: Paul RS, NC; Valcour, V; Tasima, KT, editor. HIV and the Brain: New Challenges in the Modern Era: Humana Press; 2009. p. 1-19.

[234] Brew BJ, Crowe SM, Landay A, Cysique LA, Guillemin G. Neurodegeneration and ageing in the HAART era. J Neuroimmune Pharmacol. 2009 Jun;4 (2):163-74.

[235] Sacktor N, Lyles RH, Skolasky R, Kleeberger C, Selnes OA, Miller EN, et al. HIV-associated neurologic disease incidence changes:: Multicenter AIDS Cohort Study, 1990-1998. Neurology. 2001 Jan 23;56 (2):257-60.

[236] Martin CP, Fain MJ, Klotz SA. The older HIV-positive adult: a critical review of the medical literature. Am J Med. 2008 Dec;121 (12):1032-7.

[237] Kalayjian RC, Landay A, Pollard RB, Taub DD, Gross BH, Francis IR, et al. Age-related immune dysfunction in health and in human immunodeficiency virus (HIV) disease: association of age and HIV infection with naive CD8+ cell depletion, reduced expression of CD28 on CD8+ cells, and reduced thymic volumes. J Infect Dis. 2003 Jun 15;187 (12):1924-33.

[238] Kirk JB, Goetz MB. Human immunodeficiency virus in an aging population, a complication of success. Journal of the American Geriatrics Society. 2009 Nov;57 (11): 2129-38.

[239] Butt AA, Dascomb KK, DeSalvo KB, Bazzano L, Kissinger PJ, Szerlip HM. Human immunodeficiency virus infection in elderly patients. Southern medical journal. 2001 Apr;94 (4):397-400.

[240] Manfredi R. HIV disease and advanced age: an increasing therapeutic challenge. Drugs & aging. 2002;19 (9):647-69.

[241] Goetz MB, Boscardin WJ, Wiley D, Alkasspooles S. Decreased recovery of CD4 lymphocytes in older HIV-infected patients beginning highly active antiretroviral therapy. AIDS (London, England). 2001 Aug 17;15 (12):1576-9.

[242] Thompson MA, Aberg JA, Cahn P, Montaner JS, Rizzardini G, Telenti A, et al. Antiretroviral treatment of adult HIV infection: 2010 recommendations of the International AIDS Society-USA panel. Jama. Jul 21;304 (3):321-33.

[243] Spengler U. Management of end-stage liver disease in HIV/hepatitis C virus co-infection. Curr Opin HIV AIDS. Nov;6 (6):527-33.

[244] Desquilbet L, Jacobson LP, Fried LP, Phair JP, Jamieson BD, Holloway M, et al. HIV-1 infection is associated with an earlier occurrence of a phenotype related to frailty. The journals of gerontology. 2007 Nov;62 (11):1279-86.

[245] Patel P, Hanson DL, Sullivan PS, Novak RM, Moorman AC, Tong TC, et al. Incidence of types of cancer among HIV-infected persons compared with the general population in the United States, 1992-2003. Ann Intern Med. 2008 May 20;148 (10):728-36.

[246] Zhou H, Pandak WM, Jr., Lyall V, Natarajan R, Hylemon PB. HIV protease inhibitors activate the unfolded protein response in macrophages: implication for atherosclerosis and cardiovascular disease. Molecular pharmacology. 2005 Sep;68 (3):690-700.

[247] Bozzette SA, Ake CF, Tam HK, Chang SW, Louis TA. Cardiovascular and cerebrovascular events in patients treated for human immunodeficiency virus infection. The New England journal of medicine. 2003 Feb 20;348 (8):702-10.

[248] Cherner M, Ellis RJ, Lazzaretto D, Young C, Mindt MR, Atkinson JH, et al. Effects of HIV-1 infection and aging on neurobehavioral functioning: preliminary findings. AIDS (London, England). 2004 Jan 1;18 Suppl 1:S27-34.

[249] Sacktor N, Skolasky R, Selnes OA, Watters M, Poff P, Shiramizu B, et al. Neuropsychological test profile differences between young and old human immunodeficiency virus-positive individuals. J Neurovirol. 2007 Jun;13 (3):203-9.

[250] Chang L, Yakupov R, Nakama H, Stokes B, Ernst T. Antiretroviral treatment is associated with increased attentional load-dependent brain activation in HIV patients. J Neuroimmune Pharmacol. 2008 Jun;3 (2):95-104.

[251] Gongvatana A, Cohen RA, Correia S, Devlin KN, Miles J, Kang H, et al. Clinical contributors to cerebral white matter integrity in HIV-infected individuals. J Neurovirol. Oct;17 (5):477-86.

[252] Towgood KJ, Pitkanen M, Kulasegaram R, Fradera A, Kumar A, Soni S, et al. Mapping the brain in younger and older asymptomatic HIV-1 men: frontal volume changes in the absence of other cortical or diffusion tensor abnormalities. Cortex. Feb;48 (2):230-41.

[253] Ernst T, Chang L. Effect of aging on brain metabolism in antiretroviral-naive HIV patients. AIDS (London, England). 2004 Jan 1;18 Suppl 1:S61-7.

[254] Harezlak J, Buchthal S, Taylor M, Schifitto G, Zhong J, Daar E, et al. Persistence of HIV-associated cognitive impairment, inflammation, and neuronal injury in era of highly active antiretroviral treatment. AIDS (London, England). Mar 13;25 (5):625-33.

[255] Anthony IC, Ramage SN, Carnie FW, Simmonds P, Bell JE. Influence of HAART on HIV-related CNS disease and neuroinflammation. J Neuropathol Exp Neurol. 2005 Jun;64 (6):529-36.

[256] Brew BJ. Evidence for a change in AIDS dementia complex in the era of highly active antiretroviral therapy and the possibility of new forms of AIDS dementia complex. AIDS (London, England). 2004 Jan 1;18 Suppl 1:S75-8.

[257] Anthony IC, Ramage SN, Carnie FW, Simmonds P, Bell JE. Accelerated Tau deposition in the brains of individuals infected with human immunodeficiency virus-1 before and after the advent of highly active anti-retroviral therapy. Acta Neuropathol. 2006 Jun;111 (6):529-38.

[258] Ances BM, Benzinger TL, Christensen JJ, Thomas J, Venkat R, Teshome M, et al. 11C-PiB imaging of human immunodeficiency virus-associated neurocognitive disorder. Arch Neurol. Jan;69 (1):72-7.

[259] Green DA, Masliah E, Vinters HV, Beizai P, Moore DJ, Achim CL. Brain deposition of beta-amyloid is a common pathologic feature in HIV positive patients. AIDS (London, England). 2005 Mar 4;19 (4):407-11.

[260] Rempel HC, Pulliam L. HIV-1 Tat inhibits neprilysin and elevates amyloid beta. AIDS (London, England). 2005 Jan 28;19 (2):127-35.

[261] Brew BJ, Pemberton L, Blennow K, Wallin A, Hagberg L. CSF amyloid beta42 and tau levels correlate with AIDS dementia complex. Neurology. 2005 Nov 8;65 (9): 1490-2.

[262] Esiri MM, Biddolph SC, Morris CS. Prevalence of Alzheimer plaques in AIDS. J Neurol Neurosurg Psychiatry. 1998 Jul;65 (1):29-33.

[263] Cysique LA, Maruff P, Brew BJ. Prevalence and pattern of neuropsychological impairment in human immunodeficiency virus-infected/acquired immunodeficiency syndrome (HIV/AIDS) patients across pre- and post-highly active antiretroviral therapy eras: a combined study of two cohorts. J Neurovirol. 2004 Dec;10 (6):350-7.

[264] Cysique LA, Brew BJ. Neuropsychological functioning and antiretroviral treatment in HIV/AIDS: a review. Neuropsychol Rev. 2009 Jun;19 (2):169-85.

[265] Achim CL, Adame A, Dumaop W, Everall IP, Masliah E. Increased accumulation of intraneuronal amyloid beta in HIV-infected patients. J Neuroimmune Pharmacol. 2009 Jun;4 (2):190-9.

[266] Chen CH, Vazquez-Padua M, Cheng YC. Effect of anti-human immunodeficiency virus nucleoside analogs on mitochondrial DNA and its implication for delayed toxicity. Mol Pharmacol. 1991 May;39 (5):625-8.

[267] Dalakas MC. Peripheral neuropathy and antiretroviral drugs. J Peripher Nerv Syst. 2001 Mar;6 (1):14-20.

[268] Schweinsburg BC, Taylor MJ, Alhassoon OM, Gonzalez R, Brown GG, Ellis RJ, et al. Brain mitochondrial injury in human immunodeficiency virus-seropositive (HIV+) individuals taking nucleoside reverse transcriptase inhibitors. J Neurovirol. 2005 Aug;11 (4):356-64.

[269] Dufer M, Neye Y, Krippeit-Drews P, Drews G. Direct interference of HIV protease inhibitors with pancreatic beta-cell function. Naunyn Schmiedebergs Arch Pharmacol. 2004 Jun;369 (6):583-90.

[270] Zhou H, Gurley EC, Jarujaron S, Ding H, Fang Y, Xu Z, et al. HIV protease inhibitors activate the unfolded protein response and disrupt lipid metabolism in primary hepatocytes. American journal of physiology. 2006 Dec;291 (6):G1071-80.

[271] Schutt M, Zhou J, Meier M, Klein HH. Long-term effects of HIV-1 protease inhibitors on insulin secretion and insulin signaling in INS-1 beta cells. J Endocrinol. 2004 Dec; 183 (3):445-54.

[272] Liang JS, Distler O, Cooper DA, Jamil H, Deckelbaum RJ, Ginsberg HN, et al. HIV protease inhibitors protect apolipoprotein B from degradation by the proteasome: a potential mechanism for protease inhibitor-induced hyperlipidemia. Nat Med. 2001 Dec;7 (12):1327-31.

[273] Schubert M, Gautam D, Surjo D, Ueki K, Baudler S, Schubert D, et al. Role for neuronal insulin resistance in neurodegenerative diseases. Proc Natl Acad Sci U S A. 2004 Mar 2;101 (9):3100-5.

[274] Steen E, Terry BM, Rivera EJ, Cannon JL, Neely TR, Tavares R, et al. Impaired insulin and insulin-like growth factor expression and signaling mechanisms in Alzheimer's disease--is this type 3 diabetes? J Alzheimers Dis. 2005 Feb;7 (1):63-80.

[275] Kroner Z. The relationship between Alzheimer's disease and diabetes: Type 3 diabetes? Altern Med Rev. 2009 Dec;14 (4):373-9.

[276] Moyle G. Mechanisms of HIV and nucleoside reverse transcriptase inhibitor injury to mitochondria. Antivir Ther. 2005;10 Suppl 2:M47-52.

[277] Robertson KR, Smurzynski M, Parsons TD, Wu K, Bosch RJ, Wu J, et al. The prevalence and incidence of neurocognitive impairment in the HAART era. AIDS (London, England). 2007 Sep 12;21 (14):1915-21.

[278] Cook-Easterwood J, Middaugh LD, Griffin WC, 3rd, Khan I, Tyor WR. Highly active antiretroviral therapy of cognitive dysfunction and neuronal abnormalities in SCID mice with HIV encephalitis. Exp Neurol. 2007 Jun;205 (2):506-12.

[279] Heaton RK, Clifford DB, Franklin DR, Jr., Woods SP, Ake C, Vaida F, et al. HIV-associated neurocognitive disorders persist in the era of potent antiretroviral therapy: CHARTER Study. Neurology. 2010;75 (23):2087-96.

[280] Joska JA, Gouse H, Paul RH, Stein DJ, Flisher AJ. Does highly active antiretroviral therapy improve neurocognitive function? A systematic review. J Neurovirol. Mar;16 (2):101-14.

[281] Smurzynski M, Wu K, Letendre S, Robertson K, Bosch RJ, Clifford DB, et al. Effects of central nervous system antiretroviral penetration on cognitive functioning in the ALLRT cohort. AIDS (London, England). Jan 28;25 (3):357-65.

[282] Letendre SL, McCutchan JA, Childers ME, Woods SP, Lazzaretto D, Heaton RK, et al. Enhancing antiretroviral therapy for human immunodeficiency virus cognitive disorders. Ann Neurol. 2004 Sep;56 (3):416-23.

[283] Winston A, Duncombe C, Li PC, Gill JM, Kerr SJ, Puls R, et al. Does choice of combination antiretroviral therapy (cART) alter changes in cerebral function testing after 48 weeks in treatment-naive, HIV-1-infected individuals commencing cART? A randomized, controlled study. Clin Infect Dis. Mar 15;50 (6):920-9.

Section 4

Manifestations of HIV Infection

Chapter 10

Oral Manifestations of HIV

G.A. Agbelusi, O.M. Eweka, K.A. Ùmeizudike and M. Okoh

Additional information is available at the end of the chapter

http://dx.doi.org/10.5772/52941

1. Introduction

Human Immunodeficiency Virus (HIV) was first reported in USA. In June and July of 1981, the CDC published two reports on clusters of young homosexual men who developed opportunistic infections that were chiefly detected in several immunodeficient individuals (CDC, 1993).

Acquired Immunodeficiency Syndrome (AIDS) is a complex of symptoms and infections caused by the HIV virus as it impacts the immune system. It is an acquired infection, not hereditary. AIDS since its appearance in 1981 has spread to become a major cause of premature death and so far a cure has not yet been found. The diagnosis of HIV/AIDS requires a positive HIV antibody test or evidence of HIV infection and the appearance of some very specific conditions/diseases (CDC, 1993).

AIDS is a global pandemic, 33.4 million people are currently living with the disease worldwide, and it has killed an estimated 2.4 million people, including 330,000 children (UNAIDS, 2010). Over three-quarters of these deaths occurred in Sub- Saharan Africa, retarding economic growth and destroying human capital. South Africa has the largest population of HIV patients in the world, followed by Nigeria and India (McNeil, 2007).

Oral lesions have been reported to be early clinical features of HIV infection (Greenspan et al., 1992). These lesions are often indicators of immune suppression and can be used for early testing, diagnosis and management of patients with HIV/AIDS. Oral lesions contribute to patients' morbidity, affecting the psychological and economic functioning of the individual and community (Kaminu et al., 2002).

The overall prevalence of oral manifestations of HIV infection has changed since the advent of Highly Active Anti-Retroviral Therapy (HAART). Several Studies have shown reduction in prevalence of herpes labialis and periodontal diseases along with other lesions to more than 30% after the institution of HAART (Ceballos-Salobrena et al., 1997), and in HIV-associated opportunistic infections (Septowitz, 1998).

2. Literature review

HIV has two primary strains: HIV-1 and HIV-2. HIV-1 is found throughout the world. HIV-2 is found primarily in West Africa, where the virus may have been in circulation since the 1960s–1970s (Beaupre et al., 2006).

Both HIV-1 and HIV-2 have several subtypes. The strains of HIV-1 can be classified into four groups: the "major" group M, the "outlier" group O and two new groups, N and P. These four groups may represent four separate introductions of simian immunodeficiency virus into humans. Within group M there are known to be at least nine genetically distinct subtypes (or clades) of HIV-1. These are subtypes A, B, C, D, F, G, H, J and K (Lihana et al., 2009).

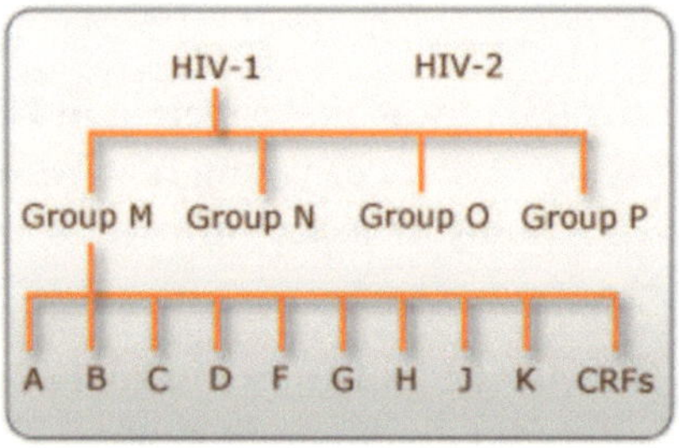

Scheme 1.

2.1. Pathophysiology

Human Immunodeficiency Virus (HIV) mainly affects white blood cells called T-lymphocytes (T-cells) by attaching to a protein on the cell surface called CD4 (Cluster of differentiation 4), it is also expressed on the surface of monocytes, macrophages, and dendritic cells (Miceli, 1993).

HIV gains entry into the body through the blood or mucosal surfaces. The virus establishes itself within the lymphoid tissue, where it replicates and makes itself available to the cells of the immune system (such as T-Lymphocytes, monocytes and macrophages).

The hallmark of HIV disease is the progressive loss of CD4+ lymphocytes. Without intervention, an average of 60 to 80 cells/mm3 is lost every year; this loss is highly variable and occurs in periods of stability and rapid decline. The level of metabolic and mitotic activity of the host CD4 cell is believed to be a factor in the rate at which the disease progresses in individual patients.

With progressive CD4 lymphocyte depletion, immunosuppression becomes increasingly more severe with the emergence of pre-AIDS opportunistic infections. Once the CD4 lymphocyte count falls below 200 cells per ml and the ratio of helper and suppressor cells is reversed, a diagnosis of AIDS is made.

3. Oral manifestations of HIV

3.1. Significance of oral lesions of HIV

Oral lesions have been reported to be early clinical features of HIV infection (Greenspan et al., 1992). They are multiple and varied, and are occasionally the first sign that patients harbour the virus. Studies have estimated that more than 90% of persons with HIV infection will have at least one oral manifestation during the course of their disease (Weinert et al., 1996). These lesions may be present in up to 50% of people with HIV infection and in up to 80% of those with a diagnosis of AIDS (Palmer et al., 1996). In cases where a person's HIV status is unknown the lesions provide a strong indication of the presence of HIV infection (Maeve et al., 2005).

Some of these lesions may have a predictive value, warning of a progression from HIV seropositivity to clinically manifest as AIDS. They are often indicators of immune suppression and can be used for early testing, diagnosis and management of patients with HIV/AIDS (Scully et al., 1991; Arendorf et al., 1998; Agbelusi and Wright, 2005). Oral lesions in HIV may serve as markers for immune deterioration and disease progression and may also indicate poor prognosis (Adurogbangba et al., 2004).

They can therefore be used as an entry or end-point in therapy and vaccine trials and can be determinants of opportunistic infection and anti- HIV therapy, staging and classification systems

Oral lesions contribute to patients' morbidity, affecting the psychological and economic functioning of the individual and community (Kaminu et al., 2002). The pain of oral lesions can lead to increased morbidity. In cases like herpes zoster of the trigeminal nerve or facial nerve palsy facial aesthetics may be compromised. Some of the oral lesions have a fatal outcome e.g. Kaposi's sarcoma. Therefore, it is important to perform oral examinations routinely in the dental and medical settings (Patel et al., 2003), in those affected with HIV and patients at risk of the disease (Maeve et al., 2005).

Predisposing factors to expression of oral lesions of AIDS include CD4 counts less than 200 cells/mm^3, viral load greater than 3000 copies/ml, xerostomia, poor oral hygiene and smoking (Greenspan et al., 2001).

3.2. Epidemiology of oral lesions of HIV

Several studies done worldwide showed varying reports of oral lesions from 40% to 93% (Mirowsky et al., 1998; Ramirez – Amardor et al., 1998; Ranganathan et al., 2000; Matee et al., 2000; Campisi et al., 2002). The prevalence of oral lesions seen in a German study showed 39% (Schmidt- Westhaunsen et al., 1997), in South Africa, 73% was reported by Kaminu and Naidoo (2002). Nigerian reports also showed a prevalence of 36.4% - 84% in various studies done in the different geopolitical zones. (Onunu et al., 2002, Anteyi et al., 2003, Wright et al., 2005; Taiwo et al., 2005; Taiwo et al., 2006; Arotiba et al., 2006; Adedigba et al., 2008).

All studies carried out showed presence of oral lesions as a manifestation of HIV/AIDS infection.

3.3. Importance of oral lesions of HIV for the dental profession

The overall growth of the global AIDS epidemic appears to have stabilized, the annual number of new HIV infections has been steadily declining since the late 1990s and there are fewer AIDS-related deaths due to the significant scale up of antiretroviral therapy over the past few years. Although the number of new infections has been falling, levels of new infections overall are still high, and with significant reductions in mortality, the number of people living with HIV (PLWA) worldwide has increased (UNAIDS, 2010). This increase in the number of PLWA translates to the fact that the likelihood of an oral health care worker particularly the dentist treating a PLWA in high incidence areas is almost certain, therefore the dental team needs to be more involved in the prevention of spread and care of infected persons.

It is also important to note that the clinical problem of HIV infection poses one of the greatest challenges to Health Care Workers all over the world.

Some oral lesions of HIV/AIDS are ulcerative and painful, and so compromise the patients' ability to eat and swallow, subsequently leading to malnutrition and emaciation which worsens the already immunocompromized state. Hence prompt and early treatment of lesions is required.

The mode of spread of HIV also poses special danger to HCW particularly the dentist who works in an environment contaminated with blood, saliva and other body fluids and has close contact with his patients.

The dentist may possibly be the first health care provider to diagnose the condition from a high index of suspicion and results of diagnostic investigations prompted by the head/neck and oral manifestations (Agbelusi and Wright, 2005). Dentists should have a good knowledge of oral lesions in HIV /AIDS and be able to recognize and accurately diagnose such lesions. Early treatment of oral lesions is also necessary to reduce morbidity and mortality in HIV-infected patients. The need to maintain oral health to prevent complications like microbial infections which may be fatal in these patients cannot be over-emphasized.

Currently, viral load and CD_4 status determination are used to initiate and monitor a patient's treatment. Diagnostic tests such as these place a greater responsibility on the dental practice team as they need to be aware of drug changes, new drugs and appropriate management of such patients. Some of the antiviral drugs may also have oral lesions as side effects.

3.4. Classification of oral lesions of HIV

Oral mucosal lesions are part of the clinical criteria in a number of HIV/AIDS classification systems currently in use. This classification can be based on the etiological factors or the strength of association. EC-Clearinghouse on Oral Problems Related to HIV Infection and

http://dx.doi.org/10.5772/52941

WHO Collaboration centre on oral manifestations of the Human Immunodeficiency Virus uses strength of association of Oral lesions with HIV infection as basis for classification (ECC/WHO, 1993)

GROUP 1: Lesions Strongly Associated with HIV infection:
Candidiasis:
Pseudomembraneous candidiasis
Erythematous candidiasis
Angular cheilitis
Hairy leukoplakia
Kaposi's sarcoma
Non- Hodgkins lymphoma
Periodontal diseases
Linear gingival erythema (LGE)
Necrotizing (ulcerative) gingivitis (NUG)
Necrotizing (ulcerative) Periodontitis (NUP)
GROUP 2: Lesions Less Commonly Associated with HIV Infection
Bacterial infections
Mycobacterium avium intra-cellulare
Mycobacterium tuberculosis
Melanotic hyperpigmentation
Necrotic (ulcerative) stomatitis
Salivary gland diseases
Xerostomia due to decreased salivary flow rate
Unilateral or Bilateral swelling of major salivary glands
Thrombocytopaenic purpura
Ulceration NOS (Not-otherwise specified)
Viral infections:
Herpes simplex virus
Human papilloma virus (HPV)
Condyloma acuminatum
Focal epithelial hyperplasia
Verruca vulgaris
Varicella zoster
Herpes zoster

3.5. Clinical characteristics and diagnosis of oral lesions of HIV

3.5.1. Oral candidiasis

This is the most common intra-oral lesion seen among HIV infected individuals. In African studies, the prevalence ranged from 15% to more than 80% in HIV+ adults. The most common organism involved with the presentation of candidiasis is *Candida albicans*. The presence of oral Candida was associated with a *CD4 count of <200 cells/microl,* cigarette smoking and heroine/methadone use (Greenspan et al., 2000). The most common organism involved with the presentation of candidiasis is *Candida albicans,* but other non- albicans species, such as *C. glabrata, C. tropicalis, C. krusei* and *C. dublinieusis* can also cause the disease.

There are 3 frequently observed forms of oral candidiasis:

- Pseudomembraneous candidiasis
- Erythematous candidiasis
- Angular Cheilitis

3.5.1.1. Pseudomembraneous candidiasis

It appears as creamy white curd-like plaques on the buccal mucosa, tongue and other oral mucosal surfaces (palate, lips etc.) that can be wiped away, leaving a red or bleeding underlying surface. The plaques consist of a mixture of fungal hyphae, desquamated epithelium, and inflammatory cells. These plaques can appear anywhere on the oral and pharyngeal mucosa.

Diagnosis: In most clinical conditions, the presumptive diagnosis of oral candidiasis is made based on the typical clinical appearance. In this situation, the presumptive diagnosis is strengthened if the patient responds to an empirical trial of anti-fungal therapy.

When the clinical diagnosis of oral candidiasis is not clear, the diagnosis can be confirmed by obtaining a direct smear and performing either a *Potassium Hydroxide* (KOH) wet mount or *a Gram's stain* (Greenspan et al., 1992). The KOH wet mount typically shows presence of yeasts or pseudo-hyphae, and the gram stain shows gram- positive staining organisms that are much larger than bacteria. Obtaining oral fungal cultures is generally reserved for situations when patients do not respond to therapy and anti-fungal resistance is suspected.

The pseudomembraneous variant was associated with severe immune suppression in several studies where these clinical parameters were available (Schoidt et al., 1990; Tukutuku et al., 1990; Hodgson, 1997; Ranganathan et al., 2000). As with other causes of oral candidiasis, recurrences are common if the underlying problem persists.

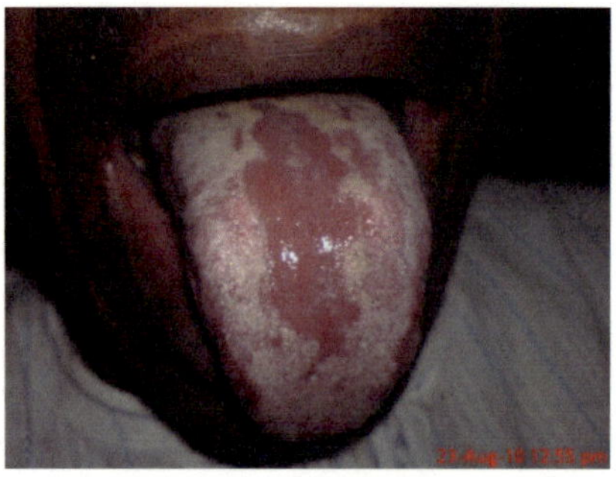

Figure 1. Pseudomembranous and erythematous candidiasis on the dorsum of the tongue

http://dx.doi.org/10.5772/52941

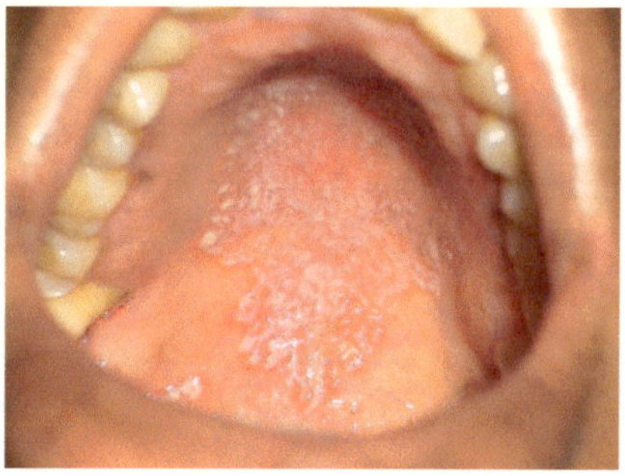

Figure 2. Pseudomembranous candidiasis on the palate

3.5.1.2. Erythematous candidiasis

This appears as a red lesion commonly located on the palate, dorsum of the tongue (as areas of depapillation) and buccal mucosa. The lesions tend to be symptomatic with patients complaining of burning mouth and change of taste, most frequently while eating salty or spicy foods or drinking acidic beverages.

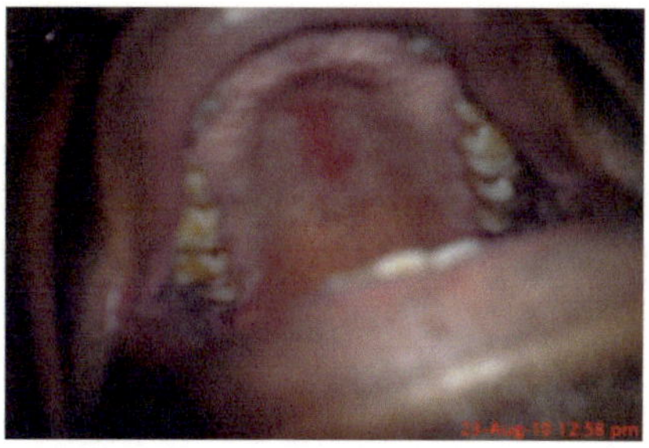

Figure 3. Erythematous candidiasis on the palate

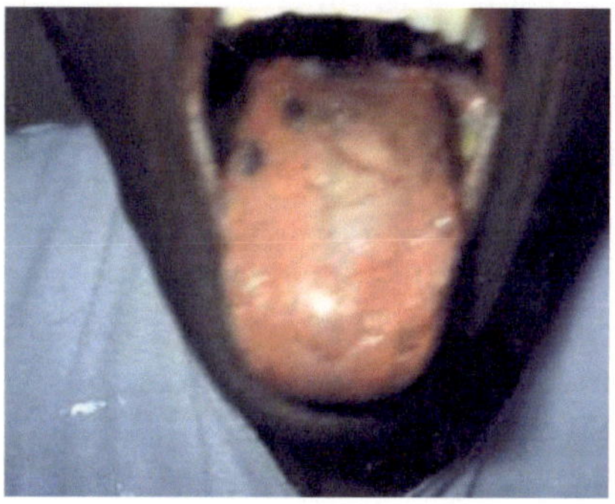

Figure 4. Erythematous candidiasis on the tongue and angular cheilitis on the lips.

3.5.1.3. Angular cheilitis

Presents as fissures or linear ulcers at the corners (commissures) of the mouth and often associated with small white plaques, could be unilateral or bilateral. It can occur with or without the presence of erythematous candidiasis or pseudomembranous candidiasis. Angular cheilitis can also exist for an extensive period of time if left untreated.

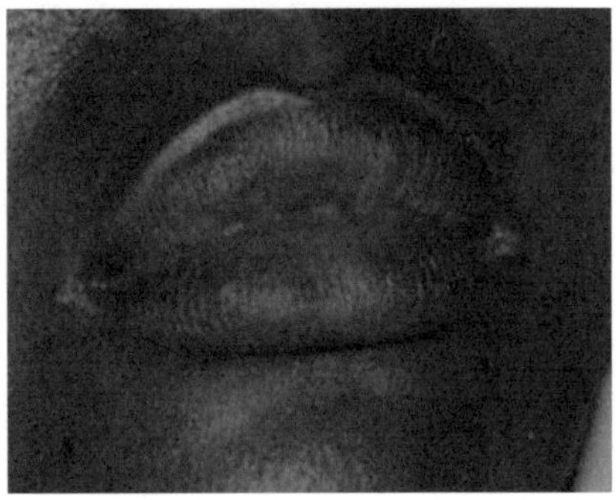

Figure 5. Angular cheilits

3.5.2. Periodontal diseases

Since the first descriptions of the HIV in 1981, a considerable number of researches have focused on the periodontal changes specifically associated with HIV infection. Earlier reports included unusual and severe forms of periodontal disease in HIV-infected individuals, particularly among homosexual males. These lesions ranged from severe gingivitis to advanced, painful periodontitis characterized by spontaneous bleeding, bone exposure and frequently bone sequestration followed by the exfoliation of several teeth (Silverman et al., 1986; Winkler et al., 1988). An increased incidence of acute necrotizing ulcerative gingivitis (ANUG) was also reported in HIV-seropositive patients (Schiodt & Pindborg, 1987; Gornitsky & Pekovie, 1987).

HIV-associated periodontal diseases were initially classified into four broad categories: HIV-associated gingivitis (HIV-G) (Winkler et al., 1988), HIV-associated periodontitis (HIV-P), ANUG and necrotizing stomatitis (NS) (Greenspan et al., 1990). Later classifications proposed that the term 'HIV-associated' be dropped in relation to periodontal disease because the conditions were also seen in non-HIV infected populations (Smith et al., 1993).

HIV-G is now known as linear gingival erythema (LGE), while HIV-P is referred to as necrotizing ulcerative periodontitis (NUP). Currently, the spectrum of periodontal diseases associated with HIV includes linear gingival erythema, necrotizing diseases (NUG and NUP), and exarcabated chronic periodontitis. LGE, necrotizing ulcerative gingivitis (NUG) and NUP are classified under lesions strongly associated with HIV infection ((ECC/WHO, 1993; Armitage, 1999; Winkler et al., 1988). The exacerbated periodontitis described in HIV infected patients is however not clinically distinguishable from that occurring in non-HIV-infected populations (Robinson et al., 2002).

http://dx.doi.org/10.5772/52941

Periodontal diseases associated with HIV infection along with some other oral lesions have important diagnostic values as they may alert the dentist to the presence of HIV infection (ECC/WHO,1993; Robinson et al., 2002). Their prognostic significance is due to their ability to predict a deteriorating immune status and progression from HIV to AIDS (Robinson et al., 1998; Soubry et al., 1995; Glick et al., 1994a; Glick et al., 1994b). Soubry et al (1995) evaluated 224 people with necrotizing periodontal disease. Overall, 81% were found to be HIV positive. When compared with the general population in their environment, the HIV prevalence was only 30% which was much lower.

3.5.2.1. Linear gingival erythema

This periodontal lesion presents as a persistent, distinct, intense, fiery red band extending 2-3mm apically from the free gingival margin. The erythema may be limited to the marginal tissue, the attached gingiva in a punctate or diffuse form, or could extend into the alveolar mucosa. These erythematous changes are usually generalized but may be confined to few teeth. Unlike conventional marginal gingivitis, the associated teeth usually have little or no plaque formation (Narani & Epstein, 2001) thus regarded as a non-plaque induced gingivitis, particularly as the degree of erythema is disproportionately intense to the amount of plaque seen (Holmstrup & Westergaard, 1998). The gingiva bleeds easily on tooth brushing or gentle probing or even spontaneously in some cases (Robinson et al., 2002). No ulceration is however present. LGE is commonly first seen earlier in the course of HIV infection and may or may not serve as a precursor to necrotizing ulcerative periodontitis (Glick & Holmstrup, 2000).

Studies have revealed a microbiota comprising *Candida albicans, Porphyromonas gingivalis, Prevotella intermedia, Actinobacillus actinomycetemcomitans, Fusobucterium nucleatum* and *Campylobacter rectus* (Murray et al., 1989; Murray et al., 1991). This microflora is consistent with that of conventional periodontitis. The Candida species isolated from some LGE lesions, suggests its possible aetiologic role (Lamster et al., 1994; Velegraki et al., 1999; Grbic et al., 1995). LGE has been classified under 'Gingival diseases of fungal origin', a separate periodontal disease entity at the 1999 International workshop for a Classification of Periodontal diseases and conditions (Armitage, 1999).

The use of tobacco has been reported to affect the extent of gingival banding which is measured by the number of affected sites (Swango et al., 1991). The relationship of LGE to severe immune suppression is variable. This condition may (Ceballos et al., 1996; Holmes et al., 2002) or may not be associated with CD4 counts < 200 cells/mm^3 (Grbic et al., 1995; Davoodi et al., 2010).

A major clinical hallmark of LGE is its non-responsiveness to conventional scaling and root planing. The differential diagnosis is conventional chronic gingivitis, a plaque-induced gingival condition which responds to conventional periodontal therapy.

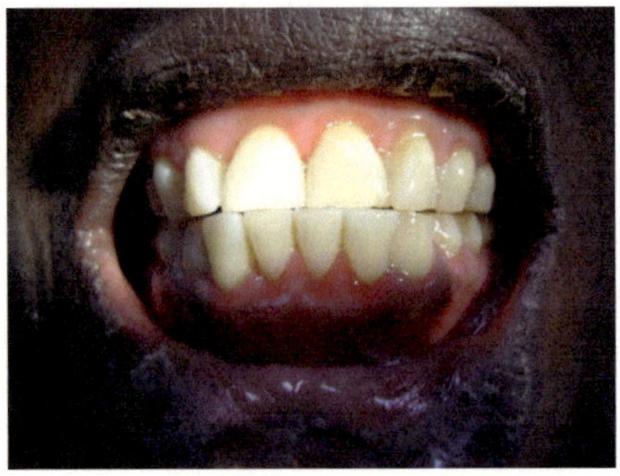

Figure 6. Linear gingival erythema

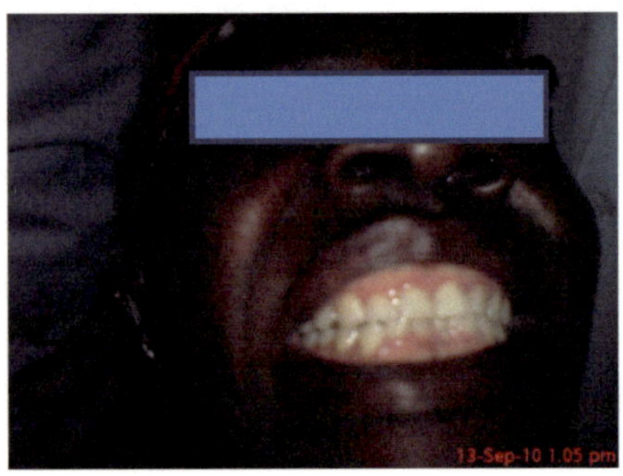

Figure 7. Linear gingival erythema in an anaemic patient

3.5.2.2. Necrotizing ulcerative gingivitis

Necrotizing ulcerative gingivitis (NUG) is defined using the presumptive diagnostic criterion (ECC/WHO, 1993) as the destruction of one or more interdental papillae. In the acute stage of the disease, ulceration, necrosis and sloughing may be accompanied by hemorrhage and a characteristic fetor. The affected gingiva may be extremely painful or asymptomatic (Robinson et al., 1998). The anterior and lower teeth are often affected (Robinson et al., 1998). The gingival ulceration may be limited to single tooth or extend to several areas of the jaws. The clinical description of NUG is only limited to lesions involving the gingiva without any loss of periodontal attachment. NUG in HIV-associated lesions represents the same spectrum of acute necrotizing ulcerative gingivitis (ANUG) seen in patients without HIV infection but in HIV-infected individuals it progresses more rapidly (Winkler and Murray, 1987). Some of the organisms isolated from NUG lesions include Borrelia, gram-positive cocci, β-hemolytic streptococci and *Candida albicans* (Reichart et al., 1987). NUG has been associated with depleted CD4 lymphocyte counts in some studies (Ceballos et al., 1996). However, others have failed to establish this association (Barr et al., 1992).

http://dx.doi.org/10.5772/52941

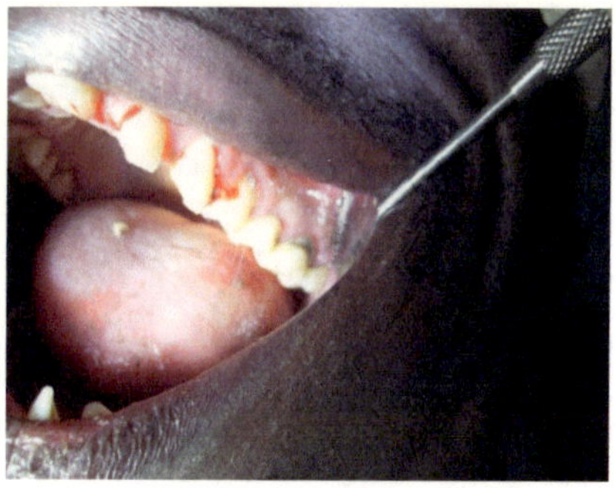

Figure 8. Necrotizing ulcerative gingivitis

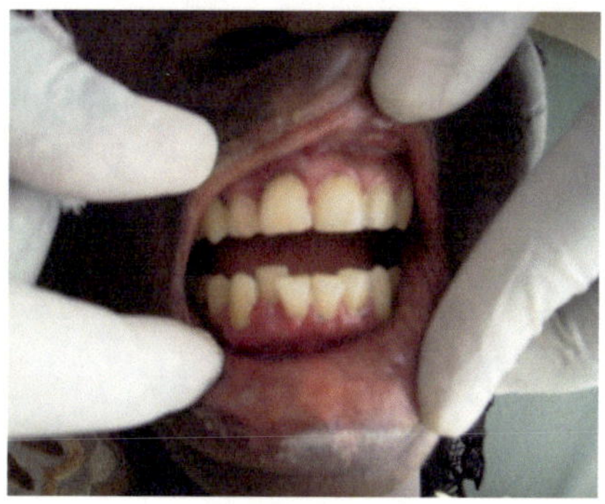

Figure 9. Necrotizing ulcerative gingivitis

3.5.2.3. Necrotizing ulcerative periodontitis

Necrotizing ulcerative periodontitis (NUP) may be an extension of NUG in HIV infected individuals. It is characterized by soft tissue loss resulting from ulceration or necrosis with rapid destruction of the periodontal attachment and interproximal bone (EC-WHO 93, Winkler & Robertson, 1992). Initially, the lesion manifests with severe, deep-seated jaw pain, interproximal necrosis and cratering. This severe pain is however not a consistent feature (Robinson et al., 1998; Masouredis et al., 1992). The bone may then be exposed, with subsequent necrosis and sequestration, resulting in loosening of the teeth (Umeizudike et al., 2011a). There is thus radiographic evidence of bone loss. Few teeth are affected in most cases in either the premolar or molar region, but the lesion may be more generalized in severe NUP cases. A characteristic fetor oris is usually present. Deep pockets are not a characteristic feature of NUP because of the extensive gingival necrosis which often coincides with loss of alveolar bone. The lesion may bleed on probing with 50% of sites bleeding spontaneously (Winkler & Robertson, 1992). Most studies report a similar microbial component in both NUP lesions associated with HIV and conventional chronic periodontitis (Glick et al., 1994b; Murray et al., 1989; Murray et al., 1991). Human herpes-viruses such as cytomegalovirus have however been identified in some NUP lesions (Slot, 2004). Homosexuals and bisexual men appear to have a higher incidence of NUP compared to other cohorts of HIV positive individuals (Glick et al., 1994b). Several studies reveal an association between NUP and HIV progression (Masouredis et al., 1992; Winkler et al., 1988). NUP has also been reported to be one of the strongest predictors of severe immune suppression, characterized by low CD4 lymphocyte counts (Glick et al., 1994a; Glick et al., 1994b). Patients with NUP may however, have CD4 counts above 200 cells/mm^3, indicating that other factors such as high viral loads may be associated (Umeizudike et al., 2011a).

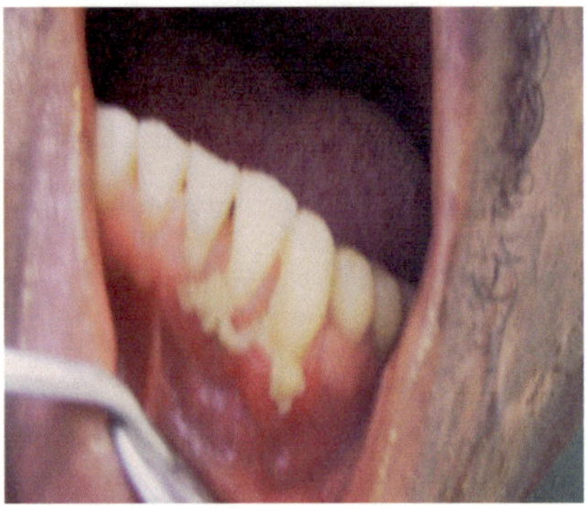

Figure 10. Necrotizing ulcerative periodontitis with sequestrum,

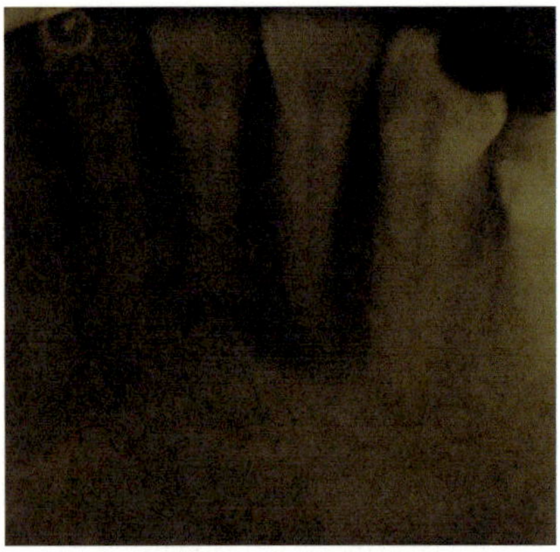

Figure 11. Radiograph of NUP showing extensive bone loss around 22.

3.5.2.4. Necrotizing ulcerative stomatitis

This is a rare condition in HIV positive patients. It is characterized by a localized, acutely painful rapidly destructive lesion which is ulcerative and necrotic. The lesion may extend from the gingiva into the adjacent oral mucosa, resulting in extensive destruction of the underlying soft tissues and osseous tissues. It may occur as a separate condition or be an extension of NUP. The condition may lead to extensive denudation and eventual sequestration of bone (Williams et al., 1990). The condition is often associated with severe immune suppression with low CD4 lymphocyte counts. This condition is similar to the cancrum oris (noma) a rare destructive condition described in nutritionally deprived individuals particularly children in Africa which progresses from ANUG (Osuji, 1990). Studies carried out by various individuals all around Nigeria did not show the presence of the disease, though the condition was seen in Lagos University Teaching Hospital in a previously undiagnosed HIV seropositive patient (Agbelusi and Eweka, 2011).

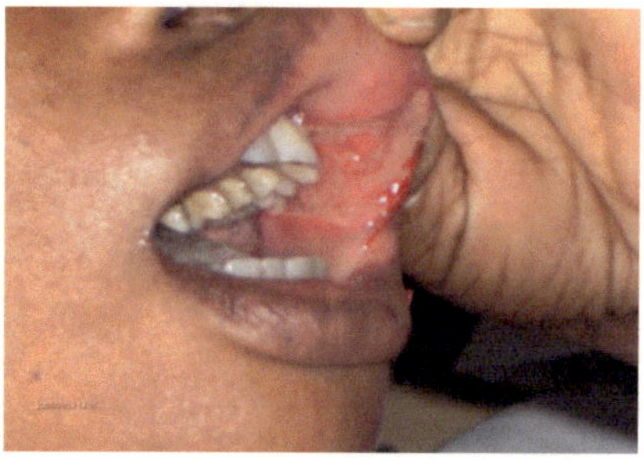

Figure 12. Necrotizing ulcerative stomatitis

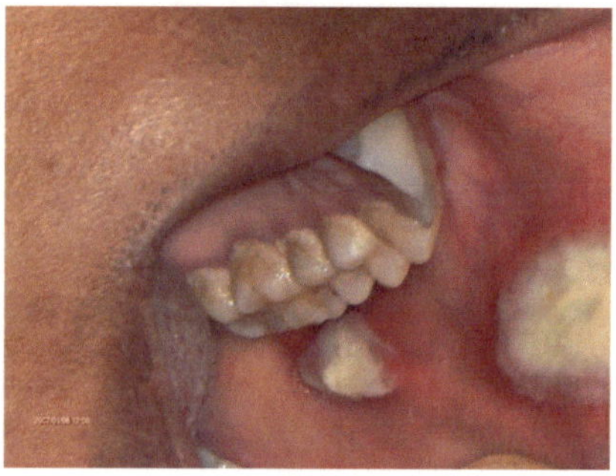

Figure 13. Necrotizing ulcerative stomatitis

3.5.2.5. Chronic periodontitis with an increased rate of attachment loss

Rapid periodontal pocket formation has been reported in HIV infection in some controlled studies (Barr et al., 1992; Yeung et al., 1993; Robinson et al., 1996; Ndiaye et al., 1997; Ranganathan et al., 2007; Umeizudike et al., 2011b). Although, this is not a consistent finding (Scheutz et al., 1997).This accelerated periodontal attachment loss reported in HIV infected individuals could be the result of severe episodes of NUP. The clinical presentation of gingivitis and chronic periodontitis in HIV-positive individuals is the same as that occurring in non HIV infected populations. It is characterized by the rapid destruction of the periodontal tissues characterized by rapid pocket formation and attachment loss. Radiographic features with evidence of alveolar bone loss are evident. The risk factors for periodontitis in HIV positive patients include age, smoking pack-years, high viral load, *Fusobacterium nucleatum, Prevotella intermedia, Actinobacillus actinomycetemcomitans,* neutrophil elastase and β-glucuronidase (Alpagot et al., 2004).

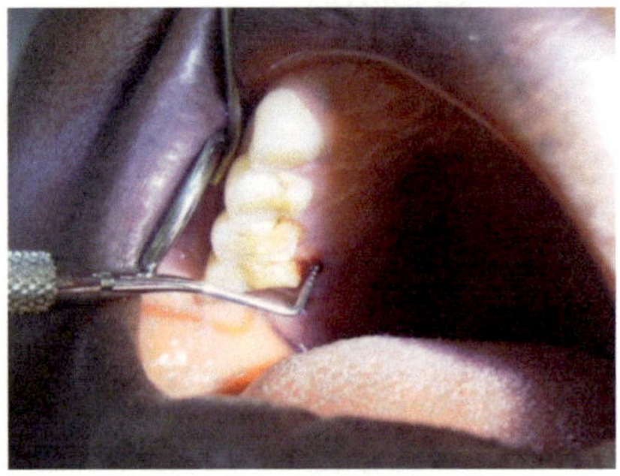

Figure 14. Deep periodontal pocket around tooth 16.

3.5.3. Oral Hairy Leukoplakia: (OHL)

This lesion usually presents as asymptomatic, white, vertical, corrugated, hair-like projections on the lateral borders of the tongue (bilaterally or unilaterally). It can spread to the dorsum of the tongue and on the ventral aspect to the floor of the mouth and occasionally on the adjacent buccal mucosa, when seen in these areas it is smooth and velvety not hair-like. Unlike candidiasis the lesion cannot be wiped off the mucosal surface (ECC/WHO, 1993).

OHL was seen and investigated in 1981 by Greenspan et al., who published the initial report of its existence among homosexual men in San Francisco in 1984 (Greenspan et al.,1984).

It is slightly less common in women than in men, and it is also rare in children. In HIV positive persons OHL heralds more rapid progressions of AIDS (Greenspan et al., 1984; Glick et al., 1994; Lifson et al., 1994).

The incidence of OHL is reported to be 20% in CDC II individuals, increasing as CD4 count falls and patient's clinical condition deteriorates (Glick et al., 1994; Lifson et al., 1994). It also appears during the late latency stages of HIV infection. Although the studies carried out by Greenspan et al in 2000, showed that the presence of OHL was not related to CD4 count but was associated with high viral load.

OHL prevalence rates ranged from 0% amongst Tanzanians (Schiodt et al., 1990) to 20% in Cape Town (Arendorf et al., 1998).

Although originally postulated to be pathognomonic for HIV infection, this lesion has subsequently been reported in other immune deficiency states as well as in immunocompetent individuals (Sirois, 1998) e.g. among organ or bone marrow recipients and those receiving long-term steroid therapy (King et al., 1994).

http://dx.doi.org/10.5772/52941

The frequency of OHL is about 20% in those with otherwise symptom- free HIV infection and increases as the CD4 count falls and the clinical condition deteriorates (Aragues et al., 1990; Feigel et al., 1991; Glick et al., 1994; Lifson et al., 1994).

Considerable research have provided a body of evidence that the *Epstein Barr virus (EBV)* is the likely cause of this lesion, which should probably now be renamed according to its aetiology as *"EBV Leukoplakia"* (Greenspan et al., 1984; Iain et al., 2000).

Histologic features of OHL shows surface corrugation, thickening of the prickle- cell layer (acanthosis) with groups or layers of ballooning cells similar to koilocytes, absence of atypia and other features of dysplasia, lack of inflammatory cells infilteration in the epithelium or adjoining connective tissues (Greenspan et al., 1984). These features are not pathognomic of OHL. Evidence of presence of EBV is required for definitive diagnosis of OHL, although presumptive diagnosis can be made on clinical appearance alone and non-response to antifungal drugs. (ECC/WHO, 1993).

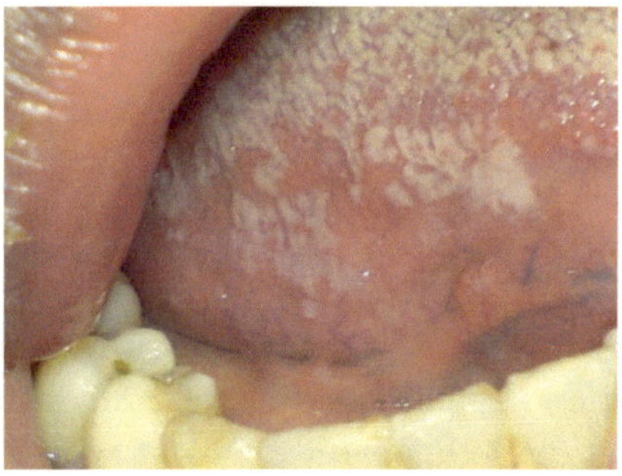

Figure 15. Hairy leukoplakia

3.5.4. Kaposi's sarcoma

This is the most common malignancy encountered in HIV/AIDS patients (Iain et al., 2000). Kaposi's sarcoma-associated herpes virus (KSHV)/Human Herpes Virus-8 (HHV-8) is the causative agent of the endothelial cell-derived tumour Kaposi's sarcoma (Sturzl et al., 2009). The lesions are commonly seen in homosexual men. The lesions are characterized by reddish, bluish or purple, single or multiple macules or nodules. These are seen on the palate or gingivae and may ulcerate, gingival involvement may lead to underlying bone destruction and tooth mobility (Iain et al., 1992). Twenty two percent of the lesions are present intraorally, with 45% of patients presenting with both skin and oral lesions (Tappero et al., 1993).

Biopsy is essential for a definitive diagnosis. It is considered pathognomonic of HIV infections.

There is evidence that oral Kaposi's sarcoma lesions are associated with patients who have lower CD4 counts than those with the skin lesions alone. (Iain et al., 2000)

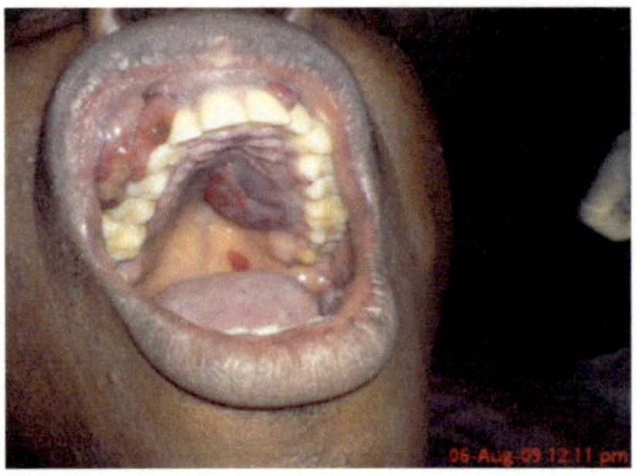

Figure 16. Kaposi's sarcoma on the palate and gingiva

3.5.5. Non- Hogdkin's Lymphoma (NHL)

This is an uncommon feature of HIV disease. It is however, the second most common malignancy in this condition, with 4% of patients developing NHL during the course of their disease (Iain et al., 2000).

NHL of the oral cavity accounts for 3% of all malignant lymphomas, which tends to occur extranodally (Epstein et al., 1992).

Characteristically, oral tumours involve the fauces and gingivae but atypically may involve other sites such as the tongue (Borring et al., 1985).

It often clinically presents as a rapidly enlarging mass with associated bony destruction. Though the presentation varies, the pathogenesis of NHL remains obscure, but there has been much interest in the role of the Epstein Barr virus, with 50% of AIDS related tumours demonstrating EBV genomes and also aetiologic role of Human Herpes Virus-8 (HHV-8) (Boshoff et al., 1997). Survival rates are low and biopsy is essential for definitive diagnosis.

3.5.6. Oral ulcers

Around 50% of AIDS patients present with oral ulcerations during the course of their disease. Recurrent aphthous ulcers (RAU) can be classified as **Minor aphthous Ulcers (MiAU) and Major Aphthous ulcers (MjAU).**

MiAU: Occur in non- keratinized mucosa and their frequency in AIDS patients is not any different from that in the general population. RAU have a prolonged course in AIDS patients as well as being more painful and difficult to treat. These ulcers are shallow in appearance, about 2-5mm in diameter, are generally covered with a whitish pseudomembrane and surrounded by an erythematous halo.

MjAU: Are generally seen in AIDS patients with severe immunodepression (median CD4 T-lymphocyte count 100 cells/mm^3or below) (Ramos-Gomez, 1997). These larger ulcers develop generally on the lateral border of the tongue, soft palate, floor of the mouth, buccal mucosa and oropharynx (occurring on both keratinized and non-keratinized surfaces). They are crater-like in appearance with elevated borders and covered with a white-yellowish

http://dx.doi.org/10.5772/52941

pseudomembrane, measuring over 1cm in diameter. These lesions are very painful and may persist for months causing difficulty in swallowing and impairment of speech and mastication. Generally, an erythematous halo can be seen surrounding the ulcer and may be accompanied by regional lymphadenopathy.

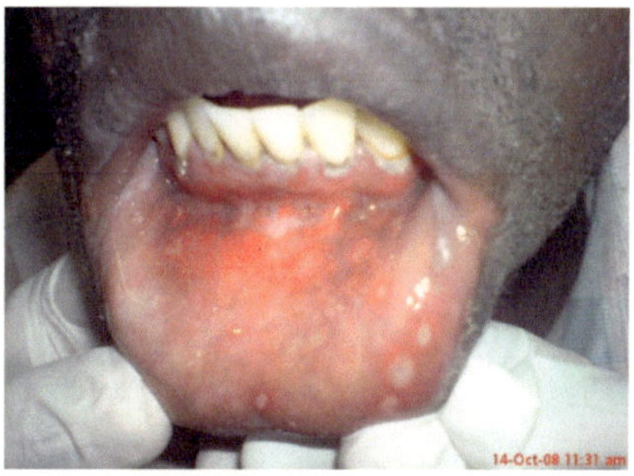

Figure 17. Minor apthous ulcers.

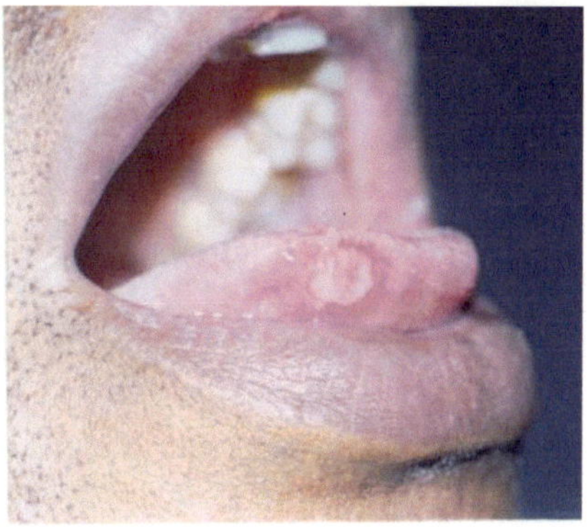

Figure 18. Major apthous ulcer.

3.5.7. *Salivary gland diseases*

Salivary gland diseases such as enlargement of the major salivary glands and xerostomia, was reported to be high in Northern Africa and Thailand (Nittayananta and Chungpanich, 1997). Malnutrition, especially in Northern Africa may play a role.

Enlargement of the salivary glands due to infilteration by CD8 lymphocytes is seen in both adult and paediatric HIV infection (Schoidt et al., 1989). Some of these glands undergo cystic change, and such benign lymphoepithelial cysts occasionally cause pain. The cause of HIV-related salivary gland diseases is unclear, for no etiological agents have been identified. It can represent a relatively beneficial host CD8 response - Diffuse Infilterative Lymphocytosis Syndrome (DILS) (Itescu et al., 1990), the lymphocytes may be anti- HIV CD8 cells. No evidence of Epstein-Barr virus or cytomegalovirus has been found in biopsies of salivary gland (Soberman et al., 1991) One report describes an association between HIV-SGD and HLA-DR5 and HLA-B35 cell-surface antigen (Schiodt et al.,1989).

Adults and children with salivary glands enlargement seem to experience slower progression of HIV disease (Katz et al., 1993).

Oral Mucoceles and ranulas are recently discovered to be oral manifestations of HIV infection. Several reports are considering it as initial symptoms and early manifestations of HIV infection (Syebele et al., 2010; Kamulegeya et al., 2012).

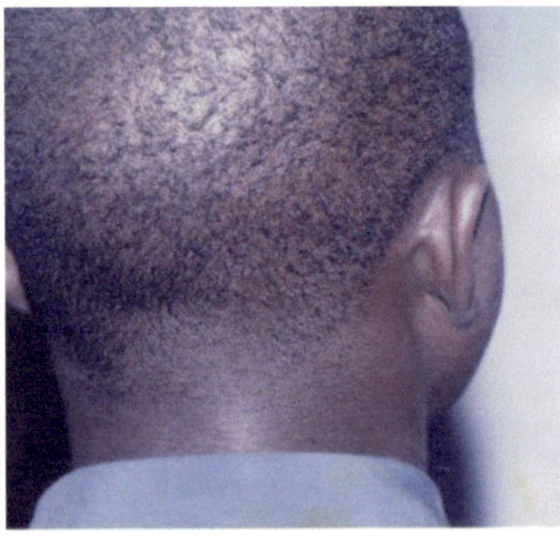

Figure 19. Salivary gland swelling

3.5.7.1. Xerostomia

This may be associated with the salivary gland enlargement but is also a common consequence of medications used by this population. Cytomegalovirus (CMV) has been demonstrated in the salivary gland of xerostomic patients (Greenspan et al., 1992). Symptomatic relief may be provided by salivary stimulants such as sugarless chewing gums or saliva substitutes. Prevention of dental caries in people with xerostomia is extremely important, and the use of topical fluoride gels and rinses should be encouraged (Greenspan et al., 1996). In addition, management of xerostomia will improve oral comfort, the quality of speech and use of any prostheses (Narani et al., 2001).

3.5.7.2. Herpes virus infections

Varicella zoster (VZV) is a herpesvirus, and, like other herpesviruses, it causes both primary and recurrent infection and remains latent in neurons present in sensory ganglia. VZV is responsible for two major clinical infections of humans: chickenpox (varicella) and shingles (herpes zoster [HZ]) (Greenburg et al., 2003).

Herpes zoster may indicate a poor prognosis of HIV infection (Scully et al., 1991). This can be an early complication of AIDS, where it is five times more common than HIV-negative persons, and potentially lethal (Cawson et al., 2002). Varicella-zoster may present with a prodrome of dental pain, preceding oral and unilateral vesicles on an erythematous base then appear in clusters, chiefly along the course of the nerve, giving the characteristic clinical picture of single dermatome involvement. Some lesions spread by viremia occur outside the dermatome. The vesicles turn to scabs in 1 week, and healing takes place in 2 to 3 weeks and condition can be life threatening in HIV disease.

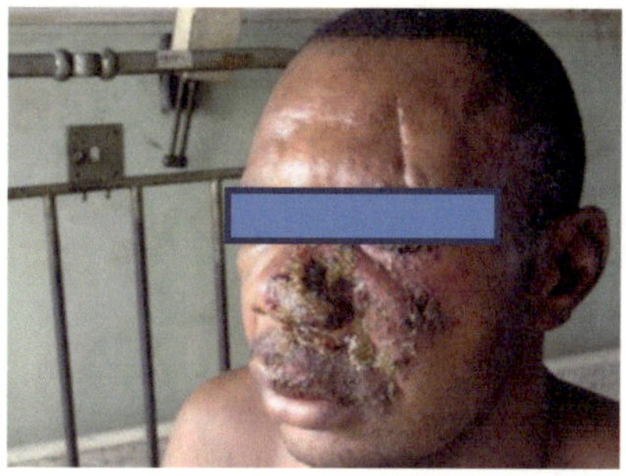

Figure 20. Herpes zoster of the left maxillary branch and the right occipital branch of the trigeminal nerve

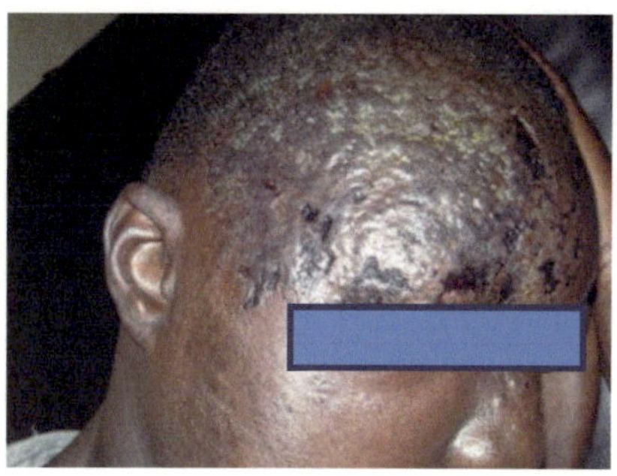

Figure 21. Herpes zoster of the left maxillary branch and the right occipital branch of the trigeminal nerve.

3.5.7.3. Melanotic hyperpigmentation

Brownish or brown black macular oral hyperpigmentation, typically associated with intraleukocytic melanin or pigment in the basal cell layer or lamina propria, with premature melanosomes has been described in HIV-infected patients (Langford et al., 1989; Porter et al., 1990). Often the cause is unknown, but identified causes include Zidovudine (AZT), Clofazimine, ketoconazole and hypoadrenocorticism as a result of adrenal Mycobacterium avium intracellulare infection (Porter et al., 1990). Usually does not respond to HAART.

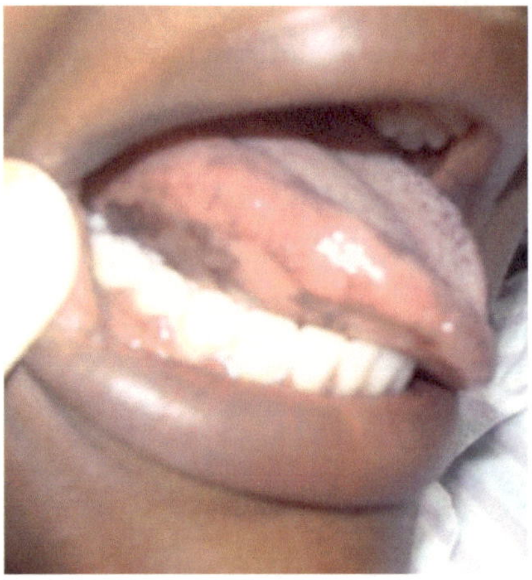

Figure 22. Melanotic hyperpigmentation

3.6. Management of oral lesions of HIV

3.6.1. Candidiasis

Treatment may be topical (using lozenges or mouth rinses) or systemic depending on the severity of the disease and other associated underlying conditions e.g. Diabetes, liver disease, xerostomia etc.

Topical:

1. Chlorhexidine (0.2%) mouth wash
2. Lozenges: e.g. Nystatin (Mycostatin) 100,000 i.u; Clotrimazole (Mycelex) 1%
3. Adhesive tablets: Miconazole 10mg
4. Miconazole oral gel- X2% daily
5. Suspension: e.g. Amphotericin B (0.5-1mg), Nystatin (100,000 i.u)

Topical treatments are preferred because they limit systemic absorption, but the effectiveness depends entirely on patient compliance. Topical medications require that the patient hold medications in the mouth for 20 to 30 minutes.

Clotrimazole is an effective topical treatment (one oral troche [10-mg tablet]) when dissolved in the mouth five times daily. Used less frequently, one vaginal troche can be dissolved in the mouth daily.

Nystatin preparations include a suspension, a vaginal tablet, and an oral pastille. Regimens are nystatin tablets (one tablet, 100,000 units, dissolved in the mouth three times a day), or nystatin oral pastille (available as a 200,000 unit oral pastille, one or two pastilles dissolved slowly in the mouth five times a day). Nystatin suspension has a high sugar content and

http://dx.doi.org/10.5772/52941

cannot be held in the mouth long enough to be effective. Topical creams and ointments containing nystatin, ketoconazole, or clotrimazole may be useful in treating angular cheilitis. For patients with initial and recurring oropharyngeal candidiasis, a topical agent is generally recommended, provided the patient has a CD4 count greater than 50 cells/mm^3 and no oesophageal involvement.

Another therapeutic choice is Amphotericin B (0.1 mg/ml). Five to 10 ml of oral solution is used as a rinse and then expectorated three to four times daily (Greenspan, 1998).

Systemic: Fluconazole 150mg daily (Diflucan) for 2 weeks or more

- Miconazole 250mg daily for 2 weeks or more
- Ketoconazole 200mg daily (Sporanox), for 2 weeks or more
- Itraconazole 100mg daily, for 2 weeks or more

Ketoconazole (Nizoral) is a 200 mg tablet taken with food once daily. Patient compliance is usually good. Careful monitoring of liver function is necessary for long-term use because of reported side effects, including hepatotoxicity. Lack of efficacy of ketoconazole may occur because of poor absorption in those with an abnormally high gastric pH.

Fluconazole (Diflucan) is a triazole antifungal agent effective in treating candidiasis (100-mg tablet taken once daily for 2 weeks (Just-Nubling et al., 1991).

Itraconazole (100 mg capsules) may be used for the treatment of oral candidiasis (200 mg daily orally for 14 days. Salivary levels of itraconazole are maintained for several hours after administration (Smith et al., 1991).

The recommendation to avoid systemic anti-fungal therapies in this setting is based on evidence that widespread use of systemic azoles is strongly linked with the development of drug-resistant candidiasis. Patients with concurrent oesophageal involvement or a CD4 count less than 50 cells/mm^3 should receive a systemic oral azole.

Ketoconazole, fluconazole, and itraconazole may interact with other medications including rifampicin, phenytoin, cyclosporin A, terfenadine, digoxin, coumarin-like medications, and oral hypoglycemic medications.

3.6.2. Linear gingival erythema

The treatment protocol for LGE is similar to that of conventional marginal gingivitis and consists of scaling and polishing of the affected sites and thorough root planing using chlorhexidine solution as an irrigant (Murray, 1994). Povidone-iodine (10%) solution may be beneficial for the irrigation because of its anaesthetic and antiseptic effects. According to Murray (1994), the rationale for scaling is to prevent the lesion from progressing to NUP, the more severe form. Typically, the patients are given oral hygiene instructions to achieve good home care, placed on chlorhexidine mouthrinses twice daily, re-assessed 2 to 3 weeks after the initial therapeutic phase, and further recalled every 3 months.

Non-responsive lesions could signal a possible candidal co-infection which may need to be treated concomitantly with topical antifungal rinses or systemic antifungal tablets such as fluconazole for 7 to 10 days (Murray, 1994). This has been shown to reduce the erythema associated with LGE. It must be borne in mind that LGE may still be refractory to treatment, hence, patient should be monitored closely for any signs of severe necrotizing periodontal conditions. The lesion has sometimes been known to undergo spontaneous remission for reasons yet unknown.

3.6.3. Necrotizing ulcerative gingivitis

The NUG lesion should be debrided thoroughly under topical anaesthesia to remove tissue slough, plaque and necrotic soft tissue in the initial phase of treatment. Irrigation should be done frequently with hydrogen peroxide or povidone iodine which is particularly advantageous because of its topical anaesthetic effect (Grassi et al., 1988). This should be accompanied by daily or alternate day visits for further debridement of affected areas for the first week with the gradual introduction of home plaque control measures to reinforce good oral hygiene. This initial phase of treatment is followed by scaling and thorough root planing if indicated. Systemic antibiotics such as metronidazole may be prescribed in severe cases of tissue loss or associated systemic effects. Topical chlorhexidine gluconate 0.12% mouthwash is prescribed. Patients are reassessed 1 month after resolution of the acute phase to determine if further therapy is needed. Most of the lesions may resolve within a week (Robinson et al., 1998).

3.6.4. Necrotizing ulcerative periodontitis

The treatment of NUP involves the gentle debridement of the affected lesions, followed by sub-gingival scaling and root planing, irrigation with chlorhexidine gluconate (Grassi et al., 1988; Umeizudike et al., 2011a) or povidone-iodine. Oral hygiene instructions should be emphasized alongside the home use of twice daily antimicrobial mouth-rinses such as 0.12% or 0.2% chlorhexidine gluconate. In severe NUP cases, systemic metronidazole 500mg loading dose and 250 mg four times daily for 5-7 days is the drug of choice. It has been shown to reduce acute pain and promote rapid healing. Metronidazole should be prescribed with caution in patients with liver alteration or history of hepatitis (Winkler & Robertson, 1992). Alternatively, penicillin may be prescribed. However, it should be used with caution to avoid the proliferation of opportunistic infections such as candidiasis. Appropriate topical or systemic antifungal treatment may be used for patients who have concurrent oral candidiasis (Holmstrup & Samaranayake, 1990). There is a need to follow up these patients after the initial phase of therapy to ensure adequate plaque control and reduce the incidence of delayed healing and continued rapid destruction (Winkler & Robertson, 1992). Oral hygiene aids such as interproximal brushes may be necessary to achieve better plaque control. Sequestra should be removed if present to facilitate wound healing (Umeizudike et al., 2011a) and may not always require antibiotic coverage (Robinson, 1991).

3.6.5. Necrotizing ulcerative stomatitis

The principles of the treatment are similar to that of necrotizing ulcerative periodontitis. It should begin with gross scaling to remove visible plaque and debridement of necrotic soft tissue. Povidone-iodine may be used for irrigation. Systemic metronidazole and chlorhexidine mouthrinses should be prescribed. Necrotic bone should be removed if present to promote wound healing (Williams et al., 1990).

3.6.6. Chronic periodontitis with an increased rate of attachment loss

This should include conservative, non-surgical periodontal therapy which basically consists of scaling and polishing of all teeth, sub-gingival scaling and root planing of affected teeth. Detailed oral hygiene instructions should be given to the patient in order to achieve effective plaque control. This should include the use of 0.2% chlorhexidine mouthwashes twice daily at home. The overall health status of the patient, the degree of immune suppression, extent of periodontal attachment loss and patient's ability to perform effective oral hygiene are all the factors that should be taken into consideration when planning for elective periodontal surgical procedures and implant placement. The hematological profile of patients may be required prior to these surgical procedures to monitor their overall health status. Periodontal maintenance recalls should be instituted at 2-3 monthly intervals initially, and later to 6 monthly intervals. Dentists should be ready to advise patients and provide dental treatments in a relaxed and calm atmosphere to minimize the patients stress and anxiety, as these HIV positive patients are prone to psychological problems (Asher et al. 1993).

In summary, it should be noted that the treatment of periodontal diseases associated with HIV should have some basic components (Winkler & Robertson, 1992).

1. Extensive debridement of necrotic tissues.
2. Antimicrobial therapy (local and systemic)
3. Immediate follow up phase
4. Regular long-term maintenance

3.6.7. Oral Hairy Leukoplakia (OHL)

OHL is usually symptomless; complaints about the discomfort and appearance sometimes justify treatment (Barr, 1995). The lesions respond to high doses of acyclovir, ganciclovir, and also podophyllin and retinoin. Treatment is usually not indicated, but improved with antiretroviral therapy e.g. AZT, Ganciclovir, acyclovir or descyclovir. Hairy leukoplakia recurs after discontinuation of therapy (Scully et al., 1992).

3.6.8. Kaposi's sarcoma

Treatment of oral kaposi's sarcoma is directed towards control of spread and palliation, for aesthetic reasons, pain or functional impairment. It is by radiotherapy or chemotherapy such as Vinblastin. Radiation therapy may be indicated for large, multiple lesions (Greenspan et al., 1984). A single dose of 800 cGy or an equivalent fractionated dose is frequently used and produces a good response. Other local therapy may involve excision of exophytic lesions or intra- lesional injection of vinblastin (Iain et al., 2000).

3.6.9. Oral ulcers

Topical steroids can be effective in the treatment of MiAUand MjAU:

i. Fluocinonide gel 0.05% with Orabase - apply to ulcers four times daily.

ii. Clobestasol 0.05% in Orabase – apply 3-4 times daily.

iii. Dexamethasone elixir 0.5mg/ml – rinse with 20ml four times daily

iv. Triamcinolone in Orabase – apply 3-4 times daily.

Ulcers are reevaluated after one week. If there is no improvement, alternative treatment should be considered, including systemic steroids e.g. Prednisolone.

Alternative forms of treatment have included **intralesional** injection with **Triamcinolone acetonide**.

Supportive therapy is necessary to aid healing of the ulcers, this includes:

- Vitamin B complex i tds
- Tabs Folic acid i daily
- Tabs Vitamin C 300mg tds
- Xylocaine gel to relieve pain and Chlorhexidine mouth wash.

3.6.10. Salivary gland diseases

No treatment is indicated for the salivary gland enlargement, although large cystic glands are sometimes removed surgically for cosmetic purposes. Radiation therapy has also been used to reduce the swelling.

3.6.11. Xerostomia

The management of xerostomia involves the use of both saliva substitutes and saliva stimulants. Patients with little or no responsive salivary gland tissue will need saliva substitutes. A properly balanced artificial saliva should be of neutral pH and contain electrolytes, including fluoride, to correspond to the composition of saliva.

Gustatory stimuli such as sugarless sweets containing citric and malic acid, chemically induce saliva production. Care must be taken that the acidic content does not result in the dissolution of tooth enamel. Controlled studies have shown that pilocarpine is an effective stimulus to saliva production (Greenspan et al., 1987; Rieke et al., 1995), side effects, mainly the result of generalised parasympathetic stimulation, are the most common reason to discontinue treatment.

http://dx.doi.org/10.5772/52941

There have been a number of studies that have shown that chewing gum increases salivary flow from patients with xerostomia of varying aetiology (Risheim et al., 1993). In some xerostomic patients, the initial stimulated salivary flow rate while chewing sugar free gum is seven times greater than the unstimulated flow rate. Chewing sugar free gum has been shown to be one of the most preferred treatments for xerostomia (Bjornstrom et al., 1990).

3.6.12. Herpes zoster

Management should be directed toward shortening the course of the disease, preventing postherpetic neuralgia in patients over 50 years of age, and preventing dissemination in immunocompromised patients. Acyclovir or the newer antiherpes drugs valacyclovir or famciclovir accelerate healing and reduce acute pain, but they do not reduce the incidence of postherpetic neuralgia. The newer drugs have greater bioavailability and are more effective in the treatment of HZ. Supportive therapy, antibiotics and analgesics are also recommended.

- Tabs Acyclovir200-400mg 5x daily for 1 week

3.7. Oral lesions and relationship with CD4 count and viral load

The hallmark of HIV disease is the progressive loss of CD4+ lymphocytes. Without intervention, an average of 60 to 80 cells/mm3 is lost every year; this loss is highly variable and occurs in periods of stability and rapid decline. High viral load is also considered to be one of the main indicators of the progression of HIV- induced immunosuppression. Several studies have shown that the higher the viral load, the quicker the progression to AIDS.

The CD4 count and viral load measure the progression of the HIV disease. Several studies have shown high prevalence of oral lesions in patients with low CD4 count, <200 cells/mm3 and high viral load: >55,000 copies/ml. CD4 count < 200 cells/mm^3 is used as criterion for initiating HAART, which is consistent with the guidelines for initiating HAART treatment by WHO (2003).

Presence of multiple lesions in infected HIV patients is also associated with severe immunosuppression and AIDS.

3.8. Oral lesions and response to HAART

The goals of HAART should be maximal and durable viral suppression. The aim is preservation and restoration of the immune system at minimal cost to the patient. This should improve the quality of life through ease of use of their regimen with minimal side-effects to enhance optimum adherence. This should translate into a reduction of HIV- related morbidity including oral manifestations. Reduction of viral burden will prevent progressive immunodeficiency, decrease the risk of the emergence of resistant viruses and possibly decrease the risk of viral transmission (Fauci et al., 2000).

It has been shown in various studies that the prevalence of HIV-related oral lesions reduces significantly with HAART. The reported percentage decrease varied from 10% in a USA study on 570 patients (Patton et al., 2000) to 50% in a Mexican study on selected 1000 HIV patients over a period of 12 years (Ramírez-Amador et al., 2003).

In a Spanish study on 154 subjects, Ceballos-Salobrena et al (2000) showed a 30% reduction of oral lesions, while Tappuni and Fleming (2001) reported a reduction of 24% in a study on 284 patients in the United Kingdom. Some looked at a particular oral manifestation (Cauda et al., 1999) as opposed to a range of oral lesions (Ceballos-Salobrena et al., 2000; Tappuni and Fleming, 2001; Eyeson et al., 2002; Ramírez-Amador et al., 2003).

Studies examining the effect of HAART on the prevalence of individual oral manifestations mainly reported on oral candidiasis, oral hairy leukoplakia, HIV-related periodontal diseases, Kaposi's sarcoma (KS), oral papilloma, and HIV-related salivary gland disease showed reduction in the prevalence (Patton et al., 2000; Schmidt-Westhausen et al., 2000; Tappuni et al., 2001).

Oral candidiasis (OC) has been shown to be one of the most common oral lesions in HIV patients. With the advent of HAART, most studies reported a decrease in the prevalence of Oral Candidiasis. In a study on 93 patients, 7% of patients on protease inhibitors (PI) had Oral Candidiasis, compared with 36% in non-PI-treated patients (Cauda et al., 1999). Schmidt-Westhausen et al (2000) detected Oral Candidiasis in 10/103 (9.7%) of their study subjects who had been on HAART for 4 weeks and in none after 6 months' therapy (n = 61). Tappuni and Fleming (2000) reported that the prevalence of Oral Candidiasis was about 50% less in patients on therapy (n = 89) compared with drug-naïve patients (n = 195). Conversely, Patton et al (2000) found no significant difference in the prevalence of Oral Candidiasis with the use of Protease Inhibitors (n = 507). In the same study, the prevalence of oral hairy leukoplakia (OHL) was found to decrease with therapy (Patton et al., 2000), in agreement with reports from other studies (Tappuni and Fleming, 2001).

The prevalence of HIV-associated periodontal diseases was reported to decrease significantly in an American cohort, from 4.8% to 1.7% with HAART (Patton et al., 2000), in concordance with findings in other studies (Ceballos-Salobrena et al., 2000; Tappuni and Fleming, 2001).

Kaposi's Sarcoma (KS) is one of the oral manifestations that is strongly associated with HIV, although its prevalence is quite low in this group (Ceballos-Salobrena et al., 2000), Studies from the USA (Patton et al., 2000) and Mexico (Ramírez-Amador et al., 2003) found no significant change in the occurrence of Kaposi Sarcoma with HAART.

Unlike most other oral manifestations of HIV, studies from the USA and the United Kingdom(UK) described an increase in the prevalence of oral warts with HAART (Patton et al., 2000; Greenwood et al., 2002), which may reach statistical significance (Greenspan et al., 2001). Others looking at a different population (Mexicans) reported similar detection rates of oral warts, papillomas, condylomas and focal epithelial hyperplasia in HIV-positive subjects on HAART compared with those not on therapy (Ramírez-Amador et al., 2003).

Other lesions that are showing a trend of rising prevalence include HIV-related salivary gland disease (Patton et al., 2000). However, this was not supported by other studies (Ramírez-Amador et al., 2003). Studies from industrialized world report a decreased frequency of

HIV-related oral manifestations of 10–50% following the introduction of HAART (Hodgson et al., 2006).

Author details

G.A. Agbelusi[1], O.M. Eweka[1], K.A. Ùmeizudike[1] and M. Okoh[2]

1 Faculty of Dental Sciences, College of Medicine, University of Lagos, Lagos State, Nigeria

2 School of Dental Sciences, College of Medicine, University of Benin, Edo State, Nigeria

References

[1] Adedigba MA, Ogunbodede EO, Jeboda SO, Naidoo S (2008): Patterns of oral manifestation of HIV/AIDS among 225 Nigerian patients. Oral Dis. 4: 314-316.

[2] Adurogbangba MI, Aderinokun GA, Odaibo GN, Olaleye OD, Lawoyin TO (2004): Oro-facial lesions and CD4 counts in an adult population in Oyo state, Nigeria. Oral Dis. 10: 319-326.

[3] Agbelusi GA, Eweka OM (2011). Necrotising Stomatitis as a presenting symptom of HIV. Scrip.org/journal/OJST. 1:1-4.

[4] Agbelusi GA, Wright AA (2005): Oral lesions as indicators of HIV infection among routine dental patients in Lagos, Nigeria. Oral Dis; 11: 370-373

[5] Alpagot T, Duzgunes N, Wolff LF, Lee A (2004): Risk factors for periodontitis in HIV positive patients. J Periodont Res; 39: 149-157.

[6] Anteyi KO, Thacher TD, Yohanna S, Idoko JI(2003): Oral manifestation of HIV/ AIDS in Nigerian patients. Int. J. AIDS; 14: 395-398.

[7] Aragues M, Sanchez Perez J, Fraga J, Burgos E, Noguerado A, Garciadiez A (1990): Hairy Leukoplakia : a clinical histopathological and ultrastructural study in 33 patients. Clin Exp Dermatol ; 15:335-339.

[8] Arendorf TM; Bredekamp B, Cloete CAC (1998): Oral manifestations of HIV infection in 600 South African patients. J. Oral Pathol Med. 27: 179-189.

[9] Armitage GC(1999): Development of a classification system for periodontal diseases and conditions. Ann Periodontol; 4:1-6.

[10] Arotiba JT, Arowojolu MO, Fasola AO, Denloye OO, Obiechina AE (2006): Oral manifestation of HIV/AIDS. Afr J Med Med Sci.;(35): 13-18.

[11] Asher RS, McDowell JD, Winquist H. (1993): HIV-related neuropsychiatric changes: concerns for dental professionals. J Am Dent Assoc 124:80.

[12] Barr C, Lopez MR, Rua-Dobles A (1992): Periodontal changes by HIV serostatus in a cohort of homosexual and bisexual men. J Clin Periodontol 19: 794-801.

[13] Bjornstrom M, Axell T, Birkhed D (1990) Comparison between saliva stimulants and saliva substitutes from patients using symptoms related to dry mouth. A multi-centre study. Swed Dent J. 14: 153-161 Boring CC, Brynes RK, Chan WC (1985): Increase in high grade lymphomas in young men. Lancet; 1: 857-859.

[14] Boring CC, Brynes RK, Chan WC (1985): Increase in high grade lymphomas in young men. Lancet; 1: 857-859.

[15] Boshoff C, Whitby D, Talbot S (1997): Aetiology of AIDS- related kaposi's sarcoma and lymphoma. Oral Dis. 3: S129-132.

[16] Campisi G, Pizzo G, Mancuso S, Margiotta V (2002): Gender differences in HIV-related oral lesions: an Italian study. Oral Surg Oral Med Oral Pathol; 93 (3): 281-286.

[17] Cauda R, Tacconelli E, Tumbarelo M, Morace G, De Bernadis et al (1999): Role of protease inhibitor in preventing recurrent oral candidosis in patients with HIV infection: a prospective case- control study. J AIDS; 21: 20-25

[18] Ceballos-Salobrena A, Aguirre-Urizar JM, Bagan-Sebastian JV (1996): Oral manifestations associated with human immunodeficiency virus infection in a Spanish population. J Oral Pathol Med: 25: 523-526.

[19] Ceballos-salobrena A, Gactan-Cepeda L A, Ceballos-Garcia L, Lezamz- Del Nalle D (1997): Oral lesions in HIV/AIDS patients undergoing Highly Active Anti-Retroviral Treatment including protease- inhibitors: a new face of oral AIDS. Oral Dis; 3 suppl 1: S46-50

[20] Centers for Disease Control and Prevention (1993): Revised classification system for HIV infection and expanded surveillance case definition for AIDS among adolescents and adults . MMWR Recomm Rep. 41:1-19.

[21] Davoodi P, Hamian M, Nourbaksh R, Motamayel FA (2010): Oral Manifestations Related To CD4 Lymphocyte Count in HIV-Positive Patients. J Dent Res Dent Clin Dent Prospect; 4(4):115-119.

[22] EC-Clearinghouse on oral Problems Related to HIV Infection and WHO Collaboration center on oral manifestations of the immunodeficiency Virus (ECC/WHO) (1993): Classification and diagnostic criteria for oral lesions in HIV infection. J Oral Pathol Med 22:289-291.

[23] Epstein JB, Silverman S (1992): Head and neck malignancies associated with HIV infection. Oral Surg. Oral Med. Oral Pathol; 73: 193-300.

[24] Eyeson JD, Tenant-Flowers M, Cooper DJ, Johnson NW, Warnakulasuriya KA (2002): Oral manifestations of an HIV positive cohort in the era of highly active anti-retroviral therapy (HAART) in South London. J Oral Pathol Med 31:169–174.

[25] Fauci AS, Bartlett JG, Goosby EP (2000): Guidelines for the use of antiretroviral agents in HIV-1 infected adults and adolescents. Panel on clinical practices for treatment of HIV infection conveyed by the department of health and Human services and the Henry J Kaiser foundation.

[26] Feigel D W, Katz MH, Greenspan D (1991): The prevalence of oral lesions in HIV- infected homosexual and bisexual men: three San-Fransisco epidemiological cohorts . AIDS; 5: 519-525.

[27] Glick M, Muzyka BC, Lurie D, Salkin LM (1994): Necrotising Ulcerative Periodontitis : a marker for immune deterioration and a predictor for the diagnosis of AIDS. J. Periodontol. 65: 393-397.

[28] Gornitsky M. Pekovie D (1987): Involvement of human immunodefiency virus (HIV) in gingival of patients with AIDS. Adv Exp Med Biol ;216: 553-62.

[29] Grassi M, Williams CA, Winkler JR et al (1988): Management of HIV-associated periodontal diseases. In Robertson, PB & GJS, ed. Perspectives on Oral Manifestations of AIDS. PSG Publishing Co., Inc., Littleton, pp. 119-130.

[30] Grbic FT, Mitchelle-Lewis DA, Fine JB (1995): The relationship of candidosis to LGE in HIV- infected homosexual men and parenteral drug users. J. Periodontol. 66: 30-37.

[31] Greenburg MS, Glick M (2003): ulcerative, vesicular and bullous lesions, Burket's oral Medicine. Diagnosis and treatment, 10th edition. 50-84.

[32] Greenspan D, Greenspan JS, Conant M, Peterson V, Silverman S, De Sonza Y (1984): Oral Hairy Leukoplakia in male homosexuals: evidence of association with both papilloma virus and a herpes group virus. Lancet 831-834.

[33] Greenspan D, Daniels TE (1987): Effectiveness of pilocarpine from postradiation xerostomia. Cancer. 59: 1123-1125

[34] Greenspan D, Greenspan JS, Schiodt M, Pindborg JJ. (1990.):In: AIDS and the mouth. Copenhagen: Munksgaard.

[35] Greenspan D, Greenspan JS (1996): HIV- related oral disease. The Lancet; 348: 729-733.

[36] Greenspan JS, Barr CE, Sciubba JJ, Winkler J R (1992): Oral manifestations of HIV infection. Oral Surg Oral Med Oral Pathol; 73: 142-144.

[37] Greenspan D (1998): Oral manifestation of HIV. HIV InSite Knowledge Base Chapter

[38] Greenspan D, Canchola AJ, MacPhail LA, Cheikh B, Greenspan JS (2001): Effect of highly active antiretroviral therapy on frequency of oral warts. Lancet 357:1411–1412.

[39] Greenwood I, Zakrzewska JM, Robinson PG (2002): Changes in the prevalence of HIV-associated mucosal disease at a dedicated clinic over 7 years. Oral Dis 8:90–94.

[40] Hodgson TA, Greenspan D, Greenspan JS (2006): Oral lesions of HIV diseases and HAART in industrialized countries. Adv. Dent. Res 19:57- 62.

[41] Holmes HK, Stephen LX (2002): Oral lesions of HIV infection in developing countries. Oral Disease; 8(2): 40-43.

[42] Holmstrup P, Westergaard J (1998): HIV infection and periodontal diseases. Periodontology 2000; (18): 37-46.

[43] Iain LC, Hamburger J(2000): The significance of oral health in HIV disease. Sex Trans infection; 76: 236-243.

[44] Itescu S, Brancato L, Buxbaum J (1990): A diffuse infiltrative CD8 lymphocytosis syndrome in HIV infection: A host immune response associated with HLA-DR5. Ann Intern Med. 112: 3-10.

[45] Just-Nubling G, Gentschew G, Meissner K (1991): Fluconazole prophylaxis of recurrent oral candidiasis in HIV-positive patients. Eur J Clin Microbiol Infect Dis;10: 917-21.

[46] Kaminu HN, Naidoo S (2002): Oral HIV lesions and oral health behavior of HIV-Positive patients attending the Queen Elizabeth II Hospital, SADJ 57:479.

[47] Katz MH, Mastrucci MT, Leggott PJ, Westenhouse J, Greenspan JS, Scott GB (1993): Prognostic significance of oral lesions in children with perinatally acquired HIV infection. Am J Dis Child 147 (1): 45-48.

[48] King GN, Healy CM, Glover MT (1994): Prevalence and risk factors associated with hairy Leukoplakia, erythematous candidiasis and gingival hyperplasia in renal transplant recipients. OralSurg Oral Med Oral Pathol; 78:18-26.

[49] Lamster IB, Begg MD, Mitchell-Lewis D, et al (1994): Oral manifestations of HIV infection in homosexual men and intravenous drug users, Oral Surg Oral Med Oral Pathol; 78: 163.

[50] Lifson AR, Hilton JF, Westenhouse JL (1994): Time from HIV seroconversion to oral candidiasis or Hairy Leukoplakia among homosexual and Bisexual men enrolled in three prospective cohorts. J AIDS; 8: 73- 79.

[51] Lihana RW, Khamadi SA , Lwembe RM, Kinyua JG, Muriuki JK et al (2009): HIV-1 subtype and viral tropism determination for evaluating antiretroviral therapy options: an analysis of archived Kenyan blood samples. BMC Infec. Dis; 9:215-217.

[52] Maeve MC, Greenspan J, Challacombe SJ (2005). Oral lesions in infection with HIV. Bulletin of the World Health Organisation. 83: 700-706.

[53] Masouredis CM, Katz MH, Greenspan D, Herrera C, Hollander H, Greenspan JS, Winkler JR (1992): Prevalence of HIV-associated periodontitis and gingivitis in HIV-infected patients attending an AIDS clinic. J Acquir Immune Defic Syndr 5: 479-483.

[54] Matee M, Scheutz F, Moshy J. (2000): Occurrence of oral lesions in relation to clinical and immunological status among HIV-infected adult Tanzanians. Oral Dis; 6: 106-111.

[55] Mckaig RG, Patton LL, Thomas JC, Strauss RP, Slade GD. (2000): Factors associated with periodontitis in an HIV infected southeast USA study. Oral dis. 6: 158-165.

[56] McNeil DG Jr (2007): "U.N. agency to say it overstated extent of HIV cases by millions". New York Times.

[57] Miceli MC, Parnes JR (1993): "Role of CD4 and CD8 in T cell activation and differentiation". Adv. Immunol. 53: 59–122.

[58] Mirowski GW, Hilton JF, Greenspan D, Canchola AJ, MacPhail LA, Maurer T, Berger TG, Greenspan JS. (1998): Association of cutaneous and oral diseases in HIV – infected men. Oral Dis. (1): 16-21.

[59] Murray PA, Grassi M, Winkler JR (1989):. The microbiology of HIV associated periodontal lesions. J Clin Periodontol 16: 636-642.

[60] Murray PA, Winkler JR, Peros WJ, French CK, Lippke JA (1991). DNA probe detection of periodontal pathogens in HIV-associated periodontal lesions. Oral Microbiol Immunol: 6: 3440.

[61] Murray PA. (1994): Periodontal diseases in patients infected by human immunodeficiency virus. Periodontology 2000. (6): 50-67.

[62] Narani N, Epstein JB (2001): classifications of oral lesions in HIV infection. J clin Periodontol ; 28: 137-145.

[63] Ndiaye CF, Critchlow CW, Leggot PJ, Kiviat NB, Ndoye I, Robertson PB, Georgas KN (1997): Periodontal status of HIV-1 and HIV-2 seropositive and HIV seronegative female commercial sex workers in Senegal. J Periodontol; 68: 827-831. West Afr J Med; 21: 9-11.

[64] Nittayananta W, Chungpanich S(1997): Oral lesions in a group of Thai people with AIDS. Oral Dis. 3:41-56.

[65] Onunu A N, Obueke N (2002): HIV- related oral diseases in Benin city,

[66] Osuji OO (1990): Necrotizing ulcerative gingivitis and cancrum oris in Ibadan, Nigeria. J Periodontol; 61: 769-772.

[67] Palmer GD, Robinson PG, Challacombe SJ, Birnbaum W, Croser D, Erridge PL et al. (1996): Aetiological factors for oral manifestation of HIV infection. Oral Dis. 2: 193-197.

[68] Patton LL, McKaig R, Strauss R, Rogers D, Eron JJ Jnr. (2000): Changing prevalence of oral manifestations of human immuno-deficiency virus in the era of protease inhibitor therapy. Oral Surg Oral Med Oral Pathol Oral Radiol Endod 89:299–304.

[69] Ramírez-Amador V, Esquivel-Pedraza L, Sierra-Madero J, Ponce-de-Leon S (1998): Oral manifestations of HIV infection by gender and transmission category in Mexico City. J Oral Pathol Med 27 (3): 135-140.

[70] Ramírez-Amador V, Esquivel-Pedraza L, Sierra-Madero J, Anaya-Saavedra G, Gonzalez-Ramírez I, Ponce-de-Leon S (2003): The changing clinical spectrum of human immunodeficiency virus (HIV)-related oral lesions in 1,000 consecutive patients: a 12-year study in a referral center in Mexico. Medicine (Balt) 82:39–50.

[71] Ramos-Gomez FJ (1997): Oral aspects of HIV disease in children. Oral Dis. 3: S31-35.

[72] Ranganathan K, Reddy BV, Kumarasamy N, Solomon S, Viswanathan R et al. (2000) Oral lesions and conditions associated with human immunodeficiency virus infection in 300 South Indian patients. Oral Diseases. 6: 152-157.

[73] Ranganathan K, Magesh KT, Kumarasamy N, Solomon S, Viswanathan R, Johnson NW (2007): Greater severity and extent of periodontal breakdown in 136 south Indian human immunodeficiency virus seropositive patients than in normal controls: A comparative study using community periodontal index of treatment needs. Indian J Dent Res. 18(2): 55-59.

[74] Reichart PA, Gelderblom HR, Becker J, Kuntz A. (1987): AIDS and the oral cavity. The HIV-infection: virology, etiology, origin, immunology, precautions and clinical observations in 110 patients. Int J Oral Maxillofac Surg; 16: 129-153.

[75] Rieke JW, Hafermann MD, Johnson JT (1995): Oral pilocarpine for radiation-induced xerostomia: integrated efficacy and safety results from two prospective randomized clinical trials. Int J Rad Onc Biol Phys. 31: 661-669

[76] Riley C, London JP, Burmester JA (1992): Periodontal health in 200 HIV positive patients. J. Oral pathol. Med. 21: 124-127.

[77] Risheim H, Arneberg P (1993) Salivary stimulation by chewing gum and lozenges from rheumatic patients using xerostomia. Scand J Dent Res. 181: 40-43

[78] Robinson PG, Sheiham A, Challacombe SJ, Wren MWD, Zakrzewska JM (1998): Gingival Ulceration in HIV infection. A case series and case control study J Clin Periodontol; 25: 260-267.

[79] Robinson PG, Adegboye A, Rowland RW, Yeung S, Johnson NW (2002): Periodontal diseases and HIV infection. Oral Diseases 8(2): 144-150.

[80] Scheutz F, Matee MIN, Andsager L, Holm AM, Moshi J et al. (1997): Is there an association between periodontal condition and HIV infection? J Clin Periodontol; 24: 580-587.

[81] Schiodt M, Pindborg JJ (1987): AIDS and the oral cavity. Epidemiology and clinical oral manifestations of HIV infection: a review. Int. J of Oral Maxillofacial surg.; 16: 1-14.

[82] Schiodt M, BakilanaPB, Haza FR (1990): Oral candidiasis and hairy leukoplakia correlate with HIV infection. Oral Surg Oral Med Oral Pathol 69:591-596.

[83] Schmidt- Westhausen AM, Priepke F, Bergman FJ, Riechart PA (2000): Decline in the rate of Oral opportunistic infections following introduction of HAART. J. Oral Pathol /Med; 29: 336-341.

[84] Scully C, McCarthy G (1992): Management of oral health in persons with HIV infection. Oral Surg Oral Med Oral Pathol; 73: 215-225.

[85] Septowitz KA (1998): Effect of HAART on natural history of AIDS- related opportunistic disorders. Lancet 351: 228-230.

[86] Silverman S Jr, Migliorati CA, Lozada-Nur F, Greenspan D, Conant MA (1986): Oral findings in people with or at high risk for AIDS: a study of 375 homosexual males. J Am Dent Assoc; 112: 187-192.

[87] Sirois DA (1998): Oral Manifestation of HIV disease. 65:322-332

[88] Slots J (2004): Update on human cytomegalovirus in destructive periodontal diseases. Oral Microbiol Immunol; 19:217.

[89] Smith DE, Midgley J, Allan M (1991): Itraconazole versus ketaconazole in the treatment of oral and oesophageal candidiasis in patients infected with HIV. AIDS; 5:1367-71.

[90] Smith GLF, Felix DH, Wray D (1993): Current classification of HIV-associated periodontal diseases. Br Dent J; 174: 102-105.

[91] Soberman N, Leonidas JC, Berdon WE, (1991): Parotid enlargement in children seropositive for human immunodeficiency virus: imaging findings. AJR;157: 553-6.

[92] Soubry R, Taelman H, Banyangiliki V et al (1995): Necrotising periodontal disease in HIV-1 infected patients: a 4 year study. In: Greenspan JS, Greenspan D, eds. Oral manifestations of HIV infection. Quintessence Publishing Co, Inc., Chicago,; 60-67.

[93] Sturzl M, Konrad A, Alkharsah KR, Jochmann R, Mathias T et al (2009): The contribution of systems biology and reverse genetics to the understanding of kaposi's sarcoma-associated herpes virus pathogenesis in endothelial cells. Thomb. Haemot.; 102: 1117-1134.

[94] Swango PA, Kleinman DV, Konzelman JL(1991): HIV and periodontal Health: a study of military personnel with HIV J. Am Dent Assoc. 122 (8): 49-54.

[95] Taiwo O, Okeke EN, Jalo PH, Danfillo IS (2006): Oral manifestation of HIV in Plateau state indigenes, Nigeria. West Afr. J. Med. (1): 32-37.

[96] Taiwo O, Okeke EN, Otoh EC, Danfillo IS (2005): Prevalence of HIV- related oral lesions in Nigerian women. Nig J. Med; 14: 132-136.

[97] Tappero JW, Conant MA, Wolfe SF (1993): Kaposi's sarcoma. J Am Acad. Dermatol; 28: 371-395.

[98] Tappuni AR, Fleming GJ (2001): The effect of antiretroviral therapy on the prevalence of oral manifestations in HIV-infected patients: a UK study. Oral Surg Oral Med Oral Pathol Oral Radiol Endod 92:623–628.

[99] Tukutuku K, Muyembe – Tamfum L, Kayembe K (1990): Oral manifestation of AIDS in a heterosexual population in a Zaire hospital. J Oral Pathol Med 19: 232-234.

[100] Umeizudike KA, Savage KO, Ayanbadejo PO, Akanmu AS (2011a) Severe presentation of Necrotizing Ulcerative Periodontitis in a Nigerian HIV Positive Patient- A Case report. Med Princ Pract. 20:374-376.

[101] Umeizudike KA, Savage KO, Ayanbadejo PO, Akanmu AS (2011b): Greater severity of periodontitis among HIV Positive Patients in Nigeria. J Dent Res 90 (Spec Iss B) 152991 AMER, www.dentalresearch.org

[102] UNAIDS: Joint United Nations Programme on HIV/AIDS (2010): Epidemiologic fact sheet on HIV and AIDS. www.UNAIDS.org

[103] Velegraki A, Nicolatou O, Theodoridou M et al (1999): Paediatric AIDS-related linear gingival erythema; a form of erythematous candidiasis? J Oral Pathol Med; 28: 178.

[104] Weinert M, Grimes RM, Lynch DP (1996): Oral manifestation of HIV infection. 125; 6:485-496.

[105] Williams CA, Winkler JR, Grassi M, Murray PA. (1990): HIV-associated periodontitis complicated by necrotizing stomatitis. Oral Surg Oral Med Oral Pathol Oral Radiol Endod 69:351-355.

[106] Winkler JR, Murray PA (1987): A potential intra-oral expression of AIDS may be rapidly progressive periodontitis. Journal of the California Dental Association; 15:20

[107] Winkler JR, Grassi M, Murray PA (1988): Clinical description and aetiology of HIV-associated periodontal disease. In: Oral manifestations of AIDS. Proceedings of 1st. international symposium on oral manifestations. AIDS eds. Robertson PB and Greenspan JS. 49-70.

[108] Winkler JR, Robertson PB (1992):Periodontal diseases associated with HIV infection Oral Med Oral pathol; 73: 145-150..

[109] Wright AA, Agbelusi GA (2005): Group II and III lesions in HIV positive Nigerians attending the general Hospital Lagos, Nigeria. Odonto- Stomatologie Tropicale; 112: 19- 23.

[110] Yeung SCH, Stewart GJ, Cooper DA, Sindhusake D (1993): Progression of periodontal disease in HIV seropositive patients. J. Periodontol; 64: 651-657.

Chapter 11

Endocrine Manifestations of HIV Infection

Bakari Adamu Girei and Sani-Bello Fatima

Additional information is available at the end of the chapter

http://dx.doi.org/10.5772/52684

1. Introduction

Human Immune deficiency Virus (HIV) infection has assumed pandemic proportion since after its identification as the causative agent of Acquired Immunodeficiency Syndrome (AIDS).The spectrum of HIV infection and AIDS is quite wide and variable. HIV infected patients have an increased risk of developing endocrine abnormalities [1]. The endocrine glands are affected in a variety of ways such as functional derangement, direct effects of HIV infection and the resultant immune suppression, effects of opportunistic infections both acute and chronic, invasion by neoplasms and the effects of the various medications used to treat HIV or any of the opportunistic infections associated with it (Table 1). While endocrine dysfunction has not been a prominent clinical feature of AIDS, all endocrine glands may be affected by the opportunistic infections and malignancies; as a result of antiretroviral treatment or indeed as a result of the direct invasion of the glands by the virus (Table 2). The introduction of anti-retroviral (ARV) drugs has significantly reduced both morbidity and mortality attributable to HIV infection [2]. The prolonged administration of these drugs however, has led to new challenges for both physicians and patients [3- 8].

Apart from the effects of acute and chronic illnesses, the relentless progression of immune dysfunction in AIDS affects endocrine function through the activation of several cytokines, chemokines and antibody formation. The use of protease inhibitors (PIs) and nonnucleoside reverse transcriptase inhibitors (NNRTIs) is associated with multiple abnormalities in glucose and lipid metabolism such as insulin resistance, increased triglycerides and increased levels of low-density lipoprotein cholesterol. These metabolic disturbances might be due to a combination of factors, including the direct effect of medications, restoration to health; HIV disease as well as individual genetic predisposition. Of the available antiretroviral medications, indinavir had been associated with causing the most insulin resistance and ritonavir with causing the most hypertriglyceridemia.

a. Destruction of endocrine tissue
• Cancer
• Infection
• Haemorrhage
• Non-specific inflammation
b. Interference with Endocrine function
• Acute illness
• Chronic illness
• Cytokines (tumour necrosis factor, interleukin-1, interferon)
• Antibodies
c. Effects of medications
• ARV's
• Anti Tuberculosis drugs.
• Antifungal drugs.
• Antiviral drugs.
• Antibiotics.

Table 1. Mechanisms of Endocrine dysfunction in patients with HIV [1]

a. Endocrinopathies as a result of direct effects of the virus.
• HIV adrenalities and impaired adrenal reserve
• Hypercorticolism
• Idiopathic adrenohypophyseal necrosis
• Hyperprolactinaemia
• Primary hypogonadism
• Growth factor
• AIDS wasting syndrome
b. Endocrinopathies as a resultof structural destruction of gland.s
• Cytomegalovirus (CMV) adrenalitis
• Pneumocystis thyroiditis
• Mycobacterial infection, cryptococcosis, toxoplasmosis(pituitary, thyroid, adrenals)
• Haemorrhages and abscesses causing insufficiency of glands (pituitary, thyroid and adrenals)

Table 2. Common Endocrine abnormalities in HIV infected patients [1].

2. The pituitary

Involvement of the pituitary gland is common in advanced HIV infection, at autopsy; varying degrees of infarction and necrosis are the most common findings occurring in nearly 10% of cases [1]. Also common are opportunistic Infections by CMV, Pneumocystis carinii, Toxoplasmosis and mycobacteria among others [9]. Furthermore, the pituitary may also be affected by neoplasms such as cerebral lymphoma with peripheral involvement of the gland.

Despite the foregoing, evaluation of anterior pituitary reserve in HIV infected patients by TSH or gonadotropin stimulation has demonstrated a normal response in nearly all patients. Suggesting that panhypopituitarism is rare in these patients.

GH deficiency does not appear to be common [1]. Posterior pituitary function may be altered in HIV patients with Hyponatremia occurring in up to 50% of inpatients and about 20% of outpatients with AIDS; two-thirds of these patients are clinically euvolemic with serum arginine vasopressin levels that are inappropriately high for the serum osmolality, consistent with the syndrome of inappropriate antidiuretic hormone secretion [10 - 12]. The presence of Pneumocystis carinii pneumonia and/ or treatment with trimethoprim appears to be the most significant risk factors for this complication. Furthermore, central diabetes insipidus has been reported in AIDS patients with herpetic meningoencephalitis.

3. Thyroid dysfunction

Although thyroid function tests are often abnormal in HIV patients, the prevalence of overt thyroid disorder is not significantly different from that of the general population [13]. Most asymptomatic patients with HIV infection have normal thyroid function. Some, however, exhibit increased serum total thyroxine (T_4) and triiodothyronine (T_3) concentrations. These increases are as a result of increases in serum thyroxine-binding globulin, the cause of which is unknown [14]. However, with progression of HIV infection and as the patients become more ill, serum T_4 and T_3 concentrations decline, as is obtained in most if not all chronically ill patients; serum thyrotropin concentrations however remain normal or slightly depressed. These changes are as a result of reduction in serum binding proteins, decreased extrathyroidal conversion of T_4 to T_3, and decreased secretion of thyrotropin [13], [14]. Cytokines may be involved in some of these; especially the reduction in the peripheral conversion of T4 to T3 [15].

An increasing number of patients taking anti-HIV drugs are presenting with thyroid disorders as a result of improved immune function (immune reconstitution syndrome). Graves' disease is the commonest among immune reconstitution syndromes; others include Hashimoto's thyroiditis and hypothyroidism. Autoimmune Thyroid Disease (AITD) occurs in 3% of women and 0.2% of men [13- 17]. Goddard proposed a staging of autoimmune manifestations related to HIV/AIDS (table 3) [18].

The prevalence of immune reconstitution Autoimmune Thyroid Disease (AITD) (Graves' disease, Hashimoto thyroiditis, and hypothyroidism) is about 3% for women and 0.2% for men. Patients with lower CD4 counts at baseline with greater increments in the CD4 counts following HAART are more likely to develop AITD.

Stage	Features
Stage I	Acute HIV infection, the immune system is intact and autoimmune diseases may develop.
Stage II	The quiescent period without overt manifestations of AIDS associated with a declining CD4 count indicative of some immunosuppression. Autoimmune diseases are not found.
Stage III	Immunosuppression with low CD4 count and the development of AIDS. CD8 T cells predominate and diseases such as psoriasis and diffuse immune lymphocytic syndrome (similar to Sjogren's syndrome) may present or even be the initial manifestation of AIDS. No autoimmune diseases are found.
Stage IV	Restoration of immune competence following HAART. In this setting, there is a resurgence of autoimmune disorders.

Table 3. Stages of autoimmune manifestations in HIV/AIDS.

Thyroid dysfunction in HIV-positive individuals can result from gland destruction by opportunistic pathogens such as Pneumocystis jirovecii which has been reported to cause a painful low uptake thyroiditis like picture with hyperthyroidism followed by hypothyroidism. Other opportunistic pathogens that could affect the thyroid gland in HIV infected individuals include Cryptococcus neoformans, Aspergillosis and cytomegaloviurs [19 - 23]. The gland may also be invaded by Kaposi Sracoma with resultant hypothyroidism [24].

Overt Hypothyroidism should be treated with levothyroxine keeping in mind that drug interactions between levothyroxine and protease inhibitors have been reported, perhaps through the shared metabolic pathway of glucuronidation. In subclinical hypothyroidism however, the TSH level should be determined again within three months as the levels normalize within a year in up to 30% of affected patients. In cases of overt hyperthyroidism, it is paramount to establish whether it is as a result of Graves' disease, or thyroiditis and the appropriate therapy instituted.

4. Adrenal dysfunction

Biochemical evidence of adrenal insufficiency is relatively common in hospitalized AIDS patients occurring in almost a fifth of such patients however, only about 4% are clinically symptomatic patients [25]. Adrenal dysfunction may be suspected in HIV-infected patients with advanced stage of AIDS. High index of suspicion is required; subtle impairment of adrenal function is manifested as fatigue, hyponatremia or rarely with clinical symptoms of adrenal insufficiency. At autopsy, the adrenal gland shows evidence of both inflammation and necrosis[1], [26 - 28]. Adrenal secretion of aldosterone and adrenal androgens may also be impaired. In fact, there appears to be a shift from adrenal androgen and aldosterone production toward glucocorticoid production. However, the secretion of aldosterone in response to assumption of the upright posture and the administration of angiotensin II is normal. The mechanisms by which HIV might affect adrenal secretion appear to be dependent on effects of cytokines and other immunomodulatory substances on the hypothalamo-pituitary-adrenal axis [29 - 32]. The potential sites of immune modulation of this is shown in this figure 1.

http://dx.doi.org/10.5772/52684

Interleukin-1 is a likely candidate as either a direct or an indirect adrenal stimulator. Its production by macrophages is stimulated by tumor necrosis factor, and the production by macrophages of both interleukin-1 and tumor necrosis factor is stimulated by HIV infection [33].

Interleukin-1 may affect the hypothalamus, pituitary, or adrenal glands in a variety of ways [29]. Interleukin-1 stimulates the release of corticotropin-releasing hormone from the hypothalamus into the portal circulation leading to the increases in corticotropin and consequently cortisol secretion. Furthermore, Interleukin-1 has been shown to directly stimulate cultured pituitary cells to release corticotropin. Cultured adrenocortical cells secrete more cortisol when cocultured with mononuclear cells most likely as a result of a response to the production of interleukin-1 by mononuclear cells [30 - 32]. Interferon, another product of HIV-infected monocytes and macrophages, is also an immunomodulator of the hypothalamo-pituitary-adrenal axis [34].

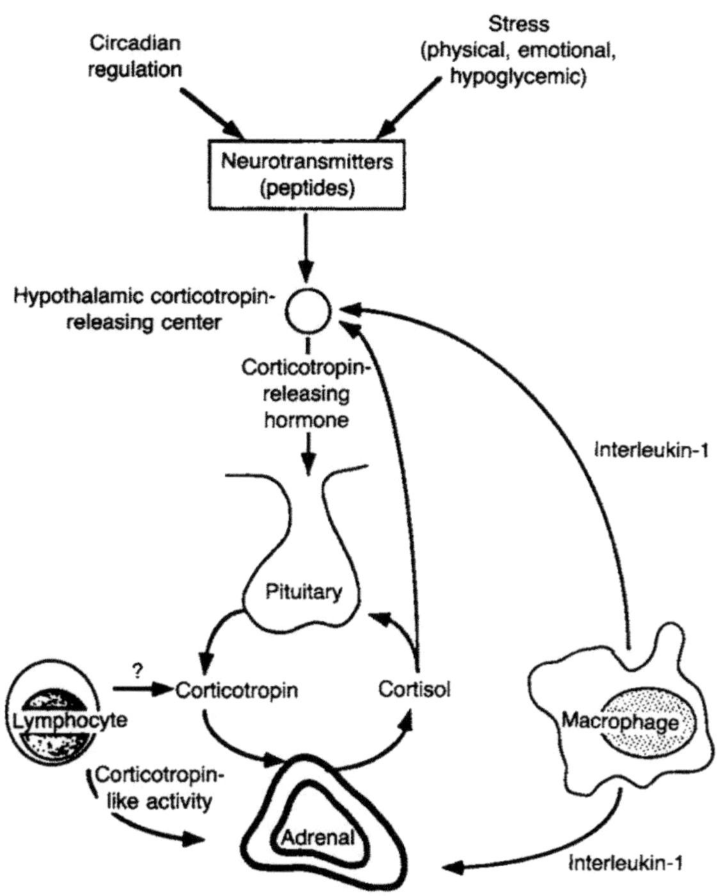

Figure 1. Effects of cytokines on the Hypothalamo-pituitary-adrenal axis.

Both interleukin-1 and interferon thus have effects that could stimulate adrenal function. Conversely, adrenal function could be inhibited in patients with HIV infection as a result of polyclonal B-cell activation and the production of anti—adrenal-cell antibodies. The specific cellular or hormonal antigenic determinants and the pathogenetic importance of these antibodies are unclear. In addition to these mechanisms of adrenal dysfunction in patients with HIV infection, drugs which impair adrenal function directly such as Ketoconazole which inhibits adrenal steroidogenesis, Rifampicin, phenytoin, and opiates which accelerate the degradation of cortisol and therefore lower serum cortisol concentrations are frequently prescribed in HIV infected patients. Although the resulting need for increased cortisol secretion is easily met in normal subjects, it may not be so in patients with HIV infection.

5. Glucocorticoids

The adrenal corticosteroids (Cortisol and Aldosterone), exert profound influences on many physiologic functions by virtue of their diverse roles in growth, development and maintenance of homeostasis [35]. The actions of these corticosteroids are mediated by intracellular receptor proteins, the glucocorticoid (GR) and mineralocorticoid (MR) receptors respectively. These receptors act as hormone-activated transcription factors which regulate the expression of the glucocorticoid and mineralocorticoid target genes respectively. The GR is ubiquitous and is found in virtually all human tissues and organs [1, 35].

Glucocorticoids are essential to maintain the integrity of central nervous system and cardiovascular function,as well as the maintenance of metabolic and immune function.

Tissue hypersensitivity to glucocorticoids was recently hypothesized in patients with Human Immunodeficiency Virus type-1 infection via the accessory proteins Vpr and Tat which enhance GR transactivation [36]. Since HIV-1 long terminal repeat (LTR) and glucocorticoid-responsive promoters use the same set of co-activators, these proteins may stimulate HIV-1-LTR and glucocorticoid-inducible genes concurrently. The former may directly stimulate viral proliferation, while the latter may indirectly enhance viral propagation by suppressing the host immune system through glucocorticoid mediated mechanisms.

6. Glucocorticoid hypersensitivity in AIDS

AIDS patients have several manifestations compatible with tissue hypersensitivity to glucocorticoids [37]. Some of the manifestations include reduction of innate and cellular immunity mediated through T helper 1 cells with resultant reduction in the secretion of interleukin (IL)-2, IL-12 and interferon and increased secretion of IL-4. These changes are similar to what obtains when exogenous glucocorticoids are administered as well as in hypercortisolemic patients with endogenous Cushing's syndrome. Furthermore, hippocampal atrophy similar to what is observed in individuals who exhibit hypercortisolism is seen in HIV infected patients especially in pediatric AIDS patients. Other features seen in HIV/AIDS patients that are similar to features of hypercortisolism include muscle wasting and myopathy, dyslipidemia and visceral obesity and insulin resistance. From the foregoing, it seems possible that some unknown factor(s) modulate tissue sensitivity to glucocorticoids in HIV infected patients.

The observed glucocorticoid hypersensitivity in HIV infected patients seem to preferentially affect the brain, fat cells, the liver, the musculoskeletal system and the immune system. It is noteworthy that the hypothalamo-pituitary-adrenal axis is not affected suggesting that appropriate negative feedback sensitivity to glucocorticoids is preserved.

There is evidence to suggest that glucocorticoid hypersensitivity in HIV/AIDS is mediated through one of the HIV-1 accessory proteins the virion-associated protein (Vpr). This is a 96 amino acid protein with multiple functions. This protein is known to act as a transcriptional activator of several viral promoters and as an enhancer of HIV-1 long terminal repeat promoter activated by Tat as well as enhances the replication of HIV-1 virus in lymphocyte- and monocyte-derived cell lines. Furthermore, the protein also increases the translocation of the HIV-1 pre-integration complex into the nucleus promoting efficient infection of non-dividing macrophages.

The protein circulates in HIV-1-infected individuals and has the capacity to penetrate cell membranes. This suggests that its effects have the potential to involve all cells including those not infected by HIV-1. It is indeed this protein that has been shown by Kino *et al* [36]to increase the tissue sensitivity to glucocorticoids by functioning as a coactivator of the GR on its responsive promoters. By inducing hypersensitivity to glucocorticoids, these proteins contribute to the proliferation of the virus indirectly by suppressing the host immune system. Extensive further clinical and basic investigations are crucial to examine the clinical importance of glucocorticoid hypersensitivity and to develop novel effective therapeutic approaches in AIDS.

Although the involvement of the adrenal gland is common in HIV patients, routine screening is not however recommended as adrenal insufficiency is a relatively rare complication of HIV infection. Its presence should however be considered, however, in those with disseminated cytomegalovirus infection or tuberculosis. It should also be suspected, in patients with otherwise unexplained symptoms and signs compatible with adrenal insufficiency, such as anorexia, nausea, weight loss, and fatigue, and especially in patients with more specific manifestations of adrenal insufficiency, such as postural hypotension, hyponatremia, or hyperkalemia. It is also reasonable to be concerned about adrenal reserve in patients who are about to undergo major stress, such as surgery. The simplest test is to measure the serum cortisol concentration in the morning, when it is highest in normal subjects. A concentration of 10 μg per deciliter (280 nmol per liter) or less suggests the presence of adrenal insufficiency. However, higher cortisol concentrations do not rule out the possibility of diminished adrenal reserve. If the basal serum cortisol concentration is low or the suspicion of adrenal insufficiency persists, provocative testing with corticotropin is indicated. Such testing involves measuring the serum cortisol concentration before and 30 and 60 minutes after the intravenous or intramuscular administration of 0.25 mg of cosyntropin. The cortisol concentration should increase by at least 7 μg per deciliter (196 nmol per liter) at 30 minutes and 11 μg per deciliter (308 nmol per liter) at 60 minutes. Alternatively, a normal response is a concentration twice the basal value at 60 minutes. Whether one considers the extent of a change in the cortisol concentration or the multiple of the basal value, the peak stimulated value should be 18 μg per deciliter (504 nmol per liter) or more for the response to be considered normal [48, 49]. Glucocorticoid therapy should be given only in cases of documented adrenal insufficiency or when there is a medical emergency in which the possibility of adrenal crisis cannot be excluded.

7. Gonadal dysfunction in male

Male gonadal dysfunction is common among AIDS patients. With more than two-thirds of male patients with advanced HIV disease exhibit of loss of libido and up to one-third of them having erective dysfunction [38, 39]. The prevalence and severity of male gonadal dysfunction is directly proportional to disease severity. In advanced disease stages, biochemical hypogonadism is found in up to half of male AIDS patients. With the advent of HAART, the prevalence of male gonal dysfunction has reduced to about 20% among those receiving HAART [40]. Gonadal dysfunction in HIV/AIDS is usually attributable to secondary causes such as the effect of under nutrition, infection-inflammation and several drugs on gonadotropin production. Other secondary causes include the role of cytokines produced in response to systemic illness may impair the secretion of gonadotropin-releasing hormone or gonadotropin [41]. Low levels of interleukin-1 enhance testicular steroidogenesis in vitro, whereas higher doses inhibit the binding of gonadotropin to Leydig cells and steroidogenesis by these cells. Ketoconazole used in the treatment of fungal infections in HIV/AIDS patients inhibits gonadal as well as adrenal steroid production and could therefore also contribute to the observed gonadal dysfunction.

Furthermore, hyperprolactinaemia and gynecomastia have been reported among HIV-infected patients [42]. Prolactin has for long been known to be an immunostimulatory hormone and is also known to be elevated in other immunostimulatory states such as systemic lupus erythematosis (SLE). Similarly, prolactin receptors are found in T and B lymphocytes as well as monocytes [43], while lymphocytes are known to produce a prolactin like protein. The men with low serum testosterone concentrations may have inappropriately normal serum gonadotropin concentrations, suggesting involvement of the pituitary gland or hypothalamus however, there is neither CT scans nor autopsy data provide evidence of pituitary or hypothalamic disease.

As sex hormone binding capacity increases in up to a third of HIV patients, the use of free testosterone assay is recommended for diagnosis. [38] Physiologic testosterone replacement that does not suppress endogenous gonadal function results in increased lean body mass, improved quality of life and reduction in depression. Standard therapy for hypogonadism has been intramuscular testosterone (enanthate or ciprionate esters) every 1–3 weeks to provide 100 mg per week. Alternate transdermal or oral routes for androgen administration are also available. Prostate-specific antigen level should be monitored in elderly patients receiving testosterone.

http://dx.doi.org/10.5772/52684

8. Gonadal dysfunction in female

Ovarian dysfunction among female AIDS patients is less common. Amenorrhoea is seen in about a quarter of women during stress of illness; while failure of ovulation is seen among half of the female patients with low CD4 counts [44]. Early menopause has been seen in up to 8% of HIV-infected female patients. Androgen deficiency has been reported especially in women with significant weight loss. The reasons for the above observations are not clear, but could be as a result of intra-adrenal shunting toward cortisol production from androgen synthesis. Human chorionic gonadotropin levels suggest intact ovarian androgen production. Delivery of low doses of testosterone using transdermal patches improves functional capacity without hirsuitism or virilisation but does not increase lean body mass [38].

9. Glucose homeostasis in HIV/AIDS

Normal glucose metabolism is largely dependent on normal insulin secretion, insulin sensitivity and to a lesser extent on the influences of other hormones and cytokines. Before the advent of highly active anti-retroviral therapy (HAART), HIV infection on its own was thought to be protective against the development of diabetes mellitus[1], this may be due to the following observations in clinically stable, symptomatic HIV-infected patients. These individuals have been shown to have higher rates of insulin clearance and increased sensitivity of peripheral tissues to insulin as well as an increase in noninsulin-mediated glucose uptake. The increase in glucose uptake is predominantly accounted for by an increase in non-oxidative glucose disposal.

Pancreatic abnormalities are common in AIDS patients as a result of opportunistic infections and malignancies[1]. However, the majority of these lesions are not extensive enough to cause clinically significant pancreatic dysfunction. Clinically significant pancreatic dysfunction is usually as a result of therapeutic interventions; noteworthy in this regard is Pentamidine [45], which is used in the management of Pneumocystis carinii and may cause pancreatic β-cell toxicity with resultant hypoglycaemia in the acute phase and some of these patients may later develop diabetes mellitus.

With the advent of HAART however, a new dysmetabolic syndrome with substantially increased risk for cardiovascular events emerged [46]. This syndrome has variable expressibility; and includes insulin resistance, visceral adiposity, peripheral lipodystrophy, dyslipidaemia and glucose intolerance. Several studies have demonstrated an increased risk of diabetes among HIV infected individual on HAART especially when protease inhibitors (PIs) are included in the regimen. Among HIV infected minority patients in the USA for example, the prevalence of diabetes after three years of PI therapy was 12%, compared to none among those not receiving PI's[4]. However, although PI's are the most frequent agents associated with metabolic complication, there are evidences to suggest that virtually all classes of agents used in ART has the potential to cause metabolic derangements. Although the mechanism by which ART drugs induce these metabolic changes are not fully clear; it has been shown that indinavir, a PI dramatically inhibits glucose uptake in a dose dependent manner in adipocytes by selectively inhibiting the Glut-4 transporter function [47]. Furthermore, there is evidence at least in laboratory studies to show that indinavir down regulates the peroxisome proliferator–activated receptor -γ (PPAγ) receptor in adipocytes [48]. Obviously some genetic predisposition could explain why not all patients on PI's develop diabetes, or any of the other metabolic complications.

10. Bone mineral dysfunction

Both osteoporosis and osteopenia are common among AIDS patients. Reduced bone mineral density is seen in almost three quarter of HIV-infected patients compared to about 30% in HIV-negative individuals of similar age [49]. Reduced vertebral bone density is associated with visceral adiposity among HIV-infected patients. Similarly, reduced bone density also occurs in HIV-infected children receiving HAART with maximum reduction seen among those with lipodystrophy. Several factors are thought to be responsible for the observed effects on the skeleton. The effects of low GH and IGF1, hypogonadism and excess visceral adiposity are possible factors as they have been found to correlate significantly with vertebral bone density [50 - 52]. Protease Inhibitors are also known to induce relative vitamin D deficiency and may also act as an additive factor.

11. Calcium and vitamin D balance

Hypocalcemia is common in HIV infected patients occurring in more than 5% of them [53]. It appears the level of calcium has an inverse relationship with the stage of the disease and its severity. Factors responsible for hypocalcaemia in these patients include vitamin D deficiency and reduced parathyroid hormone (PTH) level. The cause of the relatively reduced PTH is not known but may be as a result of the effects of cytokines; and presence of hypomagnesemia which is relatively common among HIV infected patients especially those with chronic diarhoea. On the other hand, the cause of Vitamin D deficiency is multifactorial in the setting of HIV/AIDS and may include malabsorption, decreased hydroxylation as a result of the effects of protease inhibitors. Furthermore, several therapeutic agents such as foscarnet, pentamidine, and ketoconazole, may affect calcium homeostasis [53].

Hypercalcemia is uncommon in AIDS. When present it is likely to be due to infectious, malignant, or granulomatous processes [54 - 55]. Patients with lymphoma who have hypercalcemia typically have increased serum 1,25-dihydroxyvitamin D concentrations, because the tumors contain vitamin D 1-hydroxylase and therefore convert 25-hydroxyvitamin D to 1,25-dihydroxyvitamin D. Cultured lymphoma cells infected with HIV have the same synthetic activity. Human T-cell lymphotropic virus Type I (HTLV-I), a retrovirus linked to T-cell leukemia and lymphoma may be associated with hypercalcemia. Increased bone resorption in this syndrome may be due to lymphokines such as interleukin-2 or to parathyroid hormone-related protein. A HTLV-I gene product, *tax*,has been implicated in the activation of the parathyroid hormone-related protein gene. Serum concentrations of parathyroid hormone and 1,25-dihydroxyvitamin D are not elevated in HTLV-I—related hypercalcemia.

12. AID wasting syndrome

Wasting is an age-old terminal event of AIDS, even with the advent of HAART, wasting remains common affecting more than one-third of patients [57]. Unfortunately, weight loss is a significant predictor of mortality in HIV infection. Those with a body mass index (BMI) of less than 18.4 kg/M^2 are at 2.2-fold increased risk of mortality, while those with a BMI less than 16 kg/M^2 are at 4.4-fold increased risk of mortality [58].

Currently, AIDS wasting syndrome is defined as body weight less than 90% of ideal weight or weight loss of more than 10% of body weight over 3 months. The condition is characterised by a disproportionate loss of lean body mass with a relative sparing of body fat as the disease progresses this is associated with muscle wasting, weakness, increased resting energy expenditure and hypertriglyceridemia. The exact mechanisms involved in the aetiology of this condition are not clear. However, the roles of Cytokine related increased energy expenditure and decreased appetite, diarrhoea, malabsorption and hypogonadism are likely mechanisms behind such wasting [59, 60].

Management of this condition include optimal antiretroviral therapy and adequate nutrition. Testosterone (intramuscular/transdermal) has been successfully used to increase lean body mass in men with this syndrome, whereas it has also been shown to be safe and well tolerated in women. A number of agents like anabolic steroids (oxandrolone, nandrolone), megesrtol acetate, thalidomide, human chorionic gonadotropin, pentoxyfiline, amino acid mixtures and omega 3 fatty acids have been tried in this setting with variable efficacy but potential side effects. Only testosterone administration has proved useful to increase lean body mass, especially in conjunction with progressive resistance training. Administration of supraphysiologic doses of growth hormone is currently reserved for severe wasting refractory to other treatments.

13. HIV lipodystrophy syndrome

HIV lipodystrophy syndrome is associated with metabolic derangements, changes in body composition and abnormal fat distribution. It has been most widely recognized since the era of HAART but can also be seen in antiretroviral-naïve patients [61]. It is characterized by phenotypic changes similar to those observed in Cushing’s syndrome, such as like truncal obesity, buffalo hump, peripheral fat loss, atrophy of facial fat and breast enlargement in women. Considering some physical similarities to Cushing's syndrome, it has been termed as “a pseudo-Cushing's syndrome” though no other specific stigmata of Cushing's syndrome (proximal muscle weakness, bruising and facial plethora) nor biochemical parameters are associated with this syndrome. Normal cortisol level with its normal diurnal variation and adequate suppressibility to dexamethasone are also seen in HIV lipodystrophy syndrome. However, it is very often associated with insulin resistance, hyperglycemia, and hypertriglyceridemia. In particular, dyslipidemia and diabetes mellitus are increasingly common among patients receiving HAART. management consist of exercise and lifestyle modification, switching to less-toxic NRTIs or PIs, fenofibrates to decrease serum triglyceride level, and use of insulin sensitizers like metformin to reduce visceral fat and thiazolidinediones to improve subcutaneous fat loss. Testosterone and anabolic steroids have no effect in reducing visceral fat in this syndrome.

14. Conclusion

Although HIV endocrinopathy is common, overt glandular failure is a rare clinical entity. HIV infection, acting by a number of mechanisms, may be responsible for subtle clinical and not-so-subtle biochemical abnormalities. Drug-induced endocrine toxicity is important cause of endocrinopathy in HIV infected patients.

Author details

Bakari Adamu Girei and Sani-Bello Fatima

Endocrinology Unit, Department of Medicine, Ahmadu Bello University, Zaria, Nigeria

References

[1] Sellmeyer, D. E., & Grunfeld, C. Endocrine and metabolic disturbances in Human Immunodeficiency virus infection and the acquired immune deficiency syndrome. End. Rev. (1996)., 17, 518-532.

[2] Palella FJ Jr, Delaney KM, Moorman AC, et al.Declining morbidity and mortality among patients with advanced human immunodeficiency virus infection. N Engl J Med (1998)., 338, 853-60.

[3] Deeks, S. G., Smith, M., Holodny, M., Kahn, J. O. H. I. V., proteaseinhibitors, a., review, for., & clinicians, J. A. M. JAMA (1997)., 145 EOF-53 EOF.

[4] Salehian, B., Bilas, J., Bazargam, M., & Abbasian, M. Prevalence and incidence of diabetes in HIV infected minority patients on protease inhibitors J Nat Med Ass (2005)., 97, 1088-92.

[5] Hutchinson, J., Murphy, M., Harries, R., & Skinner, C. J. Galactorrhoea and hyperprolactinoma associated with protease inhibitors. Lancet. (2000)., 356, 1003-4.

[6] Cozzolino, M., Vidal, M., Arcidiacono, M. V., Tebas, P., Yarasheski, K. E., & Dusso, H. I. HIV-protease inhibitors impair vitamin D bioactivation to 1, 25-dihydroxyvitamin D. AIDS. (2003). , 17, 513-20.

[7] Hadigan, C., Borgonha, S., Rabe, J., Young, V., & Grinspoon, S. Increased rates of lipolysis among HIV-infected men receiving highly active antiretroviral therapy. Metabolism. (2002). , 51, 1143-7.

[8] Madeddo G, Spanu A, Chessa F et al: Thyroid function in Human immunodeficiency virus patients treated with highly active antiretroviral therapy (HAART): a longitudinal study. Clinical Endocrinol 2006:64:375-83.

[9] Ferrerio, J., & Vinters, H. V. Pathology of pituitary gland in patients with acquired immune deficiency syndrome (AIDS) Pathology. (1988). , 20, 211-5.

[10] Vitting KE, Gardenswartz MH, Zabetakis PM, Frequency of hyponatraemia and non osmolar vasopressin release in the acquired immunodeficiency syndrome.JAMA (1990). , 263, 973-978.

[11] Cusano AJ, Thies HL, Siegal FP, Hyponatraemia in patients with acquired immunodeficiency syndrome.J AcquirImuneDeficSyndr HumRetrvirol(1990). , 3, 949-953.

[12] Agarwal, A., Soni, A., Ciechanowsky, M., Chander, P., & Treser, G. Hyponatraemia in patients with the acquired immunodeficiency syndrome. Nephron (1989). , 53, 317-321.

[13] Hoffman CJ, Brown TT.Thyroid function abnormalities in HIV infected patients. Clin Infect Dis. (2007). , 45, 488-94.

[14] , 5., Bourdoux, P. P., De Wit, S. A., Servais, G. M., Clumeck, N., & Bonnyns, . Biochemical thyroid profile in patients infected with human immunodeficiency virus. Thy. roid. (1991). , 1, 147-9.

[15] Jimenez C, Moran SA, Sereti I: Graves' disease after interleukin-2 therapy in patients with HIV infection : Thyroid 2004:14:1097-1102

[16] Nelson, M., et al. Thyroid dysfunction and relationship to antiretroviral therapy in HIV-positive individuals in the HAART era. J Acqu. ir Immune DeficSyndr. (1990). , 50, 113-14.

[17] Madeddo G, Spanu A, Chessa F et al: Thyroid function in Human immunodeficiency virus patients treated with highly active antiretroviral therapy (HAART): a longitudinal study. Clinical Endocrinol 2006:64:375-83.

[18] Goddard, G. Z., Shoenfeld, Y. H. I. V., autoimmunity, ., & autoimmunity, reviews. autoimmunity reviews : (2002).

[19] Ragni, M. V., Dekker, A., De Rubertis, F. R., Watson, C. G., Skolnick, M. L., Goold, S. D., Finikiotis, M. W., Doshi, S., & Myers, D. J. (1991). Pneumocystis carinii infection presenting as necrotizing thyroiditis and hypothyroidism. Am J Clin Path, 01, 95-489.

[20] Guttler, R., Singer, P. A., Pneumocystis, carinii., & thyroiditis, . Report of three cases and review of the literature. Arch Intern Med. (1993). , 153, 393-396.

[21] Frank TS, LiVolsi VA, Connor AM.Cytomegalovirus infection of the thyroid in immunocompromised adults. Yale J Biol Med (1987). S, 60, 1.

[22] Machac, J., Mejatheim, M., & Goldsmith, S. J. (1985). Gallium-67 citrate uptake in cryptococcal thyroiditis in a homosexual male. J Nucl Med Allied Sci , 29, 283-285.

[23] Martinez-Ocana, J. C., Romen, J., Llatjos, M., Sirera, G., & Clotet, B. Goiter as a manifestation of disseminated aspergillosis in a patient with AIDS. Clin Infect Dis.(1993). , 17, 953-954.

[24] Mollison, L. C., Mijch, A., Mc Bride, G., & Dwyer, B. 1991Hypothyroidism due to destruction of the thyroid by Kaposi's sarcoma. Rev Infect Dis. 1991; , 13, 826-827.

[25] Membreno, L., Irony, I., Dere, W., Klein, R., Biglieri, E. G., & Cobb, E. Adrenocortical function in acquired immune deficiency syndrome. J ClinEndocrinolMetab. (1987). , 65, 482-7.

[26] Tapper, M. L., Rotterdam, H. Z., Lemer, C. W., Al'Khafaji, K., & Seitzman, P. A. Adrenal necrosis in the acquired immunodeficiency syndrome. Ann Intern Med. (1984). , 100, 239-241.

[27] Findling, J. W., Buggy, B. P., Gilson, I. H., Brummitt, C. F., & Bernstein, Raff. H. Longitudinal evaluation of adrenocortical function in patients infected with the human immunodeficiency virus. J ClinEndocrinolMetab. (1994). , 79, 1091-1096.

[28] Verges, B., Chavanet, P., Desgres, J., Vaillant, G., Waldner, A., Brim, J. M., & Putelat, R. Adrenal function in HIV infected patients. ActaEndocrinol (Copenh). (1989). , 121, 633-637.

[29] Sapolsky R, Rivier C, Yamamoto G, Plotsky P, Vale W. Interleukin-1 stimulates the secretion of hypothalamic corticotropin-releasing factor . Science 1987;238:522–4.

[30] Woloski BM, Smith EM, Meyer WJ, Fuller GM, Blalock JE.Corticotropin-releasing activity of monokines. Science (1985). , 230, 1035-1037.

[31] Whitcomb RW, Linehan WM, Wahl LM, Knazek RA.Monocytes stimulate cortisol production by cultured human adrenocortical cells. J ClinEndocrinolMetab (1988). , 66, 33-8.

[32] Meyer, W. J. I. I. I., Smith, E. M., Richards, G. E., Cavallo, A., Morrill, achéal., & Blalock, J. E. In vivo immunoreactiveadrenocorticotropin (ACTH) production by human mononuclear leukocytes from normal and ACTH-deficient individuals. J ClinEndocrinolMetab (1987). , 64, 98-105.

[33] Merrill JE, Koyanagi Y, Chen ISY. Interleukin-1 and tumor necrosis factor α can be induced from mononuclear phagocytes by human immunodeficiency virus type 1 binding to the CD4 receptor . J Virol 1989; 63:4404–8.

[34] Szebeni, J., Dieffenbach, C., Wahl, S. M., et al. Induction of alpha interferon by human immunodeficiency virus type 1 in human monocyte-macrophage cultures. J Virol (1991). , 65, 6362-4.

[35] Guire, M. A. P., & Holbrook, N. Physiological functions of glucocorticoids in stress and their relation to pharmacological actions. Endocrinol. Rev (1984). , 5, 25-44.

[36] Kino T, Gragerov A, Kopp JB, Stauber RH, Pavlakis GN &Chrousos GP. The HIV-1 virion-associated protein vpr is a coactivator of the human glucocorticoid receptor. Journal of ExperimentalMedicine1999;189: 51–62.

[37] Kino, T., & Chrousos, G. P. Glucocorticoid and mineralocorticoid resistance/hypersensitivity syndromes. Journal of Endocrinology (2001). , 437-445.

[38] Mylonakis, E., Koutkia, P., & Grinspoon, S. Diagnosis and treatment of androgen deficiency in human immunodeficiency virus-infected men and women. Clin Infect Dis. (2001). , 33, 857-64.

[39] Dobs AS, Dempsey MA, Ladenson PW, Polk BF.Endocrine disorders in men infected with human immunodeficiency virus. Am J Med. (1988). , 84, 611-6.

[40] Rietschel, P., Corcoran, C., Stanley, T., Basgoz, N., Klibanski, A., & Grinspoon, S. Prevalence of hypogonadism among men with weight loss related to human immunodeficiency virus infection who were receiving highly active antiretroviral therapy. Clin Infect Dis. (2000). , 31, 1240-4.

[41] Calkins JH, Sigel MM, Nankin HR, Lin T. Interleukin-1 inhibits Leydig cell steroidogenesis in primary culture. Endocrinology 1988; 123:1605–10.

[42] Graff AS, Gonzalez SS, Baca VR, Ramirez ML, Daza LB etal.High serum prolactin levels in asymptomatic HIV-infected patients and in patients with Acquired Immune deficiency syndrome. ClinImuunol. Immunopath (1994). , 72, 390-3.

[43] Rusell, D. H., Matrisian, L., Kibler, R., etal, , Prolactin, receptors., on, Human. T., lymphocytes, B., their, modulation., & by, Cyclosporine. J. Immunol (1985). , 134, 3027-31.

[44] Grinspoon, S., Corcoran, C., Miller, K., Biller, Askari. H., Wang, E., et al. Body composition and endocrine function in women with acquired immunodeficiency syndrome wasting. J ClinEndocrinolMetab. (1997). , 82, 1332-7.

[45] Perronne, C., Bricaire, F., Leport, C., Assan, D., Vilde, J. L., & Assan, R. Hypoglycaemia and diabetes mellitus following parenteral pentamidinemesylate treatment in AIDS patients. Diabetic Med (1990). , 7, 585-9.

[46] Hruz PW.Molecular mechanisms for altered glucose homeostasis in HIV infection. Am J Infectious Dis. (2006). , 2, 187-192.

[47] Murata, H., Hruz, P. W., & Mueckler, M. The mechanism of insulin resistance caused by HIV protease inhibitor therapy J BiolChem (2000). , 275, 20251-4.

[48] Caron M, Auclair M, Vigouroux C et al. the HIV protease inhibitor indinavir impairs sterol regulatory element-binding protein-1 intranuclear localization, inhibits preadipocyte differentiation and induces insulin resistance. Diabetes 2001; 50:1378-88.

[49] Tebas, P., Powderly, W. G., Claxton, S., Marin, D., Tantisiriwat, W., Teitelbaum, S. L., et al. Accelerated bone mineral loss in HIV-infected patients receiving potent antiretroviral therapy. AIDS. (2000). F, 63-7.

[50] Stagi, S., Bindi, G., Galluzzi, F., Galli, L., Salti, R., & de Martino, M. Changed bone status in human immunodeficiency virus type 1 (HIV-1) perinatally infected children is related to low serum free IGF-1. ClinEndocrinol (Oxf) (2004). , 61, 692-9.

[51] Glass, A. R., & Eil, C. Ketoconazole-induced reduction in serum 1,25-dihydroxyvitamin D. and total serum calcium in hypercalcemic patients. J ClinEndocrinolMetab (1988). , 66, 934-8.

[52] Effects of growth hormone-releasing hormone on bone turnover in human immunodeficiency virus-infected men with fat accumulation. J ClinEndocrinolMetab.; ., 90, 2154-60.

[53] Kuehn EW, Anders HJ, Bogner JR, Obermaier J, Goebel FD, Schlöndorff D. Hypocalcemia in HIV infection and AIDS. J Intern Med. 1999;245:69–73.

[54] Adams JS, Fernandez M, Gacad MA, et al. Vitamin D metabolite-mediated hypercalcemia and hypercalciuria in patients with AIDS- and non-AIDS-associated lymphoma . Blood 1989;73:235–9.

[55] Dodd RC, Newman SL, Bunn PA, Winkler CF, Cohen MS, Gray TK.Lymphokine-induced monocytic differentiation as a possible mechanism for the hypercalcemia associated with adult T-cell lymph. oma. Cancer Res (1985). , 45, 2501-6.

[56] Motokura, T., Fukumoto, S., Matsumoto, T., et al. Parathyroid hormone-related protein in adult T-cell leukemia-lymphoma. Ann Intern Med (1989). , 111, 484-8.

[57] Wanke, Silva. M., Knox, T. A., Forrester, J., Speigelman, D., & Gorbach, S. L. Weight loss and wasting remain common complications in individuals infected with HIV in the era of highly active antiretroviral therapy. Clin Infect Dis. (2000). , 31, 803-5.

[58] Anthropometric indices as predictors of survival in AIDS adults. Aquitaine Cohort, France, 1985-1997. Group d'Epidemiologie Clinique du Sida en Aquitaine (GECSA) Eur J Epidemiol.; ., 16, 633-9.

[59] Grunfeld C, Pang M, Doerrler W, Shigenaga JK, Jensen P, Feingold KR. Lipids, lipoproteins, triglyceride clearance, and cytokines in human immunodeficiency virus infection and the acquired immunodeficiency syndrome . J ClinEndocrinolMetab 1992; 74:1045–52.

[60] Macallan, D. E., Noble, C., Baldwin, C., Jebb, S. A., Prentice, A. M., Coward, W. A., et al. Energy expenditure and wasting in human immunodeficiency virus infection. N Engl J Med. (1995). , 333, 83-8.

[61] Miller, K. K., Daly, P. A., Sentochnik, D., Doweiko, J., Samore, M., Basgoz, N. O., et al., & Pseudo, . Pseudo-Cushing's syndrome in human immunodeficiency virus-infected patients. Clin Infect Dis. (1998). , 27, 68-72.

Chapter 12

Lipodystrophy: The Metabolic Link of HIV Infection with Insulin-Resistance Syndrome

Paula Freitas, Davide Carvalho, Selma Souto,
António Sarmento and José Luís Medina

Additional information is available at the end of the chapter

http://dx.doi.org/10.5772/52685

1. Introduction

Human lipodystrophies are a heterogeneous group of diseases characterized by generalized or partial fat loss. If localized, they are often associated with fat hypertrophy in other depots, varying according to the type of lipodystrophy. Lipodystrophies can be genetic, which is usually uncommon, or acquired. Genetic lipodystrophy is generally related to severe metabolic alterations including insulin resistance (IR) and its associated complications, such as glucose intolerance and diabetes, dyslipidemia, hepatic steatosis, polycystic ovaries, acanthosis nigricans and early cardiovascular (CV) complications [1, 2]. The autosomal recessive congenital generalized lipodystrophy (CGL) and autosomal dominant familiar partial lipodystrophy (FPL) are the two most common types of genetic lipodystrophy [2]. Lipodystrophies have been reported in the medical literature for more than 100 years [2, 3]. However, only 13 years ago, new lipodystrophy syndromes were recognized, being associated with viral infection, specifically with the human immunodeficiency virus, in patients treated with combined antiretroviral therapy (cART) [4]. This has become the most frequent form of lipodystrophy [2]. Some first-generation antiretroviral drugs used in HIV patients are strongly related with peripheral lipoatrophy and metabolic alterations [1].

Human lipodystrophies leads to severe metabolic alterations resulting in premature CV complications. On the other hand, high adiposity, such as seen in obesity, also increases metabolic alterations and leads to increased CV risk. So, it seems that the two extremes, the absence or the excess of fat mass, are associated with the same metabolic and CV complications. The consequences of increased fat depots are markedly dependent upon their localization. Adipose tissue in the lower part of the body is able to expand and can therefore accumulate excessive energy from diet, store triglycerides, and it appears to be protective at the metabolic level [5].

By contrast, accumulation of fat in the upper part of the body is deleterious. Therefore, decreased peripheral subcutaneous adipose tissue (SAT), and even more increased visceral adipose tissue (VAT), are strongly associated with metabolic alterations and IR [1].

With regards to the HIV-associated lipodystrophy, the available data suggest that this condition is caused by a complex interaction involving side effects of cART, disease related inflammation, and individual characteristics [6]. At present, HIV-infected patients are exposed to an increased metabolic risk like the general population, resulting from ageing, increased weight and fat gain, high fat and energy food and marked sedentariness. Moreover, a number of additional factors could worsen their metabolic profile, such as the ongoing HIV infection, the presence of lipodystrophy and the continuous use of antiretroviral drugs [7]. HIV-associated lipodystrophy is also associated with premature aging [8]resembling metabolic laminopathies and progeria [1]. Premature aging of HIV-infected patients affects bone, brain, vascular wall, muscles, kidney and liver, and results of the combined effects of long-term HIV-1 infection, depleted immune responses, the toxicity of some antiretrovirals and lipodystrophy. Cellular senescence seems to result from prelamin-A accumulation induced by some antiretroviral drugs, mitochondrial dysfunction and oxidative stress. In addition, increased cytokine release in lipodystrophy further contributes to premature aging and therefore, to early CV and hepatic disease risks [9].

We focus on adipocytes dysregulation in genetic and acquired lipodystrophy, with emphasis on the most common form, HIV-lipodystrophy, fromthe etiology to its complications.

2. Adipose tissue biology –Three different adipose tissue compartments

Adipocytes are a dynamic and highly regulated population of cells. Adipose tissue is characterized by a marked cellular heterogeneity among its cellular components: adipocytes, preadipocytes, fibroblasts, macrophages, lymphocytes, endothelial cells and multipotent stem cells, able to differentiate into several cell types. Adipose tissue can release regulatory factors (adipokines, cytokines, or chemokines) or metabolites (FFAs) capable of influencing other surrounding cells, thus establishing active cross-talk among cells within adipose tissue. [9]. Overall, fat tissue consists of approximately one third mature adipocytes. The remaining two thirds are a combination of small blood vessels, nerve tissue, fibroblasts and preadipocytes in various stages of development. Preadipocytes have the ability to proliferate and differentiate into mature adipocytes, conferring a constant functional plasticity on adipose tissue [10]. Preadipocytes mature in two steps: differentiation and then hypertrophy. During the early maturation stage, an increased number of mitochondria are required [11, 12], resulting in small adipocytes, which are highly sensitive to insulin and that secrete high levels of adiponectin [12]. By contrast, older adipocytes increase in size (hypertrophy), their functional activities are lost and they become resistant to insulin. These adipocytes also exhibit decreased numbers of mitochondria with impaired mitochondrial reactive oxygen species (ROS) generated by the respiratory chain, which could have dual effects on adipocyte differentiation. New adipocytes form constantly to replace lost adipocytes, to the extent

http://dx.doi.org/10.5772/52685

that 50 % of adipocytes in the human subcutaneous fat mass are replaced approximately every eight years. Preadipocytes are recruited to become lipid-filled mature adipocytes at the same rate that adipocytes die, and in this way the fat mass is in constant flux, and adipocyte number is kept constant. Cellular death of fat cells in white adipose tissue occurs primarily by necrosis-like cell death, which involves macrophage recruitment and a subsequent inflammatory response. This has been implicated in the metabolic complications of obesity. Increased visceral fat mass leads to IR and a low-grade inflammation status in which many adipokines and other adipocyte and macrophage factors are involved [13].

Adipose tissue is not homogeneous but rather a tissue with specific regional compartments with varying roles and metabolic functions [14]. Individually considered, adipose tissue compartments have stronger associations with physiological and pathological processes than does total adipose tissue mass [15-17]. The upper-body adipose tissue, including visceral fat, is involved in fat storage after meals and the release of free fatty acids (FFA) between meals to feed the liver, muscles and other organs, therefore sparing glucose for the brain. Visceral fat has a more lipolytic profile than subcutaneous fat. Peripheral lower-body fat, in the femoro-gluteal region, is mainly used for its storage capacity, thereby buffering excess fat [7]. The femoro-gluteal fat depot is relatively insensitive to lipolytic stimuli and highly sensitive to anti-lipolytic stimuli, and may play a protective role by acting as a "sink" for circulating FFA [18]. This uptake of FFA prevents ectopic fat storage in the liver, skeletal muscle, and pancreas, which causes IR and beta-cell dysfunction [19]. The excessive lipolytic capacity of visceral fat (and probably subcutaneous upper-body depots as well) results in a condition referred as lipotoxicity (see section below on lipotoxicity) [7]. The reasons for the lower degree of expansibility of visceral adipocytes remain unknown. Visceral adipose tissue (VAT) differs histologically from subcutaneous adipose tissue (SAT): it has smaller adipocytes and a larger supply of nerves and vessels; VAT has many of the characteristics of brown adipose tissue turned into white adipose tissue [20].

3. Lipohypertrophy and lipoatrophy

Adipose tissue can be subject of different influences and undergo different transformations. SAT has a lower mitochondria content and this contributes to adipocyte apoptosis and therefore, to more lipoatrophy. VAT, with a higher number of resident macrophages [21] and more 11βhydroxysteroid dehydrogenase activity than SAT [22], is predisposed to hypertrophy. Hypertrophied VAT from HIV-infected patients demonstrates mitochondrial dysfunction but not impairment of adipogenic gene expression in comparison with SAT [23]. cART can differentially alter fat development depending on the environment and physiology of the different compartments. In the case of lipoatrophy, because peripheral subcutaneous adipocytes cannot store triglycerides, non-lipoatrophic fat depots such as VAT, probably buffers the increase in FFA, which worsens lipohypertrophy [8].

Subcutaneous adipocytes seem to be more susceptible to the deleterious effects of protease inhibitors (PIs) than visceral adipocytes [24]. Accordingly, studies performed on control human SAT explants reveal that some PIs increase FFA, interleukin – 6 (IL-6) and TNF-α production through the activation of the proinflammatory nuclear factor – kB (NFkB) pathway. This PI-induced deleterious paracrine loop, between adipocytes and macrophages, similar to the observed in obesity, is not seen in VAT. These data indicate that SAT is more sensitive to the adverse effects of some PIs than VAT [8].

4. Adipogenesis

Individuals can differ remarkably in body fat distribution and the known differences in FFA uptake of adipose tissue compartments play a role in this difference. Premenopausal female SAT takes up more FFAs than male [25] and upper-body SAT takes up FFAs more avidly than femoral fat in men, but not in women. Gene expression, mRNA transcription of FA transporters and consequently facilitated FA transport was greater in the upper body in men and in the femoro-gluteal region in women. This novel FFA disposal pathway may also play a role in the development or maintenance of body fat distribution. On the other hand, direct FFA uptake in subcutaneous fat differs from fatty acid uptake from a meal in two respects: 1) direct FFA uptake is more efficient in women than in men and 2) in men there is no preferential direct FFA uptake in upper-body subcutaneous fat compared with femoral fat in women. These gender-based differences are consistent with this process as a mechanism to develop or maintain variations of body fat distribution between men and women, both lean and obese.The greater direct FFA uptake in abdominal over femoral fat in men could be due to the greater facilitation of inward fatty acid transport. Contrary to what is generally believed, upper-body subcutaneous fat releases ~70 % of systemic FFAs in lean men and women, whereas the leg contributes only ~20%; fatty acid uptake from a meal follows a similar pattern [26]. In non-obese men, the direct uptake/storage of FFAs in upper-body and leg fat mirrors this regional difference in FFA release, whereas in lean women, direct FFA uptake was similar in upper-body and femoral adipose tissue. This imbalance between release and direct reuptake in women could redistribute fatty acids toward leg fat. In obese women, the total FFA reuptake in leg fat was also significantly greater than in upper-body fat. It may be that some populations of fat cells, such as the smaller adipocytes, take up but do not actively release FFAs, whereas larger fat cells briskly release FFAs and do not take up FFAs under post-absorptive circumstances. In summary, there is a mechanism for adipocyte fatty acid uptake and storage that has yet to be understood, but which is independent of lipoprotein lipase and it's not thought to exist in the post-absorptive state [25].

Macrophage infiltration of the human adipose organ is a well-documented phenomenon that induces a low-grade chronic inflammation that is associated with IR. This reaction appears to be related mainly to macrophage-produced cytokines (TNF-α and IL-6] capable of interfering with the normal activity of insulin receptors. The greater amount of macrophages and macrophage-secreted cytokines found in visceral fat is in line with the greater morbidity associated with these depots. Subcutaneous and visceral adipocytes have cell-autonomous properties due to inherently different progenitor cells that exhibit a different gene expression pattern. Subcutaneous white adipose tissue responds better to the anti-lipolytic effects of insulin, secretes more adiponectin and less inflammatory cytokines, and is differentially

http://dx.doi.org/10.5772/52685

affected by molecules involved in signal transduction as well as drugs, compared with visceral white adipose tissue [13].

Lipoatrophic adipose tissue is known to be characterized by smaller adipocytes, greater cell size variation, disruption of cell membranes, and signs of apoptosis as determined by immunohistochemistry staining, when compared with non-lipodystrophic adipose tissue. There is a marked difference in gene expression between dorsocervical and abdominal SAT, irrespective of the lipodystrophy status, that lies in the expression of homeobox genes involved in organogenesis and regionalization. Disparate expression of such fundamental regulators of transcription might ultimately contribute to different patterns of differentiation and affect the susceptibility of the adipose tissue depot to cART-induced toxicity, perhaps making the abdominal subcutaneous and femoro-gluteal depot more vulnerable to atrophy [27].

Morphologic alterations in lipoatrophy-prone areas of SAT have been confirmed at the level of gene expression [9]. Most studies report that these lipoatrophic areas show an abnormally low expression of the major adipogenic transcription factors peroxisome proliferator-activated receptor -γ (PPARγ), sterol-regulatory element binding protein-1 (SREBP-1), and CCAAT/enhancer-binding protein-α (C/EBPα) [28-30]. Consequently, the expression of adipogenic differentiation-related genes is also decreased. For example, there is a reduction in the expression of genes for lipoprotein lipase and for the insulin-sensitive glucose transporter GLUT 4 [28, 29], resulting in impaired fatty acid and glucose uptake, respectively, and thus leading to a deficit in the lipid-accretion capacity of SAT. Another major alteration detected, which is probably related to the impaired adipogenic gene expression, is reduced expression of the adipokine genes adiponectin and leptin [28, 29]. In addition to impaired expression of adipogenetic–related genes, adipose tissue from patients with lipodystrophy, mainly those receiving NRTIs [31, 32] also show a reduction in mitochondrial DNA (mtDNA) levels. This decrease is associated with complex alterations in mitochondrial function, such as reduced expression of mtDNA-encoded transcripts and compensatory up-regulation of dysfunctional mitochondrial mass, that likely reduce the endogenous oxidative capacity of adipose tissue [33]. Moreover, increased oxidative stress and apoptosis have also been reported in lipoatrophic SAT [34]. Lipoatrophy is also accompanied by a state of chronic low-level inflammation [35]. High levels of expression of the inflammatory markers, TNF-α, IL- 6; IL-8 and IL-18 have been reported in SAT from HIV-1-infected lipoatrophic patients [28, 30, 35-37]. Expression of TNFα and IL-6 mRNA in SAT of lipodystrophic patients correlates positively with tissue apoptosis and negatively with adipogenic marker expression, which is consistent with a role for pro-inflammatory cytokines in adipocyte viability and differentiation [30]. Unlike SAT, VAT did not exhibit impaired expression of adipogenic marker genes. However, it did show some similar changes in inflammatory markers, such as induction of TNF-α, whereas others differed from that of SAT, such as, for instance, lack of monocyte chemoattractant protein -1 (MCP-1] induction. In contrast, mitochondrial dysfunction in VAT was found to be similar to that in SAT. Therefore, mtDNA depletion and signs of altered mitochondrial function are common to atrophic (subcutaneous) and hypertrophic (visceral, dorsocervical) depots in HIV-1 lipodystrophy, indicating that mitochondrial impairment cannot explain in a simple manner the final outcome for adipose depots, either in terms of lipoatrophy or lipohypertrophy [23]. Taken together, these observations indicate that different responses occurring in subcutaneous and visceral fat depots in lipodystrophic patients are likely to be related to intrinsic differences in fat physiology and/or capacity to react to the same insult. One adipose depot (visceral) enlarges in size and approaches its fat storage capacity threshold (as in obesity) merely because another adipose depot (subcutaneous) cannot [38]. A direct role for HIV-1 infection has been proposed by analyzing SAT from untreated HIV-1-infected patients ("naïve") as compared to healthy controls. Early histological studies did not indicate clear mitochondrial or inflammatory-related disturbances [39], but subsequent gene expression studies have shown a significant decrease in the expression of the adipocyte differentiation controller PPARγ and some impairment in the expression of genes encoding mitochondrial proteins and proteins specifically related to adipocyte metabolism, including adiponectin and 11β-steroid dehydrogenase type-1, the enzyme responsible for glucocorticoid activation [9, 29]. Some signs of inflammatory response have also been reported [29]. All these alterations are further enhanced in SAT oflipodystrophic patients. Therefore, it appears that HIV-1 infection initiates a first wave of alterations in adipose tissue that is amplified by cART and ultimately results in lipoatrophy [9].

5. Congenital generalized lipodystrophies

Generalized lipodystrophies are rare disorders that may be congenital or acquired. The genetic lipodystrophies have been reported in about 1000 patients [2]. The congenital generalized lipodystrophy (CGL) Berardinelli-Seip syndrome (BSCL), is an autosomal recessive disorder initially reported by Berardinelli [3] and Seip [40] with frequent parental consanguinity [41-44]. It has been proposed that Berardinelli-Seip syndrome could be a Portuguese disease, later spread by the Portuguese across the world [45].

Patients with CGL are recognized at birth or soon thereafter due to a near-total lack of body fat and prominent muscularity that causes a severe and striking phenotype (Figure 2A and 2B). Diabetes develops during infancy or most often during the teenage years. Hepatosplenomegaly, umbilical prominence or hernia, acanthosis nigricans, voracious appetite and accelerated growth can occur. Female patients develop hirsutism, may have clitoromegaly, oligomenorrhea and polycystic ovaries. Other uncommon manifestations include hypertrophic cardiomyopathy, mild mental retardation, and focal lytic lesions in the appendicular bones after puberty [41, 42]. Diabetes and its complications, hyperlipidemia and recurrent attacks of acute pancreatitis, hepatic steatosis and occasionally cirrhosis are the causes of morbidity and mortality [2].

At least 4 molecularly distinct forms of congenital lipodystrophy have been defined, with the mutations of the enzyme acyltransferase 1-acylglycerol-3-phosphate O- acyltransferase 2 (AGPAT2) or (BSCL1- locus 1) and Berardinelli-Seip (BSCL2 - locus 2) being both responsible for 95 % of gene mutations. AGPAT2 has been mapped in chromosomes 9q34. AGPATs are critical enzymes involved in the biosynthesis of triglycerides and phospholipids from glycerol-3-phosphate. They catalyze acylation of fatty acids at the sn-2 position of glycerol moiety and convert lysophosphatidic acid to phosphatidic acid [2, 46]. AGPAT2 is highly expressed in the adipose tissue, and its deficiency may cause lipodystrophy by limiting triglyceride or phospholipid biosynthesis [47].

http://dx.doi.org/10.5772/52685

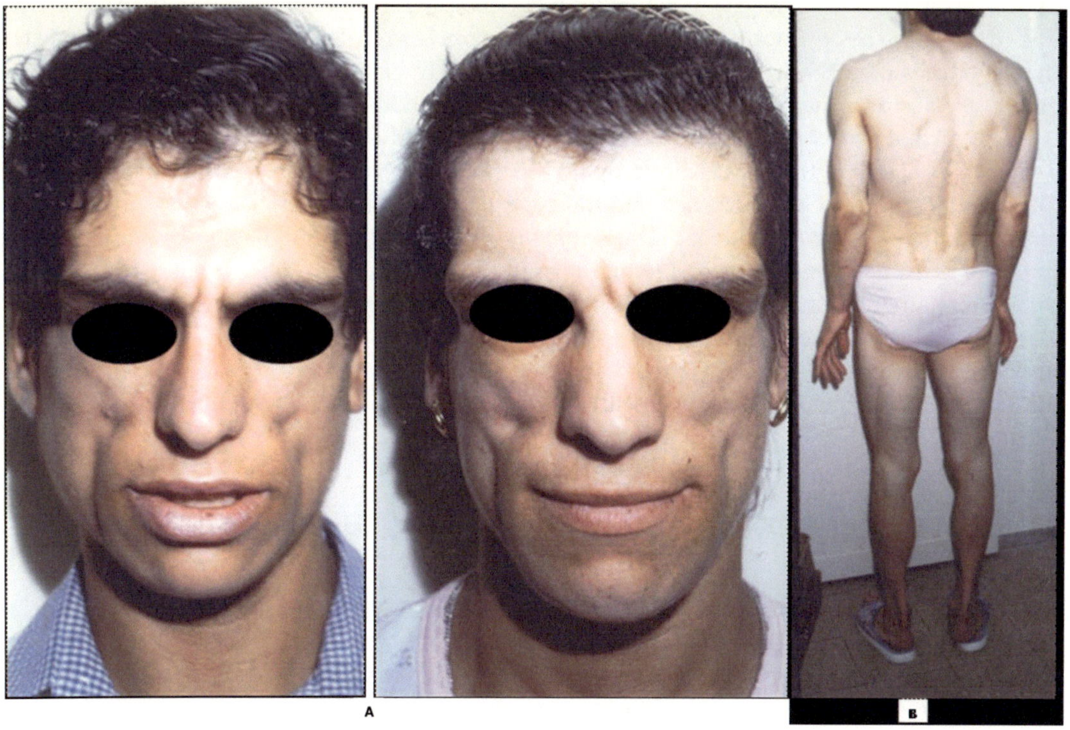

Figure 1. A: Two sisters with Berardinelli-Seip syndrome B: Women with Berardinelli-Seip syndrome

Type 2 CGL is due to BSCL2 gene mutations. This gene is located in chromosome11q13 and encodes a protein called seipin [48]. Seipin appears to play a role in lipid droplet formation and may also be involved in adipocyte differentiation [49-51].

Patients with BSCL2 mutations have the most severe variety of CGL and are born without any body fat [2]. Two other genes were identified for CGL: caveolin 1 (CAV1) [52] and polymerase I and transcript release factor (PTRF) [53]. Caveolin 1 is the main component of caveolae, specialized microdomains seen in abundance on adipocyte membranes [54]. It binds fatty acids and translocates them to lipid droplets. PTRF (also known as cavin) is involved in biogenesis of caveolae and regulates expression of caveolins 1 and 3 [53].

6. Mortality in generalized lipodystrophies

Patients with generalized lipodystrophies are predisposed to develop acute pancreatitis, cirrhosis, endstage diabetic renal disease requiring transplantation, and blindness due to diabetic retinopathy. Many patients with FPL die of coronary heart disease or cardiomyopathy and rhythm disturbances [55-57]. Sudden death has been reported during childhood in CGL, type 4, likely due to arrhythmias [58]. Patients with HIV-lipodystrophy are predisposed to developing coronary heart disease [59]. Patients with congenital Berardinelli-Seip lipodystrophy frequently develop hypertrophic cardiomyopathy that can lead to death from cardiac failure [41]. In individuals with BSCL, ventricular dysfunction and hypertrophic cardiomyopathy are often observed. In cardiac biopsies performed in eight individuals with BSCL, the presence of subendocardial fibrosis and an abnormal architecture in the left ventricular lumen was observed [60, 61]. Hypertrophic cardiomyopathy in BSCL patients has been correlated with high plasmatic insulin levels, which activate the type 1 insulin-like growth receptors, present in large quantities in the myocardial tissue, that stimulate cell growth [62, 63]. In addition, the presence of IR and hypertriglyceridemia in individuals with BSCL may predispose them to premature atherosclerosis. Individuals who have mutations on chromosome 11 (BSCL2) seemed to present more severe symptoms than those who had mutations in BSCL1, with a high incidence of premature deaths. Cardiomyopathy was three times more frequent in those with BSCL2 mutations than in individuals with alterations in BSCL1 [42].

7. Mandibuloacral Dysplasia (MAD)-associated lipodystrophy

MAD is characterized by skeletal abnormalities such as mandibular and clavicular hypoplasia and acroosteolysis [64], progeroid manifestations, partial or generalized lipodystrophy and metabolic complications, among other clinical features [65, 66]. Patients with MAD harbor mutations in lamin A/C (LMNA) or zinc metalloproteinase (ZMPSTE24) [67, 68]. ZMPSTE24 is involved in post-translational proteolytic processing of prelamin A to mature laminA [2].

8. Autoinflammatory syndromes

A syndrome of joint contractures, muscle atrophy, microcytic anemia, and panniculitis-induced (JMP) lipodystrophy was reported by Garg in three patients, belonging to two pedigrees, who were from Portugal and Mexico [69]. Three other patients have been reported from Japan [70, 71]. Mutations in PSMB8 may trigger an autoinflammatory response resulting in infiltration of adipose tissue with lymphocytes and other immune cells and adipocytes [2]. The other autoinflammatory syndrome is the chronic atypical neutrophilic dermatosis with lipodystrophy and elevated temperature (CANDLE) syndrome. The mode of inheritance seems to be autosomal recessive, but the molecular basis remains unknown [2, 72, 73].

9. Familial Partial Lipodystrophy(FPL)

FPL is characterized by the onset of fat loss from the limbs and other regions of the body, usually during childhood, adolescence or adulthood. Many regions of the body, such as the face, neck, and intra-abdominal region are spared, and patients accumulate excess body fat in the non-lipodystrophic regions [74-76]. Metabolic complications, acanthosis nigricans, oligoamenorrhea, hirsutism, polycystic ovarian syndrome, mild to moderate myopathy, cardiomyopathy, and conduction system abnormalities indicative of multisystem dystrophy can occur [2, 55, 56, 77]. The identification of the first gene for FPL, Dunnigan variety, i.e. LMNA, on chromosome 1q21-22 [2, 78-81], an integral component of nuclear lamin, was made in 1998. Thereafter, four other genes were identified: PPARγ [82-84], a key transcription factor involved in adipocyte differentiation; v-AKT murine thymoma oncogene homolog 2 (AKT2) [85], involved in downstream insulin signaling; and cell death-inducing DNA fragmentation factor a-like effector c (CIDEC) [86] and perilipin 1 (PLIN1) [87], both involved in lipid droplet formation [2, 88]. Adipocyte loss is due to premature cell death resulting from disruption of the nuclear envelope [87, 89]. Defective adipocyte differentiation seems to be the cause of the lipodystrophy of PPARγ and AKT2 mutations. Fibrosis of adipose tissue with small adipocytes is responsible for the lipodystrophy of PLIN1 mutations [2, 87].

There are other rare genetic syndromes whose molecular basis remains unknown, namely atypical progeroid syndrome [90], Hutchinson-Gilford progeria syndrome [91], SHORT-associated lipodystrophy [92], and Wiedemann-Rautenstrauch syndrome [93].

Patients with FPL syndromes display mixed lipodystrophy with subcutaneous lipoatrophy and central fat accumulation. Those with FPLD2 also have an increased amount of fat in the cervico-facial area compared to patients without these mutations. Therefore, a single protein mutation leads to two opposing fat localization phenotypes [8]. Importantly, mutations in LMNA are also responsible for metabolic laminopathies resembling the metabolic syndrome (MS) and Hutchinson-Gilford progeria, a severe syndrome of premature aging [94]. Prelamin A is implicated in increased oxidative stress and in the occurrence of cellular senescence [8].

10. Acquired lipodystrophies

10.1. Acquired Generalized Lipodystrophy(AGL) – Lawrence syndrome

The onset of subcutaneous fat loss in patients with AGL usually occurs during childhood [95]. The pattern and extent of fat loss is quite variable and most patients have generalized loss of fat, but a few of them have areas such as intra-abdominal and bone marrow fat spared. AGL patients are highly likely to develop severe hepatic steatosis and fibrosis, diabetes, and hypertriglyceridemia [2]. The pathogenesis of fat loss remains unknown. Panniculitis may precede loss of fat. Lipodystrophy can be associated with autoimmune diseases such as juvenile dermatomyositis [95]. Chronic hepatitis with autoimmune features and low serum complement 4 levels, suggesting involvement of the classical complement pathway in the pathogenesis of fat loss, has been reported [96].

10.2. Acquired partial lipodystrophy–Barraquer-Simons syndrome

Fat loss occurs gradually in a symmetric fashion, first affecting the face and then spreading downward. Most patients lose fat from the face, neck, upper extremities, and trunk, and subcutaneous fat from the lower abdomen and legs is spared. Many patients accumulate excess subcutaneous fat in the hips and legs. Metabolic complications are rare. Misra et al suggest that the fat loss involves autoimmune-mediated destruction of adipocytes because the patients have low serum levels of complement 3 and complement 3-nephritic factor, which blocks degradation of the enzyme C3 convertase [95]. It is possible that the C3-nephritic factor induces lysis of adipocytes expressing factor D [97].

10.3. Localized lipodystrophy

Localized lipodystrophies present focal loss of subcutaneous fat, usually causing one or more dimples, and in general occurs due to subcutaneous injection of various drugs (Figure 4), panniculitis, pressure, and other mechanisms [98].

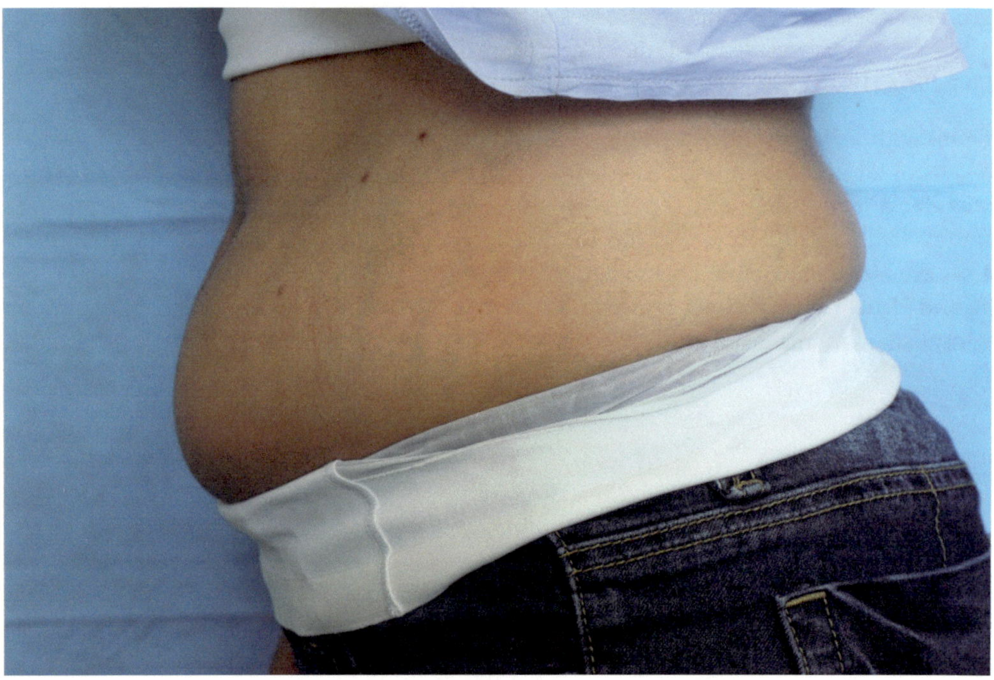

Figure 2. Patient with lipohypertrophy related to subcutaneous administration of pegvisomant.

10.4. Lipodystrophy associated with HIV-infection

The impressive progress resulting from the discovery of drugs able to control HIV infection on a long-term basis, has offered most patients a prolonged lifespan, possibly as long as that observed in non-infected subjects [7]. Suppression of viral replication has become a treatment goal that can be reached with the use ofcART. After the introduction of protease inhibitors (PIs) in 1996, as a component of highly active antiretroviral therapy, the morbidity and mortality associated with HIV has dramatically been reduced [99]. However, patients develop a syndrome of fat redistribution with peripheral fat loss (face, upper limbs and femoro-gluteal) and visceral fat accumulation, generally associated with metabolic abnormalities [4, 100-103] and increased risk of CV diseases [104, 105], similar to what occurs in congenital lipodystrophies [4, 59]. Lipohypertrophy usually represents a central visceral fat accumulation in the abdomen and trunk, but can also be found in breasts (in women), dorsocervical region ("buffalo hump"), double chin, lipomas, and within the muscle and liver [59, 106]. Lipoatrophy and lipohypertrophy are frequently associated (mixed form), but they also can occur independently of each other [59]. This HIV-associated lipodystrophy has been proposed to be a age-related fat redistribution condition that could amplify age-related co-morbidities and lead to their earlier occurrence [8]. Also, hyperlactenemia and bone demineralization can occur [107, 108].

Owing to a lack of a consensus on the definition of lipodystrophy and lipodystrophy syndrome in HIV-infected patients, its exact prevalence is not known [6]. In the early 2000s, about half of HIV-infected patients undergoing cART were diagnosed as lipodystrophic (20-80%) [109]. Abnormalities in peripheral and central fat masses are clinically evident in 20-35 % of patients after approximately 12-24 months of cART [59, 107, 110, 111]. With the new anti-retroviral agents, the probability of developing lipoatrophy has decreased in western countries as the pattern of cART prescription has significantly changed [112]. In the study of Nguyen, lipodystrophy has become less frequent since 2003 [112]. Two widely used thymidine analogs from the first class of ART, stavudine and zidovudine, are responsible for lipoatrophy and now they have been replaced by a new generation of potent NRTIs. Although metabolic toxicity of boosted PIs is far less than of first-generation protease inhibitors (PIs), they are still considered responsible for increased CV risk. The new classes of ART, fusion inhibitors (F20), integrase inhibitors (raltegravir) or entry inhibitors (anti-CCR5, maraviroc) have not yet been shown to alter metabolic parameters or fat distribution [8, 112-117].

HIV-infected patients can have 4 different phenotypes of body fat composition: no lipodystrophy, isolated peripheral lipoatrophy, isolated central fat accumulation and a mixed form of lipodystrophy (or redistribution syndrome) [100]. About 50% of patients with HIV-associated lipodystrophy display mixed forms, with the loss of limb fat and marked expansion of VAT [113]. The high frequency of this association suggests that these two opposite phenotypes could be, at least in part, causally related [8]. Also, HIV patients may have a picture similar to partial lipodystrophy patients with peripheral fat atrophy and hypertrophied central fat depots. Thus, there are similarities between HIV lipodystrophy and genetic forms.

11. HIV-lipodystrophy and related factors

There is a possible role of the virus contribution for lipodystrophy i.e. the HIV or hepatitis infection affects fat tissue before any ART. Monocytes are relatively resistant to HIV infection, but differentiated macrophages are highly susceptible and tissue macrophages have been found to harbor HIV-1 [118]. Infected macrophages release pro-inflammatory cytokines. Systemic inflammation associated with HIV infection might promote monocyte migration across the vascular endothelium, leading to an increased number of activated macrophages in fat

[118]. Several studies reported that the severity of HIV infection is associated with an increased prevalence of lipodystrophy [59, 119], probably as a consequence of persistent HIV-infected macrophages in adipose tissue, which could enhance local inflammation.

ART-naïve HIV-positive patients have increased TNF-α expression compared with uninfected controls [29], which is consistent with increased inflammation. TNF-α alters adipocyte function and differentiation, in part through the inhibition of PPARγ expression [120]. Infected macrophages might also release viral proteins (such as Vpr and Nef) that can impact on adjacent adipocytes and lead to decreased PPARγ activity and inhibition of adipogenesis [121, 122]. Although lipodystrophy is uncommon in ART-naïve patients [113], the HIV infection of macrophages could itself result in low-grade fat inflammation and lead to the release of viral proteins that affect neighboring adipocytes and decrease their differentiation.

The development of lipodystrophy and metabolic toxicities is partially related to the individual drugs included in cART regimens, associated with other risk factors [123] such as gender and pre-HIV-infection body composition, disease-specific factors such as the nadir levels of CD4+ lymphocytes and the duration of HIV infection [110, 123, 124]. The most significant risk factors associated with lipoatrophy are exposure to and duration of nucleoside thymidine analogues (most commonly stavudine), age, severity of disease markers (CD4 lymphocyte count and plasma HIV viral load), therapy duration, and belonging to the Caucasian race. On the other hand, the most common statistically significant risk factors for lipohypertrophy are therapy duration, PI administration, markers of disease severity, and age. We cannot forget that along the years, patients have done multiple regimes and combinations of antiretroviral drugs, which makes it difficult to identify different risks with different drugs, and studies therefore report conflicting results [6].

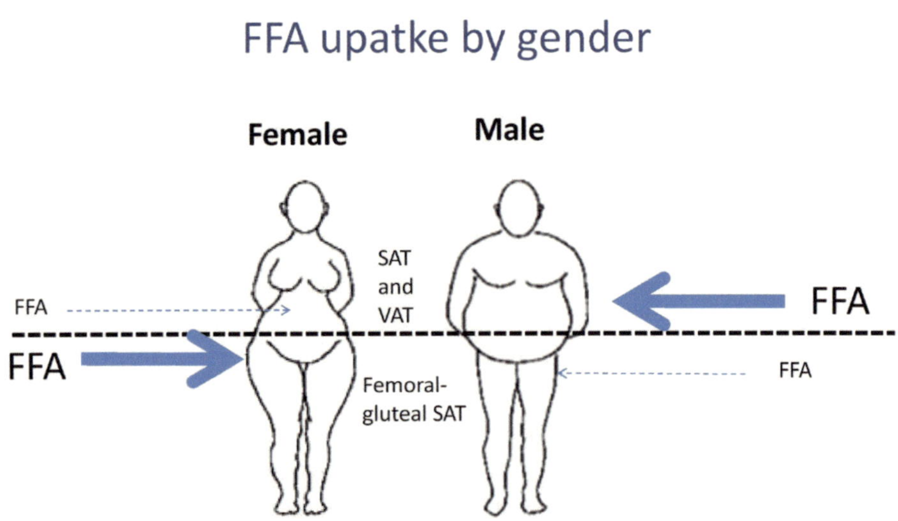

Figure 3. FFA uptake by gender (SAT - abdominal subcutaneous adipose tissue; VAT – visceral adipose tissue; FFA – free fat acids)

12. Protease inhibitors

PIs affect multiple metabolic pathways and are associated with lipohypertrophy, lipoatrophy, atherogenic dyslipidemia and IR, [125, 126]. Studies in-vitro reported that PIs are able to alter a number of adipocyte functions, including differentiation, expression of transcriptase factors involved in adipogenesis, cell survival, cytokine production, mitochondrial function and IR [127]. PIs may cause lipodystrophy by inhibiting ZMPSTE24, resulting in accumulation of toxic farnesylated prelamin A [128], increased oxidative stress and altered adipokine and cytokine production [89, 127, 129]. The adverse effect of PIs could also result from the induction of endoplasmic reticulum stress or the inhibition of the proteasome [130, 131].

Different PIs might affect key intranuclear genes, causing reduction in levels of RNA encoding SREBP-1, which changes the expression of PPAR γ [28]. The levels reduction of intranuclear SREBP-1 leads to a decreased adipocyte differentiation and an altered release of adipocytokines [132]. PIs can inhibit lipogenesis and stimulate lipolysis [28, 132-135], and may induce IR by inhibiting glucose transporter 4 expression (GLUT4) [136].

13. Nucleoside and Nucleotide Reverse Transcriptase Inhibitors (NRTIs)

NRTIs are analogs that inhibit the viral reverse transcriptase enzyme. The thymidine NRTIs (zidovudine, stavudine and didanosine) cause mitochondrial toxicity by mitochondrial DNA polymerase inhibition and by causing DNA mitochondrial mutations [31, 137, 138]. These disturbances result in apoptosis of peripheral adipocytes and lead to lipoatrophy [31]. NRTIs are also associated with fat hypertrophy in visceral depots [113, 139, 140]. Nucleoside analogues may inhibit adipogenesis and adipocyte differentiation, promote lipolysis, and exert synergistic toxic effects when associated to PIs [31, 141-143]. Moreover, NRTIs promote lipolysis and the subsequent efflux of non-esterified fatty acids from adipose tissue [142, 144].

14. Mitochondrial toxicity and fat redistribution

In western countries, long-term HIV-infected patients present several age-related comorbidities earlier than the general population [145], and display signs of premature aging [8]. New hypotheses were recently suggested about the pathophysiology of fat redistribution, proposing that mitochondrial toxicity was involved in lipoatrophy and in fat hypertrophy. HIV-associated lipodystrophy could be an age-related fat redistribution that could amplify age-related comorbidities and their earlier occurrence [8]. Mitochondria play an important role in adipocyte differentiation and function. At physiological low levels, ROS could act as secondary messengers to activate adipogenesis and lipogenesis, resulting in increased adipocyte number and size. In hepatic cells, oxidative stress activates the transcription factor SREBP1c, which is highly expressed in adipocytes and increases lipogenesis and lipid accumulation [146]. At higher levels, ROS could inhibit differentiation [8].

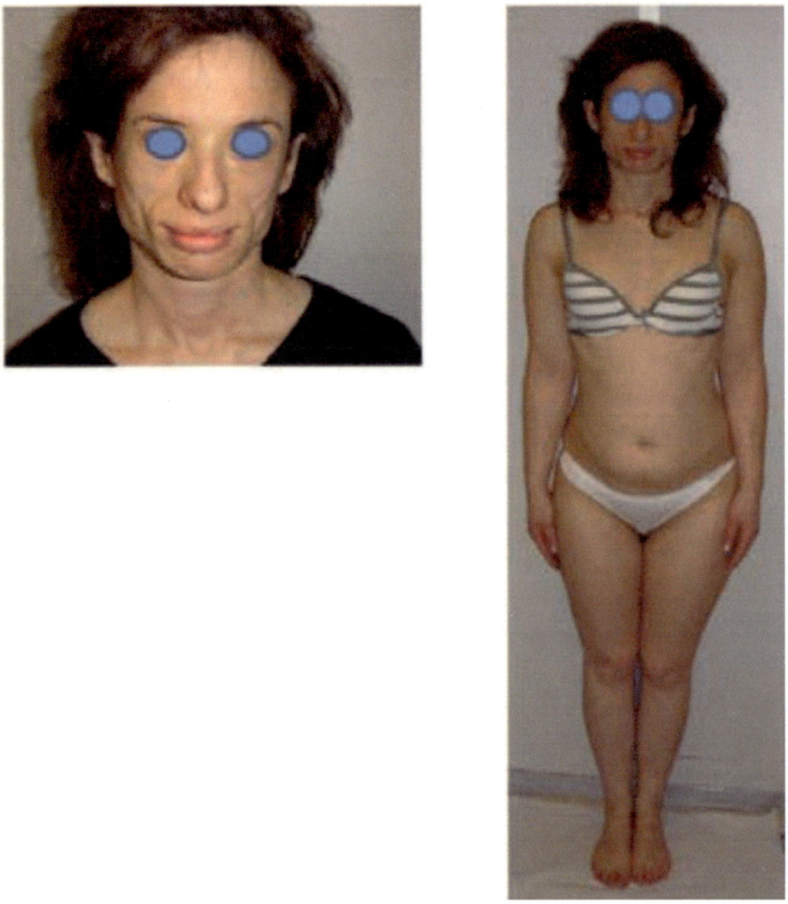

Figure 4. Acquired partial lipodystrophy - Barraquer-Simons syndrome

Excessive VAT releases increased visceral adipocyte-FFAs, adipokines and cytokines. Indeed, activated macrophages, which have an M1 proinflammatory phenotype, invade expanded adipose tissue; upon invasion, their production of proinflammatory cytokines and chemokines increases. This could lead to the decreased secretion of adiponectin by adipocytes in response to TNF-α [36]. Increased abdominal fat lipolysis increases ectopic fat deposition within tissues (liver, skeletal muscle and heart). Subsequently, these derivatives overwhelm mitochondrial oxidative capacity and activate stress kinases, leading to IR. This situation, known as lipotoxicity, associates ectopic depots of triglycerides in non-adipose tissues that buffer excess fatty acid derivatives [147]. Moreover, a paracrine loop is present between adipocytes and macrophages; macrophage-secreted cytokines (TNF-α and IL-6] activate the NFkB pathway in adipocytes, resulting in increased IL-6 and FFA production. Saturated FFA can, in turn, activate the Toll-like receptor-4 (TLR-4) on macrophages and adipocytes, thereby increasing the proinflammatory loop. This paracrine loop has been reported in obesity as a result of macrophages infiltrating fat [148].

http://dx.doi.org/10.5772/52685

15. Cortisol and fat redistribution

Patients with hypercortisolism also have an acquired form of lipodystrophy [1], characterized by fat hypertrophy in the upper body with increased VAT and decreased limb fat. Cortisol can activate adipocyte differentiation and hypertrophy, mainly in visceral fat depots, because of the higher expression of glucocorticoid receptors (GR-α) and the 11β-hydroxysteroid dehydrogenase type 1 (11β-HSD-1) that transforms inactive cortisone into active cortisol in adipocytes from central depots [22]. In addition, cortisol induces IR and increases lipolysis in adipocytes [22]. It has been hypothesized that glucocorticoid activation is involved in cART-linked central fat hypertrophy [8]. Higher ratios of urinary cortisol:cortisone metabolites and higher subcutaneous 11β-HSD-1 expression are observed in patients with severe lipodystrophy compared with those without [149]. In cART-naïve patients, 11β-HSD-1 expression increases in both abdominal and thigh SAT after 12 months of ART, but only in patients with lipohypertrophy or without lipoatrophy [150]. Because TNF-α expression in fat is related to that of 11β-HSD-1 [149], inflammation is linked to glucocorticoid activation [8]. TNF-α activates 11-β-hydroxysteroid dehydrogenase (HSD)-type 1, and this enzyme's activity is higher in visceral fat compared with subcutaneous fat. Visceral fat is able to locally produce cortisol, which could act inside the adipocytes and increase lipid accumulation [151]. Other hormones, such as growth hormone and testosterone, can modulate the activity of 11β-HSD-1. It is interesting to note that HIV-infected patients with lipodystrophy often present with a relative decrease in growth hormone [152] and testosterone levels. Moreover, when patients with visceral fat hypertrophy are treated with growth hormone, a reduced amount of visceral fat is reported, together with improved metabolic status [153].

16. Aging

In the general population, age is associated with central fat redistribution, mitochondrial impairment and increased levels of pro-inflammatory cytokines [154]. Aging adipocytes release more pro-inflammatory cytokines than young ones [155]. Aging is physiologically associated with fat redistribution, oxidative stress and low-grade inflammation. In the general population, the interaction between the proinflammatory state and genetic background potentially triggers the onset of age-related inflammatory diseases such as atherosclerosis, sarcopenia and frailty. Decreased immune response leading to immunosenescence is also probably involved in early aging [8, 156]. Aging and some cARTs result in mitochondrial dysfunction and oxidative stress, which lead to cellular senescence. Moreover, some PIs induce the accumulation of the pro-senescent protein prelaminA [8].

17. Genetic factors and HIV-lipodystrophy

A role for genetics is also probable in HIV-lipodystrophy. TNF-α gene promoter polymorphism is associated with lipodystrophy, but this association has not been confirmed in larger studies [157]. Interestingly, stavudine-induced lipoatrophy is linked to the HLA-B100*4001 allele, which is located in close proximity to the TNF-α gene; this observation further supports the theory that there is a role for inflammation in lipoatrophy [158]. Apo C3-455 also plays a role in lipoatrophy, and two variants of the adipogenic β2 receptor seems to be involved in fat accumulation, whereas PPARγ variants are not involved [159]. The toxicity of ART also depends on a patient's metabolism, in part genetically determined.

18. Role of inflammation

Even if infectivity of adipocytes by HIV has been contested, the ability of the virus to modify adipocyte phenotype has been shown in some studies [160, 161]. Moreover, macrophages and dendritic cells present in lipodystrophic adipose tissue could be infected, which could modify their characteristics [7]. Macrophage infiltration is observed in adipose tissue from patients with HIV-related lipodystrophy together with decreased adipokine and increased pro-inflammatory cytokine production [162]. Some anti-retrovirals increase oxidative stress and generation of reactive species, which results in decreased production of adiponectin and leptin by adipocytes and increased production of pro-inflammatory cytokines [7].

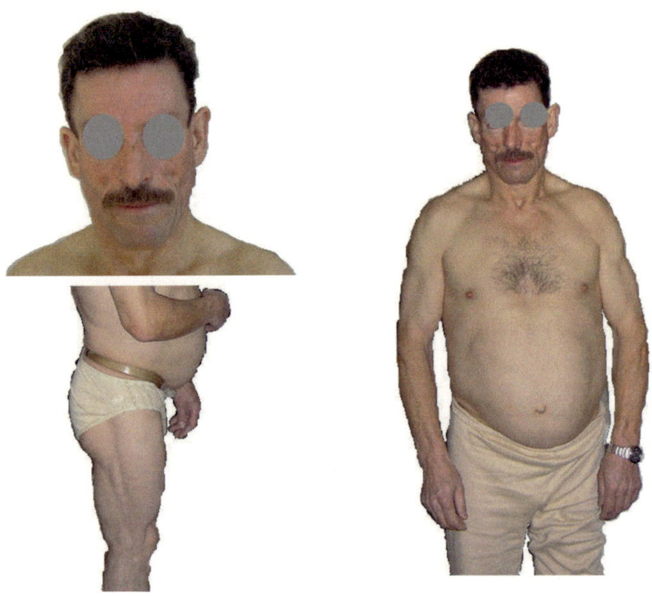

Figure 5. Patient with mixed lipodystrophy (absence of subcutaneous peripheral fat in arms, legs and face and increased abdominal fat mass)

http://dx.doi.org/10.5772/52685

19. Lipotoxicity

Lipotoxicity is a possible explanation for the development of metabolic syndrome (MS) and diabetes in multiple pathological situations, from obesity to lipodystrophies of distinct origin. According to the lipotoxicity theory, excess availability of fatty acids or a limited capacity to metabolize them in organs and tissues elicits most of the alterations that are characteristic of MS, especially IR. The toxicity of fatty acids toward β-cells may lead to altered insulin production. Actually, high FA levels can induce a reduction in GLUT2 on β cell surfaces and induce a decrease in insulin secretion [19]. Increased availability and, ultimately, increased accumulation of fat into skeletal muscle tends to promote IR; and fatty acid levels in liver that exceed the capacity of this organ to oxidize or export them, lead to the increased accumulation of fat that is often associated with MS. All of these events could result from alterations in fat metabolism or excess intake of fat-enriched nutrients, but they could also arise as a result of intrinsic alterations in the capacity of adipose tissue to store and thereby buffer the excessive accumulation of fatty acids in other tissues and organs [163]. One hypothesis consistent with the appearance of MS in ART-associated lipodystrophy syndrome is lipotoxicity resulting from limitations in the capacity of subcutaneous fat to store the appropriate amounts of fat and the subsequent diversion of fatty acids to ectopic sites [164]. Several arguments in support of lipotoxicity as a major contributor to MS in distinct human pathologies come from the paradoxically common metabolic alterations found in the obesity and in lipodystrophies of genetic origin. According to the lipotoxicity theory, the fat stored in adipose tissue is biologically inert and the observed metabolic alterations are primarily caused by the increased exposure of cells to non-esterified fatty acid. Thus, in obese patients, it is not the amount of fat stored in adipose tissue that elicits metabolic dysfunctions, but rather the balance between the availability of those fatty acids to tissues and organs and the capacity of the organs to eliminate them through triglyceride storage in adipose tissue, or oxidation [165]. A complementary concept is the idea that there is a threshold for adipose tissue expansibility; once it's reached, as it occurs in obese individuals, appropriate storage of fatty acids inside adipocytes in their inert and esterified form is impaired, determining the extent of lipotoxicity [164]. Either a total or partial lack of adipose tissue storage capacity causes an increase in circulating lipid levels and is associated with ectopic lipid accumulation in non-fat tissues such as liver, skeletal muscle and pancreas. These alterations lead to non-alcoholic fatty liver diseases, hepatic and muscle IR and development of type 2 diabetes. Adipokine deficiency further contributes to metabolic alterations (e.g. hyperphagia) owing to an associated leptin deficiency, which also contributes to positive energy balance and potential lipotoxicity through increased fat intake [94].

20. Insulin resistance

IR occurs in about one-third of patients on certain PI-based regimens, although the thymidine NRTIs have also been associated [166]. Asymptomatic type 2 diabetes mellitus is diagnosed in 5-10 % of patients [126]. The new-generation PIs appear to have a milder IR effect and the prevalence of diabetes is lower than described in the early 2000s. Its prevalence, however, remains higher than in the general population at the same age. In particular, patients with severe lipodystrophy are more prone to develop IR [7]. The pathogenesis of glucose metabolism disorders is still unclear and, although a direct effect of potent antiretroviral combinations is certainly involved, it is likely that multiple factors play a role, including genetic predisposition, cytokine and hormonal alterations, changes in the immune system, non-antiretroviral drug-induced toxic effects, opportunistic diseases, and perhaps the HIV infection itself [167]. Risk factors for the development of IR in HIV-positive population include duration of ART, PI treatment, concurrent fat redistribution syndrome, dyslipidemia, increasing age, hepatitis C virus co-infection, as well as pharmacological treatment with pentamidine or megestrol acetate [100, 167-169].

PIs (including indinavir, amprenavir, nelfinavir, and ritonavir) have been shown to induce IR in vitro by reducing glucose transport mediated by the glucose transporter 4, a receptor involved in glucose uptake [136]. The deleterious impact of some PIs on adipocytes through the inhibition of GLUT4 transporters was directly demonstrated in healthy controls, after given these molecules for a few weeks [169-171]. Several PIs can interfere with nuclear transcription factors, leading to decreased adiponectin levels, which also leads to IR [123]. Some PIs might also cause mitochondrial toxicity [172]. Additionally, the increase in FFA levels associated with PIs, as well as with fat redistribution, might also have a role in the development of IR (*see* lipotoxicity) [173].

21. Dyslipidemia

A number of HIV-infected patients present dyslipidemia, increased cholesterol, low-density lipoprotein (LDL)-cholesterol and triglycerides together with decreased HDL. This profile has been associated with the presence of a MS, resulting from an increased visceral fat amount with IR [7].

In patients receiving cART, the prevalence of hyperlipidemia ranges from 28 to 80% in different studies [167, 174], and it includes hypertriglyceridemia in the majority of cases [123]. Dyslipidemia is frequently, but not always, associated with fat redistribution syndrome: although lipid and glucose metabolism alterations are more common in patients with body-fat abnormalities, they are also observed in those without these morphological changes [167].

Several pathogenetic mechanisms have been proposed to explain cART-associated hyperlipidemia, which seems to result from a complex and multifactorial pathologic process: possibly HIV infection itself, leading in some cases to permanent low grade inflammation with abnormal levels of some pro-inflammatory cytokines; lipodystrophy itself, as in the genetic forms, with decreased lower-body fat depots and increased visceral fat; and antiretroviral molecules (PIs, NNRTIs and some NRTIs) [7].

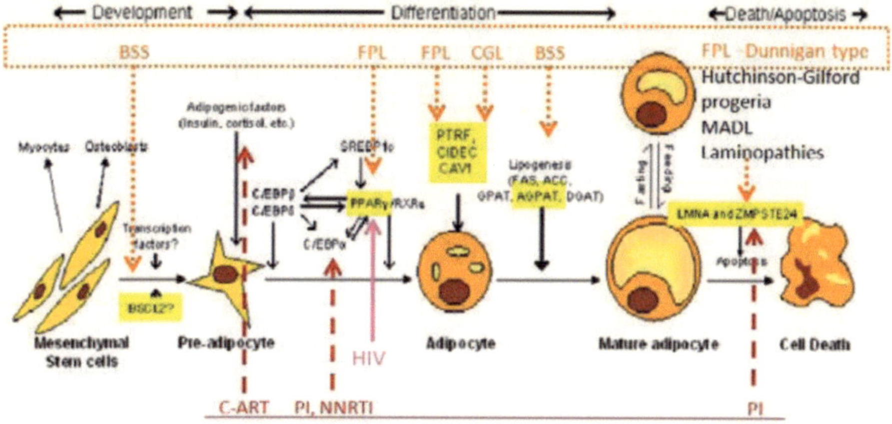

Figure 6. Genetic and adquiredlipodystrophies (CGL – congenital generalized lipodystrophy; BSS – Berardinelli-Seip syndrome; cART- combined antiretroviral therapy; NRTI – nucleoside and nucleotide reverse transcriptase inhibitors; PI - protease inhibitors; FPL- familiar partial lipodystrophy; MADL- mandibuloacral dysplasia associated lipodystrophy; adapted from Agarwal&Garg. Ann Rev Genomics Human Genet 2006; 7: 175-199]

Various mechanisms involved in ART-related dyslipidemia have been described: reduction in the catabolism of VLDL, increased VLDL production, impaired catabolism of FFA, increased liver triglyceride synthesis, increased secretion of apolipoprotein B-containing lipoproteins, reduced expression of LDL receptors, reduced degradation of SREBP, and reduction in FXR (farnesoid X receptor) [175]. The first hypothesized mechanism is based upon the structural similarity between the catalytic region of HIV-1 protease and two human proteins involved in lipid metabolism: the cytoplasmic retinoic acid-binding protein type 1 (CRABP-1) and the low-density lipoprotein-receptor-related protein (LRP). PIs probably bind to CRABP-1 and erroneously inhibit the formation of cis-9-retinoic acid, leading to increased apoptosis of peripheral adipocytes, decreased lipid storage and increased lipid release into the bloodstream. Similarly, PIs may inhibit the normal functioning of LRP and interfere with fatty acid storage in the adipocytes [167, 176]. Furthermore, data from in vitro and in vivo studies suggest that PIs may prevent proteasomal degradation of nascent apolipoprotein B, a key protein component of circulating triglycerides, leading to increased production of VLDL particles. An upregulation of metabolic pathways leading to an excessive production of VLDL can also be caused by the PI-induced intra-hepatocyte accumulation of nuclear transcription factors involved in the metabolism of apolipoprotein B, such as SRBPs. In addition, the levels of lipoprotein particles containing apolipoprotein C-III and apolipoprotein E are increased in PI-treated patients [176-179].

22. Metabolic syndrome

In the general population, MS is described as an association of increased upper-body fat, particularly in the visceral area, with IR responsible for and revealed by metabolic alterations, including increased LDL, decreased HDL, increased triglycerides, increased glycemia or diabetes and increased blood pressure [180-182]. All these parameters constitute a constellation of major CV risk factors [180]. This situation also includes low-grade inflammation and a prothrombotic state [7].

The pathophysiology of MS is complex – genetic factors, aging and weight gain associated with sedentariness and food habits constitute major risk factors. Also, decreased mitochondrial function related to aging [183] and an age-related redistribution of fat towards the central, visceral areas are involved, leading to IR and metabolic abnormalities [7].

The components of the HIV lipodystrophy syndrome(s) bear a striking resemblance to those of MS [123]. Both can present hyperinsulinemia, glucose intolerance, central or abdominal obesity, hypertension, atherogenic lipid profile, hyperuricemia, prothromboticand proinflammatory states [123].

Liver lesions of nonalcoholic steatohepatitis (or NASH) are a complication of MS, with a possible evolution towards severe liver complications such as cirrhosis. HIV-infected patients, with IR in the context of a severe lipodystrophy, present an increased risk of liver lesions [184]. Moreover, as HCV infection has been associated with steatosis and hepatic IR resulting from viral or metabolic effects, HCV co-infection could aggravate the metabolic and liver status of HIV-infected patients [185]. HIV-infected patients with MS are more likely to have higher values of carotid intima-media thickness (cIMT) and detectable coronary artery calcium score [186].

23. Clinical sequelae associated with HIV and HIV-lipodystrophy

Different studies suggest that the CV risk is increased among HIV-infected patients on cART and the responsible mechanisms are complex: in addition to the direct effect of the virus on the vasculature, the toxicity of antiretroviral drugs and the set of metabolic alterations aggregated in the MS are involved [187]. Whether the increased CV risk is due to HIV infection itself, to ART, or to a synergistic interaction between these factors, remains to be established [167]. HIV infection itself may increase CV risk. The HIV surface glycoprotein gp120 can stimulate endothelial cell production of tissue factor, an early step in the development of atherosclerosis [188]. Both HIV infection and ART promote atherosclerosis and its clinical manifestations through inflammatory mechanisms involving endothelial cells, either directly or indirectly, and also by inducing lipid alterations [189, 190].

Furthermore, some data suggest that endothelial dysfunction, impaired fibrinolysis, and excess inflammation are more common in HIV-positive patients than in general population, which may contribute to an increased CV risk [191]. At the same time, cIMT and coronary calcification assessments suggest increased incidence of atherosclerotic disease and premature occurrence of arterial atherosclerotic lesions among HIV-infected individuals [192]. Surrogate markers of atherosclerosis, including abnormal cIMT [193, 194], altered endothelial reactivity [195], abnormal coronary calcium scores [196], higher than expected C-reactive protein levels and abnormal proinflammatory and prothrombotic indices [197], all suggest a state of increased atherosclerotic risk [123].

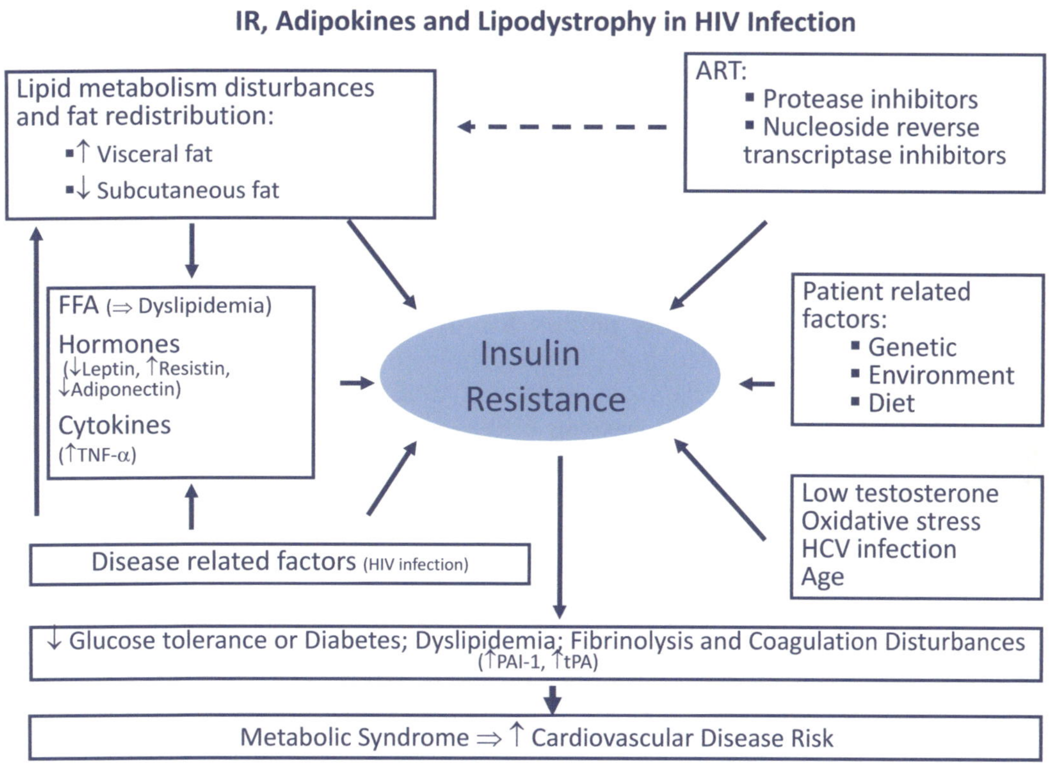

Figure 7. The relationship between HIV infection, lipodystrophy, ART, insulin resistance, adipokines, metabolic alterations, metabolic syndrome and cardiovascular disease risk

Endothelial cells have been shown to be variably permissive for HIV infection. The HIV virus itself is able to penetrate coronary artery and brain microvascular endothelial cell membranes and to initiate inflammatory and biochemical intracellular reactions [198, 199]. The activation of endothelium induced by either HIV infection itself or by a leukocyte-mediated inflammatory cascade triggered by the same virus leads to an increased expression of endothelial cellular adhesion molecules, such as intercellular adhesion molecule 1 (ICAM-1), vascular adhesion molecule 1 (VCAM-1], E-selectin, P-selectin, thrombomodulin, tissue plasminogen activator (tPA), and PAI-1. A significant association between increasing serum concentrations of adhesion molecules and risk of future myocardial infarction has been shown in apparently healthy men and women, and these molecules are now considered as soluble biomarkers of endothelial inflammation and early atherosclerosis [200, 201]. Increased serum levels of ICAM-1, VCAM-1, E-selectin, and thrombomodulin were demonstrated in patients with advanced HIV infection and opportunistic diseases. A correlation between ICAM-1 concentrations and the progression of disease as well as the reduction of CD4 lymphocyte count was also reported. If circulating adhesion molecules indicate vascular endothelium injury, it seems clear that endothelium injury is associated with the progression and severity of HIV disease [202]. cART should reduce the endothelial damage by controlling HIV infection, but it would also contribute to stimulating endothelial activation by deranging both lipid and glucose metabolism [167]. Some PIs, as ritonavir and indinavir are able to directly cause endothelial dysfunction, with mitochondrial DNA damage and cell death, independently of lipid profile [203]. cART may promote atherosclerosis both by direct effects on endothelial cells and by indirect effects associated with metabolic disturbances [167].

Elevated serum levels of PAI-1, tPA, and CRP, as well as reduced serum levels of adiponectin could be considered biochemical markers of endothelial dysfunction, metabolic alterations, and CV risk in HIV-infected patients [192]. Some authors suggested that the pathogenetic mechanism responsible for carotid lesions associated with HIV infection may be more similar to an inflammatory process than to the classical atherogenesis [204, 205]. Some retrospective and prospective studies have shown that the incidence of myocardial infarction in HIV-positive subjects treated with ART tends to be higher than in the general population, particularly in those receiving a PI-based treatment [206]. However, reports from large observational studies demonstrate that there is still considerable controversy regarding the association of cART, particularly PI-based combinations, with increased incidence of coronary heart disease risk [167].

Moreover, prospective studies involving large cohorts of HIV-infected patients have documented an increased incidence of myocardial infarction and cerebrovascular diseases in association with a prolonged exposure to cART. However, the absolute risk of CV events remains low, and should be balanced against the remarkable benefits ofcART in terms of improvement in immune function and related morbidity and mortality [167].

In other words, incidence of CV disease in successfully cART-treated HIV-infected patients is low. However, the risk of CV disease is increased compared with that of uninfected people. This fact is due in great part to a higher prevalence of underlying traditional CV risk factors that are mostly host dependent. HIV may additionally contribute through immune activation, inflammation, and immunodeficiency. In a more modest way than HIV infection, the type of ART may also contribute, mainly through the impact on metabolic and body fat parameters, and possibly through other factors that are currently unclear. From the CV perspective, the benefits of ART outweigh any potential risk [207, 208].

24. Conclusions

Human lipodystrophies are a heterogeneous group of diseases with generalized or partial fat loss. They include rare genetic conditions or more frequent acquired forms, and may be old, or more recent, such as HIV-related lipodystrophy. Almost all lipodystrophies are associated with metabolic alterations including IR, diabetes, dyslipidemia and early CV disease. In this new context of increased aging of HIV-infected patients, increased metabolic and CV complications are to be expected due to high incidences of smoking status, over-nutrition

http://dx.doi.org/10.5772/52685

and reduced exercise, lipodystrophy, dyslipidemia, altered glucose tolerance with IR and low-grade infection with the ongoing drug-induced inflammation. It is important to be aware of these alterations and to apply risk-modification strategies to reduce CV risk in the HIV-infected patients.

Author details

Paula Freitas*, Davide Carvalho, Selma Souto, António Sarmento and José Luís Medina

*Address all correspondence to: paula_freitas@sapo.pt

Department of Endocrinology, Centro Hospitalar São João and University of Porto Medical School, Porto, Portugal

References

[1] Capeau J, Magre J, Caron-Debarle M, Lagathu C, Antoine B, Bereziat V, et al. Human lipodystrophies: genetic and acquired diseases of adipose tissue. Endocr Dev. 2010;19:1-20.

[2] Garg A. Lipodystrophies: Genetic and Acquired Body Fat Disorders. J Clin Endocrinol Metab. 2011 Aug 24.

[3] Berardinelli W. An undiagnosed endocrinometabolic syndrome: report of 2 cases. J Clin Endocrinol Metab. 1954 Feb;14 [2]:193-204.

[4] Carr A, Samaras K, Burton S, Law M, Freund J, Chisholm DJ, et al. A syndrome of peripheral lipodystrophy, hyperlipidaemia and insulin resistance in patients receiving HIV protease inhibitors. AIDS. 1998 May 7;12 [7]:F51-8.

[5] Snijder MB, Dekker JM, Visser M, Bouter LM, Stehouwer CD, Yudkin JS, et al. Trunk fat and leg fat have independent and opposite associations with fasting and postload glucose levels: the Hoorn study. Diabetes Care. 2004 Feb;27 [2]:372-7.

[6] Tershakovec AM, Frank I, Rader D. HIV-related lipodystrophy and related factors. Atherosclerosis. 2004 May;174 [1]:1-10.

[7] Capeau J. From lipodystrophy and insulin resistance to metabolic syndrome: HIV infection, treatment and aging. Curr Opin HIV AIDS. 2007 Jul;2 [4]:247-52.

[8] Caron-Debarle M, Lagathu C, Boccara F, Vigouroux C, Capeau J. HIV-associated lipodystrophy: from fat injury to premature aging. Trends Mol Med. 2010 May;16 [5]: 218-29.

[9] Giralt M, Domingo P, Villarroya F. Adipose tissue biology and HIV-infection. Best Pract Res Clin Endocrinol Metab. 2011 Jun;25 [3]:487-99.

[10] Sethi JK, Vidal-Puig AJ. Thematic review series: adipocyte biology. Adipose tissue function and plasticity orchestrate nutritional adaptation. J Lipid Res. 2007 Jun;48 [6]: 1253-62.

[11] De Pauw A, Tejerina S, Raes M, Keijer J, Arnould T. Mitochondrial (dys)function in adipocyte (de)differentiation and systemic metabolic alterations. Am J Pathol. 2009 Sep;175 [3]:927-39.

[12] Koh EH, Park JY, Park HS, Jeon MJ, Ryu JW, Kim M, et al. Essential role of mitochondrial function in adiponectin synthesis in adipocytes. Diabetes. 2007 Dec;56 [12]: 2973-81.

[13] Gil A, Olza J, Gil-Campos M, Gomez-Llorente C, Aguilera CM. Is adipose tissue metabolically different at different sites? Int J Pediatr Obes. 2011 Sep;6 Suppl 1:13-20.

[14] Despres JP, Nadeau A, Tremblay A, Ferland M, Moorjani S, Lupien PJ, et al. Role of deep abdominal fat in the association between regional adipose tissue distribution and glucose tolerance in obese women. Diabetes. 1989 Mar;38 [3]:304-9.

[15] Kelley DE, Thaete FL, Troost F, Huwe T, Goodpaster BH. Subdivisions of subcutaneous abdominal adipose tissue and insulin resistance. Am J Physiol Endocrinol Metab. 2000 May;278 [5]:E941-8.

[16] Schoen RE, Evans RW, Sankey SS, Weissfeld JL, Kuller L. Does visceral adipose tissue differ from subcutaneous adipose tissue in fatty acid content? Int J Obes Relat Metab Disord. 1996 Apr;20 [4]:346-52.

[17] Ross R, Shaw KD, Rissanen J, Martel Y, de Guise J, Avruch L. Sex differences in lean and adipose tissue distribution by magnetic resonance imaging: anthropometric relationships. Am J Clin Nutr. 1994 Jun;59 [6]:1277-85.

[18] Frayn KN. Adipose tissue as a buffer for daily lipid flux. Diabetologia. 2002 Sep;45 [9]:1201-10.

[19] Ohtsubo K, Chen MZ, Olefsky JM, Marth JD. Pathway to diabetes through attenuation of pancreatic beta cell glycosylation and glucose transport. Nat Med. 2011 Sep;17 [9]:1067-75.

[20] Cinti S. Between brown and white: novel aspects of adipocyte differentiation. Ann Med. 2011 Mar;43 [2]:104-15.

[21] Aron-Wisnewsky J, Tordjman J, Poitou C, Darakhshan F, Hugol D, Basdevant A, et al. Human adipose tissue macrophages: m1 and m2 cell surface markers in subcutaneous and omental depots and after weight loss. J Clin Endocrinol Metab. 2009 Nov; 94 [11]:4619-23.

[22] Morton NM. Obesity and corticosteroids: 11beta-hydroxysteroid type 1 as a cause and therapeutic target in metabolic disease. Mol Cell Endocrinol. 2010 Mar 25;316 [2]: 154-64.

[23] Villarroya J, Giralt M, Villarroya F. Mitochondrial DNA: an up-and-coming actor in white adipose tissue pathophysiology. Obesity (Silver Spring). 2009 Oct;17 [10]: 1814-20.

[24] Kovsan J, Osnis A, Maissel A, Mazor L, Tarnovscki T, Hollander L, et al. Depot-specific adipocyte cell lines reveal differential drug-induced responses of white adipocytes--relevance for partial lipodystrophy. Am J Physiol Endocrinol Metab. 2009 Feb; 296 [2]:E315-22.

[25] Shadid S, Koutsari C, Jensen MD. Direct free fatty acid uptake into human adipocytes in vivo: relation to body fat distribution. Diabetes. 2007 May;56 [5]:1369-75.

[26] Nielsen S, Guo Z, Johnson CM, Hensrud DD, Jensen MD. Splanchnic lipolysis in human obesity. J Clin Invest. 2004 Jun;113 [11]:1582-8.

[27] Sevastianova K, Sutinen J, Greco D, Sievers M, Salmenkivi K, Perttila J, et al. Comparison of dorsocervical with abdominal subcutaneous adipose tissue in patients with and without antiretroviral therapy-associated lipodystrophy. Diabetes. 2011 Jul; 60 [7]:1894-900.

[28] Bastard JP, Caron M, Vidal H, Jan V, Auclair M, Vigouroux C, et al. Association between altered expression of adipogenic factor SREBP1 in lipoatrophic adipose tissue from HIV-1-infected patients and abnormal adipocyte differentiation and insulin resistance. Lancet. 2002 Mar 23;359 [9311]:1026-31.

[29] Giralt M, Domingo P, Guallar JP, Rodriguez de la Concepcion ML, Alegre M, Domingo JC, et al. HIV-1 infection alters gene expression in adipose tissue, which contributes to HIV- 1/HAART-associated lipodystrophy. Antivir Ther. 2006;11 [6]:729-40.

[30] Jan V, Cervera P, Maachi M, Baudrimont M, Kim M, Vidal H, et al. Altered fat differentiation and adipocytokine expression are inter-related and linked to morphological changes and insulin resistance in HIV-1-infected lipodystrophic patients. Antivir Ther. 2004 Aug;9 [4]:555-64.

[31] Nolan D, Hammond E, Martin A, Taylor L, Herrmann S, McKinnon E, et al. Mitochondrial DNA depletion and morphologic changes in adipocytes associated with nucleoside reverse transcriptase inhibitor therapy. AIDS. 2003 Jun 13;17 [9]:1329-38.

[32] Pace CS, Martin AM, Hammond EL, Mamotte CD, Nolan DA, Mallal SA. Mitochondrial proliferation, DNA depletion and adipocyte differentiation in subcutaneous adipose tissue of HIV-positive HAART recipients. Antivir Ther. 2003 Aug;8 [4]: 323-31.

[33] Villarroya F, Domingo P, Giralt M. Mechanisms of antiretroviral-induced mitochondrial dysfunction in adipocytes and adipose tissue: in-vitro, animal and human adipose tissue studies. Curr Opin HIV AIDS. 2007 Jul;2 [4]:261-7.

[34] McComsey GA, Libutti DE, O'Riordan M, Shelton JM, Storer N, Ganz J, et al. Mitochondrial RNA and DNA alterations in HIV lipoatrophy are linked to antiretroviral therapy and not to HIV infection. Antivir Ther. 2008;13 [5]:715-22.

[35] Lagathu C, Kim M, Maachi M, Vigouroux C, Cervera P, Capeau J, et al. HIV antiretroviral treatment alters adipokine expression and insulin sensitivity of adipose tissue in vitro and in vivo. Biochimie. 2005 Jan;87 [1]:65-71.

[36] Lihn AS, Richelsen B, Pedersen SB, Haugaard SB, Rathje GS, Madsbad S, et al. Increased expression of TNF-alpha, IL-6, and IL-8 in HALS: implications for reduced adiponectin expression and plasma levels. Am J Physiol Endocrinol Metab. 2003 Nov;285 [5]:E1072-80.

[37] Sevastianova K, Sutinen J, Kannisto K, Hamsten A, Ristola M, Yki-Jarvinen H. Adipose tissue inflammation and liver fat in patients with highly active antiretroviral therapy-associated lipodystrophy. Am J Physiol Endocrinol Metab. 2008 Jul;295 [1]:E85-91.

[38] Villarroya F, Domingo P, Giralt M. Drug-induced lipotoxicity: lipodystrophy associated with HIV-1 infection and antiretroviral treatment. Biochim Biophys Acta. 2010 Mar;1801 [3]:392-9.

[39] Nolan D, Hammond E, James I, McKinnon E, Mallal S. Contribution of nucleoside-analogue reverse transcriptase inhibitor therapy to lipoatrophy from the population to the cellular level. Antivir Ther. 2003 Dec;8 [6]:617-26.

[40] Seip M. Lipodystrophy and gigantism with associated endocrine manifestations. A new diencephalic syndrome? Acta Paediatr. 1959 Nov;48:555-74.

[41] Van Maldergem L, Magre J, Khallouf TE, Gedde-Dahl T, Jr., Delepine M, Trygstad O, et al. Genotype-phenotype relationships in Berardinelli-Seip congenital lipodystrophy. J Med Genet. 2002 Oct;39 [10]:722-33.

[42] Agarwal AK, Simha V, Oral EA, Moran SA, Gorden P, O'Rahilly S, et al. Phenotypic and genetic heterogeneity in congenital generalized lipodystrophy. J Clin Endocrinol Metab. 2003 Oct;88 [10]:4840-7.

[43] Pardini VC, Victoria IM, Rocha SM, Andrade DG, Rocha AM, Pieroni FB, et al. Leptin levels, beta-cell function, and insulin sensitivity in families with congenital and acquired generalized lipoatropic diabetes. J Clin Endocrinol Metab. 1998 Feb;83 [2]:503-8.

[44] Magre J, Delepine M, Van Maldergem L, Robert JJ, Maassen JA, Meier M, et al. Prevalence of mutations in AGPAT2 among human lipodystrophies. Diabetes. 2003 Jun;52 [6]:1573-8.

[45] Van Maldergem L, Da Silva H, Freitas P, D' Abronzo FH. Berardinelli-Seip Syndrome: a new Portuguese disease? Eur J Hum Genet. 1998 [6]:74A.

[46] Garg A, Wilson R, Barnes R, Arioglu E, Zaidi Z, Gurakan F, et al. A gene for congenital generalized lipodystrophy maps to human chromosome 9q34. J Clin Endocrinol Metab. 1999 Sep;84 [9]:3390-4.

[47] Agarwal AK, Garg A. Congenital generalized lipodystrophy: significance of triglyceride biosynthetic pathways. Trends Endocrinol Metab. 2003 Jul;14 [5]:214-21.

[48] Magre J, Delepine M, Khallouf E, Gedde-Dahl T, Jr., Van Maldergem L, Sobel E, et al. Identification of the gene altered in Berardinelli-Seip congenital lipodystrophy on chromosome 11q13. Nat Genet. 2001 Aug;28 [4]:365-70.

[49] Szymanski KM, Binns D, Bartz R, Grishin NV, Li WP, Agarwal AK, et al. The lipodystrophy protein seipin is found at endoplasmic reticulum lipid droplet junctions and is important for droplet morphology. Proc Natl Acad Sci U S A. 2007 Dec 26;104 [52]:20890-5.

[50] Fei W, Shui G, Gaeta B, Du X, Kuerschner L, Li P, et al. Fld1p, a functional homologue of human seipin, regulates the size of lipid droplets in yeast. J Cell Biol. 2008 Feb 11;180 [3]:473-82.

[51] Payne VA, Grimsey N, Tuthill A, Virtue S, Gray SL, Dalla Nora E, et al. The human lipodystrophy gene BSCL2/seipin may be essential for normal adipocyte differentiation. Diabetes. 2008 Aug;57 [8]:2055-60.

[52] Kim CA, Delepine M, Boutet E, El Mourabit H, Le Lay S, Meier M, et al. Association of a homozygous nonsense caveolin-1 mutation with Berardinelli-Seip congenital lipodystrophy. J Clin Endocrinol Metab. 2008 Apr;93 [4]:1129-34.

[53] Hayashi YK, Matsuda C, Ogawa M, Goto K, Tominaga K, Mitsuhashi S, et al. Human PTRF mutations cause secondary deficiency of caveolins resulting in muscular dystrophy with generalized lipodystrophy. J Clin Invest. 2009 Sep;119 [9]:2623-33.

[54] Garg A, Agarwal AK. Caveolin-1: a new locus for human lipodystrophy. J Clin Endocrinol Metab. 2008 Apr;93 [4]:1183-5.

[55] Garg A, Speckman RA, Bowcock AM. Multisystem dystrophy syndrome due to novel missense mutations in the amino-terminal head and alpha-helical rod domains of the lamin A/C gene. Am J Med. 2002 May;112 [7]:549-55.

[56] Subramanyam L, Simha V, Garg A. Overlapping syndrome with familial partial lipodystrophy, Dunnigan variety and cardiomyopathy due to amino-terminal heterozygous missense lamin A/C mutations. Clin Genet. 2010 Jul;78 [1]:66-73.

[57] Hegele RA. Familial partial lipodystrophy: a monogenic form of the insulin resistance syndrome. Mol Genet Metab. 2000 Dec;71 [4]:539-44.

[58] Rajab A, Straub V, McCann LJ, Seelow D, Varon R, Barresi R, et al. Fatal cardiac arrhythmia and long-QT syndrome in a new form of congenital generalized lipodystrophy with muscle rippling (CGL4] due to PTRF-CAVIN mutations. PLoS Genet. 2010 Mar;6 [3]:e1000874.

[59] Grinspoon S, Carr A. Cardiovascular risk and body-fat abnormalities in HIV-infected adults. N Engl J Med. 2005 Jan 6;352 [1]:48-62.

[60] Afifi AK, Mire-Salman J, Najjar S. The myopahtology of congenital generalized lipodystrophy light and electron microscopic observations. Johns Hopkins Med J. 1976 Dec;139 SUPPL:61-8.

[61] Bjornstad PG, Foerster A, Ihlen H. Cardiac findings in generalized lipodystrophy. Acta Paediatr Suppl. 1996 Jun;413:39-43.

[62] Chandalia M, Garg A, Vuitch F, Nizzi F. Postmortem findings in congenital generalized lipodystrophy. J Clin Endocrinol Metab. 1995 Oct;80 [10]:3077-81.

[63] Bhayana S, Siu VM, Joubert GI, Clarson CL, Cao H, Hegele RA. Cardiomyopathy in congenital complete lipodystrophy. Clin Genet. 2002 Apr;61 [4]:283-7.

[64] Young LW, Radebaugh JF, Rubin P, Sensenbrenner JA, Fiorelli G, McKusick VA. New syndrome manifested by mandibular hypoplasia, acroosteolysis, stiff joints and cutaneous atrophy (mandibuloacral dysplasia) in two unrelated boys. Birth Defects Orig Artic Ser. 1971 Jun;7 [7]:291-7.

[65] Simha V, Agarwal AK, Oral EA, Fryns JP, Garg A. Genetic and phenotypic heterogeneity in patients with mandibuloacral dysplasia-associated lipodystrophy. J Clin Endocrinol Metab. 2003 Jun;88 [6]:2821-4.

[66] Freidenberg GR, Cutler DL, Jones MC, Hall B, Mier RJ, Culler F, et al. Severe insulin resistance and diabetes mellitus in mandibuloacral dysplasia. Am J Dis Child. 1992 Jan;146 [1]:93-9.

[67] Novelli G, Muchir A, Sangiuolo F, Helbling-Leclerc A, D'Apice MR, Massart C, et al. Mandibuloacral dysplasia is caused by a mutation in LMNA-encoding lamin A/C. Am J Hum Genet. 2002 Aug;71 [2]:426-31.

[68] Agarwal AK, Fryns JP, Auchus RJ, Garg A. Zinc metalloproteinase, ZMPSTE24, is mutated in mandibuloacral dysplasia. Hum Mol Genet. 2003 Aug 15;12 [16]: 1995-2001.

[69] Garg A, Hernandez MD, Sousa AB, Subramanyam L, Martinez de Villarreal L, dos Santos HG, et al. An autosomal recessive syndrome of joint contractures, muscular atrophy, microcytic anemia, and panniculitis-associated lipodystrophy. J Clin Endocrinol Metab. 2010 Sep;95 [9]:E58-63.

[70] Horikoshi A, Iwabuchi S, Iizuka Y, Hagiwara T, Amaki I. [A case of partial lipodystrophy with erythema, dactylic deformities, calcification of the basal ganglia, immunological disorders and low IQ level (author's transl]. Rinsho Shinkeigaku. 1980 Mar; 20 [3]:173-80.

[71] Tanaka M, Miyatani N, Yamada S, Miyashita K, Toyoshima I, Sakuma K, et al. Hereditary lipo-muscular atrophy with joint contracture, skin eruptions and hyper-gamma-globulinemia: a new syndrome. Intern Med. 1993 Jan;32 [1]:42-5.

[72] Torrelo A, Patel S, Colmenero I, Gurbindo D, Lendinez F, Hernandez A, et al. Chronic atypical neutrophilic dermatosis with lipodystrophy and elevated temperature (CANDLE) syndrome. J Am Acad Dermatol. 2010 Mar;62 [3]:489-95.

[73] Ramot Y, Czarnowicki T, Maly A, Navon-Elkan P, Zlotogorski A. Chronic Atypical Neutrophilic Dermatosis with Lipodystrophy and Elevated Temperature Syndrome: A Case Report. Pediatr Dermatol. 2010 Jun 9.

[74] Dunnigan MG, Cochrane MA, Kelly A, Scott JW. Familial lipoatrophic diabetes with dominant transmission. A new syndrome. Q J Med. 1974 Jan;43 [169]:33-48.

[75] Kobberling J, Dunnigan MG. Familial partial lipodystrophy: two types of an X linked dominant syndrome, lethal in the hemizygous state. J Med Genet. 1986 Apr;23 [2]: 120-7.

[76] Garg A, Peshock RM, Fleckenstein JL. Adipose tissue distribution pattern in patients with familial partial lipodystrophy (Dunnigan variety). J Clin Endocrinol Metab. 1999 Jan;84 [1]:170-4.

[77] Garg A. Gender differences in the prevalence of metabolic complications in familial partial lipodystrophy (Dunnigan variety). J Clin Endocrinol Metab. 2000 May;85 [5]: 1776-82.

[78] Peters JM, Barnes R, Bennett L, Gitomer WM, Bowcock AM, Garg A. Localization of the gene for familial partial lipodystrophy (Dunnigan variety) to chromosome 1q21-22. Nat Genet. 1998 Mar;18 [3]:292-5.

[79] Cao H, Hegele RA. Nuclear lamin A/C R482Q mutation in canadian kindreds with Dunnigan-type familial partial lipodystrophy. Hum Mol Genet. 2000 Jan 1;9 [1]: 109-12.

[80] Shackleton S, Lloyd DJ, Jackson SN, Evans R, Niermeijer MF, Singh BM, et al. LMNA, encoding lamin A/C, is mutated in partial lipodystrophy. Nat Genet. 2000 Feb;24 [2]:153-6.

[81] Speckman RA, Garg A, Du F, Bennett L, Veile R, Arioglu E, et al. Mutational and haplotype analyses of families with familial partial lipodystrophy (Dunnigan variety) reveal recurrent missense mutations in the globular C-terminal domain of lamin A/C. Am J Hum Genet. 2000 Apr;66 [4]:1192-8.

[82] Agarwal AK, Garg A. A novel heterozygous mutation in peroxisome proliferator-activated receptor-gamma gene in a patient with familial partial lipodystrophy. J Clin Endocrinol Metab. 2002 Jan;87 [1]:408-11.

[83] Hegele RA, Cao H, Frankowski C, Mathews ST, Leff T. PPARG F388L, a transactivation-deficient mutant, in familial partial lipodystrophy. Diabetes. 2002 Dec;51 [12]: 3586-90.

[84] Semple RK, Chatterjee VK, O'Rahilly S. PPAR gamma and human metabolic disease. J Clin Invest. 2006 Mar;116 [3]:581-9.

[85] George S, Rochford JJ, Wolfrum C, Gray SL, Schinner S, Wilson JC, et al. A family with severe insulin resistance and diabetes due to a mutation in AKT2. Science. 2004 May 28;304 [5675]:1325-8.

[86] Rubio-Cabezas O, Puri V, Murano I, Saudek V, Semple RK, Dash S, et al. Partial lipodystrophy and insulin resistant diabetes in a patient with a homozygous nonsense mutation in CIDEC. EMBO Mol Med. 2009 Aug;1 [5]:280-7.

[87] Gandotra S, Le Dour C, Bottomley W, Cervera P, Giral P, Reznik Y, et al. Perilipin deficiency and autosomal dominant partial lipodystrophy. N Engl J Med. 2011 Feb 24;364 [8]:740-8.

[88] Olofsson SO, Bostrom P, Andersson L, Rutberg M, Levin M, Perman J, et al. Triglyceride containing lipid droplets and lipid droplet-associated proteins. Curr Opin Lipidol. 2008 Oct;19 [5]:441-7.

[89] Caron M, Auclair M, Donadille B, Bereziat V, Guerci B, Laville M, et al. Human lipodystrophies linked to mutations in A-type lamins and to HIV protease inhibitor therapy are both associated with prelamin A accumulation, oxidative stress and premature cellular senescence. Cell Death Differ. 2007 Oct;14 [10]:1759-67.

[90] Garg A, Subramanyam L, Agarwal AK, Simha V, Levine B, D'Apice MR, et al. Atypical progeroid syndrome due to heterozygous missense LMNA mutations. J Clin Endocrinol Metab. 2009 Dec;94 [12]:4971-83.

[91] Merideth MA, Gordon LB, Clauss S, Sachdev V, Smith AC, Perry MB, et al. Phenotype and course of Hutchinson-Gilford progeria syndrome. N Engl J Med. 2008 Feb 7;358 [6]:592-604.

[92] Sensenbrenner JA, Hussels IE, Levin LS. A low birthweight syndrome, ? Rieger syndrome. Birth Defects Orig Artic Ser. 1975;11 [2]:423-6.

[93] O'Neill B, Simha V, Kotha V, Garg A. Body fat distribution and metabolic variables in patients with neonatal progeroid syndrome. Am J Med Genet A. 2007 Jul 1;143A [13]:1421-30.

[94] Garg A, Agarwal AK. Lipodystrophies: disorders of adipose tissue biology. Biochim Biophys Acta. 2009 Jun;1791 [6]:507-13.

[95] Misra A, Garg A. Clinical features and metabolic derangements in acquired generalized lipodystrophy: case reports and review of the literature. Medicine (Baltimore). 2003 Mar;82 [2]:129-46.

[96] Hegele RA, Cao H, Liu DM, Costain GA, Charlton-Menys V, Rodger NW, et al. Sequencing of the reannotated LMNB2 gene reveals novel mutations in patients with acquired partial lipodystrophy. Am J Hum Genet. 2006 Aug;79 [2]:383-9.

[97] Mathieson PW, Wurzner R, Oliveria DB, Lachmann PJ, Peters DK. Complement-mediated adipocyte lysis by nephritic factor sera. J Exp Med. 1993 Jun 1;177 [6]:1827-31.

[98] Garg A. Lipodystrophies. Am J Med. 2000 Feb;108 [2]:143-52.

[99] Palella FJ, Jr., Delaney KM, Moorman AC, Loveless MO, Fuhrer J, Satten GA, et al. Declining morbidity and mortality among patients with advanced human immunodeficiency virus infection. HIV Outpatient Study Investigators. N Engl J Med. 1998 Mar 26;338 [13]:853-60.

[100] Carr A, Samaras K, Thorisdottir A, Kaufmann GR, Chisholm DJ, Cooper DA. Diagnosis, prediction, and natural course of HIV-1 protease-inhibitor-associated lipodystrophy, hyperlipidaemia, and diabetes mellitus: a cohort study. Lancet. 1999 Jun 19;353 [9170]:2093-9.

[101] Walli R, Herfort O, Michl GM, Demant T, Jager H, Dieterle C, et al. Treatment with protease inhibitors associated with peripheral insulin resistance and impaired oral glucose tolerance in HIV-1-infected patients. AIDS. 1998 Oct 22;12 [15]:F167-73.

[102] Thiebaut R, Daucourt V, Mercie P, Ekouevi DK, Malvy D, Morlat P, et al. Lipodystrophy, metabolic disorders, and human immunodeficiency virus infection: Aquitaine Cohort, France, 1999. Groupe d'Epidemiologie Clinique du Syndrome d'Immunodeficience Acquise en Aquitaine. Clin Infect Dis. 2000 Dec;31 [6]:1482-7.

[103] Dube MP, Johnson DL, Currier JS, Leedom JM. Protease inhibitor-associated hyperglycaemia. Lancet. 1997 Sep 6;350 [9079]:713-4.

[104] Carr A. HIV lipodystrophy: risk factors, pathogenesis, diagnosis and management. AIDS. 2003 Apr;17 Suppl 1:S141-8.

[105] Hawkins T. Appearance-related side effects of HIV-1 treatment. AIDS Patient Care STDS. 2006 Jan;20 [1]:6-18.

[106] Chen D, Misra A, Garg A. Clinical review 153: Lipodystrophy in human immunodeficiency virus-infected patients. J Clin Endocrinol Metab. 2002 Nov;87 [11]:4845-56.

[107] Mallon PW, Miller J, Cooper DA, Carr A. Prospective evaluation of the effects of antiretroviral therapy on body composition in HIV-1-infected men starting therapy. AIDS. 2003 May 2;17 [7]:971-9.

[108] John M, Moore CB, James IR, Nolan D, Upton RP, McKinnon EJ, et al. Chronic hyperlactatemia in HIV-infected patients taking antiretroviral therapy. AIDS. 2001 Apr 13;15 [6]:717-23.

[109] Carr A, Cooper DA. Adverse effects of antiretroviral therapy. Lancet. 2000 Oct 21;356 [9239]:1423-30.

[110] Martinez E, Mocroft A, Garcia-Viejo MA, Perez-Cuevas JB, Blanco JL, Mallolas J, et al. Risk of lipodystrophy in HIV-1-infected patients treated with protease inhibitors: a prospective cohort study. Lancet. 2001 Feb 24;357 [9256]:592-8.

[111] Heath KV, Hogg RS, Singer J, Chan KJ, O'Shaughnessy MV, Montaner JS. Antiretroviral treatment patterns and incident HIV-associated morphologic and lipid abnor-

malities in a population-based chort. J Acquir Immune Defic Syndr. 2002 Aug 1;30 [4]:440-7.

[112] Nguyen A, Calmy A, Schiffer V, Bernasconi E, Battegay M, Opravil M, et al. Lipodystrophy and weight changes: data from the Swiss HIV Cohort Study, 2000-2006. HIV Med. 2008 Mar;9 [3]:142-50.

[113] Miller J, Carr A, Emery S, Law M, Mallal S, Baker D, et al. HIV lipodystrophy: prevalence, severity and correlates of risk in Australia. HIV Med. 2003 Jul;4 [3]:293-301.

[114] Mallon PW. Antiretroviral therapy-induced lipid alterations: in-vitro, animal and human studies. Curr Opin HIV AIDS. 2007 Jul;2 [4]:282-92.

[115] van Leuven SI, Sankatsing RR, Vermeulen JN, Kastelein JJ, Reiss P, Stroes ES. Atherosclerotic vascular disease in HIV: it is not just antiretroviral therapy that hurts the heart! Curr Opin HIV AIDS. 2007 Jul;2 [4]:324-31.

[116] Saves M, Raffi F, Capeau J, Rozenbaum W, Ragnaud JM, Perronne C, et al. Factors related to lipodystrophy and metabolic alterations in patients with human immunodeficiency virus infection receiving highly active antiretroviral therapy. Clin Infect Dis. 2002 May 15;34 [10]:1396-405.

[117] Calmy A, Hirschel B, Cooper DA, Carr A. A new era of antiretroviral drug toxicity. Antivir Ther. 2009;14 [2]:165-79.

[118] Crowe SM, Westhorpe CL, Mukhamedova N, Jaworowski A, Sviridov D, Bukrinsky M. The macrophage: the intersection between HIV infection and atherosclerosis. J Leukoc Biol. 2010 Apr;87 [4]:589-98.

[119] Jacobson DL, Knox T, Spiegelman D, Skinner S, Gorbach S, Wanke C. Prevalence of, evolution of, and risk factors for fat atrophy and fat deposition in a cohort of HIV-infected men and women. Clin Infect Dis. 2005 Jun 15;40 [12]:1837-45.

[120] Bastard JP, Maachi M, Lagathu C, Kim MJ, Caron M, Vidal H, et al. Recent advances in the relationship between obesity, inflammation, and insulin resistance. Eur Cytokine Netw. 2006 Mar;17 [1]:4-12.

[121] Otake K, Omoto S, Yamamoto T, Okuyama H, Okada H, Okada N, et al. HIV-1 Nef protein in the nucleus influences adipogenesis as well as viral transcription through the peroxisome proliferator-activated receptors. AIDS. 2004 Jan 23;18 [2]:189-98.

[122] Shrivastav S, Kino T, Cunningham T, Ichijo T, Schubert U, Heinklein P, et al. Human immunodeficiency virus (HIV)-1 viral protein R suppresses transcriptional activity of peroxisome proliferator-activated receptor {gamma} and inhibits adipocyte differentiation: implications for HIV-associated lipodystrophy. Mol Endocrinol. 2008 Feb;22 [2]:234-47.

[123] Falutz J. Therapy insight: Body-shape changes and metabolic complications associated with HIV and highly active antiretroviral therapy. Nat Clin Pract Endocrinol Metab. 2007 Sep;3 [9]:651-61.

[124] Lichtenstein KA, Ward DJ, Moorman AC, Delaney KM, Young B, Palella FJ, Jr., et al. Clinical assessment of HIV-associated lipodystrophy in an ambulatory population. AIDS. 2001 Jul 27;15 [11]:1389-98.

[125] Periard D, Telenti A, Sudre P, Cheseaux JJ, Halfon P, Reymond MJ, et al. Atherogenic dyslipidemia in HIV-infected individuals treated with protease inhibitors. The Swiss HIV Cohort Study. Circulation. 1999 Aug 17;100 [7]:700-5.

[126] Grinspoon S. Mechanisms and strategies for insulin resistance in acquired immune deficiency syndrome. Clin Infect Dis. 2003;37 Suppl 2:S85-90.

[127] Caron M, Vigouroux C, Bastard JP, Capeau J. Adipocyte dysfunction in response to antiretroviral therapy: clinical, tissue and in-vitro studies. Curr Opin HIV AIDS. 2007 Jul;2 [4]:268-73.

[128] Hudon SE, Coffinier C, Michaelis S, Fong LG, Young SG, Hrycyna CA. HIV-protease inhibitors block the enzymatic activity of purified Ste24p. Biochem Biophys Res Commun. 2008 Sep 19;374 [2]:365-8.

[129] Lagathu C, Eustace B, Prot M, Frantz D, Gu Y, Bastard JP, et al. Some HIV antiretrovirals increase oxidative stress and alter chemokine, cytokine or adiponectin production in human adipocytes and macrophages. Antivir Ther. 2007;12 [4]:489-500.

[130] Flint OP, Noor MA, Hruz PW, Hylemon PB, Yarasheski K, Kotler DP, et al. The role of protease inhibitors in the pathogenesis of HIV-associated lipodystrophy: cellular mechanisms and clinical implications. Toxicol Pathol. 2009;37 [1]:65-77.

[131] Djedaini M, Peraldi P, Drici MD, Darini C, Saint-Marc P, Dani C, et al. Lopinavir co-induces insulin resistance and ER stress in human adipocytes. Biochem Biophys Res Commun. 2009 Aug 14;386 [1]:96-100.

[132] Caron M, Auclair M, Vigouroux C, Glorian M, Forest C, Capeau J. The HIV protease inhibitor indinavir impairs sterol regulatory element-binding protein-1 intranuclear localization, inhibits preadipocyte differentiation, and induces insulin resistance. Diabetes. 2001 Jun;50 [6]:1378-88.

[133] Dowell P, Flexner C, Kwiterovich PO, Lane MD. Suppression of preadipocyte differentiation and promotion of adipocyte death by HIV protease inhibitors. J Biol Chem. 2000 Dec 29;275 [52]:41325-32.

[134] Lenhard JM, Furfine ES, Jain RG, Ittoop O, Orband-Miller LA, Blanchard SG, et al. HIV protease inhibitors block adipogenesis and increase lipolysis in vitro. Antiviral Res. 2000 Aug;47 [2]:121-9.

[135] Caron M, Auclair M, Sterlingot H, Kornprobst M, Capeau J. Some HIV protease inhibitors alter lamin A/C maturation and stability, SREBP-1 nuclear localization and adipocyte differentiation. AIDS. 2003 Nov 21;17 [17]:2437-44.

[136] Murata H, Hruz PW, Mueckler M. The mechanism of insulin resistance caused by HIV protease inhibitor therapy. J Biol Chem. 2000 Jul 7;275 [27]:20251-4.

[137] Brinkman K, Smeitink JA, Romijn JA, Reiss P. Mitochondrial toxicity induced by nucleoside-analogue reverse-transcriptase inhibitors is a key factor in the pathogenesis of antiretroviral-therapy-related lipodystrophy. Lancet. 1999 Sep 25;354 [9184]: 1112-5.

[138] McComsey G, Bai RK, Maa JF, Seekins D, Wong LJ. Extensive investigations of mitochondrial DNA genome in treated HIV-infected subjects: beyond mitochondrial DNA depletion. J Acquir Immune Defic Syndr. 2005 Jun 1;39 [2]:181-8.

[139] van Vonderen MG, van Agtmael MA, Hassink EA, Milinkovic A, Brinkman K, Geerlings SE, et al. Zidovudine/lamivudine for HIV-1 infection contributes to limb fat loss. PLoS One. 2009;4 [5]:e5647.

[140] Boothby M, McGee KC, Tomlinson JW, Gathercole LL, McTernan PG, Shojaee-Moradie F, et al. Adipocyte differentiation, mitochondrial gene expression and fat distribution: differences between zidovudine and tenofovir after 6 months. Antivir Ther. 2009;14 [8]:1089-100.

[141] Reiss P, Casula M, de Ronde A, Weverling GJ, Goudsmit J, Lange JM. Greater and more rapid depletion of mitochondrial DNA in blood of patients treated with dual (zidovudine+didanosine or zidovudine+zalcitabine) vs. single (zidovudine) nucleoside reverse transcriptase inhibitors. HIV Med. 2004 Jan;5 [1]:11-4.

[142] Hadigan C, Borgonha S, Rabe J, Young V, Grinspoon S. Increased rates of lipolysis among human immunodeficiency virus-infected men receiving highly active antiretroviral therapy. Metabolism. 2002 Sep;51 [9]:1143-7.

[143] Roche R, Poizot-Martin I, Yazidi CM, Compe E, Gastaut JA, Torresani J, et al. Effects of antiretroviral drug combinations on the differentiation of adipocytes. AIDS. 2002 Jan 4;16 [1]:13-20.

[144] van Vonderen MG, Blumer RM, Hassink EA, Sutinen J, Ackermans MT, van Agtmael MA, et al. Insulin sensitivity in multiple pathways is differently affected during zidovudine/lamivudine-containing compared with NRTI-sparing combination antiretroviral therapy. J Acquir Immune Defic Syndr. 2010 Feb 1;53 [2]:186-93.

[145] Guaraldi G, Baraboutis IG. Evolving perspectives on HIV-associated lipodystrophy syndrome: moving from lipodystrophy to non-infectious HIV co-morbidities. J Antimicrob Chemother. 2009 Sep;64 [3]:437-40.

[146] Sekiya M, Hiraishi A, Touyama M, Sakamoto K. Oxidative stress induced lipid accumulation via SREBP1c activation in HepG2 cells. Biochem Biophys Res Commun. 2008 Oct 31;375 [4]:602-7.

[147] Szendroedi J, Roden M. Ectopic lipids and organ function. Curr Opin Lipidol. 2009 Feb;20 [1]:50-6.

[148] Suganami T, Tanimoto-Koyama K, Nishida J, Itoh M, Yuan X, Mizuarai S, et al. Role of the Toll-like receptor 4/NF-kappaB pathway in saturated fatty acid-induced in-

flammatory changes in the interaction between adipocytes and macrophages. Arterioscler Thromb Vasc Biol. 2007 Jan;27 [1]:84-91.

[149] Sutinen J, Kannisto K, Korsheninnikova E, Nyman T, Ehrenborg E, Andrew R, et al. In the lipodystrophy associated with highly active antiretroviral therapy, pseudo-Cushing's syndrome is associated with increased regeneration of cortisol by 11beta-hydroxysteroid dehydrogenase type 1 in adipose tissue. Diabetologia. 2004 Oct;47 [10]:1668-71.

[150] Kratz M, Purnell JQ, Breen PA, Thomas KK, Utzschneider KM, Carr DB, et al. Reduced adipogenic gene expression in thigh adipose tissue precedes human immunodeficiency virus-associated lipoatrophy. J Clin Endocrinol Metab. 2008 Mar;93 [3]:959-66.

[151] Gougeon ML, Penicaud L, Fromenty B, Leclercq P, Viard JP, Capeau J. Adipocytes targets and actors in the pathogenesis of HIV-associated lipodystrophy and metabolic alterations. Antivir Ther. 2004 Apr;9 [2]:161-77.

[152] Rietschel P, Hadigan C, Corcoran C, Stanley T, Neubauer G, Gertner J, et al. Assessment of growth hormone dynamics in human immunodeficiency virus-related lipodystrophy. J Clin Endocrinol Metab. 2001 Feb;86 [2]:504-10.

[153] Lo JC, Mulligan K, Noor MA, Schwarz JM, Halvorsen RA, Grunfeld C, et al. The effects of recombinant human growth hormone on body composition and glucose metabolism in HIV-infected patients with fat accumulation. J Clin Endocrinol Metab. 2001 Aug;86 [8]:3480-7.

[154] Franceschi C, Capri M, Monti D, Giunta S, Olivieri F, Sevini F, et al. Inflammaging and anti-inflammaging: a systemic perspective on aging and longevity emerged from studies in humans. Mech Ageing Dev. 2007 Jan;128 [1]:92-105.

[155] Wu D, Ren Z, Pae M, Guo W, Cui X, Merrill AH, et al. Aging up-regulates expression of inflammatory mediators in mouse adipose tissue. J Immunol. 2007 Oct 1;179 [7]:4829-39.

[156] Effros RB, Fletcher CV, Gebo K, Halter JB, Hazzard WR, Horne FM, et al. Aging and infectious diseases: workshop on HIV infection and aging: what is known and future research directions. Clin Infect Dis. 2008 Aug 15;47 [4]:542-53.

[157] Tarr PE, Taffe P, Bleiber G, Furrer H, Rotger M, Martinez R, et al. Modeling the influence of APOC3, APOE, and TNF polymorphisms on the risk of antiretroviral therapy-associated lipid disorders. J Infect Dis. 2005 May 1;191 [9]:1419-26.

[158] Wangsomboonsiri W, Mahasirimongkol S, Chantarangsu S, Kiertiburanakul S, Charoenyingwattana A, Komindr S, et al. Association between HLA-B*4001 and lipodystrophy among HIV-infected patients from Thailand who received a stavudine-containing antiretroviral regimen. Clin Infect Dis. 2010 Feb 15;50 [4]:597-604.

[159] Zanone Poma B, Riva A, Nasi M, Cicconi P, Broggini V, Lepri AC, et al. Genetic polymorphisms differently influencing the emergence of atrophy and fat accumulation in HIV-related lipodystrophy. AIDS. 2008 Sep 12;22 [14]:1769-78.

[160] Maurin T, Saillan-Barreau C, Cousin B, Casteilla L, Doglio A, Penicaud L. Tumor necrosis factor-alpha stimulates HIV-1 production in primary culture of human adipocytes. Exp Cell Res. 2005 Apr 1;304 [2]:544-51.

[161] Sankale JL, Tong Q, Hadigan CM, Tan G, Grinspoon SK, Kanki PJ, et al. Regulation of adiponectin in adipocytes upon exposure to HIV-1. HIV Med. 2006 May;7 [4]:268-74.

[162] Hammond E, Nolan D. Adipose tissue inflammation and altered adipokine and cytokine production in antiretroviral therapy-associated lipodystrophy. Curr Opin HIV AIDS. 2007 Jul;2 [4]:274-81.

[163] Unger RH, Clark GO, Scherer PE, Orci L. Lipid homeostasis, lipotoxicity and the metabolic syndrome. Biochim Biophys Acta. 2010 Mar;1801 [3]:209-14.

[164] Giralt M, Diaz-Delfin J, Gallego-Escuredo JM, Villarroya J, Domingo P, Villarroya F. Lipotoxicity on the basis of metabolic syndrome and lipodystrophy in HIV-1-infected patients under antiretroviral treatment. Curr Pharm Des. 2010 Oct;16 [30]:3371-8.

[165] Virtue S, Vidal-Puig A. Adipose tissue expandability, lipotoxicity and the Metabolic Syndrome--an allostatic perspective. Biochim Biophys Acta. 2010 Mar;1801 [3]:338-49.

[166] Brown TT, Li X, Cole SR, Kingsley LA, Palella FJ, Riddler SA, et al. Cumulative exposure to nucleoside analogue reverse transcriptase inhibitors is associated with insulin resistance markers in the Multicenter AIDS Cohort Study. AIDS. 2005 Sep 2;19 [13]: 1375-83.

[167] Calza L, Manfredi R, Pocaterra D, Chiodo F. Risk of premature atherosclerosis and ischemic heart disease associated with HIV infection and antiretroviral therapy. J Infect. 2008 Jul;57 [1]:16-32.

[168] Behrens GM, Boerner AR, Weber K, van den Hoff J, Ockenga J, Brabant G, et al. Impaired glucose phosphorylation and transport in skeletal muscle cause insulin resistance in HIV-1-infected patients with lipodystrophy. J Clin Invest. 2002 Nov;110 [9]: 1319-27.

[169] Noor MA, Flint OP, Maa JF, Parker RA. Effects of atazanavir/ritonavir and lopinavir/ ritonavir on glucose uptake and insulin sensitivity: demonstrable differences in vitro and clinically. AIDS. 2006 Sep 11;20 [14]:1813-21.

[170] Schambelan M, Benson CA, Carr A, Currier JS, Dube MP, Gerber JG, et al. Management of metabolic complications associated with antiretroviral therapy for HIV-1 infection: recommendations of an International AIDS Society-USA panel. J Acquir Immune Defic Syndr. 2002 Nov 1;31 [3]:257-75.

[171] Hruz PW. Molecular Mechanisms for Altered Glucose Homeostasis in HIV Infection. Am J Infect Dis. 2006;2 [3]:187-92.

[172] Mukhopadhyay A, Wei B, Zullo SJ, Wood LV, Weiner H. In vitro evidence of inhibition of mitochondrial protease processing by HIV-1 protease inhibitors in yeast: a possible contribution to lipodystrophy syndrome. Mitochondrion. 2002 Oct;1 [6]:511-8.

[173] Meininger G, Hadigan C, Laposata M, Brown J, Rabe J, Louca J, et al. Elevated concentrations of free fatty acids are associated with increased insulin response to standard glucose challenge in human immunodeficiency virus-infected subjects with fat redistribution. Metabolism. 2002 Feb;51 [2]:260-6.

[174] Calza L, Manfredi R, Chiodo F. Hyperlipidaemia in patients with HIV-1 infection receiving highly active antiretroviral therapy: epidemiology, pathogenesis, clinical course and management. Int J Antimicrob Agents. 2003 Aug;22 [2]:89-99.

[175] Estrada V, Portilla J. Dyslipidemia related to antiretroviral therapy. AIDS Rev. 2011 Jan-Mar;13 [1]:49-56.

[176] Liang JS, Distler O, Cooper DA, Jamil H, Deckelbaum RJ, Ginsberg HN, et al. HIV protease inhibitors protect apolipoprotein B from degradation by the proteasome: a potential mechanism for protease inhibitor-induced hyperlipidemia. Nat Med. 2001 Dec;7 [12]:1327-31.

[177] Riddle TM, Schildmeyer NM, Phan C, Fichtenbaum CJ, Hui DY. The HIV protease inhibitor ritonavir increases lipoprotein production and has no effect on lipoprotein clearance in mice. J Lipid Res. 2002 Sep;43 [9]:1458-63.

[178] Riddle TM, Kuhel DG, Woollett LA, Fichtenbaum CJ, Hui DY. HIV protease inhibitor induces fatty acid and sterol biosynthesis in liver and adipose tissues due to the accumulation of activated sterol regulatory element-binding proteins in the nucleus. J Biol Chem. 2001 Oct 5;276 [40]:37514-9.

[179] Zaera MG, Miro O, Pedrol E, Soler A, Picon M, Cardellach F, et al. Mitochondrial involvement in antiretroviral therapy-related lipodystrophy. AIDS. 2001 Sep 7;15 [13]: 1643-51.

[180] Grundy SM, Cleeman JI, Daniels SR, Donato KA, Eckel RH, Franklin BA, et al. Diagnosis and management of the metabolic syndrome: an American Heart Association/ National Heart, Lung, and Blood Institute Scientific Statement. Circulation. 2005 Oct 25;112 [17]:2735-52.

[181] Gazzaruso C, Sacchi P, Garzaniti A, Fratino P, Bruno R, Filice G. Prevalence of metabolic syndrome among HIV patients. Diabetes Care. 2002 Jul;25 [7]:1253-4.

[182] Wand H, Calmy A, Carey DL, Samaras K, Carr A, Law MG, et al. Metabolic syndrome, cardiovascular disease and type 2 diabetes mellitus after initiation of antiretroviral therapy in HIV infection. AIDS. 2007 Nov 30;21 [18]:2445-53.

[183] Petersen KF, Shulman GI. Etiology of insulin resistance. Am J Med. 2006 May;119 [5 Suppl 1]:S10-6.

[184] Lemoine M, Barbu V, Girard PM, Kim M, Bastard JP, Wendum D, et al. Altered hepatic expression of SREBP-1 and PPARgamma is associated with liver injury in insulin-resistant lipodystrophic HIV-infected patients. AIDS. 2006 Feb 14;20 [3]:387-95.

[185] Howard AA, Lo Y, Floris-Moore M, Klein RS, Fleischer N, Schoenbaum EE. Hepatitis C virus infection is associated with insulin resistance among older adults with or at risk of HIV infection. AIDS. 2007 Mar 12;21 [5]:633-41.

[186] Mangili A, Jacobson DL, Gerrior J, Polak JF, Gorbach SL, Wanke CA. Metabolic syndrome and subclinical atherosclerosis in patients infected with HIV. Clin Infect Dis. 2007 May 15;44 [10]:1368-74.

[187] Triant VA, Grinspoon SK. Vascular dysfunction and cardiovascular complications. Curr Opin HIV AIDS. 2007 Jul;2 [4]:299-304.

[188] Schecter AD, Berman AB, Yi L, Mosoian A, McManus CM, Berman JW, et al. HIV envelope gp120 activates human arterial smooth muscle cells. Proc Natl Acad Sci U S A. 2001 Aug 28;98 [18]:10142-7.

[189] de Gaetano Donati K, Rabagliati R, Iacoviello L, Cauda R. HIV infection, HAART, and endothelial adhesion molecules: current perspectives. Lancet Infect Dis. 2004 Apr;4 [4]:213-22.

[190] Thomas CM, Smart EJ. How HIV protease inhibitors promote atherosclerotic lesion formation. Curr Opin Lipidol. 2007 Oct;18 [5]:561-5.

[191] Koppel K, Bratt G, Schulman S, Bylund H, Sandstrom E. Hypofibrinolytic state in HIV-1-infected patients treated with protease inhibitor-containing highly active antiretroviral therapy. J Acquir Immune Defic Syndr. 2002 Apr 15;29 [5]:441-9.

[192] Kamin DS, Grinspoon SK. Cardiovascular disease in HIV-positive patients. AIDS. 2005 Apr 29;19 [7]:641-52.

[193] Mercie P, Thiebaut R, Aurillac-Lavignolle V, Pellegrin JL, Yvorra-Vives MC, Cipriano C, et al. Carotid intima-media thickness is slightly increased over time in HIV-1-infected patients. HIV Med. 2005 Nov;6 [6]:380-7.

[194] Currier JS, Kendall MA, Henry WK, Alston-Smith B, Torriani FJ, Tebas P, et al. Progression of carotid artery intima-media thickening in HIV-infected and uninfected adults. AIDS. 2007 May 31;21 [9]:1137-45.

[195] Stein JH, Klein MA, Bellehumeur JL, McBride PE, Wiebe DA, Otvos JD, et al. Use of human immunodeficiency virus-1 protease inhibitors is associated with atherogenic lipoprotein changes and endothelial dysfunction. Circulation. 2001 Jul 17;104 [3]: 257-62.

[196] Meng Q, Lima JA, Lai H, Vlahov D, Celentano DD, Strathdee SA, et al. Coronary artery calcification, atherogenic lipid changes, and increased erythrocyte volume in black injection drug users infected with human immunodeficiency virus-1 treated with protease inhibitors. Am Heart J. 2002 Oct;144 [4]:642-8.

[197] Fisher SD, Miller TL, Lipshultz SE. Impact of HIV and highly active antiretroviral therapy on leukocyte adhesion molecules, arterial inflammation, dyslipidemia, and atherosclerosis. Atherosclerosis. 2006 Mar;185 [1]:1-11.

[198] Stefano GB, Salzet M, Bilfinger TV. Long-term exposure of human blood vessels to HIV gp120, morphine, and anandamide increases endothelial adhesion of monocytes: uncoupling of nitric oxide release. J Cardiovasc Pharmacol. 1998 Jun;31 [6]:862-8.

[199] Ren Z, Yao Q, Chen C. HIV-1 envelope glycoprotein 120 increases intercellular adhesion molecule-1 expression by human endothelial cells. Lab Invest. 2002 Mar;82 [3]: 245-55.

[200] Hwang SJ, Ballantyne CM, Sharrett AR, Smith LC, Davis CE, Gotto AM, Jr., et al. Circulating adhesion molecules VCAM-1, ICAM-1, and E-selectin in carotid atherosclerosis and incident coronary heart disease cases: the Atherosclerosis Risk In Communities (ARIC) study. Circulation. 1997 Dec 16;96 [12]:4219-25.

[201] Jager A, van Hinsbergh VW, Kostense PJ, Emeis JJ, Nijpels G, Dekker JM, et al. Increased levels of soluble vascular cell adhesion molecule 1 are associated with risk of cardiovascular mortality in type 2 diabetes: the Hoorn study. Diabetes. 2000 Mar;49 [3]: 485-91.

[202] Galea P, Vermot-Desroches C, Le Contel C, Wijdenes J, Chermann JC. Circulating cell adhesion molecules in HIV1-infected patients as indicator markers for AIDS progression. Res Immunol. 1997 Feb;148 [2]:109-17.

[203] Zhong DS, Lu XH, Conklin BS, Lin PH, Lumsden AB, Yao Q, et al. HIV protease inhibitor ritonavir induces cytotoxicity of human endothelial cells. Arterioscler Thromb Vasc Biol. 2002 Oct 1;22 [10]:1560-6.

[204] Maggi P, Perilli F, Lillo A, Carito V, Epifani G, Bellacosa C, et al. An ultrasound-based comparative study on carotid plaques in HIV-positive patients vs. atherosclerotic and arteritis patients: atherosclerotic or inflammatory lesions? Coron Artery Dis. 2007 Feb;18 [1]:23-9.

[205] Coll B, Parra S, Alonso-Villaverde C, Aragones G, Montero M, Camps J, et al. The role of immunity and inflammation in the progression of atherosclerosis in patients with HIV infection. Stroke. 2007 Sep;38 [9]:2477-84.

[206] Stein JH. Managing cardiovascular risk in patients with HIV infection. J Acquir Immune Defic Syndr. 2005 Feb 1;38 [2]:115-23.

[207] Martinez E, Larrousse M, Gatell JM. Cardiovascular disease and HIV infection: host, virus, or drugs? Curr Opin Infect Dis. 2009 Feb;22 [1]:28-34.

[208] Sabin CA, d'Arminio Monforte A, Friis-Moller N, Weber R, El-Sadr WM, Reiss P, et al. Changes over time in risk factors for cardiovascular disease and use of lipid-lowering drugs in HIV-infected individuals and impact on myocardial infarction. Clin Infect Dis. 2008 Apr 1;46 [7]:1101-10.

Chapter 13

HIV/AIDS: Vertical Transmission

Enrique Valdés Rubio

Additional information is available at the end of the chapter

http://dx.doi.org/10.5772/53204

1. Introduction

In The Eight Millennium Development Goals, the World Health Organization proposed to attempt at reverting the world negative HIV/AIDS epidemics through disease prevention and treatment for the year 2015. Attaining virtual elimination of Vertical Transmission (Prevention of mother-to-child transmission, PMTCT) worldwide is one of such aims [1].

The current chapter will address topics related to epidemiologic, pathophysiological, diagnostic and therapeutic aspects of vertical transmission of the Human Immunodeficiency Virus (HIV). Such information will enable the reader to understand how the health strategies aiming at preventing transmission to the fetus have turned into a paradigm of Perinatal Medicine, since the implementation of a series of biomedical interventions has proven to be successful to prevent transmission of HIV from an infected pregnant mother to her child.

2. Epidemiology

World Epidemiological Status

Prevalence of Vertical Transmission (VT) in the different regions of the world varies with geographic location and, specifically, with the economic resources invested by the different countries to support various strategies applied to health care policies that aim at the prevention and treatment of infected mothers. Proof of thereof is the fact that in countries with government programs in which the economic support is sufficient to implement the planned strategies for VT prevention, the prevalence of perinatal infection is under 2% [2,3].

HIV epidemics are showing a trend towards stabilization worldwide. Thus, in 2009 approximately 2.6 million persons became newly infected by the virus, representing 19% fewer than the newly infected in 1999 and more than a fifth less (21%) of the estimates in 1997. In fact, in 33 countries the incidence of infection has fallen by 25%. This includes 22 countries of the Sub-Saharan African region, the zone with the highest number of new cases worldwide (Ethiopia, Nigeria, South Africa, Zambia and Zimbabwe). In Eastern, Central and Western Europe, Central and Northern Asia the incidence of HIV infection has remained stable for the past five years. However in some high income countries infection rates have increased due to sex practices between homosexuals. Central Asia and Eastern Europe continue with high transmission rates among drug addicts and their sexual partners [4].

Regarding vertical transmission, an estimate of 370,000 children became infected with HIV during perinatal and lactation periods in 2009. Such figure is quite lower than the estimated 500,000 newly infected children in 2001. The latter has been possible thanks to Vertical Transmission (VT) prevention healthcare strategies that have been planned and implemented. Accordingly, the WHO and the UNAIDS proposed to virtually eliminate such transmission route by 2015. To accomplish such goal, besides the efforts already implemented, they stated the importance of controlling the infection among youngsters. It is estimated that more than half of seropositive persons are girls and women [1,4].

In the Sub-Saharan African region, there are 8 times more infected women than men among persons aged between 15 and 24. Most of women are infected during unsafe heterosexual sexual activity. Such situation is the main responsible for the fact that such countries are assembling 90% of the children infected worldwide. Despite of the latter, the incidence of subjects with a carrier status among children under 15 years of age has declined in 32% in South Africa, the country in which AIDS is the main cause of maternal death and that accounts for 35% of deaths in children under 5 years of age. Accordingly, worldwide data show that only 15% of women in whom the carrier status had been detected during their perinatal period stayed subsequently on lifelong antiretroviral therapy [4].

It is estimated that approximately 4.9 million people in Asia were seropositive during 2009. Such figure is similar to those reported in the previous years, thus reflecting that the epidemics has stabilized. In such continent, the number of infected children under the age of 15 has increased marginally, from 140,000 in 2005 to 160,000 in 2009 and AIDS-related deaths have dropped in 15% since 2004 [4].

In Western Europe, epidemiology indicators regarding maternal carrier status have evolved favorably. The estimated prevalence of infection among pregnant women in the United Kingdom is 0.2% and HIV screening coverage in gestating women is 90%. The latter has resulted in a sustained decline of VT from 12% in 1999 to 2% in 2007 [4,5].

In North America the carrier status has reached stability and VT has evidenced a dramatic decrease. In Canada, infection of the newborn has decreased from 5.2% in 1997 to 2.7% in 2012, and when the seropositive mother was administered HAART, such figure reached 0.4% [4,6].

In Central and South America the number of affected children under 15 years of age is still low, with approximately 4000 new cases during 2009, in spite of the fact that the coverage of

VT prevention programs is only marginally superior to that reported in countries with low or moderate income [4].

According to reports from 2006, the estimated number of seropositive subjects in Latin America is 1.7 millions, with 140,000 new cases and 65,000 deaths. Two thirds of the infected individuals live in four countries: Argentina, Brazil, Colombia and Mexico. The main agent responsible for the infection is HIV-1. The most commonly isolated genotype is type B, followed by types F and A [2].

In the American countries that compose the Southern Cone, HIV/AIDS epidemiological surveillance is carried out through mandatory notification (passive mechanism) and in some, through active surveillance by means of sentinel centers [2].

Most of such Latin American countries have implemented, since the second half of the 90s, an Antenatal Prevention of Mother To Child Transmission (APMTCT) program, consisting of the early voluntary diagnosis of HIV infection in the gestating population, universal access to antiretroviral therapy (ART) for the mother-child binomial, the C-section surgery and suppression of lactation, a program that aims at eliminating vertical transmission as a route of infection [2,3].

The main route of transmission in Latin America is represented by sex between men. There has been a significant increase in transmission through heterosexual intercourse since 1990. With the exception of Argentina, where initially transmission was mainly represented by needle sharing during drug injection, with a current dramatic drop, estimates of new cases of transmission through such route in 2005 do not exceed 5%. On the other hand, there is concern in the area, regarding the relationship between HIV and drug addition, since it has been demonstrated that illicit drug abuse, regardless of the route of administration, favors risk behaviors [2].

In view of the above stated, it is possible to conclude that the features of the epidemics in the Southern Cone have varied, showing a trend to impoverishment, feminization, and shift towards homosexual and scholar populations. Moreover, the fact of the most affected age group is between 20 and 39 years is of great importance, since it demonstrates that the mostly affected population is that representing the childbearing age, a situation that has a direct impact on VT risk. The latter warrants the importance of implementing human sexuality education to all levels of the population, providing the necessary information and recognizing the right of women to be informed to enable them to take the appropriate measures to protect themselves and prevent HIV infection. [2-4].

The rate of HIV seropositive pregnant women fluctuates in the different countries of the Region, between 3 and 7/1000. It is estimated that more than 2 million HIV (+) women get pregnant and 90% of them belong to developing countries, thus between 370,000 and 500,000 infected children are born annually, that die mostly because of the disease [4]. Pregnancy would play a protective role for maternal mortality among HIV (+) women. Such effect would be related to the low pregnancy rates achieved among women at advanced stages of the disease. [2]. Conversely, in developed countries, the rate of maternal mortality has decreased significantly since the introduction of the Highly Active Antiretroviral Therapy (HAART). Moreover, the latter has increased the probability of achieving pregnancy, thus decreasing the rate of stillbirths and gestation-related diseases [7].

Since the beginning of the pandemics, the importance of VT as transmission route has been clear. However, not even the most optimistic would have thought that PMTCT would turn into an example of effective biomedical intervention to prevent HIV transmission. It is important to point that most of Latin American countries have healthcare programs aiming at decreasing VT (PMTCT) that are based on the early prenatal voluntary screening for infection, the offering of antiretroviral therapies (ARVT), the C-section [8], substitution of breastfeeding [9] and multidisciplinary management during pregnancy. Regarding antenatal carrier status diagnosis, it is important to note that there are studies that reveal that between 25 and 55% of the total number of pregnant women who accept the test do not schedule a subsequent visit to know the results, thus they do not receive therapy. The latter suggests that fast intrapartum tests should be implemented on pregnant women unaware of their serologic condition. This is supported by a recent study carried out in Peru. The study concluded that the use of fast result tests (oral or blood) is a strategy advisable to decrease VT risk, in populations where PMTCT coverage does not reach the expected goals [10].

Pharmacological measures that have been implemented to decrease VT in the Southern region of America, were based on the ACTG 076 protocol [11] involving therapeutic antiretroviral management aiming at obtaining low or undetectable maternal viral loads, without toxic and/or teratogenic fetal effects. Such protocol consisted on the administration of Zidovudine to the mother during pregnancy and delivery, as well as to the newborn until the 6th week of life, together with indication of an elective C-section operation and contraindication of breastfeeding. Such scheme managed to decrease VT in the region, from 29% to 5.6% during 2001. [2] Subsequently, due to the emergence of new evidence supporting that triple-drug therapy was even more effective than monotherapy for VT prevention, a protocol was designed using a combination of reverse transcriptase and protease inhibitors. Such schemes were named together HAART. Thanks to such therapy, VT has dropped to figures close to 1% [2].

Because of the implementation and coverage of healthcare government programs in countries of the region, only few pregnant women have viral loads higher than 1000 copies/ml in the proximity of delivery. The latter is responsible for the VT drop estimated as 1%. [2] A recent study assessed the risk of VT in pregnant women who were administered PMTCT and concluded that the VT risk was 0.097 (95% IC; 0.030-0.163). This reflects a reduction of transmission risk related to such route in almost 40% regarding VT before the implementation of such program [12].

Chile, where an early detection program and timely treatment are currently being carried out, is probably one of the countries in the region having reached the best VT rates. This is a result of healthcare strategies aiming an adequate and permanently updated diagnosis of the behavior of the epidemics in the country. The proportion of female HIV carriers has increased as compared to that of males, due to the fact that the main transmission route is sex (93.6%). Such figure together with the impact of viral transmission both through homosexual as well as bisexual intercourse (46.1%), positions the monogamous heterosexual woman as the highest risk population (51.1%). Moreover, there is a sustained increase of cases transmitted through sex between men and women as compared to those transmitted through homosexual intercourse. This has shifted the epidemics towards heterosexual population groups, with a higher impact among female populations [2,3].

To summarize, HIV VT in the region is responsible for a low percentage of people reported with HIV/AIDS, but is accountable for most of the children affected by the infection in the Southern Cone. An important reduction of transmission by means of such exposition route, reaching levels very close to the proposed goals, has been evidenced. Such decline might probably be explained by the wide coverage and effectiveness of the measures propounded by the health authorities to tackle the issue [2,3].

3. Virology and Natural History of the Infection

The Human Immunodeficiency Virus (HIV) is a lentivirus that belongs to the Retroviridae family. Two types of HIV have been identified: HIV-1, the most common, results in acquired immunodeficiency syndrome and death, and HIV-2, affecting mainly inhabitants or visitors from Western Africa, is transmitted less effectively and results in a more indolent disease with subsequent AIDS and death. They share less than 50% sequence homology. Through phylogenetic analysis, HIV-1 strains can be divided into two large groups: The M (Major) group in turn divided into 10 subtypes (from A to J) and the O (Outlier) group. The eventual importance of HIV-1 typification lies in developing antibody screening techniques, diagnosing the infection in the newborn, and in the quantification of plasma viral RNA for follow up of infected patients [13, 14,15].

This monostranded RNA virus incorporates its genetic material into the host cell DNA, infecting cells that express CD4 antigen on their surface, such as helper T cells, macrophages, central nervous system cells and even placental cells [13,16,17].

Once the infection has occurred, the patient may present a primoinfection characterized by mononucleosis–like non-specific symptoms, where antibody production is triggered. Subsequently the patient undergoes a silent carrier phase. The latter used to last between 9 and 11 years before the emergence of antiretroviral therapy. As the immune system is being progressively involved, the host becomes more susceptible to suffer opportunistic infections, cancers and dementia / encephalopathy, which are complications that enable labeling such stage as AIDS stage. In further consensus, the following findings were added: CD4 count under $200/mm^3$, uterine cervix cancer, lung tuberculosis and recurrent pneumonia [13,16,17].

4. Viral Replication Mechanism

The genome of HIV-1 is relatively small, and composed of genes coding for structural, regulatory and accessory proteins. The viral particle joins the cells of the susceptible host, among which are T cells, monocytes, macrophages, follicular dendritic cells and microglial cells. A high affinity bond is generated between the gp 120 of the viral surface and the CD4 receptor molecule on the host cell. Cell membranes fuse together and the virus enters the cell, uncovering its RNA. It is propounded that after infection, it is the downregulation of CD4 expression on the infected cell surface that prevents a superinfection, enables an efficacious replication of the virus, and decreases the possibility of early cell death or apoptosis. During an early stage, the viral reverse transcriptase is activated together with other factors, and complete double stranded DNA copies are formed from the viral RNA. Such DNA copy is transported to the cell nucleus and binds to the host cell DNA through the viral integrase, generating the so-called provirus. The provirus may remain latent during a period of time. The host factors that influence the latency period duration are unknown. In activated cells, proviral transcription generates genomic RNA for its incorporation into new virions and messenger RNA that will be translated into structural proteins and several regulator and accessory proteins that facilitate viral replication, assembling and release [13,16,17].

The adult immune system has several components that are critical for HIV infection, such as B and T cells, antigen-presenting cells, major histocompatibility antigens (types I and II), natural killer cells, cytokines and complement. Before an infection or antigenic stimulation, B cells are always "naïve". Following their stimulation, they generate two HIV specific subgroups that actively secrete antibodies against the virus. Likewise, there are "innocent" and other T cells with specific memory as a result of a prior exposure to the virus. In the great majority of the infected people HIV invasion disrupts normal immune reactions and induces a chronic progressive, polymorphic dysfunction that, at a given time, makes the individual susceptible to opportunistic infections, cancers, neurological disorders and premature death. The initial HIV infection in adults is frequently followed 2 to 6 weeks later by an acute viral syndrome that manifests with fever, pharyngitis, myalgia, tender lymphadenopathies, nonspecific rash and lasts from 7 to 14 days. There is an acute drop of circulating lymphocyte counts, with a fairly rapid normalization of figures. However, CD4+ T cell counts do not fully regain baseline values. During such period viral replication and dissemination to lymph nodes and mononuclear / macrophagic cells occur speedily [13,16,17].

The circulating viral load is high in the initial absence of an effective antibody response. Typically, IgM appear one or two months after HIV exposure, followed by IgG (specifically anti-gp 120/41) and the development of an anti-p24 response that fades out in more advanced stages of the infection. Shortly afterwards, anti-gp120 and gp41 antibodies emerge, and persist for a lifetime. As anti–HIV antibody titers increase, the circulating viral load decreases and the infected subjects initiate an asymptomatic phase that commonly lasts from 3 to 11 years. During such asymptomatic phase viral replication is extremely intense, as well as is the destruction and replacement of CD4+ T cells. It should be taken into consideration that before causing a gradual CD4+ T cell depletion, HIV infection causes a CD4+ T cell dysfunction. Chemoprophylaxis, antibody-related cell-mediated cytotoxicity, intracellular antimicrobial activity and disorders of cytokine production also occur due to monocyte and macrophage dysfunction caused by the HIV infection [13,16,17].

During pregnancy, the mother undergoes a modulation of her immune response characterized by a TH2 response (humoral type) more prominent than TH1-type (cellular) response

http://dx.doi.org/10.5772/53204

that renders her more susceptible to certain infections. Based on the latter, it has been postulated that pregnancy might influence the course of the infection. Such hypothesis has been thoroughly discussed, and currently the conclusion is that gestation does not have adverse effects on survival or on the expression of the disease. Such conclusion is supported by the fact that the absolute CD4 count and the viral load remain stable during pregnancy in untreated pregnant women [7,13,16 -18].

Almost all clinical disorders described in HIV-infected adults may appear in infants, however their rates of onset might be different in both life periods. The evolution of disease among infants infected during the perinatal stage is faster than in adults. This has raised questions such as if the developing immune system in fetuses and newborns represents a better ground for viral replication or is less efficient for infection control. Immaturity of the immune system of fetuses, newborns and infants causes two pathophysiological differences between adults and children: B cells are seldom susceptible to HIV infection and their circulating values remain normal; however such cells show abnormalities in infected children as compared to infected adults. As the infant has been exposed to few external antigens (and thus has a limited immune memory), the resulting immune dysfunction is more severe than in adults. Because of the poor development of T and B cell memory, children infected in perinatal stages are more vulnerable to antibody-mediated pyogenic infections than infected adults [13,16,17].

Almost as soon as the infected cells die, they are replaced, until the degree of the immune dysfunction is such as to make the immune control of the virus inefficient. Thus, the clinical conditions defining AIDS are progressively met.

5. HIV behavior in women

The main HIV transmission risk factor for females worldwide is sexual intercourse. More than 90% of HIV-AIDS-infected women have acquired the infection through heterosexual transmission. In most of the cases, such women had sexual intercourse only with their stable spouse, thus attesting for their vulnerability to transmission, which is directly related to their sexual partner's behavior (bisexuality, drug addictions, promiscuity) [3].

The reasons explaining why women are more susceptible to be infected by HIV than men are varied. Thus, healthcare staff must be aware of such factors and therefore generate a sympathetic and empathic environment to achieve a good physician-patient relationship. Among such reasons, the following should be considered:

- Sexual transmission of the virus is several times more common from men to women than vice versa. Women with thinned vaginal mucosa or lacking the physiological defense mechanisms (pubertal and postmenopausal women) are at higher risk.

- Asymptomatic sexually transmitted vaginosis is commonly underdiagnosed and results in a disturbance of the indemnity of the vaginal mucosa.

- Women depend economically, socially and emotionally on men and such situation makes rejection of high-risk sexual intercourse difficult.

- Cultural norms encourage promiscuity among males, thus increasing transmission risk among monogamous females.

- There is a lack of easy access to woman-controlled-preventive methods (female condoms).

Regarding the last point and aiming at identifying other prevention methods, recent studies have demonstrated that the use of tenofovir gel might be a useful tool to prevent infection. In fact, a South African study concluded that the pre and post-coital prophylactic use of such microbicide among women aged between 18 and 40 reduced HIV infection in 39% and HSV-2 infection in 51%. [19] On the other hand, circumcision in adults has proven to be effective to prevent infection among seronegative males with an HIV+ partner. The latter has led the UNAIDS and WHO to recommend such intervention in countries with high prevalence [4]. Finally, there are also studies that propose the use of tenofovir prior to sexual intercourse in infected or high-risk couples. All these prophylactic measures should be assessed with further adequately designed studies.

Probably due to such reasons and in light of the pooled data in developing and developed countries, the proportion of HIV carrier women has increased as compared to that of men. The cause is that the main transmission route is sex. The latter together with the impact of viral transmission route in homo and heterosexual mode, have transformed heterosexual monogamous women into the highest risk population. Moreover, there is a sustained increase of cases transmitted by sexual intercourse between men and women as compared to those transmitted through homosexual intercourse. This has shifted the epidemics towards population groups with a lower social-economic level and with a clear decrease of females in higher school education levels [2, 3, 16,17].

Epidemiology studies suggest that the observed prevalence among women in childbearing age is comparable to prevalence in pregnant women. On the other hand, pregnancy rates in seropositive women that have not developed AIDS are comparable to those seen among uninfected women, while among women who developed the disease the probability of getting pregnant is quite lower [13-15].

6. Management of seropositive pregnant woman for Vertical Transmission Prevention

Most of women discover their carrier status or their disease during pregnancy or subsequently after birth upon screening of their offspring. With regard to the need for screening of all women during their pre and/or post-conception consultation, the American College of Obstetricians and Gynecologists recommends carrying it out on a routine basis, which is a conduct commonly adopted in many countries of the world. In fact, in most of these countries, such screening is performed together with the mandatory pre-test counseling act, with the informed consent and with the willfulness of individuals in the decision to undergo the

http://dx.doi.org/10.5772/53204

test. Therefore, screening requires the participation of staff trained in "counseling", which has reinforced the decision to undergo the test among women. This has shown to be of most importance for the generation of awareness about the disease, adherence to therapy and the incorporation of behaviors by the carrier to prevent transmission to her personal environment [20-24]. Pre and post-conceptional counseling is understood as a "confidential dialogue between a questioner and a counselor aiming at empowering women to face stress, decision making regarding HIV/AIDS during pregnancy and discussion of the elements for prevention of vertical transmission". It is important to recommend the following topics to be addressed upon counseling:

- Impact of HIV on pregnancy.

- Vertical Transmission risk and impact of prophylactic measures.

- Risks and benefits of antiretroviral therapy.

- Prognosis for children who become infected.

– Breastfeeding-related risks.

7. Diagnosis

The most popular methods worldwide are tests that screen for specific antibodies against viral antigens. The most used technique for screening is Enzyme Linked Immunosorbent Assay (ELISA). The most used technique for infection confirmation is the Western blot technique [25].

The ELISA test uses antigens derived from the intact virus and binds them to microtitration wells. The serum or plasma from the patient is added into the wells and if there are antibodies against HIV they bind to the antigen present. A chromogen substrate is also provided to evidence the potentially bound enzyme and the intensity of the color generated is read on a spectrophotometer. Color reading is proportional to the amount of the enzyme-antibody complex that bound the HIV antigen present in the wells. Commercially available tests have sensitivity and specificity rates between 98 and 100%. The disadvantage of such tests is they detect antibodies and thus may yield false positive results if transmission occurred shortly before the test. Such time lapse is known as window period, which may last between 3 and 6 months. For such reason, fourth generation ELISA is recommended. Such test is able to detect simultaneously Ag p24 and its respective antibodies, and therefore it can shorten the window period to approximately 30 days, with 99.9% sensitivity and 99.5% specificity. Despite the latter, it is important to point that the positive predictive value of this test during pregnancy is approximately 50%, because it is applied to a low prevalence population, and therefore a confirmation test is mandatory (Western blot) [16].

Additionally, in pregnant women with unknown serology status and attending consultation for labor or medical situations where pregnancy termination is imminent, services should have rapid diagnostic techniques. Despite their non-optimal specificity and sensitivity, positive results on such tests should be able to generate the recommendation of preventive measures during the peripartum period, with prior patient informed consent [5,10].

The confirmation Western blot technique is carried out with a nitrocellulose strip to which HIV shell proteins are added. Patient serum is applied on the strips: any antibody against such virus present in serum will bind to its specific antigen. This generates a series of dark bands. By comparing the band position with a control, it is possible to determine if the patient's blood contains HIV-specific antibodies [16].

On occasions, individuals with recent infection or in the process of structuring a complete antibody response yield undetermined responses. In such cases, the test should be repeated within one to two months.

PCR tests are sensitive and useful to confirm the infection status. They are able to detect very small amounts of virus and they do not rely on an antibody response to infection. PCR is used in clinical practice to establish the infection status on infants born to infected mothers and potentially within the window period between infection and presence of detectable specific antibodies. PCR and other amplification techniques have been improved to quantify HIV RNA. There is considerable interest on perfecting reliable tests to detect the virus in oral fluids or urine, since they are easy to collect without causing either disturbance to the patient or risks to the collector. Moreover, they can be especially helpful in children and adults in whom vein access can be difficult [16].

Assessment of HIV infection status is complex in children under the age of 6 months because of gestation and early lactation immunology. The most commonly used tests in adults are based on the detection of IgG antibodies against the virus. During pregnancy, maternal IgG crosses easily the placenta towards fetal circulation, where it remains until 18 months after birth. For such reason, assessment of the HIV infection status in infants requires testing other than ELISA and Western blot. The options are virus cultures and PCR, as well as detection of IgA antibodies directed against HIV [14,16].

8. HIV and Pregnancy

According to epidemiological studies, pregnancy rates among seropositive women that have not presented AIDS are comparable to rates in uninfected women. The probability of becoming pregnant is quite lower among women who develop AIDS. Despite of certain contradictory evidence, latest studies seem to confirm that pregnancy does not affect the course or the complications of the disease [26].

As for the role played by the viral load or the immune condition of the pregnant woman, there is evidence supporting a close relationship between high viral loads and higher VT risk. However there is not a viral load warranting a virus-free neonate. Mother-to-child transmission is possible despite viral levels being undetectable in the mother. On the other hand, maternal CD4 concentrations < 700 cells/mm relate to a higher VT risk [27].

Nevertheless, opportunistic infections (Pneumocystis jirovecii, Herpes Zoster, etc.) and prevalent diseases such as tuberculosis and malaria are those with more aggressive course in seropositive pregnant women and increase significantly maternal and perinatal morbidity and mortality. [28]

Vertical transmission is one of the mostly studied transmission routes, thus it is possible to share some conclusions regarding the moment of transmission to the fetus or newborn and the factors that increase VT risk [14,16].

Moment of transmission to the product of conception:

- During pregnancy: up to 35%.

- During delivery: up to 65%.

- During lactation: up to 14%.

Obstetric factors that favor VT:

- Premature Rupture of Membranes of more than 4 hours.

- Premature delivery.

- Low Birth Weight (under 2,500 g).

- Ovular infection.

- Direct contact of the fetus with cervical and vaginal secretions and/or blood in the birth canal.

Fortunately, the gravid status does not seem to have an impact on the course or the natural history of HIV infection, since although a decrease in CD4+ T cell counts has been described during pregnancy, they return to baseline values after delivery [17]. In the absence of complications such as drug addictions or chronic medical diseases, the incidence of obstetric pathology does not increase; spontaneous abortion, intrauterine growth restriction, preterm delivery and stillbirth are within the expected prevalence range. However, the risk of infectious complications increases among pregnant women with a significant impairment of the immune system (CD4 < 300/dl) [18].

A seropositive gestating woman should be clinically addressed based on a multidisciplinary and thorough assessment of her initial health status. The latter should include a full physical examination, especially observing those signs that guide diagnosis towards an opportunistic infectious pathology and assessing the current immune status. Upon indicating the therapeutic and/or prophylactic antiretroviral treatment, a risk versus benefit assessment should be carried out to evaluate the effectiveness of the pharmacological scheme and the eventual teratogenic and toxic effects on mother and fetus.

The following laboratory tests might be performed in addition to the routine tests that should be requested for pregnant women at the beginning of their prenatal follow-up [4,16]:

Infectious parameters:

- Rubella serology

- Urine culture

- Hepatitis B surface antigen Hepatitis B core antigen for Hepatitis B virus.

- Serology for the detection of Syphilis (RPR or VDRL).

- Serology for Hepatitis C.

- PPD (skin test for tuberculosis).

- Serology for certain parasitoses depending on their geographic prevalence (Toxoplasma gondii, Chagas disease, Malaria, etc.).

- Serology for cytomegalovirus.

- Culture for gonococcus, Chlamydia, Mycoplasma and Ureaplasma.

Immunological parameters:

- CD4+ T cell counts

- Viral load assessment (PCR).

Sequential detection of the viral load and CD4 counts are used to predict the risk of a rapid disease progression in the pregnant woman and the eventual VT in such patient group. However, as an intent to identify a more cost-effective test than the latter, the role of HIV typification through sequential study of specific bands offered by the Western blot technique has been studied recently. Such preliminary studies demonstrated that the absence of anti pol antibodies was associated with an acute infection. Although it is true that the lack of anti gag p39 antibodies was related to a rapid disease progression and a higher probability of infection of the newborn, such absence was not as statistically significant to predict a higher risk for VT. Therefore, such diagnostic tool needs still to be upheld by further studies before it becomes indicated for clinical use. [29]

All antenatal diagnostic assessments may be carried out without contradictions, except for those involving invasive techniques that imply an additional infection risk to the fetus (chorionic villus biopsy, amniocentesis, cordocentesis).

9. Antiretroviral therapy during pregnancy

The aim of antiretroviral therapy during pregnancy is to decrease the maternal viral load to undetectable levels without causing deleterious or teratogenic effects on the product of conception, and on the other hand, to decrease the risk of vertical transmission. To attain such goal, there are currently 14 antiretroviral drugs available (Table 1). Such drugs must be used within schemes individually adapted for each patient. Drug selection should be based on the prior treatment of the woman (if she were under any), the current status of the patient and her motivation, the viral load, drug resistance, CD4+ T cell counts, and associated toxic and teratogenic effects (Table 2). The use of Zidovudine is recommended within the scheme. Zidovudine has been the only drug to enter a protocol and that has demonstrated efficacy in the protection of the fetus from vertical transmission. However, new studies have demonstrated the efficacy of other antiretroviral drugs in VT reduction.

Generic name	FDA Classs
Abacavir	C
Didanosine (ddI)	B
Lamivudine (3TC)	C
Lamivudine + Zidovudine (Convivir)	C
Stavudine (d4T Zalcitabine)	C
Zidovudine (ZDZ, AZT)	C
Non-nucleosidic reverse transcriptase Inhibitors	
Delavirdine	C
Efavirenz *	X
Nevirapine	C
Protease inhibitors	
Amprenavir *	X
Indinavir	C
Nelfinavir	X
Ritonavir	B
Saquinavir	B

Table 1. ANTIRETROVIRAL AGENTS,Nucleosidic reverse transcriptase inhibitors

A: Controlled studies show no risk
B: No evidence of risks in humans
C: Risks cannot be ruled out. However, a potential benefit might justify its use.
D: Positive evidence of risk.
X: Contraindicated in pregnancy.

Table 2. FDA Drug Category Rankings (Drugs and pregnancy)

10. Management Protocol in the Prevention of Vertical Transmission (ACTG 076)

The first formalized intent in prevention of VT was that assessed by a joint study carried out in France and the United States, attempting at the evaluation of a management protocol (Clinical Group Protocol 076-ACTG 076) [11], consisting of a study and follow up of HIV+ pregnant women that had a gestational age between weeks 14 and 34, without antiretroviral therapy or indications for such therapy, with CD4+ T cell count > or equal to 200 cells/mm^3.

The group that was administered placebo was compared to the group receiving AZT (orally during pregnancy, injectable during delivery and as syrup to the newborn for 6 weeks). Results showed that transmission was 8.3% with AZT and 25% with placebo, which is equivalent to a reduction in 67% (p= 0,00006). (Table 3)

Prepartum: AZT between weeks 14 and 34: AZT 100 mg po 5 times per day or AZT 200 mg po 3 times per day or AZT 300 mg po 2 times per day
Intrapartum: AZT 2 mg/kg intravenous during one hour,Followed by continuous infusion of 1 mg/kg until delivery
Postpartum: AZT to the neonate from 8 to 12 hours after birth in 2 mg/kg doses (syrup) every 6 hours during the first 6 weeks of life

Table 3. ACTG 076 PROTOCOL

11. High Activity Antiretroviral (ART) Therapy (HAART)

The first attempt at a successful pharmacological scheme to control VT was achieved by the ACTG 076 protocol. Such protocol together with elective C-section and suppression of lactation (biomedical measures) achieved a decrease in VT from 29% to 5.6% [11]. Although the latter is true, new evidence demonstrated that the triple drug therapy was more effective than monotherapy or bitherapy to prevent Vertical Transmission (VT). A protocol, that combined the biomedical preventive measures already mentioned and the indication of three antiretroviral drugs was designed. Such drugs included nucleosidic and non-nucleosidic reverse transcriptase inhibitors (NRTI and NNRTI respectively) and Protease inhibitors (PI), and together formed a series of schemes known as highly active antiretroviral therapy (HAART). It is by virtue of the latter that VT has decreased to values close to 1.0 [2-6, 30-34].

It is a known fact that VT may occur among seropositive pregnant women during pregnancy (35%), delivery (65%) and lactation (14%-29%) and that there are factors that increase the risk of fetal infection (Primoinfection, Sexually transmitted diseases and CD4+ T cell counts). The most important of such factors is maternal viral load [27]. Loads under 1000 copies/ml have significantly lower risks of VT, however there is no evidence pointing to the minimal load that exempts from risk. The latter supports the need to use a highly active antiretroviral therapy (HAART) with the highest effectiveness and safety to reach, hopefully, undetectable viral load levels. With such purpose, and considering that most of transmissions to the newborn occur during the peripartum period, an attempt at reaching the lowest viral loads during the third trimester of gestation (weeks 34-36) should be made. However, due to the potential toxic effects of therapeutic drugs, it is suggested their use is limited to the periods of maximum effectiveness considering risks and benefits of such exposure to the mother-child binomial. Anyway, AZT should be added to the therapeutic scheme if possible, even in cases in which such drug was not used during the antepartum period, since it has proven to be helpful to decrease vertical transmission even in abbreviated schemes (intrapartum and postpartum) [4,5,34].

Based on the above-mentioned, HAART type ART should be indicated in the following situations: [34]

1. In seropositive pregnant women without prior treatment from week 24
2. In pregnant women with viral loads higher than 100,000 copies/ml from 14 weeks
3. In case of seroconversion during pregnancy it should be indicated at once

Within the HAART concept, the selection of the NRTI combination to be used should follow the efficacy of the latter in reducing VT, considering the potential teratogenic effects and the eventual toxicity to the mother-child binomial. Based on the teratogenesis risk classification of the FDA, NRTI are classed as B or C. The largest experience involves Zidovudine (AZT or ZDV) that has demonstrated being quite a safe drug, with low resistance and high efficacy to prevent VT. In addition, the association of ZDV and Lamivudine (ZDV/3TC) has demonstrated to be more effective than ZDV as monotherapy in mother-to-child transmission prevention. Such combination does not imply higher toxicity or risk of teratogenesis [2-6, 30-34].

Regarding the search for the third drug, Lopinavir-Ritonavir has demonstrated efficacy and safety in VT prevention. The association of Saquinavir reinforced with Ritonavir has gathered enough evidence to suggest that such combination is a good supplementary alternative to render the pharmacological therapy more effective [26].

Although Nevirapine (NVP) has been widely indicated and has demonstrated being effective in the prevention of mother-to-child transmission mostly in developing countries with low economical resources, the use of such drug has been related to the development of viral resistance both in mothers as in children who were infected despite the received prophylaxis. Moreover, mothers who were administered Nevirapine had a higher incidence of toxic effects (hepatic, hypersensitivity) in particular pregnant women with CD4+ T cell counts higher than 250 cells/ml. The above mentioned suggests that such indication should be considered among patients never having received Nevirapine and with CD4+ T cell counts under 250 cells/ml. When such drug is used in the intrapartum period, it is advisable to indicate ZDV y Lamivudine (3TC) for 7 days both to the mother as well as to the newborn, to reduce the risk of viral resistance to Nevirapine and other NNTRI [30-34].

The following are among the drugs that should not be indicated during pregnancy: Efavirenz, Nelfinavir and the association of d4T (Stavudine) and ddI (Didanosine). All share teratogenicity and toxicity risk for the mother-child binomial [30-36].

In 2010 the World Health Organization stressed the importance of offering a lifelong antiretroviral therapy to patients with a carrier condition recognized during pregnancy. The

WHO proposed two prophylactic treatment schemes (A and B) for pregnant women who did not meet the criterion of a certain CD4+ T cell count (<350/ mm^3). A third option (B+) as appeared recently, aiming at implementing the HAART for a lifetime to all seropositive pregnant women regardless of their CD4+ T cell count (Table 4). This new option has the following advantages: it simplifies drug supply, since it relates drugs to national antiretroviral therapy programs, protects against VT, prevents transmission to seronegative partners and prevents discontinuation of the follow up of therapies already implemented by the patients. It finally suggests that such new option should be evaluated depending on the reality of each country [31].

	Woman Receives:		
	Treatment	**Prophylaxis**	**Infant receives:**
	(for CD4 count ≤ 350 cells/mm^3)	(for CD4 count > 350 cells/ mm^3)	
Option Aa	Triple ARVs starting as soon as diagnosed, *continued for life*	*Antepartum*: AZT starting as early as 14 weeks gestation *Intrapartum*: at onset of labour, single-dose NVP and first dose of AZT/3TC *Postpartum*: daily AZT/3TC through 7 days postpartum	Daily NVP from birth until 1 week after cessation of all breastfeeding; or, if not breastfeeding or if mother is on treatment, through age 4–6 weeks
Option B$_a$	*Same initial ARVs for both$_b$:* Triple ARVs starting as soon as diagnosed, *continued for life*	*Same initial ARVs for both$_b$:* Triple ARVs starting as early as 14 weeks gestation and continued intrapartum and through childbirth if not breastfeeding or until 1 week after cessation of all breastfeeding	Daily NVP or AZT from birth through age 4–6 weeks regardless of infant feeding method
Option B+	*Same for treatment and prophylaxis$_b$:* Regardless of CD4 count, triple ARVs starting as soon as diagnosed,c continued for life	*Same for treatment and prophylaxis$_b$:* Regardless of CD4 count, triple ARVs starting as soon as diagnosed,c continued for life	Daily NVP or AZT from birth through age 4–6 weeks regardless of infant feeding method

Table 4. Note: "Triple ARVs" refers to the use of one of the recommended 3-drug fully suppressive treatment options. For the drug abbreviations in the table: AZT (azidothymidine, zidovudine [ZDV]); NVP (nevirapine); 3TC (lamivudine).a Recommended in WHO 2010 PMTCT guidelines b True only for EFV-based first-line ART; NVP-based ART not recommended for prophylaxis (CD4 >350) c Formal recommendations for Option B+ have not been made, but presumably ART would start at diagnosis. Options for PMTCT programs

11.1. Toxic and Side effects of ART

The eventual toxic effect of such medications on the mother-child binomial is among the aspects that need to be assessed for the election of the pharmacological treatment. According to study reports, approximately 80% of gestating women under treatment developed some side effect such as anemia, nausea, vomiting, hepatic enzyme disorders or hyperglycemia [26,35-37]. Because of this, it is important to know which are the side and toxic effects of the drugs that are commonly used, in order to identify them and treat them accordingly.

11.2. Protease inhibitors and hyperglycemia

In non-pregnant women, the use of protease inhibitors has been related to the development of different degrees of carbohydrate Intolerance. This should be considered when they are used during pregnancy since they may trigger gestational diabetes [26,35-37].

11.3. Mitochondrial toxicity and nucleosidic reverse transcriptase inhibitors

Reverse transcriptase nucleoside inhibitors are recognized for their induction of mitochondrial dysfunction due to their affinity for mitochondrial DNA-polymerase gamma. Such effect is more intense for Stavudine (d4T), ddI (Didanosine) and less intense for ZDV (Zidovudine), 3TC (Lamivudine), ABC (Abacavir) and TDF (Tenofir). Additionally, these drugs are also related to lactic acidosis in cases with concomitant hepatic steatosis. Such association would be higher with the use of d4T (Stavudine) with an estimated rate of 0,8% and 1,2% per year per treated patient. [26, 35-37]. Clinical manifestations of this condition are varied and include polyneuritis, myopathies, cardiopathies, hepatic steatosis and lactic acidosis. Not uncommonly patients develop a condition similar to the HELLP Syndrome that should be considered when addressing differential diagnoses. Finally, there are reports about uninfected children, born to seropositive mothers that received ZDV or ZDV/Lamivudine (ZDV/3TC) during pregnancy, who developed mitochondrial dysfunction –related symptoms during the first months of life. Such finding was not confirmed with the protocol assessment ACTG 076 [11].

Regarding the mode of delivery in seropositive pregnant women who did not receive ART or had partial indication of ART, elective C-section at week 38 (a surgical procedure carried out before the initiation of labor and without premature rupture of membranes) has demonstrated a decrease of VT risk in one half. [8,38]. Recent studies propose the option of vaginal delivery to be used according to the obstetric conditions in seropositive women with viral load under 1000 copies/ml and prior patient consent. Such indication is supported by the fact that C-section benefits are indeed difficult to evaluate and moreover, data retrieved from a large number of patients did not evidence a higher reduction of VT among patients with viral loads < 1000 copies/ml that underwent C-section. Furthermore, C-section increased infectious morbidity between 7 and 10 fold [33].

When facing the vaginal delivery option, episiorrhaphy and forceps or spatulas should be avoided. Invasive procedures such as amniocentesis, chorionic villus biopsy and invasive monitoring might increase fetal exposure to infected maternal blood, and thus should also be avoided. The use of oxytocin has no contraindications, as opposed to ergot-derivatives that might present an eventual synergic action in association to Protease Inhibitors that would exaggerate vasoconstriction and ischemia, and therefore are contraindicated [39].

During delivery (C-section or vaginal delivery), the indication of intravenous administration of ZDV to the mother should be the rule, since fetal plasma levels of such drug, reached by transplacental route, ensure an adequate pre-exposition prophylaxis. Such indication together with the administration of ZDV suspension orally to the newborn during six weeks increases the preventive effect on infection transmission. This is regardless of the mother being administered ZDV within the therapeutic scheme or even in the event of resistance to ZDV. Finally, the use of Nevirapine (200 mg one time only dose) should only be indicated to patients with late initiation of the prevention protocol, on patients with a viral load > 1000 copies/ml or in the case of diagnosis of maternal carrier status during labor [4,5,33,34].

There is evidence pointing that among patients that are not treated within an antiretroviral management protocol, transmission to the newborn through breastfeeding ranges between 5% and 14% [9,40]. Free and cell-bound virus has been isolated from breast milk through PCR techniques and viral culture. Such cells are more numerous in the colostrum and in breast milk secreted during the immediate puerperium. The latter, in association with the immature immune system of the newborn, make transmission through breastfeeding higher during the first month of life. All the above-mentioned, warrant the recommendation to suppress lactation in countries where infantile malnutrition and diarrheic syndrome - related mortality are low [34].

12. Summary of Mother-to-child Prevention Management

1. Every pregnant woman should be offered the possibility of undergoing HIV testing not later than upon the second pregnancy follow-up visit within the first trimester of gestation, and depending on resources, also within the third trimester.
2. A quick HIV test for HIV diagnosis enabling immediate action to be taken should be offered to women who arrive to delivery without having their test results available, even if tests have been carried out. Counseling and consent are mandatory.
3. ART is recommended to prevent HIV vertical transmission in pregnant women without prior therapy between gestation weeks 20 and 28. The use of ZDV in association with Lamivudine is recommended.
4. Viral loads should be followed up 6 weeks after initiation of ART during gestation and subsequently on a monthly basis until gestation weeks 34 and 36.
5. Elective C-section should be indicated at 39 weeks in HIV+ women without ART over pregnancy, in women that do not have a viral load result upon weeks 34-36, in those with a viral load > 1.000 copies/ ml or in women co-infected with Hepatitis C virus.
6. In the event a pregnant woman meets the conditions for a vaginal delivery, her consent should be obtained after being informed about the eventual associated risks. Epis-

iorrhaphy and all procedures involving the use of instruments should be avoided (forceps or spatulas).

7. Intrapartum intravenous ZDV should be used regardless of the delivery mode chosen.

8. ZDV suspension should be administered orally for 6 weeks starting from 8 to 12 hours from birth, to all newborns to HIV+ mothers. The recommended ZDV dose for term newborns is 2 mg/Kg/dose every 6 hours p.o. or 1.5 mg/Kg/dose every 6 hours intravenous. The same dose should be administered every 12 hours in preterm newborns of less than 35 weeks gestational age.

9. If Nevirapine is administered intrapartum, ZDV/3TC must be associated for 7 days after delivery to reduce the risk of developing NVP resistance.

10. Lactation should be suppressed with cabergoline or bromocriptin.

11. The newborn should be administered ZDV suspension, orally, for 6 weeks starting from 8 to 12 hours after birth. The recommended AZT dose for term newborns is 2 mg/ Kg/ dose every 6 hours orally or 1.5 mg/Kg/dose every 6 hours intravenous. The same dose should be administered every 12 hours in preterm newborns of less than 35 weeks gestation.

12. Newborns to mothers who received NVP as part of mother-to-child transmission prevention should receive, besides ZDV, 2 doses of 2 mg/Kg of NVP oral solution. The first dose should be administered the earliest as possible postpartum and the second should be administered at 48 to 72 hours of life.

13. The newborns to mothers who did not receive the mother-to-child transmission prevention protocol, or who just received intrapartum prophylaxis, should be administered the AZT scheme and 1 to 2 NVP doses.

13. Conclusion

A seropositive gestating woman should be clinically addressed based on a multidisciplinary and thorough assessment of her initial health status. The latter should include a full physical examination, especially observing those signs that guide diagnosis towards an opportunistic infectious pathology and assessing the current immune status.Once the effectiveness of biomedical healthcare provisions for the prevention of MTCT (mother-to-child-transmission) is demonstrated, it is important to ensure collection of epidemiological history in order to achieve an adequate report, key data to reassess the design and the effectiveness of preventive programs. To achieve such aims, it is critical to maintain and improve diagnosis and primary prevention of the infection among women in childbearing age. ON the other hand, it is important to prevent high rates of unwanted pregnancies and abortions that are direct indicators of risk behaviors in such population group. Likewise, one should aim at achieving 100% screening during the first trimester, also at the possibility of repeating it during the third trimester and at training maternity staff on rapid testing for carrier status detection during labor, for those pregnant women without having accessed an AMTCPP (Antenatal Mother-to-Child Prevention Program).

Finally, MTCT prevention strategy has been based on the ongoing revision of the pooled evidence, therefore it is of key importance to continue evaluating new conducts that enable identification of other aspects: the eventual induction of antiviral resistance and toxicity on the pregnant woman and the newborn and their potential impacts on further quality of life, the use of micronutrients and their impact on MTCT decrease, assessment of the vaginal delivery option in gestating women with low viral load, and sperm wash as an element to reduce MTCT [40].

Nomenclature

VT: Vertical Transmission:

HIV: Human Immunodeficiency Human

AIDS: Acquired Immune Deficiency Syndrome

PMTCT: Prevention of mother-to-child transmission

AMTCPP: Antenatal Mother-to-Child Prevention Program

UNAIDS: Joint United Nations Program on HIV/AIDS

ART: Antiretroviral Therapy

HAART: Highly Active Antiretroviral Treatment

NRTI: Nucleoside reverse transcriptase inhibitor

NNRTI: Non nucleoside reverse transcriptase inhibitor

PI: Protease inhibitor

AZT or ZDV: zidovudine

NVP: Nevirapine

3TC: Lamivudine

d4T: Stavudine

ddI: Didanosine

Author details

Enrique Valdés Rubio*

Address all correspondence to: evaldes@vtr.net

Maternal –Fetal Medicine Unit. Obstetrics and Gynecology Department. Hospital Clínico Universidad de Chile. Santiago, Chile

References

[1] The Millennium Development Goals. (2012). Eight goals for 2015. Found in: http://www.who.int/topics/millennium_development_goals/diseases/es/index.html Access on June 30th.

[2] Valdés, E., Candia, P., & Lattes, K. (2009). Transmisión Vertical de VIH y SIDA: Realidad epidemiológica del Cono Sur Progr Obstet Ginecol. 52(12), 719-24.

[3] Valdés, E., Sepúlveda, A., Candia, P., Sepúlveda, C., & Lattes, K. (2011). VIH/SIDA: Comportamiento epidemiológico de la transmisión vertical en el contexto general de la infección en Chile. *Rev Chil Obstet Ginecol*, 76(1), 52-57.

[4] UNAIDS. (2010). Global Report. Found in: http://www.unaids.org/globalreport/global_report.htm Access on June 30th 2012.

[5] Royal College of Obstetricians and Gynaecologists. (2010). Management of HIV in pregnancy. Green-top Guideline N°39 June. Found in: http://www.rcog.org.uk/womens-health/clinical-guidance/management-hiv-pregnancy-green-top-39 Access on June 30th 2012.

[6] Forbes, J., Alimenti, A., Singer, J., Brophy, J., Bitnun, A., Sanson, L., et al. (2012). A national review of vertical HIV transmission. *AIDS*, 26(6).

[7] Blair, J. M., Hanson, D. L., Jones, J. L., et al. (2004). Trends in pregnancy rates among women with human immunodeficiency virus. *Obstet Gynecol*, 103, 663-668.

[8] M5 The European Mode of Delivery Collaboration. (1999). Elective caesarean-section versus vaginal delivery in prevention of vertical HIV-1 transmission: a randomized clinical trial. *Lancet*, 353, 1035-9.

[9] Coutsoudis, A., Pillay, K., Spooner, E., Kuhn, L., & Coovadia, H. M. (1999). Influence of infant feeding patterns on early mother to child transmission of HIV-1 in Durban South Africa: A prospective cohort study. *Lancet*, 354(9177), 471-477.

[10] Melvin, Z., Alarcon, A. J., Velasquez, J. C., et al. (2004). Rapid HIV type 1 testing of women presenting in late pregnancy with unknown HIV status in Lima, Peru. *Aids Research- Human retroviruses*, 20(10), 1046-1052.

[11] Connor, E. M., Sperling, R. S., & Gelber, R. (1994). Reduction of maternal- infant transmission of human immunodeficiency virus type 1 with zidovudine treatment. *N Engl J Med*, 331(18), 1173-80.

[12] Read, J., Cahn, P., Losso, M., Pinto, J., et al. (2007). Management of Human Immunodeficiency Virus-Infected Pregnant Women at Latin American and Caribbean Sites. *Obstet Gynecol J*, 109(6), 1358-1367.

[13] Valdés, E. (2002). VIH-SIDA y embarazo: actualización y realidad en Chile. *Rev Chil Obstet Ginecol*, 67, 160-6.

[14] Burns, D. N., Nourjah, P., Minkoff, H., Korelitz, J., Biggar, R. J., Landesman, S., Rubinstein, A., Wright, D., & Nugent, R. P. (1996). Changes in CD4+ and CD8+ cell levels during pregnancy and post partum in women seropositive and seronegative for human immunodeficiency virus-1. *Am J Obstet Gynecol*, 174, 1461-8.

[15] Minkoff, H. L., Willoughby, A., Mendez, H., Moroso, G., Holman, S., Goedert, J. J., & Landesman, S. H. (1990). Serious infections during pregnancy among women with advanced HIV infection. *Am J Obstet Gynecol*, 162, 30-4.

[16] Capítulo "VIH- SIDA y embarazo". (2006). E. Valdés. Libro "Urgencias y complicaciones en Obstetricia" M García Huidobro. *J Hasbún. Editorial Mediterráneo*, 447.

[17] "Mujer y VIH". (2002). *E. Herane, E. Valdés. Libro SIDA. C. Sepúlveda A. Afani. Editorial Mediterráneo. Tercera edición*, 721.

[18] French, R., & Broklehurst, P. (1998). The effect of pregnancy on survival in women infected with HIV: a systematic review of the literature and meta-analysis. *Br. J Obstet Gynecol*, 105, 827-35.

[19] Wade, A.S, et al. (2005). HIV infection and sexually transmitted infections among men who have sex with men in Senegal. *AIDS*, 19, 2133-2140.

[20] De Bruyn, M., & Paxton, S. (2005). HIV testing of pregnant women-what is needed to protect positive women's needs and rights? *Sex Health*, 2, 143-51.

[21] Dhai, A., & Noble, R. (2005). Ethical issues in HIV. *Best Pract Res Clin Obstet Gynaecol*, 19, 255-67.

[22] Bowden, FJ. (2005). Reconsidering HIV testing-consent is still the key. *Sex Health*, 2, 165-7.

[23] Chou, R., Smits, A. K., Huffman, L. H., Fu, R., & Korthuis, P. T. (2005). US Preventive Services Task Force. Prenatal screening for HIV: A review of the evidence for the U.S. Preventive Services Task Force. *Ann Intern Med*, 143, 38-54.

[24] Campos-Outcalt, D. (2007). Time to revise your HIV testing routine. *J Fam Pract*, 56, 283-4.

[25] Winn, H., & Hobbins, J. (2000). Clinical Maternal-Fetal Medicine. Parthenon Publish Group; Cap 26.

[26] Abarzúa, F. (2012). VIH y Embarazo. Capítulo 21. pag Found in: www.acog.cl/educación.php?sort=ddAccess on June 30th., 413-23.

[27] The European Collaborative Study. (1999). Maternal viral load and vertical transmission of HIV-1: an important factor but not the only one. *AIDS*, 13, 1377-1385.

[28] Khan, M., Pillay, T., Moodley, J. M., et al. (2001). Maternal mortality associated with tuberculosis-HIV-1 co-infection in Durban, South Africa. *AIDS*, 15, 1857-1863.

[29] Duri, K., Müller, F., Gumbo, F., Kurewa, N., Rusakaniko, S., Chirenje, M., et al. (2011). Human Immunodeficiency Virus (HIV) types Western blot (WB) band profiles as potential surrogate markers of HIV disease progression and predictors of vertical transmission in a cohort of infected but antiretroviral therapy naïve pregnant women in Harare, Zimbabwe. *BMC infectious Diseases*, 11, 7.

[30] El Beitune, P., Duarte, G., Quintana, S. M., Figueiro-Filho, E. A., Marcolin, A. C., & Abduch, R. (2004). Antiretroviral therapy during pregnancy and early neonatal life: consequences for HIV-exposed uninfected children. *Braz J Infect Dis*, 8, 140-50.

[31] Use of antiretroviral drugs for treating pregnant women and preventing HIV infection in infants Programmatic update. (2012). Abril. Found in: http://www.who.int/hiv/pub/mtct/programmatic_update2012/en/index.html Access on June 30th.

[32] Abarzúa, F., Pérez, C., Callejas, C., Yombi, J. C., & Vandercam, B. (2004). Ausencia de transmisión perinatal de VIH en 40 embarazadas tratadas con terapia anti-retroviral de alta potencia. *Rev Chil Obstet Ginecol*, 69, 232-8.

[33] Abarzúa, F., Nuñez, F., Hubinont, C., Bernard, P., Yombi, J. C., & Vandercam, B. (2005). Human immunodeficiency virus (HIV) infection in pregnancy: antiretroviral treatment (ART) and mode of delivery. *Rev Chil Infectol*, 22, 327-37.

[34] Guía Clínica (2010). Síndrome de Inmunodeficiencia Adquirida. VIH/SIDA. Found in : www.redsalud.gov.cl/portal/url/item/7220fdc4340c44a9e04001011f0113b9.pdf Access on June 30th 2012

[35] Poirier, M. C., Olivero, O. A., Walker, D. M., & Walker, V. E. (2004). Perinatal genotoxicity and carcinogenicity of anti-retroviral nucleoside analog drugs. *Toxicol Appl Pharmacol*, 199(2), 151-61.

[36] Brogly, S. B., Ylitalo, N., Mofenson, L. M., Oleske, J., Van Dyke, R., Crain, M. J., Abzug, M. J., Brady, M., Jean-Philippe, P., Hughes, M. D., & Seage, G. R. 3rd. (2007). In utero nucleoside reverse transcriptase inhibitor exposure and signs of possible mitochondrial dysfunction in HIV-uninfected children. *AIDS*, 21, 929-38.

[37] Lorenzini, P., Spicher, V. M., Laubereau, B., Hirschel, B., Kind, C., Rudin, C , et al. (1998). Antiretroviral therapies in pregnancy: maternal, fetal and neonatal effects. Swiss HIV Cohort Study, the Swiss Collaborative HIV and Pregnancy study, and the Swiss Neonatal AHIV study. *AIDS*, 12(18), F241-7.

[38] Read, J. S., & Newell, M. K. (2005). Efficacy and safety of cesarean delivery for prevention of mother-to-child transmission of HIV-1. *Cochrane Database Syst Rev* [4], CD005479.

[39] Safety and Toxicity of individual Antiretroviral Agents in pregnancy. (2012). Found in: http://img.thebody.com/hivatis/pdfs/pregnancy_guide.pdf Access on June 30th.

[40] Semprini, A. E., Vucetich, A., & Hollander, L. (2004). Sperm washing, use of HAART and role of elective caesarean section. *Curr Opin Obstet Gynecol*, 16, 465-70.

Chapter 14

Reproductive Health Challenges of Living with HIV-Infection in Sub Saharan Africa

O. Erhabor, T.C. Adias and C.I. Akani

Additional information is available at the end of the chapter

http://dx.doi.org/10.5772/52682

1. Introduction

The human immunodeficiency Virus (HIV) pandemic is one of the most serious health crisis faced by the world today. An estimated 34 million people were living with HIV/AIDS as at 2010 [1]. A disproportionate burden has been placed on women and children who continue to experience high rates of new infection and HIV-related illness and death. Availability and use of antiretroviral drugs has changed the landscape of HIV/AIDS bringing about a change in the perception of HIV from an incurable deadly disease to a chronic manageable illness. As effective HIV treatments become more widespread, HIV-infected individuals in sub Saharan Africa are living longer, healthier lives. Many HIV-affected couples (sero-discordant and sero-concordant) are now considering long-term life projects including options for safer reproduction or procreation. There has also been increase in advocacy to expand the capacity for the health care system particularly in Africa to provide the sexual and reproductive health services that HIV infected persons in Africa desperately need [2]. This decade has witnessed greater commitment to sexual and reproductive health and HIV linkages particularly in the developed world. More recent opportunities include policy developments within the Global Fund to Fight AIDS, Tuberculosis and Malaria to accept proposals that form linkages with sexual and reproductive health within the overall frameworks of HIV, tuberculosis (TB) and malaria. There has also been a renewed commitment by the United States of America to international sexual and reproductive health through support of the United Nations Population Fund and the repeal of the Mexico City Policy, also known as the "global gag rule", a United States government policy that hitherto prohibited non-governmental organizations from receiving federal funding for performing or promoting abortion services in other countries. A large body of evidence suggests that reproductive technologies can help HIV-affected couples to safely conceive with minimal risk of HIV transmission to their partner and baby. However, for most couples particularly in low income countries in sub Saharan Africa, such technologies are neither geographically nor economically accessible. In sub-Saharan Africa where HIV is endemic, 63% of women have an unmet need for sexual and reproductive health services, there is a high incidence of unintended pregnancies, a significant number of women do not know their HIV status, many women have limited access to sexual and reproductive health information and services (family planning, management of sexually transmitted diseases, HIV prevention and maternal health) to help them protect themselves from the triad of unwanted pregnancy, HIV infection and HIV transmission to their sexual partners and their children. With HIV now considered to be a chronic manageable disease, attention is shifting to offering and improving quality of life particularly by the provision of reproductive health options/care to men and women living with HIV-1.

A healthcare workforce that is highly motivated and well informed on the evidence –based practices in sexual and reproductive health options for persons living with HIV/AIDS is crucial to meeting the sexual and reproductive needs of PLWHA in Africa. A high morale and productive workforce are the driving force for the success of any reproductive health programme. Unless these staffs are motivated and have high morale, they may become a stumbling block to the success and scaling –up of sexual and reproductive health services [3]. There are several challenges associated with meeting the sexual and reproductive health needs of persons living with HIV/AIDS in Africa; suboptimal antenatal care, absence of evidence-based and affordable assisted reproductive technologies, inadequate number of appropriately trained healthcare workers, suboptimal health infrastructure, lack of enabling legislation and policies on sexual and reproductive health of HIV-infected persons, challenge of stigmatization and discrimination, unprofessional negative attitudes towards PLWHA desiring to procreate. The aim of this chapter is to highlight the reproductive health concerns associated with living with HIV infection in sub Saharan Africa.

2. History of Africa

Africa is the world's second-largest and second-most-populous continent in the planet, after Asia. With 1,032,532,874 billion people as at 2011 [4]. It accounts for about 14.72% of the world's human population. At about 30.2 million km^2 (11.7 million sq miles) including adjacent islands, it covers 6% of the Earths' total surface area and 20.4% of the total land area [5]. It is made up of 54 member states. Western Sahara although a member of the African union, its sovereignty is being disputed by Morocco. South Sudan has become Africa newest nation having recently separated from North Sudan. The population of Africa is estimated at greater than one billion people. Africa account for a significant 14% of the world's population. Africa contains the Nile River system which is the worlds longest. It also prides itself as the continent with the world's largest Sahara desert. Africa is surrounded by the Mediterranean Sea (north) and the Suez Canal and the Red sea (northwest), the Indian Ocean (east) and the Atlantic Ocean (west). Although endowed with abundant natural resources, Africa remains the world's poorest and most underdeveloped continent, the result of a variety of causes that may include the spread of deadly

http://dx.doi.org/10.5772/52682

viruses and diseases (HIV/AIDS, malaria and tuberculosis), corruption in government that have often committed serious human right abuses and violations, failed central planning, high levels of illiteracy, lack of access to foreign capital, and frequent tribal and military conflict (ranging from guerrilla warfare to genocide). According to the United Nation's Human Development Report in 2003, the bottom 25 ranked nations (151st to 175th) were all African [6].Poverty, illiteracy, malnutrition and inadequate water supply and sanitation, as well as poor health, affect a large proportion of the people who reside in the African continent. About 80.5% of the Sub-Saharan Africa population lives on less than $2.50 per person per day in 2005 [7]. Africa faces several daunting challenges with regards to access to basic health services like their counterparts in most developed countries of the world. The healthcare system and infrastructure are suboptimal. This is often due to fundamental limitations in funding, lack of adequate qualified health professional and equipment as well as deep rooted, institutionalized and chronic corruption among the political class and bureaucratic compensation and corruption among civil servants [8]. Africa remains the world's most corrupt continent. Corruption is the abuse of entrusted power for private gain, in public and private sectors [9]. This vice has contributed to a large extent to the stunted development and impoverishment seen in many African states. The African union estimates that corruption among the political class is costing the continent more than $150 billion dollars per year. These are funds that could be used to improve the health infrastructure and quality of life of people of people in the continent but rather are laundered out of developing countries to banks in the developed world thus perpetrating poverty among African people. Industrialized countries have continued to encourage corruption in Africa and perpetuation of poverty among people in the African continent by providing crooked African leaders with a safe haven for their looted funds rather than repatriating such funds back and ensuring that they are used to enhance the infrastructural development of the continent. Corruption is endemic and continues to thrive in the African continent for several reasons; institutional weakness and criminal collaboration between the executive and the legislative and judicial arms of government, non-existence of the principle of rule of law, political god fatherism, institutional failure and criminal collaboration between civil servants and politicians. Corruption is a cankerworm that continues to weaken societies, ruins lives, and impedes development in the African continent [10]. This is further compounded by the high incidence of infectious diseases (HIV, TB and Malaria). Africa is plagued by poverty, malnutrition, poor sanitation, disease, high mortality rate, conflict, wars and crime. These challenges have a significant negative effect on life expectance in the continent. The continent has the world's shortest life expectancy. Citizens of Sub-Saharan African countries are much more likely to die prematurely, than people in wealthier parts of the world. Children under- the age of 5 years are more likely to die from malaria, respiratory tract infections, diarrhoea, perinatal conditions, measles and HIV/AIDS while those who survive the first 5 years of life are likely to die before their 60th birthday from HIV/AIDS, tuberculosis, and maternal mortality (for women as a result of pregnancy-related mortality). According to the CIA World Fact book 2009 [11], the life expectancy at birth of the world is 67.2 years (65.0 years for males and 69.5 years for females). The United Nations World Population Prospects 2006 Revision put the world's life expectancy at birth at 66.57 years (64.52 years for males and 68.76 years for females).Women on the average are found to live longer than men with the exception of Zimbabwe, Afghanistan, Swaziland and Lesotho [12].Countries in Africa particularly those with a high HIV/AIDS prevalence have must lower life expectancies [11]. Provision of low technology, safer, affordable and readily available reproductive health options particularly for PLWHA in Africa is a crucial but often unaddressed component of HIV prevention programme. The aim of this chapter is to evaluate the sexual and reproductive health challenges associated with HIV infection in sub Saharan Africa.

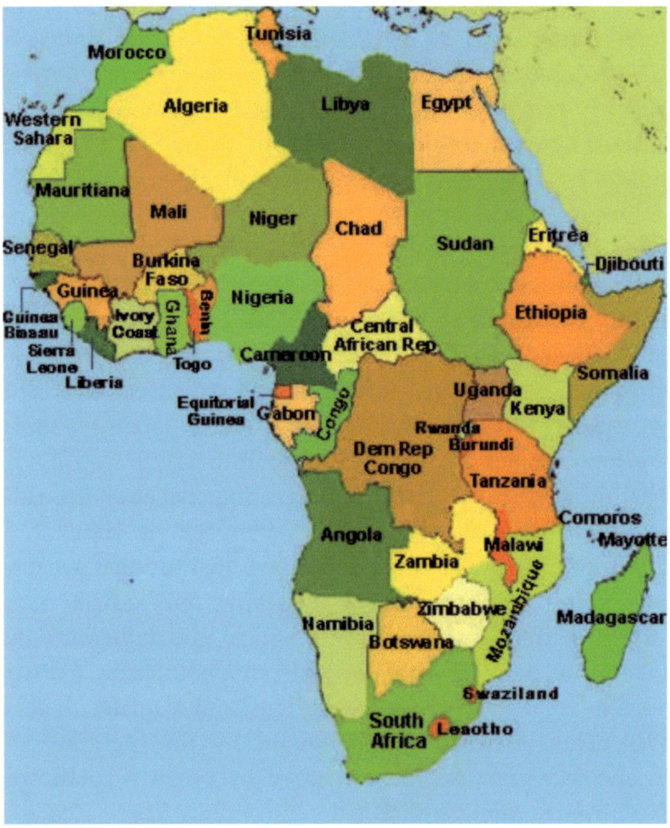

Figure 1.

3. Challenge of suboptimal antenatal services in Africa

Organized preventive screening programmes for antenatal care were first introduced in Western Europe in the twentieth century with the hope that routine antenatal care would contribute to a reduction in maternal and infant mortality rates. Figures on maternal mortality in the developed world show that the risk of death as a result of pregnancy and child birth is approximately 1 in 7000 compared to 1 in 23 for women living in many parts of Africa where antenatal care is poor or non-existent [13]. Antenatal care is an opportunity to reach the mothers and young girls in a safe non-stigmatising environment. The importance of developing links between sexual and reproductive health and HIV services is widely recognized. Four priority areas for linkages has been identified– learning about one's HIV status, promoting safer sex, optimizing links between HIV and sexually transmitted infection services and integrating HIV with maternal and infant health. These priorities could lead to significant public health benefits and improve efficient use of resources particularly in resource –constrained settings in Africa. There are many challenges and issues that affect reproductive health choices particularly for persons living with HIV in Africa. They include; paucity of evidenced-based information regarding safe pregnancy and Prevention of Mother To Child Transmission (PMTCT) of HIV, absence of universal access to Voluntary Counselling and Testing (VCT) services, negative attitudes by society and un-informed healthcare workers towards PLWHA desiring to have children, lack of universal access to condoms, contraceptives medications and Highly Active Antiretroviral Therapy (HAART), sup-optimal levels of skilled sexual and reproductive health staffs, lack of service infrastructures and absence of legislation on the reproductive health right of PLWHA. All these factors negatively affects and complicates the ability of PLWHA to make evidenced based reproductive health choices particularly in many sub Saharan African settings.

Antenatal care creates an opportunity for women to access HIV testing and counselling. It is the port of entry to accessing HIV prevention and care. In 2001, CDC modified the recommendations for pregnant women to emphasize HIV screening as a routine part of prenatal care, simplification of the testing process so that pre-test counselling would not pose a barrier, and flexibility of the consent process to allow multiple types of informed consent [14].Many pregnant women particularly in Africa do not know their HIV serostatus. Many particularly those in rural settings lack adequate information on the benefit of antenatal care for themselves and their babies. High level of illiteracy, inequalities in access to healthcare services, being pregnant at an early age, women dependence economically on men, limited mobility, poverty, religious and cultural restrictions, being a member of a marginalized community or population remains major barriers or stumbling blocks that militate against access to effective antenatal particularly in resource-constrained settings in sub Saharan Africa [15]. Women all over the world will most likely accept VCT services if it is offered especially in settings where there is universal access to HAART and evidenced-based effective sexual and reproductive services rendered by staff who are appropriately trained to render the best possible evidenced-based counselling about HIV and other STIs as well as affordable and readily available reproductive health options with empathy rather than being judgemental. Humiliating and stigmatising attitudes and breaches of confidentiality of antenatal women can create a barrier that can potentially prevent women from accessing sexual and reproductive health services even when they are available.

There are several ways to possibly enhance the uptake of VCT services in Africa. They include approaches such as the "opt-out" approach, use of traditional voluntary counselling and testing strategies as well as making antenatal visit as interactive and activity based. These approaches are more likely to provide the much needed coverage [16]. There has been argument as to whether the "opt-out" approach negates the principle of informed consent [17] particularly in African settings where many antenatal women are reluctant to challenge health care procedures. It is important however to note that "opt-out" approach does not in any way compromise the principle of informed consent. This approach assumes that testing is an intrinsic part of an effective and holistic antenatal care. The women are informed about what test is required as well as the importance of testing to the mother and the developing baby with an opportunity given to women to refuse testing if they so desire.

There is also the need to foster more male involvement in antenatal care in Africa. Evidence has shown that involving men in the reproductive health care of their partners rather than basing antenatal care exclusively on women can potentially enhance the pregnancy experience, reduces incidence of gender-based violence, promote the likelihood of getting a joint consent, facilitate HIV prevention, compliance to HAART in partner in which it is indicated as well as enables a holistic uptake of sexual and reproductive health service for couples. There are several challenges that militate against male-gender involvement in antenatal care particularly in Africa; cultural and religious beliefs, obstacles of working fathers, prevalence of polygamy and maintenance by men of multiple sex partners [18-19].

When HIV infection is diagnosed, health-care providers should strongly encourage patients to disclose their HIV status to their spouses, current sex partners, and previous sex partners and recommend that these partners be tested for HIV infection. Health departments can assist patients by notifying, counselling, and providing HIV testing for partners without disclosing the patient's identity [20]. Policy allowing providers to inform patients who receive a new diagnosis of HIV infection that they might be contacted by health department staff for a voluntary interview to discuss notification of their partners may play a beneficial role and facilitate uptake of sexual and reproductive health services in Africa. A disproportionate burden has been placed on women and children who continue to experience high rate of new HIV infection and HIV-related illness and death. Most children living with HIV acquire the infection through Mother to Child Transmission (MTCT) which can occur during pregnancy, during delivery or during breastfeeding.

3.1. A strong cultural and religious attachment to having children puts PLWHA under pressure to procreate

Being HIV positive has been shown to modify but not remove the reproductive desires of individuals. Diversity existed in reproductive intentions among PLWHA. Some HIV positive individuals wished to avoid pregnancy. Fears of partner and infant infection and having a previously infected baby were important factors deterring some individuals from considering having children. There is also strongly perceived community disapproval associated with HIV and reproduction. Strong desires to experience parenthood, mediated by prevailing social and cultural norms that encouraged childbearing in society have also been reported. Motherhood is seen as an important component of married women's identity and important for women's social status in Africa. Family, husbands and societal expectations for childbearing have significant influences on the African woman's reproductive intentions [21]. Availability and use of antiretroviral drugs has changed the landscape of HIV/AIDS bringing about a change in the perception of HIV from an incurable deadly disease to a chronic manageable illness. As effective HIV treatments become more widespread, HIV-infected individuals are living longer, healthier lives. Many HIV-affected couples (sero-discordant and sero-concordant) are considering options for safer reproduction. A large body of evidence suggests that reproductive technologies can help HIV-affected couples to safely conceive with minimal risk of HIV transmission to their partner and baby. However, for most couples particularly in low income countries in sub Saharan Africa, such technologies are neither geographically nor economically accessible. With HIV now considered to be a chronic manageable disease, attention is shifting to offering and improving quality of life particularly by the provision of reproductive health options/care to men and women living with HIV-1. Many HIV-infected men and women are now expressing their desire to father or mother a child. Assisted reproductive technologies, including intrauterine insemination (IUI), in vitro fertilisation (IVF) and intracytoplasmatic sperm injection (ICSI) in combination with semen washing have been used to decrease the risk of HIV -1 transmission in HIV-1-infected discordant couples with an HIV-1-infected man. Previous report indicates that in HIV-positive men taking HAART, seminal viral load is decreased but not eliminated and fertilization should be achieved through sperm washing to offer maximum protection for the uninfected female. Pregnant HIV-positive women on antiretroviral medication have a reduced risk of transmitting the virus, but should still be counselled about the possibility to further limit the chances of infecting their infant through elective Caesarean section. HIV sero-discordant couples with strong desire for childbearing have a dilemma of risking HIV infection or infecting their spouse. Some risk transmission of HIV infection to reproduce. Over two-thirds of 104 surveyed couple wanting to procreate reported unprotected sex with their partner in the past 6 months. Most respondents, regardless of serostatus, said that viral load testing and awareness of post-exposure prevention had no effect on their condom use. A paucity of interventions targeting sero-discordant couples on contraceptive choices is at odds with a strong cultural importance in Africa attached to having children. HIV discordance in Africa creates a serious dilemma for fertility decision-making in couples. Stigma, discrimination, and non-disclosure fuel HIV transmission between partners. A previous study [22] in Nigeria a country in the Western part of Africa that investigated the reproductive health concerns among persons living with HIV/AIDS in the Niger Delta of Nigeria has shown that a significant number of PLWHA in Nigeria have conception dreams. The main reasons for wanting to procreate included: ensuring lineage continuity and posterity (52.3%), securing relationships (27.0%) and pressure from relatives to reproduce (20.7%). Single subjects were more inclined to have children (76.3%) compared to married (51.5%), widowed (18.2%) and separated/divorced (11.1%) ($p=0.03$). Of the 111 subjects that indicated their desire to have children, women were more inclined to have children (64.5%) compared to men (47.7%). The major concern among the 84 (43.1%) subjects not desiring more children were the fear of infecting sero-discordant partner and baby (57.1%), fear of dying and leaving behind orphans (28.6%) and the fear that they may become too ill and unable to financially support the child (14.3%). Persons with no formal education were more likely to have children irrespective of their positive HIV status (66.7%) compared to persons educated to tertiary education level (37.0%) (p=0.01). Out of the 111 subjects that desired to have more children, only 58% had gone for reproductive health counselling with HIV counsellors. Reasons for not seeking advice were anticipated negative reactions and discrimination from the counsellors. A significant number of subjects were only aware of some reproductive health options available to reduce risk of infecting their partners and or baby such as artificial vaginal insemination, intrauterine insemination, caesarean section, avoidance of breast feeding and offering prenatal pre-exposure prophylaxis to the foetus. They were unaware of other options such as sperm washing, IVF and ICSI. Of the 43.1% not anticipating more children, 36.9% were anticipating adoption.

A significant number of PLWHA in Africa desire to have children irrespective of the HIV positive status. Women are more inclined to have children compared to men. Persons with no formal education are more inclined to have children irrespective of their positive HIV status compared to persons educated to tertiary education level. The main reasons for wanting a child included: ensuring lineage continuity and posterity, securing relationships and pressure from relatives to reproduce. There may be several reasons for this association, including the fact that better educated people generally having greater access to information particularly the mode of transmission of HIV than those who have less formal education, and are more likely to make informed decisions and act on information given. In addition, better educated people generally have better jobs and greater access to money and other resources which can help them lead healthier lives. Also single persons living with HIV are more likely to want to have children compared to married, separated and widowed subjects. Regardless of interpersonal and public health concerns, studies in both resource-rich and resource-limited settings suggest that HIV-infected men and women desire children [23 – 25]. In addition, in resource limited settings, couples often desire larger families. The reasons for this are debated but likely include among others, the strong cultural attachment to having children, stigmatization associated with childlessness, role of children with inheritance, the importance of children in agricultural economies, the importance of childbearing on the status of women, the role of children as caretakers of the elderly, and high rates of infant mortality [26]. Previous report indicated that forty percent of HIV infected women desired more children and women with fewer children were more likely to become pregnant [27].

PLWHA are often not wanting to procreate because of the fear of infecting sero-discordant partner and baby, fear of dying and living behind orphans and the fear that they may become too ill and unable to financially support the child.Previous report indicates that the major challenges faced by HIV-infected subjects not desiring to procreate included: risk of HIV transmission to partner and child and failure of health systems to offer safe methods of reproduction [28]. Identifying the determinants of the decision to have children among sero-discordant couples will help in setting reproductive intervention priorities in resource-poor countries. The gender of the positive partner affects the factors associated with a desire for children. Interventions targeting sero-discordant couples should explore contraceptive choices, the cultural importance of children, and partner communication [29].

http://dx.doi.org/10.5772/52682

Given the importance of procreation in African settings and the lack of low –technology and affordable assisted reproduction services, HIV-infected couples are faced with a serious dilemma about making an informed decision to procreate. Many PLWHA in Africa who have a desire to have children do not seek reproductive health counselling from HIV counsellors. Reasons for not seeking counselling were anticipated negative reactions and stigmatization from the counsellors resulting from their negative attitude towards unprotected sexual activity and child bearing by HIV-infected couples. HIV-infected individuals and their partners are requiring education and counselling regarding HIV disease and reproduction and HIV counsellors particularly in Africa do not seem to have access to evidenced -based information that the HIV-infected population desperately need to enable them make informed reproductive health decisions. Previous report suggest that there is need to draw up a protocol for reproductive counselling of HIV infected that have a desire for conception [30]. HIV counsellors need to come to terms with the fact that simply encouraging HIV- infected couples to abstain from procreation may no longer be a realistic strategy, particularly in sub Saharan Africa where there is strong cultural attachment to having children. In the absence of counselling that recognizes the desire and importance of having children, couples may knowingly take on the risks of transmission in order to have children. Sharing our evidenced- based best practices about HIV transmission and reproductive health options while recognizing patient goals may help couples minimize risk and reduce the harm of unprotected sex. However, the great risks taken by HIV –infected persons desiring to procreate could be minimized through counselling and close monitoring by reproductive health care provider.

Reproductive health knowledge among HIV-infected subjects desiring to procreate in Africa is poor. Most PLWHA in Africa are unaware of reproductive health options such as sperm washing, in vitro fertilization (IVF) and intracytoplasmic sperm injection (ICSI) available to reduce risk of infecting their partners and or baby. A significant number of men taking HAART have lower seminal concentration of HIV, and sexual transmission may be reduced. However, a certain percentage of aviraemic men retain viral presence in semen, and unprotected intercourse to achieve fertilization must be discouraged as it carries the risk of sexual transmission of the virus. HIV-discordant couples should be informed that sperm washing can remove HIV from semen, allowing conception without the risk of infection for the seronegative female and eventually the child. In HIV-positive women, perinatal transmission of HIV can be curtailed to less than 2% by using HAART to decrease maternal viral load and offering prenatal pre-exposure prophylaxis of the foetus, and elective Caesarean section. Each intervention carries specific risks and benefits. The contribution of each preventive arm in achieving foetal protection can only be crudely measured and optimal obstetric management must involve discussion with the pregnant woman of the pros and cons of each strategy. HIV-affected couples who want to have children is presented with at least three distinct and daunting clinical challenges. The first is dealing with stigma arising from many health care providers' negative attitude towards sexual activity and child bearing by HIV infected couples [31] and stigmatization from immediate family members and society [32]. The second is maintaining the mother's health before, during and after pregnancy. The third is preventing vertical transmission from mother to child as well as preventing HIV transmission to the partner in sero-discordant relationship. Several approaches have been suggested to reduce risk of horizontal transmission for HIV-affected couples who want to conceive children. These approaches includes the use of ; male sperm washing, IUI, ICSI, screening and pre-treatment for Sexually Transmitted Infections (STI's), Delay in procreation until viral load is controlled, limited, timed unprotected sexual encounters, female artificial insemination, self-insemination and circumcision. Experience among couples in whom the male was (HIV) seropositive who underwent assisted reproductive technologies (ART) in order to attain family goals while minimizing the risk of HIV transmission indicated that all female recipients tested seronegative for HIV at 3 and 6 months post-embryo transfer. All delivered babies (n = 8) tested seronegative for HIV at birth and 3 months postpartum and that ART should be considered for HIV serodiscordant couples who desire to have children in order to minimize the risk of viral infection [33]. Several people play a role in reproductive health decision making of PLWHA; the relatives who used traditional norms to encourage procreation; the health workers who violates the autonomy and human rights of HIV-infected by using their medical knowledge to dissuade clients from childbearing by preaching mandatory contraception [34] and the health care system that do not recognize and meet the sexual and reproductive health needs of their clients [35]. Health care providers in Africa must realize that it is their responsibility to offer information to enable HIV-infected persons arrive at their own informed decisions on their reproductive and sexual health needs regardless of the health professional's opinion. Similarly, there may be need to offer additional training to enable counsellors' particularly in sub Saharan Africa offer evidenced- based sexual and reproductive health information to their clients. Reproductive health policies in this HIV/AIDS era are lacking in most African settings. It is recommended that sero-discordant couples who desire to have children should undergo assisted fertility treatment such as sperm washing, intra uterine insemination and in-vitro fertilization to avoid HIV transmission to their partners [36]. However cost implication is a major issue affecting the feasibility of offering assisted fertility treatment such as sperm washing, intra uterine insemination and in-vitro fertilization particularly among low socioeconomic people. There is a major challenge with the development of evidenced- based, cost- effective and best-practice guidelines in most settings in Africa to optimize the sexual and reproductive health service rendered to persons living with HIV/AIDS. In resource-limited settings, couples should be counselled on ovulation cycles and may engage in timed unprotected sex only during the fertile period of the woman's monthly cycle to facilitate conception while reducing number of exposures. If the man is HIV-negative with a positive partner, partners can be taught artificial insemination, timed to the woman's fertile period. For couples in which both partners are positive, there may be need for a careful and informed natural conception when their viral loads have fallen to below the level of detection.

4. Lack of integration between sexual and reproductive, family planning and existing HIV /AIDS services

There is increasing concern that Sub-Saharan Africa is the region where more women are infected by HIV than men. About 60 per cent of people living with HIV infections in Africa are women. Among young men and women aged 15 to 24 years, for every one man, four women are infected with HIV. There were 12-13 infected women to 10 infected men in 2001 [37]. Biological, cultural and socio-economic factors contribute to women's greater vulnerability to HIV/AIDS. Women are 4 times more at risk of becoming infected with HIV during unprotected vaginal intercourse than men. The vagina's greater area of susceptible tissue and micro trauma that occurs during sexual intercourse makes women more physiologically more vulnerable [38]. Semen has higher viral load than vaginal fluids and the semen stays longer in the female genital tract after sexual intercourse which increases the chances of HIV transmission. The synergy between HIV and sexually transmitted infection (STIs) is another biological factor that makes women more vulnerable to HIV. This is especially significant among African women. Most STI cases in women often go untreated, symptoms are often latent, women diagnosed with STIs are often stigmatised and majority have no access to medical treatments [39]. Socio-economic factors including women's lack of access to education, personal income, and economic dependence on men perpetuate women's lower status. Moreover widespread poverty often drives these vulnerable women into commercial sex work. Furthermore men control over condom use- the main tool for reducing the risk of sexual transmission of HIV puts women at risk of HIV. Cultural practices inherent in Africa such as forced marriage, polygamy, female genital mutilation and older men's preferences for sex with younger women, Sexual violence coercion at home and in the work place during job hiring, promotion and to avoid dismissal are common practices, use of women as bait by companies to secure contracts, sexual abuse of orphans and domestic workers further complicates female gender vulnerability to HIV [40]. Moreover, women are more subjected to HIV stigma and discrimination. In Africa, the HIV virus that causes AIDS is transmitted through two major routes. The first, which accounts for 80 per cent of the cases, is through unprotected sex between men and women. This is followed by HIV transmission from mother to child during pregnancy, labour and breastfeeding, which is responsible for about 20 per cent of the cases. There are several biological, social and cultural reasons why women and girls in Africa are more vulnerable to HIV infection. Gender inequalities that exist in African society, women have less access to information than men, they are less likely to make informed decisions and act on information given, they have less access to education, and better jobs, money and other resources which can help them lead healthier lives. During vaginal sex, which is commonly practiced in Africa, the chance of HIV transmission from a man to a woman is two to three times greater than transmission from a woman to a man. This is due to the biological make up of the female genital tract. The female genital tract has a larger area of exposed tissue. Young girls are especially vulnerable when they have sex with older men because because the genital tract of young girls are immature, prone to tear and invasion by HIV.

There has never been a better time than this to target and integrate sexual and reproductive health, family planning and HIV/AIDS services particularly in Africa. Most sceptics erroneously often consider reproductive health to be a euphemism for abortion services. It is worthy to note that reproductive health covers a broad range of women's health issues including detecting and treating sexually transmitted infections and supporting HIV-infected women's desire to have children safely. Integration of HIV and reproductive health has the potential to produce important HIV-related outcomes. Recent international consensus statements have urged the strengthening of these linkages [41]. In order to reduce HIV-infected births, infant and child mortality, the number of children orphaned by AIDS and maternal mortality, adding family planning and reproductive health to PMTCT, VCT and ARV programmes makes a logical and a programmatic sense.

5. HIV–infected need information and services on safe procreation and the health system is unable to provide evidenced-based answers

Data from most settings in Africa increasingly demonstrate that some HIV-infected women particularly those on ARVs as they begin to feel better and function more normally due to the effect of treatment on reduction on viral load, would like to become pregnant [42]. It is a growing expectation that the health system should have the ability to counsel HIV-positive women on the risk and benefits of child bearing and to respect the reproductive intentions, choices and rights including access to contraception and other reproductive health services. Previous report [22] indicates that reproductive health knowledge among HIV-infected subjects desiring to procreate was poor. Subjects were unaware of reproductive health options such as sperm washing, in vitro fertilization (IVF) and intracytoplasmic sperm injection (ICSI) available to reduce risk of infecting their partners and or baby. A significant number of men taking HAART have lower seminal concentration of HIV, and sexual transmission may be reduced. However, a certain percentage of aviraemic men retain viral presence in semen, and unprotected intercourse to achieve fertilization must be discouraged as it carries the risk of sexual transmission of the virus. HIV-discordant couples should be informed that sperm washing can remove HIV from semen, allowing conception without the risk of infection for the seronegative female and eventually the child. In HIV-positive women, perinatal transmission of HIV can be curtailed to less than 2% by using HAART to decrease maternal viral load and offering prenatal pre-exposure prophylaxis of the foetus, and elective Caesarean section. Each intervention carries specific risks and benefits. The contribution of each preventive arm in achieving foetal protection can only be crudely measured and optimal obstetric management must involve discussion with the pregnant woman of the pros and cons of each strategy. Several approaches have been suggested to reduce risk of horizontal transmission for HIV-affected couples who want to conceive children. These approaches includes the use of ; male sperm washing, IUI, ICSI, screening and pre-treatment for Sexually Transmitted Infections (STI's), delay in procreation until viral load is controlled, limited, timed unprotected sexual encounters, female artificial insemination, self-insemination and circumcision. Accurate and accessible information to make informed choices and safe, pleasurable sexual relationships possible is best delivered through peer education and health professionals trained on empathetic approaches to sensitive issues [43]. Interventions based on positive prevention, which combine protection of personal health with avoiding HIV/STI transmission to partners, are recommended.

http://dx.doi.org/10.5772/52682

6. Non-protection of the reproductive rights of PLWHA in Africa

It is increasing clear particularly that a significant majority of PLWHA in Africa are of reproductive age, that conception and reproductive options for this population are important issues for health care delivery and research and that HIV-seropositive individuals deserve full reproductive rights like every other person [44]. International reproductive guidelines shifted a decade ago from recommending avoidance of pregnancy to recognizing conception and parenting as realistic options and rights for people with HIV infection and their partners [45]. Mindful of this indisputable fact, US Centers for Disease Control and Prevention (CDC) has encouraged information and support for HIV-affected couples who want to explore their reproductive options [14]. There are many persons who plays a role in reproductive health decision making of persons living with HIV/AIDS: The relatives who used traditional norms to encourage procreation; the health workers who violates the autonomy and human rights of HIV-infected by using their medical knowledge to dissuade clients from childbearing by preaching mandatory contraception [34] and health care system that does not recognize and meet the sexual and reproductive health needs of their clients [35].Health care providers in Africa must realize that it is their responsibility to offer information to enable HIV-infected persons arrive at their own informed decisions on their reproductive and sexual health needs regardless of the health professional's opinion. Similarly, there may need to offer additional training to enable counsellors' offer evidenced- based sexual and reproductive health information to their clients. Reproductive health policies in this HIV/AIDS era are lacking in most African settings. It is recommended that sero-discordant couples who desire to have children should undergo assisted fertility treatment such as sperm washing, intra uterine insemination and *in-vitro* fertilization to avoid HIV transmission to their partners [36, 46]. However cost implication is a major issue affecting the feasibility of offering assisted fertility treatment such as sperm washing, intra uterine insemination and *in-vitro* fertilization particularly among low socioeconomic people. There is a major challenge with the development of evidenced- based, cost effective and best-practice guidelines locally in most African setting to help optimize the sexual and reproductive health service rendered to persons living with HIV/AIDS particularly in the Africa. Like it is in other developed countries in the world. HIV-infected couples wanting to procreate in Africa should be counselled on ovulation cycles, timed sex only during the fertile period of the woman's monthly cycle to facilitate conception while reducing number of exposures. If the man is HIV-negative with a positive partner, partners can be taught artificial insemination, timed to the woman's fertile period. For couples in which both partners are positive, there may be need for a careful and informed natural conception when their viral loads have fallen to below the level of detection. There is the need to support the sexual and reproductive rights of HIV-infected individuals. Additional training needs to be offered to HIV counsellors on evidence- based best and affordable practices regarding reproductive health issues among persons living with HIV. Policies that support the availability and accessibility to relevant reproductive and sexual health services including contraception and procreation needs to be developed. Public enlightenment programmes on HIV is needed to reduce the stigmatization that HIV-infected persons face from family members and their communities. Developing and testing safer conception methods that reduce HIV transmission to HIV-seronegative partners in serodiscordant couples and reduce superinfection in HIV-seroconcordant couples is a crucial component of HIV prevention programme that needs to be urgently addressed in Africa [47].

7. Challenge of HIV-related stigma and discrimination

HIV-related stigma and discrimination remains an enormous barrier to the fight against AIDS. Fear of discrimination often prevents people from getting tested, seeking treatment and admitting their HIV status publicly. Since laws and policies alone cannot reverse the stigma that surrounds HIV infection, AIDS education in Africa needs to be scaled-up to combat the ignorance that causes people to discriminate. The fear and prejudice that lies at the core of HIV and AIDS discrimination needs to be tackled at both community and national levels. There is strong ethical imperative to support the sexual and reproductive health needs of HIV-infected individuals allowing them to make informed decisions about their reproductive health. Increasingly, fertility clinics in developed countries are offering their services to HIV-serodiscordant couples where the woman is seropositive and in HIV-seroconcordant relationships. Reproductive health care workers in Africa can learn from the evidenced- based best practices in the developed world to ensure that like their counterparts in most developed countries, HIV infected persons particularly in Africa can access the best quality reproductive and sexual health service. Recent advances in HIV clinical care and assisted reproduction technique (ART) procedures directed at reducing the risk of viral transmission during gamete transfer particularly where good healthcare is available has significantly reduced the risk of transmission of HIV among discordant couples to 1-2%. Promotion of risk reduction counselling, screening for sexually transmitted diseases and lower genital tract disease, assessment of options for birth control, and pre-conception counselling should be integral components of gynaecologic health care for HIV-infected women.

Since the beginning of the human immunodeficiency virus (HIV) epidemic, stigma and discrimination (SAD) have been identified as the major obstacles to effective responses to HIV [48]. HIV-affected couples who desire sexual and reproductive health services are faced with at least three distinct and daunting challenges. The first is dealing with stigma arising from many health care providers' negative attitude towards sexual activity and child bearing by HIV infected couples [49] and stigmatization from immediate family members and society [32]. The second is maintaining the mother's health before, during and after pregnancy. The third is preventing vertical transmission from mother to child as well as preventing HIV transmission to the partner in sero-discordant relationship. HIV/AIDS-related SAD has been extensively documented among health care providers. There have been many reports from health care settings of HIV testing without consent, breaches of confidentiality, labelling, gossip, verbal harassment, differential treatment, and even denial of treatment. HIV-infected-individuals who feel stigmatized by health care providers face problems accessing HIV testing and other sexual and reproductive health care services [50]. The fear of stigma impedes prevention efforts, including discussions of safer sex and the prevention of mother-to-child transmission [51].

Sexually transmitted infection including HIV have always been imbued with stigma and discrimination particularly in Africa particularly due to their negative association with behaviour considered by society as deviant or immoral [52]. Stigma generally refers to negatively perceived defining characteristics either tangible or intangible. It is an attribute used to set the infected person or group from the normalized social order. It has a way of devaluing a person [53]. Similarly; societies have historically reacted with fear to disfiguring, debilitating, and fatal diseases and have translated this aversion into discriminatory actions against the infected [54]. The HIV/AIDS pandemic has presented the world with a condition that combines these characteristics – and it has frequently been met with stigma and discrimination, a reaction dubbed "the second epidemic" [55]. HIV infection affects women and men's view of parenthood. It has a negative impact on their ability to have children, related not only to psychosocial aspects such as stigma and discrimination and decreased sexual activity, but also to the clinical impact of HIV infection and sexually transmitted infections (STIs) on fertility [56-57]. Learning more about stigma is important given the growing assertions that testing is a 'critical gateway' to HIV prevention and treatment. As access to HIV testing and treatment improves, providers increasingly need to understand and address how stigma acts as a barrier to services. There is need to develop programs to address the negative service provider attitudes towards HIV-positive women, especially those wanting children. Stigma and discrimination is a population and health system level barrier that discourages HIV-infected women and men from seeking reproductive health counselling and other sexual and reproductive health counselling.

HIV-related stigmatization, discrimination and denial continue to characterize the pandemic in Africa and present a major challenge to the effectiveness of prevention, sexual and reproductive care and treatment programmes. Much of the societal and individual reaction towards people with HIV/AIDS is stigma and discrimination oriented. Stigmatization and discrimination occurs in a variety of forms. It ranges from societal level responses such as coercive government policies and laws, to apathy and denial of the HIV epidemic. At the individual level, the internalization of these societal responses may result in an individual's self-exclusion from information, treatment and care. Stigmatization and discrimination are often explored through socio-cultural understandings of illness and disease transmission and its manifestations at societal and individual level. Contexts of discrimination include employment, health care systems, and travel and migration restrictions. Although there are widespread reports of HIV-related discrimination throughout the world there has also been significant progress towards reducing these practices. In addition to what is being done there is still much that we need to understand about the forms and contexts of stigmatization and discrimination if we are to succeed in our efforts to control the HIV epidemic particularly in Africa [58]. Stigma and discrimination in Africa can be challenged. One way to reduce their impact is at the legislative level, it is also vital to focus on community-based interventions. These projects target stigmatization manifested in a wide range of community contexts, including: family and immediate community, workplace, health services, religion and the media.

8. Need for the development and implementation of affordable, readily available, low technology and safer conception services

Many HIV-infected men and women are now expressing their desire to have children. Although no conception methods are 100% risk -free of HIV infection other than those that use fresh sperm from an HIV negative donor or adoption. The strong desire among Africans to have their own biological children makes these options untenable for many PLWHA. However there is several risk reduction method for safer conception in which the HIV infected partner is on antiretroviral therapy to achieve a significant reduction of viral load and increase in CD4 count. Assisted reproductive technologies, including intrauterine insemination (IUI), in vitro fertilisation (IVF) and intracytoplasmatic sperm injection (ICSI) in combination with semen washing have been used to decrease the risk of HIV -1 transmission in HIV-1-infected discordant couples with an HIV-1-infected man particularly in developed countries. Previous report indicates that in HIV-positive men taking HAART, seminal viral load is decreased to undetectable limits but not eliminated and fertilization should be achieved through sperm washing to offer maximum protection for the uninfected female. Pregnant HIV-positive women on antiretroviral medication have a reduced risk of transmitting the virus, but should still be counselled about the possibility to further limit the chances of infecting their infant through elective Caesarean section. HIV sero-discordant couples with strong desire for childbearing have a dilemma of risking HIV infection or infecting their spouse. Some risk transmission of HIV infection to reproduce. Majority of HIV –infected couples wanting to procreate are having unprotected sex with their partners. Most persons living with HIV infection need information on viral load testing, awareness of post-exposure prevention and condom use. A paucity of interventions targeting HIV sero-discordant couples on contraceptive choices is at odds with a strong cultural importance in Africa attached to having children. HIV discordance creates a serious dilemma for fertility decision-making in couples. However, majority of these risk reduction method for safer conception are either unavailable regionally in Africa or unaffordable. Other low-technology and readily available and affordable option that could be used in Africa and other resource- constrained settings include; timed unprotected sexual intercourse for HIV concordant couples, vaginal insemination of fresh semen into the vagina via a disposable pipette or syringe, for HIV positive men with sero negative partners, the use of antiretroviral drugs by the HIV-infected male partner to lower HIV viral load in seminal plasma to undetectable levels, use of pre-exposure prophylaxis (PrEP) by the HIV sero-negative female partner prior to and following timed unprotected sex at the female partners ovulation period. It is vital that couples practice safer sex practices after conception and throughout the pregnancy. Previous report [59] has shown that HIV horizontal seroconversion occurred in couples who reported unsafe sex practices during pregnancy after conception. American researchers and clinicians have advocated the possibilities of using PrEP for safer conception [60]. A Recent study has indicated the potential role of PrEP in the prevention of heterosexual HIV transmission [61]. Similarly, the Pre-exposure Prophylaxis Initiative (IPrEx) trial using tenofovir/ emtricitabine has shown that PrEP is safe and capable of producing a reduction in HIV infection risk in HIV-seronegative men who have sex with men [62]. Also the CAPRISA 004 trial showed that the use of 1% tenofovir topical gel reduced the rate of HIV acquisition by 39% in heterosexual seronegative women [63]. The use of PrEP is rapidly growing as an important component of safer conception programs for HIV-serodiscordant couples [47, 64]. In the face of the high HIV prevalence in most African setting, it is expedient that low –technology, safer conception methods that is feasible, affordable and are acceptable is implemented.

8.1. Sperm washing with intrauterine insemination

Several studies have reported on the efficacy of sperm washing in combination with IUI in terms of pregnancy rates, live birth rates, and HIV transmission incidence [65- 67]. However, evaluation of the efficacy of this safer conception strategy is limited by methodological issues, including small sample sizes, lack of standardized protocols, and non-rigorous study designs. For example, most studies reported only on retrospective data and very few used control groups. Sperm washing and insemination lower transmission risk for HIV-negative women who want to have children with HIV-positive men. Data from the European experience which included a 14 years of follow up for 1,036 sero-discordant couples with an HIV-positive male resulted in 580 pregnancies and no HIV sero conversions [68].

Intracytoplasmic sperm injection (ICSI).ICSI is a high-technology in vitro fertilization procedure in which a single sperm is injected into an egg. It is a popular assisted reproduction technique used as a safe conception technique in HIV seropositive men and their partners. Previous reports have shown that ICSI is particularly useful and effective in the prevention of HIV among serodiscordant couples in which the man is HIV-seropositive [46, 69]. However there are a number of challenges associated with its utility particularly in Africa. These include high cost, increased risk of multiple pregnancies and the risk of use of an HIV-infected gamete [68]. It is crucial to introduce harm-reduction methods and safer conception methods for people with HIV infection in settings where assisted reproductive technologies are unavailable and unaffordable. However, these strategies are not feasible on a widespread basis in resource-constrained settings. Sperm washing and ICSI is not feasible in most resource-constrained settings. Its high cost, the invasive nature of the procedure, the high number of cancelled cycles, increased risk of multiple pregnancies and potential danger of using an HIV-infected gamete all militate against the use of ICSI. The most practicable method in most settings in Africa is vaginal insemination with an uninfected male partner's sperm during the fertile time of the woman's menstrual cycle. Several studies in Africa have evaluated the outcome of natural concention in HIV sero-discordant couples. Ryder and colleagues [70] studied 178 married HIV sero-discordant couples in the Democratic Republic of Congo between 1987 to 1990. Couples engaged in unprotected sex during the moment ovulation period and resulted in the birth of 24 children and one sero -conversion. Similarly a cross sectional study [71] involving 55 HIV-positive Nigeria women on antiretroviral therapy married to HIV-sero-negative men indicated that younger women compared to older women were more likely to pursue natural conception options than assisted reproduction.

9. Factors to consider before implementation of safer conception in sub Saharan Africa

National medical societies such as the American Society of Reproductive Medicine and the American College of Obstetricians /Gynaecologist has re-affirmed that it is unethical to refuse to provide safer conception services to PLWHA [72].The protection of the sexual and reproductive health of all people including PLWHA has been recognized as a fundamental human right. PLWHA particularly in Africa have the right to choose to have children and to access non-judgemental, non-stigmatised and non-discriminatory evidenced-based quality sexual and reproductive services. There are however factors that need to be considered in implementing safer conception intervention; the feasibility, availability and affordability of the intervention, the need for antiretroviral therapy to ensure a low viral load, high CD4 count, absence of AIDS defining symptoms and STIs, the need for couple anticipating conception to be in a stable relationship [73], consideration of fertility problems in HIV-infected population, concomitant low success rate with assisted reproductive technologies in PLWHA, low pregnancy rate and high fetal death rates among HIV-infected women [74].

10. Conclusion

Sustained and increased investment in sexual and reproductive health services in Africa promises tremendous benefits to women, families and societies. In addition to improved health, sexual and reproductive health services contribute to economic growth, societal and gender equity, and democratic governance. Evidence has shown that a significant number of HIV-infected persons in Africa desire to have children irrespective of their positive sero status. There is the need to support the sexual and reproductive rights of HIV-infected individuals. Additional training needs to be offered to HIV counsellors on evidenced- based best and affordable practices regarding reproductive health issues among persons living with HIV. There is the urgent need to develop policies that support the availability and accessibility to relevant reproductive and sexual health services including contraception and procreation. There is also the need for public enlightenment programmes on HIV to reduce the stigmatization that HIV-infected persons in sub Saharan Africa face from family members and their communities. Implementation of explicit policies recognizing reproductive rights and choice of HIV-infected in Africa as well as support for health counselling and service interventions that advance safer and healthier reproductive options for HIV positive individuals is advocated. Intrauterine insemination (IUI) and Intracytoplasmic sperm injection ICSI does not seem a cost-effective option in Africa and other resource-constrained settings. However vaginal insemination with the sperm of an HIV-seronegative male partner is highly feasible and has been found to be reasonably acceptable to both men and women and reduces the risk of transmission of HIV from infected women to their uninfected partners. This may be a practicable, affordable, low- technology, safer conception option that may need to be implemented in Africa and other resource-limited settings. There is increasing advocacy that timed, limited, unprotected sex for HIV-seroconcordant couples, and timed,

http://dx.doi.org/10.5772/52682

unprotected sex accompanied by periconceptionPrEP for the HIV seronegative female partner in serodisconcordant relationship could form part of a harm-reduction strategy to reduce exposure to HIV when planning conception in resource-limited settings. There is the need to increase the awareness, understanding, and acceptability of readily available, affordable, evidenced-based, low-technology and safer conception strategies among PLWHA in Africa. Evidenced based –best practices needs to be implemented in Africa to avoid HIV transmission enabling HIV-affected couples to embark on safer childbearing and to prevent the risk of mother-to-child HIV transmission as well as infection of the uninfected partners particularly in sero-discordance relationships. Countries in Africa must now come to terms that failure of the health system to engage HIV-seropositive women and men in fertility management and denying safer conception services to PLWHA who want to conceive a child is unethical and a deprivation of their fundamental reproductive right.

Author details

O. Erhabor[1*], T.C. Adias[2] and C.I. Akani[3]

*Address all correspondence to: n_osaro@yahoo.com

1 Department of Medical Laboratory Science, Usmanu Danfodio University Sokoto, Nigeria

2 Bayelsa State College of Health Technology, Bayelsa State, Nigeria

3 Department of Obstetrics and Gynaecology, University of Port Harcourt Teaching Hospital, Nigeria

References

[1] UNAIDS (2011). Report of the global AIDS epidemic. November 2011.

[2] Stratchan, M., Kwateng-Addo, A., Hardel, K., et al. (2004). An analysis of family planning content in HIV/AIDS, VCT and PMTCT policies in 16 countries. Policy Working Paper Series, Washington DC Policy Project, 2004.(9)

[3] Kober, K,van., & Damme, W. (2004). Access to antiretroviral treatment in Southern Africa: WHO will do the job? Lancet; , 364(982), 103-107.

[4] Sayre AP. Africa, Twenty-First Century Books. (1999). 0-76131-367-2.

[5] Richard Sandbrook (1985). The Politics of Africa's Economic Stagnation. Cambridge University Press, Cambridge, 1985 passim.

[6] The developing world is poorer than we thought, but no less successful in the fight against poverty.World Bank.

[7] Couch JF, Atkinson KE, Shughart WF (1992). Ethics Laws and the Outside Earnings of Politicians: The Case of Alabama's `Legislator-Educators'" Public Choice. , 73(2), 135-45.

[8] Transparency International, The anti-corruption catalyst: realising the MDGs by (2015). Transparency International, and www.transparency.org.

[9] Transparency International. Corruption PerceptionsIndex, TransparencyInternational, www.transparency.org.

[10] CIA World Fact book 2009.

[11] CIA-The World Fact book (2008). Rank order HIV/AIDS-Adult prevalence rate.

[12] United Nations. (2006). revision of the United Nations World Population Prospects report, for. , 2005-2010.

[13] Carroli, G., Rooney, C., & Villar, J. (2001). How effective is antenatal care in preventing maternal mortality and serious morbidity? An overview of the evidence. PaediatrPerinatEpidemiol ; , 15(1), 1-42.

[14] CDC ((2001).). Revised recommendations for HIV screening of pregnant women. MMWR; 50 ( ):63-85.(RR-19)

[15] Almeida SD, Barros MB (2005). Equity and access to health care for pregnant women in Campinas (SP), Brazil. RevistaPanamericana de SaludPublica; , 17(1), 15-25.

[16] O', Connor. K. E., & Mac, Donald. S. E. (2002). Aiming for zero: preventing mother-to-child transmission of HIV. Canadian Medical Association Journal; , 166(7), 909-910.

[17] IPAS (2005). Reproductive rights for women affected by HIV/AIDS.

[18] Mullick, S., Kunene, B., & Wanjiru, M. Involving men in maternity care: health service delivery issues. Agenda: Special focus on Gender, Culture and Rights (Special (124-135), 124-135.

[19] UNAIDS/02.31E (2002). Keeping the promise. Summary of the Declaration of Commitment on HIV/AIDS. United Nations General Assembly Special Session on HIV/AIDS (UNGASS), June 2001.Geneva: UNAIDS., 25-27.

[20] CDC (1998). HIV partner counselling and referral services guidance. Atlanta, GA: US Department of Health and Human Services, CDC.

[21] Cooper, D., Harries, J., Myer, L., Orner, P., & Bracken, H. (2007). Life is still going on. Reproductive intentions among HIV-positive women and men in South Africa. Social Science and Medicine; , 65(2), 274-278.

[22] Erhabor, O., Akani, C. I., & Eyindah, . (2012). Reproductive health options among HIV-infected persons in the low-income Niger Delta of Nigeria. HIV AIDS (Auckl); , 4, 29-35.

[23] Frodsham, L. C., Boag, F., Barton, S., & Gilling-Smith, C. (2006). Human immunodeficiency virus infection and fertility care in the United Kingdom: Demand and supply. *Fertility and Sterility*, 285 EOF-289 EOF.

[24] Myer, L., Morroni, C., & Rebe, K. (2007). Prevalence and determinants of fertility intentions of HIV-infected women and men receiving antiretroviral therapy in South Africa. *AIDS Patient Care and STDs*, 278 EOF-285 EOF.

[25] Matthews LT, Mukherjee JS (2009). Strategies for harm reduction among HIV-affected couples who want to conceive. AIDS Behav; , 1, 5-11.

[26] Sonko SI. (1994). Fertility and culture in Sub-Saharan Africa: A review. *International Social Science Journal*.

[27] Allen, S., Meinzen-Derr, J., Kautzman, M., Zulu, I., Trask, S., Fideli, U., et al. (2003). Sexual behaviour of HIV discordant couples after HIV counselling and testin. g. AIDS

[28] Beyeza-Kashesya, J., Kaharuza, F., Mirembe, F., Neema, S., Ekstrom, A. M., & Kulane, A. 2 EOF-12 EOF.

[29] Beyeza-Kashesya, J., Ekstrom, A. M., Kaharuza, F., Mirembe, F., Neema, S., & Kulane, A. (2010). My partner wants a child: a cross-sectional study of the determinants of the desire for children among mutually disclosed sero-discordant couples receiving care in Uganda. BMC Public Health; 13, 10, 247.

[30] Barreiro, P., Duerr, A., Beckerman, K., & Soriano, V. (2006). Reproductive options for HIV-serodiscordant couples. AIDS Rev; 8(3), , 158 EOF-70 EOF.

[31] de Bruyn, M. (2004). Living with HIV: Challenges in reproductive health care in South Africa. African Journal of Reproductive Health; , 8(1), 92-98.

[32] Kalichman SC, Simbayi LC (2003). HIV testing attitudes, AIDS stigma and voluntary HIV counselling and testing in a black township in Cape Town, South Africa. Sex TransmInfec; , 79, 42-447.

[33] Peña, J. E., Klein, J., Thornton, M. H., & 2nd, Sauer. M. V. (2003). Providing assisted reproductive care to male haemophiliacs infected with human immunodeficiency virus: preliminary experience. *Haemophilia*, 9(3), 309-316.

[34] Stern AM (2005). Sterilized in the name of public health: race, immigration and reproductive control in modern California. Am J Public Health, 2005; , 95, 1128-1138.

[35] Sauer M V (2003). Providing fertility care to those with HIV: Time to re-examine healthcare policy. The American Journal of Bioethics , 3(1), 33-40.

[36] Semprini, A. E., Levi-Setti, P., Bozzo, M., et al. (1992). Insemination of HIV-negative women with processed semen of HIV-positive partners. *Lancet*, 340, 1317-1319.

[37] Geeta RG (2002). How men's power over women fuel the HIV epidemics.Br Med J; , 324(7331), 183-184.

[38] Peter, K. L., Kristen, R., Willard, C., (2002, , & , H. I. V. A. I. D. (2002). HIV/AIDS evolving impact on global health. In: Ron Valdisiern (ed). Dawning answers: How the HIV/AIDS epidemic has strengthened public health. New York. Oxford press.

[39] UNAIDS (1997). Women and AIDS. UNAIDS point of view. UNAIDS. Geneva.

[40] Gomez AC, Marin VB (1996). Gender, culture and power: Barriers to HIV-prevent. ion strategies for women. Journal of Sex Research; , 33(4), 355-362.

[41] The Glion Call to Action on family planning and HIV/AIDS in women and children" a consensus advocacy statement from a consultation in May 2004.

[42] Coopera, D., et al. (2005). Reproductive intentions and choices among HIV-infected individuals in Cape Town, South Africa. Lessons for reproductive policy and service provision from a qualitative study", Policy Brief, Women's Health Research Unit and Infectious Diseases epidemiology Unit, University of Cape Town, South Africa and the population council, New York, September 2005.

[43] Shapiro, K., & Ray, S. (2007). Sexual health for people living with HIV. Reproductive Health Matter; , 15(29), 67-92.

[44] Mantell JE, Smit JA, Stein ZA (2009). The right to choose parenthood among HIV-infected women and men. J Public Health Policy. ; , 30, 367-378.

[45] Fakoya, A., Lamba, H., Mackie, N., et al. (2008). British HIV Association, BASHH and FSRH guidelines for the management of the sexual and reproductive health of people li. ving with HIV infection 2008. HIV Med; , 9, 681-720.

[46] Ohi, J. P. M., Wittemer, C., et al. (2003). Assisted reproduction techniques for HIV serodiscordant couples: 18 months of experience. Hum Reprod; , 18, 1244-1249.

[47] Chadwick, R. J., Mantell, J. E., Moodley, J., Harries, J., Zweigenthal, V., & Cooper, D. (2011). Safer conception interventions for HIV-affected couples: implications for resource-constrained settings. Top AntivirMed ; , 19(4), 148-55.

[48] Nyblade, L., & Mac, Quarrie. K. (2006). Can We Measure HIV/AIDS-related Stigma and Discrimination? Current Knowledge about Quantifying Stigma in Developing Countries. Washington, DC: United States Agency for International Development.

[49] Shelton JD, Peterson EA. (2004). The imperative for family planning in ART therapy in Africa. *Lancet*, 364, 1916-1918.

[50] Sayles, J. N., Wong, Kinsler. J. J., Martins, D., & Cunningham, W. E. (2009). The association of stigma and self-reported access to medical care and antiretroviral therapy adherence in persons living with HIV/AIDS. J Gen Intern Med; , 24(10), 1101-1108.

[51] Obermeyer, C. M., & Osborn, M. (2007). The utilization of testing and counselling for HIV: a review of the social and behavioural evidence. Am J Public Health; , 97(10), 1762-1774.

[52] Goldin, C. (1994). Stigmatization and AIDS: Critical issues in public health." Social Science and Medicine; , 39(9), 1359-1366.

[53] Norbert, G., & Somerville, M. (1994). Stigmatization, scapegoating and discrimination in sexually transmitted diseases: Overcoming them and us. Social Science and Medicine; , 39(3), 1359-1366.

[54] Angelo, A., & Reynolds, N. (1995). Stigma, HIV and AIDS: An exploration and elaboration of a stigma trajectory." Social Science and Medicine; , 41(3), 303-315.

[55] Somerville, Margaret and Andrew Orkin ((1989).). "Human rights, discrimination and AIDS: Concepts and issues."AIDS; 3(1): S -S287., 283.

[56] Zaba, B., & Gregson, S. (1998). Measuring the impact of HIV on fertility in Africa..HIV-related stigma and discrimination have been shown to impede prevention, care and treatment. AIDS; , 12(1), 341-350.

[57] Paiva, V., Filipe, E. V., Santos, N., Lima, T. N. ., & Segurado, A. (2003). The right to love: The desire for parenthood among men living with HIV. *Reproductive Health Matters*, 11(22), 91-100.

[58] Malcolm, A., Aggleton, P., Bronfman, M., Galvão, J., Mane, P., & Verrall, J. (1998). HIV-related stigmatization and discrimination: Its forms and contexts.Critical Public Health; , 8(4), 347-370.

[59] Mandelbrot, L., Heard, I., Henrion, E., & Henrion, R. (1997). Natural conception in HIV-negative women with HIV-infected partners.*Lancet* . 13, 2314-2315.

[60] Lampe MA, Smith DK, Anderson GJ, Edwards AE, Nesheim SR (2011). Achieving safe conception in HIV-discordant couples: the potential role of oral pre-exposure prophylaxis (PrEP) in the United States. Am J Obstet Gynecol.204: 488.

[61] Baeten, J., Celum, C., et al. (2011). The partners PrEP Study Team. Antiretroviral pre-exposure prophylaxis for HIV-1 prevention among heterosexual African men and women: the Partners PrPE Study(Abstract MOAX01) 6th IAS Conference on HIV Pathogenesis, Treatment and Prevention. July Rome Italy., 17-20.

[62] Grant RM, Lama JR, Anderson PL, et al (2011). Pre-exposure chemoprophylaxis for HIV prevention in men who have sex with men. N Engl J Med; , 363, 2587-2599.

[63] Abdool, Karim. Q., Abdool, Karim. S. S., Frohlich, J. A., et al. (2010). Effectiveness and safety of tenofovir gel, an antiretroviral microbicide, for the prevention of HIV infection in women. Science; 329: 1168.

[64] Mathews, L. T., Baeten, J. M., Celum, C., & Bangsberg, D. R. (2010). Periconception pre-exposure prophylaxis to prevent HIV transmission: benefits, risks and challenges to implementation.AIDS; , 24, 1975-1982.

[65] Semiprini AE (2000). Viral transmission in ART risks for patients and healthcare providers. Hum Reprod; 15:69.

[66] Manigart, Y., Rozenberg, S., Barlow, P., Ge-rard, M., Bartrand, E., & Delvigne, A. (2006). ART out-come in HIV-infected patients. Hum Reprod; , 21, 2935-2940.

[67] Savasi, V., Ferrazzi, E., Lanzani, C., Oneta, M., Parrilla, B., & Persico, T. (2007). Safety of sperm washing and ART outcome in 741 HIV-1 sero-discordant couples. Hum Reprod; , 22, 772-777.

[68] Bujan, L., Hollander, L., Coudert, M., Gilling-Smith, C., Vucetich, A., Guibert, J., Vernazza, P., Ohl, J., Weigel, M., Englert, Y., Semprini, A. E., Th, C. R. E. A., & network, E. (2007). Safety and efficacy of sperm washing in HIV-1-serodiscordant couples where the male is infected: results from the European CREAThE network. AIDS; , 21(14), 1909-14.

[69] Kashima, K., Takakuka, K., Suzuki, M., et al. (2009). Studies of assisted reproduction techniques (ART) for HIV-1 discordant couples using washed sperm and the nested PCR method: a comparison of the pregnancy rates in HIV-1 discordant couples and control couples. Jpn J Infec Dis.2009; , 62, 173-176.

[70] Ryder, R. W., Kamenga, C., Jinju, M., Mbuyi, N., Mbu, l., & Behets, F. (2005). Pregnancy and HIV-1 incidence in 178 married couples with discordant HIV-1 serostatus: additional experience at an HIV-1 counselling centre in the Democratic Republic of the Congo. Trop Med Int Health: , 482-487.

[71] Ezeanochie, M., Olagbuji, B., Ande, A., & Oboro, V. (2009). Fertility preferences, condom use and concerns among HIV-positive women in serodiscordant relationships in the era of antiretroviral therapy. Int J GynaecolObstet; , 10, 97-98.

[72] Kambin, S., & Batzer, F. (2004). Assisted reproductive technology in HIV serodiscordant couples. Sexuality, Reproduction and Menopause.2004; , 2, 92-100.

[73] Gilling-Smith, C., Nicopoullos, Semprini. A. E., Frodsham, L. C., (2006, , & , H. I. (2006). HIV and reproductive care-a review of current practice; , 113, 869-878.

[74] Englert, Y., Lesage, B., Van Vooren, J. P., et al. (2004). Medically assisted reproduction in the presence of chronic viral disease. Hum Reprod Update; , 10, 149-162.

Section 5

Prevention and Treatment of HIV Infection

Chapter 15

The Downside of an Effective cART: The Immune Restoration Disease

Claudia Colomba and Raffaella Rubino

Additional information is available at the end of the chapter

http://dx.doi.org/10.5772/53352

1. Introduction

The prognosis of patients infected with human immunodeficiency virus (HIV) type 1 has dramatically improved since the advent of the highly active antiretroviral therapy (HAART), which have enabled sustained suppression of HIV replication and recovery of CD4+ T cells count [1-3]. However, many patients in resource-poor settings still start HAART at a late stage of HIV infection when they already have advanced immunodeficiency [4,5]. Immune reconstitution in HIV infected patients is characterized by replenishment of immune cells depleted directly or indirectly by HIV infection, by regeneration of primary and secondary lymphoid organs, by restoration of pathogen-specific T, B and NK cells and by a regulation of the reconstituted immune system [2]. It is unclear whether complete immune reconstitution ever occurs but individuals with human immunodeficiency virus infection starting antiretroviral therapy when they are very immunodeficient are susceptible to immune reconstitution disorders. This phenomenon is known as a multitude of names including "immune reconstitution inflammatory syndrome (IRIS)", "immune reconstitution or restoration disease" (IRD) or immune reconstitution syndrome" and includes various forms of a clinical deterioration as a consequence of a rapid and dysregulated restoration of antigen specific immune responses causing an exuberant inflammatory reaction and a cytokines storm [1-3]. This was first noted following the introduction of zidovudine monotherapy in the early 1990s, when localized forms of *Mycobacterium avium intracellulare* (MAI) infection where observed in association with the recovery rather than failure of cellular immune response [6]. Later, in 1992, *French MA et al* showed that the disease associated with Mycobacterium avium complex (MAC) infection occurred after nucleoside analogue therapy and correlated with restoration of delayed hypersensitivity (DTH) responses to mycobacterial antigens [7].

2. Definition and epidemiology

IRIS is a well established entity still lacking of a consistent definition due to a wide variety of pathogens and disease processes involved. It has been associated with herpetic, mycobacterial and cryptococcal infections, Kaposi's sarcoma, non – Hodgkin lymphoma and progressive multifocal leukoencephalopathy. Non AIDS defining pathologies such as sarcoidosis, Graves disease and rheumatic disease can also occur [1-3]. General case definitions have been proposed by *Shelburne et al* (2009), *French MA et al* (2004) and by *Robertson J et al* (2006) [8,9,10] but diagnostic criteria for IRIS have not been standardized except for TB-IRIS [3, 11]. This syndrome can be elicited by infectious and non infectious antigens and may arise in two different settings, depending on whether HAART was started in a patient treated for an ongoing opportunistic infection or in a clinically stable patient with or without requiring primary prophylaxis [2]. "Unsmasking IRIS" is an immune response against an infection that was subclinical before the initiation of HAART whereas "paradoxical IRIS" indicates a condition in which the opportunistic infection is present and treated at the time of initiation of HAART and worsens on therapy. Unmasking IRIS usually presents within the first three months of therapy and viable pathogens may be isolated from samples obtained from affected body sites, particularly when there is tissue necrosis. Paradoxical IRIS is common during the first three months of HAART but may present later and frequently immune response is against non viable pathogens. It occurs in 8-43% of patients with treated tuberculosis and in 4-66% of patients with treated cryptococcal infection becoming an important concern in poor resources countries [1-3]. Paradoxical IRIS is also exemplified by immune recovery, which occurs in eyes previously affected by cytomegalovirus (CMV) retinitis. Particularly in paradoxical IRIS, clinicians need to exclude alternative explanations for deterioration, such as failure to treat the opportunistic infection or failure of HAART because of poor adherence or drug resistance [3].

Some authors suggested using terms of "simultaneous IRIS" for patients who develop IRIS and a newly diagnosed opportunistic infection (OI) at the same time and "delayed IRIS" for those with an OI in which IRIS manifests sometimes thereafter [12].

However, although several case definitions for IRIS have been proposed, certain minimum criteria should be fulfilled in order to diagnose it. First of all, there must be the temporal association between initiation of HAART and subsequent development of symptoms of an inflammatory localized or systemic process, characterized by worsening of clinical or laboratory parameters despite "favorable" evolution of the HIV surrogate markers [1,2]. A rise in blood CD4 + T cells is commonly seen in IRIS but it is not an essential element for the diagnosis and is only a supportive criterion in both of the general case definitions for IRIS [9,10]. *Philips P et al* found that about 10% of patients with Mycobacterium avium complex immune restoration disease haven't an increased CD4+ T cells count [13]. Neverthless, a lack of rise in blood CD4 + T cells doesn't indicate that there has been no restoration of functional T lymphocyte response. On the other hand, IRIS has been described at higher CD4 + T cells count, suggesting that functional status of cells has a role in the pathogenesis of IRIS too. Therefore a falling plasma viral load is a more important indicator than CD4 T cells count recovery [14].

The immune restoration outcomes range from minimal morbidity to fatal progression [15]. The immune restoration shows a biphasic pattern and is demonstrated by a decrease in plasma HIV RNA levels by more than 1 $\log_{10}$ copies/ml and an increase in CD4 + T cells count from baseline [1,2,16]. Initial recovery of the immune system consists in an increase in memory T cells followed by an increase in thymic production of naïve T cells [1,2,16-20]. In addition there is the recovery of reduced or damaged secondary lymphoid organs such as the gut and the mesentheric associated lymphoid tissue, which are often lost due to chronic HIV- mediated inflammation [21]. The initial and rapid rise of CD4 + T memory cells released from compartments into circulation can be detrimental and a mild OI can appear as an overwhelming infection because memory T cells respond to their antigens more readily than naïve T cells [2,22].

CD8 + T cells also increase during the first two months of HAART and then tend to return to baseline [18].

Differentiation between an opportunistic infection with normal presentation and a disorder with a presentation compatible with unmasking IRIS is particularly difficult and the differences between intended HAART – associated immune reconstitution and undesired manifestations of IRIS is probably a continuum [3].The damage may indicate a failure of the immune system to properly regulate the potency of the immune response [23].

The differential diagnosis includes failure of the antimicrobial therapy in patient with active infection, manifestations of a new opportunistic infection, unmasking of an ongoing, previously undiagnosed infection or manifestation of a diagnosed, ongoing infection in a previously unrecognized site of involvement [1-3,16]. Drug toxicity must be ruled out. For example, hepatitis flares in patients coinfected with hepatitis B virus or hepatitis C virus may be the result of IRIS in the liver or of HAART- associated hepatotoxicity [2, 24].In occurring IRIS, inflammation is atypical in presentation or more exaggerated than in immunodeficiency disease being characterized by pain, suppuration and necrosis and examination of affected tissue or body fluids samples reveals evidence of an immune response with scarcity of pathogens, infiltrating lymphocytes and granulomatous reaction [1-3].

IRIS may be estimated to occur in 10% to 50 % of patients starting HAART with similar percentages occurring in children and the incidence varies with the AIDS-defining illness [1-3]. Differences reported in the incidence of IRIS between opportunistic infections seem to be related to CD4+ T cells count at baseline [3]. IRIS is common in patients starting HAART with a low CD4 + T cells count and a CMV retinitis or cryptococcal meningitis whereas Kaposi's sarcoma and TB-IRIS have also been described at an high count of CD4 + T cells count [3,25].

Moreover, the variation reported in frequency is due to differences in case definitions and, above all, to differences in study populations with heterogeneous risk profiles and underlying burden of opportunistic infections [1,2]. In a recent meta-analysis and systematic review including 54 cohort studies and 13.103 patients starting HAART of whom 1699 develope IRIS, the lowest to highest incidence of IRIS by previously diagnosed opportunistic illness resulted 6,4% in patients with Kaposi's sarcoma (based on two studies), 12,2% in patients with Herpes Zoster (based on one study), 15,7% in patients with tuberculosis (based on 16 studies), 16,7% in patients with progressive multifocal leukoencephalopathy (based on two studies), 19,5% in patients with cryptococcal meningitis (based on six studies) and 37,7% in patients with cytomegalovirus retinitis (based on ten studies). In the same review IRIS developed in 16,1% of unselected patients starting HAART and the incidence of IRIS associated with tuberculosis and cryptococcal meningitis seemed to be lower in cohorts from low and middle income countries probably due to limited diagnostic capacity in these settings. The strength of this affirmation is supported by the evidence of an high incidence of IRIS associated uveitis in all settings: inflammatory reactions, even if moderate, are more likely to be recognized in the eye than in other organs [3].

Risk factors for IRIS are difficult to establish because of the cohorts differ with regards to the study populations and the type of IRIS examined. Anyway, several risk factors for IRIS has been identified and, first of all, the presence of an opportunistic infection at the time of initiation of HAART, specially for TB and cryptococcal diseases [1,2]. *Müller M et colleagues* reported an analysis stratified by median CD4+ T cells count at the beginning of HAART showing the different incidence of IRIS [Tab. 1, 3]. Male sex and younger age have been identified as significant predictors too [15,26].

Initiation of HAART soon after treatment for an opportunistic infection is considered a risk factor too [1-3,15].

A shorter interval between the treatment of an opportunistic infection and the initiation of HAART is associated with a higher risk of IRIS in these patients [1-3,15].

3. Pathogenesis

The immunopathological process is still poorly understood but is strictly related with the provoking pathogen and with host. In fact, some people develop IRIS and others, with similar clinical status and risk factors, do not. It remains unclear if the disease mechanisms associated with IRIS are the same for each OI or if there are microbial-driven specific immune responses that result in different pathologies for each pathogen [12]. Several studies using a simian immunodeficiency virus model indicate differential expression of viral peptides by distinct MHC alleles, which could influence the aggressiveness of the immune response directed toward SIV [27].

Essentially any pathogen that can cause an opportunistic infection in patients with impaired cellular immune responses can provoke IRIS. It also appears that HIV infection itself can cause IRIS [28]. Two patients were reported with HIV encephalitis after effective HAART. Neuropathological features consisted in massive CD8+/CD4- lymphocytes brain infiltration and in a diffuse microglial hyperplasia [28].

The antigenic stimulus in infectious conditions are either intact viable organism or dead organism and their residual antigens whereas autoimmunity to innate antigens are involved in the non-infectious causes of the syndrome [1-3].

If the pathogen is viral, i.e. CMV or JC, CD8 + - T lymphocytes predominate in inflammatory cells infiltrates whereas if the pathogen is tuberculous or non tuberculous mycobacteria, a

http://dx.doi.org/10.5772/53352

protozoan as Leishmania species or a fungus as Cryptococcus neoformans granulomatous CD4 + - T helper cells type 1 inflammation predominates [1-3].

Price P et al suggested a genetic predisposition and certain genes have been associated with an increased susceptibility to development of IRIS in presence of mycobacteria and herpes-viruses. The TNF α-308*2 carried in linkage disequilibrium with HLA-A2,-B44,-DR4 and without BAT1 (intron 10)*2 is more common in patients with herpesvirus-associated IRIS and is not present in any patients who has experienced mycobacterial IRIS. Therefore TNF α polymorphisms should be considered in the context of the adjacent MHC alleles. The absence of C allele of IL6-174 together with TNF α - 308*1 confers an increased relative risk for mycobacterial IRIS probably due to a limited TNF-mediated bactericidal activity and to a lower TNFα production in monocytes [29]. The CMV retinitis IRD patients have over 4 years on HAART progressively increased plasma levels of bioavailable IL-6 and of soluble CD30, a type 2 (T2) immune response marker and 92% of them result homozygous for IL12B-3'UTR* 1 suggesting a dysregulation of the T1/T2 balance [30,31]. Th1 cells are characterized by the production of interferon γ and elicit proinflammatory responses. Th2 cells produce antiinflammatory and immunosuppressive cytokines (i.e. interleukin 10). [31,32]. These considerations suggest that IRIS could be sustained form several immunopathological mechanisms and that further studies need to better establish the role of cytokines in the different forms of IRIS [31].

In addition to the reconstitution of immune cell numbers and function, redistribution of lymphocytes, defects in regulatory function, changes in Th cell profile are also involved [23]. Mycobacterial IRIS usually presents with suppuration of lympho nodes or other organ affected because of an activation of Th 17 lymphocytes inducing inflammation mediated by neutrophils [33]. Production of cytokines inducing cellular proliferation is the main mechanism of IRIS-Kaposi [34]. An unbalanced immune reconstitution of effector and regulatory T cells in patients receiving HAART has been noted. In particular, two types of T cells seem to take part to the development of the disease: the proinflammatory Th 17 lymphocytse and the T regulatory cells. The latter are implied in preventing collateral damage from exuberant inflammatory responses and may be defective in number and function during IRIS [1,2,23,31]. A role has been hypotized for NK cells by killer immunoglobulin-like receptors activity. Macrophages are inappropriately activated in IRIS-TB [1].

Actually serological markers for IRIS diagnosis are lacking. Inflammatory markers, cytokines and chemokines are shown to be elevated in IRIS, specially IL 6. Paradoxical TB-IRIS has been associated with elevation of interleukin(IL) -4, IL -6, IL-7, IFN (interferon) γ and tumor necrosis factor alpha (TNF-α) and cryptococcal meningitis with increased pre-HAART levels of C reactive protein (CRP), IL-4 e IL-17 and lower levels of vascular endothelial growth factor (VEGF), granulocytes colony-stimulating factor (G-CSF) and TNF-α during clinical events [1,31,35].

To sum up, IRIS has been associated with certain human leucocyte antigen (HLA) profiles and regulatory cytokine genes polymorphisms but further research is needed to evaluate their potential role in identifying patients at risk, developing better therapeutics and monitoring response to therapy.

4. Clinical settings

Lots of clinical manifestation have been described in occurring IRIS.

Several pathogens have been associated with IRIS, including JC virus, herpes viruses, BK virus, Parvovirus B19, human T lymphotropic virus type 2, Epstein Barr virus, HHV 8, Cytomegalovirus, Cryptococcus neoformans, Toxoplasma gondii. Mycobacterium tuberculosis, Mycobacterium leprae and Mycobacterium avium complex (MAC) contribute too [1-3,15]. The antigens driving IRIS often belong to opportunistic pathogens but sometimes IRIS can be a result of HIV- specific responses [1-3,15].

TB-IRIS manifestations include worsening respiratory symptoms, fever, lymphonode enlargement and suppuration, appearance of new infiltrates and mediastinal lymphoadenopathy on chest radiograph, visceral or cutaneous abscesses, pleural and pericardial effusion and rarely intracranial tubercoloma, acute renal failure, meningitis and cognitive impairment. Moreover abdominal TB-IRIS can present with non-specific abdominal pain and obstructive jaundice. Differential diagnosis from drug-resistant tuberculosis is difficult [15,36-39]. MAC remains the most reported atypical mycobacterium and the most common manifestation in MAC-IRIS is fever with suppurative painful lymphadenitis followed by pulmonary disease but involvement of joints, spine, skin and soft tissue has also been reported. In contrast to disseminated MAC disease of advanced AIDS, MAC-IRIS usually presents as localized disease [40]. Mycobacterial IRIS has to be distinguished from sarcoidosis that can also occur in the context of IRIS [1]. Measurement of a delayed-type hypersensitivity response to tuberculin by a skin test may help to differentiate immune reconstitution-associated sarcoidosis from mycobacterial IRIS, because a response is absent in patients with sarcoidosis but is often present in patients with mycobacterial IRIS [1,2,7, 41,42].

Patients with Pneumocystis jirovecii IRIS manifest recurrence of fever, worsening hypoxia and fresh pulmonary infiltrates on chest radiograph. In addition to the general risk factors, $PaO_2 < 70$ mmHg and a recent completion of steroid therapy for Pneumocystis jirovecii pneumonia promote IRIS [1, 43,44].

CNS-IRIS occurs at much lower frequencies with about 0,9-1,5% of patients developing some CNS-IRIS after initiating HAART [45-47]. The heightened immune response in a relatively closed space leads to raised intracranial pressure, with potentially irreversible damage. Diagnosis of CNS-IRIS is difficult because CNS is a region of limited access and requires pathological confirmation and invasive procedures. A worsening of clinical neurological status can be accompanied by new neuroradiological findings or by deterioration of previous findings with T cell infiltrates into the CNS. Depending on the severity of CNS-IRIS it may be classified as asymptomatic, symptomatic and catastrophic. Asymptomatic CNS-IRIS consists in radiological changes only, such as increased enhancement. Symptomatic CNS-IRIS is characterized by clinical deterioration in neurological function with new changes on MRI scan of brain. In the catastrophic CNS-IRIS severe neurological deficits occur such as coma and imminent signs of cerebral herniation [12, 45-48]. JC virus is the causative agent of PML and one of the most devastating of the OIs associated with IRIS leading to a 42% mortality. Of the approximate 5% of HIV + patients who develop PML up to 19% are PML-IRIS patients. Differential diagnosis between PML and PML-IRIS can be done by MRI:

the presence of contrast enhancement suggest an inflammatory response and is indicative of PML-IRIS. The response to steroids confirms the diagnosis. The prognosis of delayed PML-IRIS is worse than the form that begins simultaneously [49,50].

A stroke occurring after initiation of HAART can be due to a vasculitis in the context of a VZV-IRIS [51]. Genital ulceration related to Herpes Simplex virus and genital warts related to human papillomavirus are frequently observed [1]. Most commonly CMV is associated with CMV-IRIS retinitis, vitreitis and uveitis with loss of visual acuity and floaters [1, 52]. CMV ventriculitis without retinal damage has been described [53].

Cryptococcus neoformans is frequently involved in IRIS development. It can provoke a CNS associated IRIS and a non-CNS IRIS: the first results in an aseptic recurrence of meningitis or rarely in a cryptococcoma; the second is more common and is a lymphoadenitis or a mediastinitis or rarely a cavitary pneumonia. In a patient with cryptococcal meningitis rapidly worsening because of headache, nausea and vomiting after HAART initiation IRIS has to be considered above all in presence of sterile inflammation of the CSF, residual cryptococcal antigens and absence of viable yeast on culture. Patients with Cryptococcus neoformans associated IRIS has usually higher opening pressure, white cell count and glucose levels than patients with Cryptococcus neoformans infection only. Neuroimaging is usually not useful in cryptococcal meningitis diagnosis but in occurring IRIS evidence of meningeal or choroid plexus enhancement or linear perivascular enhancement in the sulci at CT scan is frequent and represent a sign of inflammation [54-57]. Patients with cryptococcal meningitis particularly with IRIS are likely to develop a communicating idrocephalus due to blockage of CSF absorption at the arachnoid villi by cryptococcal antigens and by the inflammatory cells. This is a serious condition that may require drainage by repeated lumbar punctures [48].

There is only a case report of immune reconstitution syndrome occurring in a patient with Candida meningitis in the literature and a case report of visual loss and detection of EBV in CSF by PCR after initiation of HAART [12, 58]. In few cases Toxoplasma gondi is the responsible agent of CNS-IRIS [59].

Some patients may develop a severe progressive encephalitis after initiation of HAART with seizures, altered mental status, coma and death. HIV may be detectable in CSF even when results undetectable in blood. MRI can show diffuse multifocal white matter changes with associated cerebral edema [12,28].

Given the known associations of Kaposi's sarcoma with human herpesvirus 8 and non Hodgkin lymphoma with Epstein Barr virus it is not surprising to observe these cancers occurring or worsening in the context of IRIS [12,60-63]. Both clinical sudden progression of established lesions and new Kaposi sarcoma have been described after HAART initiation [12, 60-62]. HIV-infected patients starting HAART may present manifestations of autoimmune disease like most frequently sarcoidosis and Graves disease but also systemic lupus erythematosus, rheumatoid arthritis, Reiter's syndrome, polymyositis and Guillain-Barrè syndrome [1-3, 64-70]. At last, high levels of CNS inflammation have been demonstrated in the hippocampus of patients successfully treated with HAART and IRIS could contribute to pathogenetic mechanism leading to a cognitive impairment [12].

5. Treatment and prevention

Till now, on the grounds of available data, it appears prudent that HAART should be initiated before the onset of severe immunodeficiency. A detailed evaluation should be done for identification of opportunistic infections before HAART initiation. Patients with high risk features for the development of IRIS should be identified and OIs should be optimally treated if present [1-3, 71-73]. In the context of opportunistic infections, the benefit of reducing the likelihood of IRIS by deferring HAART must be balanced with the risk of delaying HAART, above all if patients are severely immunodeficient. The ACTG 5164 is a randomized trial comparing immediate versus deferred antiretroviral therapy initiation in patients presenting with acute OIs. Significant reduction in clinical progression or death among patients who received antiretroviral therapy within 14 days of presenting with acute OI versus those who deferred antiretroviral therapy until after OI had been treated was found and the incidence of immune reconstitution events resulted similar between groups [73].

To date, literature is lacking about the optimal time of HAART initiation following a treatment of opportunistic infections with exception of tuberculosis/HIV coinfection. Regarding this concern the most recent WHO and DHHS guidelines recommend the initiation of HAART between 2 and 8 weeks after starting treatment against tuberculosis for patients with a CD4 count < 200/µl [71,72].

Actually management of patients with IRIS was founded upon clinical observations and expert opinions only. In general non steroidal anti-inflammatory drugs should be reserved for milder manifestations and steroids for cases with severe inflammation. Interruption of HAART is rarely necessary but could be considered in life threatening situations or when pathogens involved are not controllable by specific antimicrobial therapy, as JC virus [15]. Stopping HAART may improve symptoms but there is no guarantee that the condition will not recur once HAART is resumed [74]. In a randomized controlled trial, *Meintjes G et al* reported the utility of prednisolone (1.5 mg/kg per day for two weeks followed by 0.75 mg/kg per day for further two weeks) in the treatment of paradoxical tuberculosis-IRIS with worsening chest radiograph, enlarging lymph node, serous effusion and cold abscess, CNS manifestations, tracheal compression due to lymphadenopathy and acute respiratory distress syndrome (ARDS). For atypical mycobacterial – IRIS treatment is similar to TB-IRIS. Surgical excision of profoundly enlarged nodes or debridement of necrotic areas is anecdotally reported [75,76]. Cryptococcal meningoencephalitis IRIS requires prompt control of raised intracranial pressure and hydrocephalus by serial lumbar punctures. Corticosteroids are indicated for cerebral oedema and ARDS in pulmonary cryptococcosis [48,77-78]. The development of PCP-IRIS after discontinuation of steroid therapy suggest a role for the reintroduction of steroids in these patients [44]. In cases of ocular CMV-IRIS systemic or periocular steroid injections have been used bur a clear benefit has not been demonstrated. The role of corticosteroids in PML-IRIS is not clear and a long term treatment may be necessary until T memory cells and a more directed immune response against JC virus predominates [50,79]. Unfortunately increased risk of progression of herpes zoster and Kaposi's sarcoma and reactivation of latent infections have also been reported with corticosteroids.

6. Conclusions

The majority of patients with IRIS have a self-limiting disease course but associated morbidity places a considerable burden on the health care system. Morbidity and mortality rates vary according to the pathogen and organ involved. Mortality is usually uncommon with the exception of the setting of opportunistic infections involving the CNS [1]. Lethality ranges from about 3% in patients with tuberculosis to more than 20% in patients with cryptococcal meningitis, with an higher early mortality in resource-limited settings due to probable underdiagnoses [3]. The occurrence of IRIS and its contribution to mortality in a given setting is affected by the relative importance of different infections, the degree of access to facilities for diagnosis of such illnesses and the extent of screening for and treatment of opportunistic infections before starting HAART [80].Research efforts should be focused on increasing knowledge about IRIS so that diagnostic tests and prevention and treatment strategies could be improved.

	CD4 < 50 μl	CD4 > 50 μl
IRIS-TB	20,7%	17,7%
IRIS-cryptococcal meningitis	28,3%	2%
IRIS- CMV retinitis	37,7%	No studies

Table 1. Development of IRIS in analysis stratified by median CD4+ cells count at the start of HAART [3]

Author details

Claudia Colomba and Raffaella Rubino

*Address all correspondence to: claudia.colomba@libero.it

Dipartimento di Scienze per la Promozione della Salute, Università di Palermo, Via del Vespro, Palermo, Italy

References

[1] Surendra KS et al. HIV & immune reconstitution inflammatory syndrome (IRIS). Indian J Med Res 2011; 134: 866-877.

[2] French MA. Immune reconstitution inflammatory syndrome: a reappraisal. Clin Infect Dis 2009; 48: 101-107.

[3] Müller M et al. Immune reconstitution inflammatory syndrome in patients starting antiretroviral therapy for HIV infection: a systematic review and meta-analysis. Lancet Infect Dis 2010; 10: 251-261.

[4] The Antiretroviral Therapy in Lower Income Countries (ART-LINC) Collaboration and ART Cohort Collaboration (ART-CC) groups. Mortality of HIV-1-infected patients in the first year of antiretroviral therapy: comparison between low-income and high-income countries. Lancet 2006; 367: 817-824.

[5] Keiser O et al. Antiretroviral therapy in resource limited settings 1996-2006: patients characteristics, treatment regimens and monitoring in Sub-saharan Africa, Asia and Latin America. Trop Med Int Health 2008; 13: 870-879.

[6] French MA et al. Zidovudine – induced restoration of cell mediated immunity to mycobacteria in immunodeficient HIV- infected patients. AIDS 1992; 6: 1293-1297.

[7] French et al. Immune restoration disease after the treatment of immunodeficient HIV-infected patients with highly active antiretroviral therapy. HIV Med 2000; 1: 107-115.

[8] Shelburne ISA et al. Immune reconstitution inflammatory syndrome: emergence of a unique syndrome during highly active antiretroviral therapy. Medicine 2002; 81: 213-217.

[9] French MA et al. Immune restoration disease after antiretroviral therapy. AIDS 2004; 18: 1615-27.

[10] Robertson J et al. Immune reconstitution syndrome in HIV: validating a case definition and identifying clinical predictors in person initiating antiretroviral therapy. Clin Infect Dis 2006; 42: 1639-1646.

[11] Meintjes G et al. Tuberculosis associated immune reconstitution inflammatory syndrome: case definition for use in resource limited settings. Lancet Infect Dis 2008; 8: 516-523.

[12] Johnson T et al. Neurological complications of immune reconstitutio in HIV-infected populations. Ann N Y Acad Sci 2010; 1184: 106-120.

[13] Philips P et al. Non tuberculous mycobacteria immune reconstitution syndrome in HIV- infected patients: spectrum of disease and long-term follow up. Clin Infect Dis 2005; 41: 1483-97.

[14] Lawn SD et al. Immune reconstitution disease associated with mycobacterial infections in HIV- infected individuals receiving antiretrovirals. Lancet Infect Dis 2005; 5: 361-373.

[15] Murdoch DM et al. Immune reconstitution inflammatory syndrome (IRIS): review of common infectious manifestations and treatment options. AIDS Research and Therapy 2007; 4:9.

[16] Hirsch HH et al. Immune Reconstitution in HIV-infected patients. Clin Infect Dis 2004; 38: 1159-1166.

[17] Bucy RP et al. Initial increase in blood CD4(+) lymphocytes after HIVantiretroviral therapy reflects redistribution from lymphoid tissues. J Clin Invest 1999; 103: 1391-1398.

[18] Pakker NG et al. Biphasic kinetics of peripheral blood T cells after triple combination therapy in HIV-1 infection: a composite of redistribution and proliferation. Nat Med 1998; 4: 208-214.

[19] Kauffmann GR et al.CD4-T lymphocyte recovery in individuals with advanced HIV-1 infection receiving potent antiretroviral therapy for 4 years: the Swiss HIV Cohort Study. Arch Intern Med 2003; 163: 2187-2195.

[20] Battegay M et al. Immunological recovery and antiretroviral therapy in HIV-1 infection. Lancet Infect Dis 2006; 6: 280-287.

[21] Guadalupe M et al. Severe CD4 + T cell depletivo in gut lypmphoid tissue during primary human immunodeficiency virus type 1 infection and substantial delay in restoration following highly active antiretroviral therapy. J Virol 2003; 77: 11708-11717.

[22] Berard M et al. Qualitative differences between naïve and memory T cells. Immunology 2002; 106: 127-138.

[23] Seddiki N et al. Proliferation of weakly suppressive regulatory CD4 + T - cells is associated with over-active CD4 + T – cell responses in HIV-positive patients with mycobacterial immune restoration disease. Eur J Immunol 2009; 39: 391-402.

[24] Soriano V et al. Antiretroviral drugs and liver injury. AIDS 2008; 22: 1-13.

[25] Crowe SM et al. Predictive value of CD4 lymphocyte numbers for the development of opportunistic infections and malignancies in HIV infected persons. J Acquir Immune Defic Syndr 1991; 4: 770-776.

[26] Ratnam I et al. Incidence and risk factors for immune reconstitution inflammatory syndrome in an ethnically diverse HIV type 1 infected cohort. Clin Infect Dis 2006; 42(3): 418-427.

[27] Mankowski JL et al. Natural host genetic resistance to lentiviral CNS disease: a neuroprotective MHC class I allele in SIV-infected macaques. PLoS ONE 2008; 3: e3603.

[28] Miller RF et al. CD8 + lymphocytosis in HIV-1 infected patients with immune restoration induced by HAART. Acta Neuropathol 2004; 108 (1): 17-23.

[29] Price P et al. Polymorphisms in cytokine genes define subpopulations of HIV-1 patients who experienced immune restoration diseases. AIDS 2002; 16: 2043-2047.

[30] Stone SF et al. Cytomegalovirus (CMV) retinitis immune restoration disease occurs during HAART- induced restoration of a CMV specific immune responses within a predominant Th2 cytokine environment. J Infect Dis 2002; 185 (12): 1813-1817.

[31] Kestens L et al. Immunopathogenesis of the immune reconstitution disease in HIV patients responding to antiretroviral therapy. Curr Opinion HIV AIDS 2008; 3: 419-424.

[32] Singh N et al. Immune reconstitution syndrome associated with opportunistic mycoses. Lancet Infect Dis 2007; 7: 395-401.

[33] French MA. The immunopathogenesis of mycobacterial immune restoration disease. Lancet Infect Dis 2006; 6: 461-2.

[34] Tamburini J et al. Cytokine pattern in Kaposi's sarcoma associated with immune restoration disease in HIV and tuberculosis co-infected patients. AIDS 2007; 21: 1980-1983.

[35] Stone SF et al. Plasma bioavailable interleukin-6 is elevated in human immunodeficiency virus infected patients who experience herpesvirus associated immune restoration disease after start of highly active antiretroviral therapy. J Inf Dis 2001; 184:1073–1077.

[36] Lawn SD et al. Immune reconstitution disease associated with mycobacterial infections in HIV- infected individuals receiving antiretrovirals. Lancet Infect Dis 2005; 5(6): 361-373.

[37] Jehle AW et al. Acute renal failure on immune reconstitution in an HIV-positive patient with miliary tuberculosis. Clin Infect Dis 2004; 38(4): e32-35.

[38] Narita M et al. Paradoxical worsening of tuberculosis following antiretroviral therapy in patients with AIDS. Am J Respir Crit Care Med 1998; 158: 157-161.

[39] Vidal JE et al. Paradoxical reaction during treatment of tuberculous brain abscess in a patient with AIDS. Rev Inst Med Trop Sao Paulo 2003; 45(3): 177-178.

[40] Philip P et al. Non tuberculous mycobacterial immune reconstitution syndrome in HIV- infected patients: spectrum of the disease and long-term follow up. Clin Infect Dis 2005; 41: 1483-97.

[41] Haramati LB et al. Newly diagnosed pulmonary sarcoidosis in HIV-infected patients. Radiology 2001; 218: 242-246.

[42] Foulon G et al. Sarcoidosis in HIV-infected patients in the era of highly active antiretroviral therapy. Clin Infect Dis 2004; 38: 418-425.

[43] Wislez M et al. Acute respiratory failure following HAART introduction in patient treated for Pneumocystis carinii pneumonia. Am J Respir Crit Care Med 2001; 164: 847-851.

[44] Jagannathan P et al. Life-threatening immune reconstitution inflammatory syndrome after Pneumocystis pneumonia: a cautionary case series. AIDS 2009; 23: 1794-1796.

[45] McCombe JA et al. Neurologic immune reconstitution inflammatory syndrome in HIV/AIDS: outcome and epidemiology. Neurology 2009; 72: 835-841.

[46] Torok ME et al. Immune reconstitution disease of the central nervous system. Curr Opin HIV AIDS 2008; 438-445.

[47] Gray F et al. Central nervous system immune reconstitution disease in acquired immunodeficiency syndrome patients receiving highly active antiretroviral treatment. J Neurovirol 2005; 11 (3): 16-22.

[48] Venkataramana A et al. Immune reconstitution inflammatory syndrome in the CNS of HIV- infected patients. Neurology 2006; 67: 383-388.

[49] Wyen C et al. Progressive multifocal leukencephalopathy in patients on highly active antiretroviral therapy: survival and risk factors of death. J Acquir Immune Defic Syndr 2004; 37: 1263-1268.

[50] Tan K et al. PML-IRIS in patients with HIV infection. Clinical manifestation and treatment with steroids. Neurology 2009; 72: 1458-1464.

[51] Newsome SD et al. Varicella-zoster virus vasculopathy and central nervous system immune reconstitution inflammatory syndrome with human immunodeficiency virus infection treated with steroids. J neurovirol 2009; 15: 288-291.

[52] Jacobson MA et al. Cytomegalovirus retinitis after initiation of highly active antiretroviral therapy. Lancet 1997; 349 (9063): 1443-1445.

[53] Janowicz DM et al. Successful treatment of CMV ventriculitis immune reconstitution syndrome. J Neurol Neurosurg Psychiatry 2005; 76: 891-892.

[54] Bicanic T et al. Immune reconstitution inflammatory syndrome in HIV-associated cryptococcal meningitis: a prospective study. J Acquir Immune Defic Syndr 2009; 51: 130-134.

[55] Jarvis JN et al. HIV-associated cryptococcal meningitis. AIDS 2007; 21: 2119-2129.

[56] York J et al. Raised intracranial pressure complicating cryptococcal meningitis: immune reconstitution inflammatory syndrome or recurrent cryptococcal disease? J Infect 2005; 51: 165-171.

[57] Boelaert JR et al. Relapsing meningitis caused by persistent cryptococcal antigens and immune reconstitution after the initiation of highly active antiretroviral therapy. AIDS 2004; 18: 1223-1224.

[58] Berkeley JL et al. Fatal immune reconstitution inflammatory syndrome with human immunodeficiency virus infection and Candida meningitis: case report and review of literature. J neurovirol 2008; 14: 267-176.

[59] Tsambiras PE et al. Case report. Toxoplasma encephalitis after initiation of HAART. AIDS Read 2001; 11: 608-610, 615-616.

[60] Connick E et al. Immune reconstitution inflammatory syndrome associated with Kaposi sarcoma during potent antiretroviral therapy. Clin Infect Dis 2004; 39: 1852-1855.

[61] Leidner RS et al. Recrudescent Kaposi's sarcoma after initiation of HAART: a manifestation of immune reconstitution syndrome. AIDS Patient Care STDs 2005; 19: 635-644.

[62] Bower M et al. Immune reconstitution inflammatory syndrome associated with Kaposi's sarcoma. J Clin Oncol 2005; 23: 5224-5228.

[63] Jaffe HW et al. Immune reconstitution and risk of Kaposi sarcoma and non-Hodgking lymphoma in HIV-infected adults. AIDS 2011; 25: 1395-1403.

[64] Crum NF et al. Graves disease: an increasingly recognized immune reconstitution syndrome. AIDS 2006; 20: 466-469.

[65] Knysz B et al. Graves' disease as an immune reconstitution syndrome in an HIV-1 positive patient commencing effective antiretroviral therapy: case report and review of literature. Viral Immunol 2006; 19: 102-107.

[66] Vos F et al. Graves' disease during immune reconstitution in HIV infected patients treated with HAART. Scand J Infect Dis 2006; 38: 124-126.

[67] Calza L et al. Systemic and discoid lupus erythematosus in HIV-infected patients treated with highly active antiretroviral therapy. Int J STD AIDS 2003; 14: 356-359.

[68] Bell C et al. A case of immune reconstitution rheumatoid arthritis. Int J STD AIDS 2002; 13: 580-581.

[69] Piliero PJ et al. Guillain-Barrè syndrome associated with immune reconstitution. Clin Infect Dis 2003; 36: e 111-114.

[70] Neuman S et al. Reiter's syndrome as manifestation of immune reconstitution syndrome in an HIV infected patient: successful treatment with doxycycline. Cli Infect Dis 2003; 36: 1628-1629.

[71] Panel on Antiretroviral Guidelines for the Use of Antiretroviral Agents in HIV-1 infected Adults and Adolescents. Department of Health and Human Services. March 2012.

[72] Center for Disease Control and Prevention. Guidelines for Prevention and Treatment of Opportunistic Infections in HIV-1 Infected Adults and Adolescents. MMWR 2009.

[73] Zolopa A et al. Immediate vs deferred ART in the setting of acute AIDS-related opportunistic infection: final results of a randomized strategy trial. ACTG A5164. Program and abstracts of the 15th Conference on Retroviruses and Opportunistic Infections 2008; Boston, Massachusetts. Abstract 142.

[74] Lipman M et al. Immune reconstitution inflammatory syndrome in HIV. Curr Opin Infect Dis 2006; 19: 20-25.

[75] Lawn SD et al. Pyomyositis and cutaneous abscesses due to Mycobacterium avium: an immune reconstitution manifestation in a patient with AIDS. Clin Infect Dis 2004; 38 (3): 461-463.

[76] Aberg JA et al. Localized osteomyelitis due to Mycobacterium avium complex in patient with human immunodeficiency virus receiving highly active antiretroviral therapy. Clin Infect Dis 2002; 35 (1): e 8-13.

[77] Perfect JR et al. Clinical practice guidelines for the management of cryptococcal disease: 2010 update by the infectious diseases society of America. Clin Infect Dis 2010. 50: 291-322.

[78] McComsey GA et al. Placebo-controlled trial of prednisone in advanced HIV-1 infection. AIDS 2001; 15: 321-327.

[79] Du Pasquier RA et al. Inflammatory reaction in progressive multifocal leukencephalopathy: harmful or beneficial?. J Neurovirol 2003; 9 (1): 25-31.

[80] Davies MA et al. Assessing the contribution of the immune reconstitution inflammatory syndrome to mortality in developing country antiretroviral therapy programs. Clin Infect Dis 2009; 49:973-975.

Chapter 16

HIV Infection and Viral Hepatitis in Drug Abusers

Arantza Sanvisens, Ferran Bolao, Gabriel Vallecillo,
Marta Torrens, Daniel Fuster, Santiago Pérez-Hoyos,
Jordi Tor, Inmaculada Rivas and Robert Muga

Additional information is available at the end of the chapter

http://dx.doi.org/10.5772/53074

1. Introduction

The epidemiology of HIV infection and viral hepatitis among injection drug users (IDUs) is changing in western countries; reductions in the epidemic of blood-borne infections, such as HIV infection, and viral hepatitis among drug users are probably related to the generalization of harm-reduction interventions and to the treatment of both HIV/AIDS and substance abuse. Opioid substitution therapy for the treatment of patients with heroin dependence, needle exchange programmes, access to Highly Active Antiretroviral Therapy (HAART) and supervised injecting facilities, among other preventive interventions, have contributed to reduce the impact of the HIV epidemic among drug users.

Surveillance of HIV infection in Spain is available in 15 out of the country's 17 autonomous regions. According to the National AIDS Programme, 2,264 new HIV infections were diagnosed in 2009, which represents 79 cases per million of the population [1].

As previously reported [2], the beginning of the HIV epidemic in Spain was largely driven by IDUs and the initial decrease in the rates of infection were reported more than a decade ago [3]. In 2009, 77% of new HIV infections were reported as sexually transmitted and IDUs represented less than 8% of cases [1].

The HIV epidemic among IDUs continues to develop differently across different parts of Europe. In the European Union, the reported rates of newly diagnosed cases of HIV infection in IDUs are mostly stable or in decline [4]. Data on newly reported cases of HIV infection in IDUs for 2009 suggest that rates of infection are still declining in Europe, following a peak in 2002, which was due to outbreaks in eastern countries. Reductions in the rates of HIV infection in IDUs are partially the result of better preventive interventions and access to care

[5,6], however, Spain is one of the western European countries reporting high rates of newly diagnosed HIV infection among IDUs between 2004 and 2009 (Figure 1)[4].

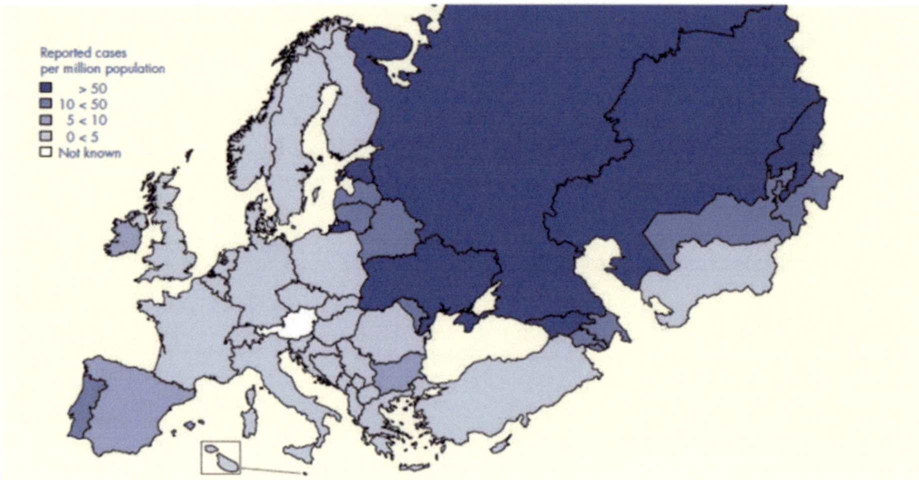

Figure 1. Newly diagnosed HIV infections among IDUs from Europe and central Asia in 2009. Source: *Annual Report 2011*, European Monitoring Centre for Drugs and Drug Addiction(4).

Several studies have shown that IDUs are at increased risk of sexually transmitted HIV infection [7,8] and other authors have shown higher rates of HIV infection among recent and younger IDUs [9,10].

Non-injecting drug users (non-IDUs) are not exposed to blood-borne infections, but remain at risk of sexually transmitted diseases including HIV. Some studies have found a relationship between non-IDU and the increased risk of HIV and other sexually transmitted diseases [11,12]. Moreover, there have been reports on the causal relationship between alcohol drinking and the risk of HIV infection [13-15].

1.1. Hepatitis B and C

About 80% of individuals exposed to hepatitis C virus (HCV) infection and 5% of adults exposed to hepatitis B virus (HBV) infection develop chronic liver disease. Cirrhosis and hepatocellular carcinoma are the most important sequelae of these infections [16].

It is well known that HCV infection is highly prevalent among drug users and that many IDUs contract the infection early in the course of injecting drugs; this implies that there may be only a small time window for initiating preventive interventions to reduce transmission of HCV infection.

About 10 million IDUs (range 6.0-15.2 million) worldwide were anti-HCV positive in 2010 and 1.2 million IDUs (range 0.3-2.7 million) were HBV infected (HBsAg positive). Geographical differences exist in the distribution of blood-borne infections among drug users and eastern Europe, east Asia and southeast Asia have the largest populations of IDUs infected with viral hepatitis [4,17].

Two major risk factors for HBV infection include the IDU his/herself and unprotected sex [18-21]. Studies among drug users from the United States have shown that 70% of cases are infected within five years of initiating drug use [22] and that 38%-89% of IDUs from Europe and North America have markers of HBV infection in cross-sectional studies [23].

In 2004, 16% of acute viral hepatitis reported to the Center for Disease Control in the United States had recent use of injected drugs as a risk factor [24].

In any case, the epidemiology of hepatitis B virus infection in drug users and other subpopulations at risk may vary according to the extent of preventive immunization; in Spain, the first selective hepatitis B vaccination programme began in 1984 [25].

In this study among IDUs and non-IDUs seeking treatment of substance abuse in Barcelona, Spain, we aimed to analyse trends in the epidemiology of HIV, HCV and HBV infections.

2. Patients and methods

2.1. Setting and study population

Prospective study in a cohort of patients admitted to substance abuse treatment programmes in three teaching hospitals between January 1997 and December 2006. The treatment units are located in Barcelona (Hospital del Mar), Badalona (Hospital Universitari Germans Trias i Pujol) and L'Hospitalet de Llobregat (Hospital Universitari de Bellvitge).

Patients admitted to treatment were referred from primary care centres and the principal criterion for admission was the severity of addiction. Patients were required to be older than 18 years and the main objective of admission was to control signs and symptoms of withdrawal. Upon admission, we collected socio-demographic characteristics, the history of substance abuse (main drug, age at first drug use, route of administration, history of opioid substitution treatment) and blood samples to test for HIV infection, HCV infection and HBV (HBcAb) infection, as previously reported [26,27].

The blood samples were tested by Enzyme ImmunoAssay (EIA) for antibodies to HIV infection and the results were confirmed by Western blot.

At discharge, patients were referred to their primary care providers. Pharmacological treatment was recommended in the majority of cases and all patients were advised to continue with medical visits at the outpatient clinics.

For the purposes of this study, patients who were admitted more than once between 1997 and 2006 were analysed only with regard to the first admission. Similarly, data from two hospitals were controlled so that no duplicate patients existed.

All the participants gave their consent for the determination of HIV and hepatitis serology. The methods utilized to perform this study complied with ethical standards for medical research and with principles of good clinical practice.

2.2. Statistical analysis

Bivariate analyses were performed on the characteristics of patients according to the route of drug administration: 1) non-IDU patients were defined as those individuals without a history of injection drug use; 2) IDU patients were defined as those with current or past use of intravenous drug use. The bivariate analyses included the χ^2 Pearson test for categorical variables and Student's t test for continuous variables.

Prevalent cases correspond to patients that tested HIV, HCV or HBV-positive at admission.

Incident cases were defined as those HIV-seronegative patients at admission that subsequently became HIV-positive during follow-up.

We carried out a direct measurement of HIV incidence based on the follow-up of the initially HIV-seronegative patients. However, due to the relatively low percentage (44%) of patients that underwent new HIV tests, we used a sensitivity analysis in a scenario based on the absence of new infections among those not re-tested for HIV infection during follow-up. Sensitivity analysis is useful in predicting the outcome of a decision if a situation turns out to be different compared to that which was previously assumed. By creating a given set of scenarios, the method can determine how changes in one variable will impact on the results.

All incidence rates were calculated in person-years with the number of HIV infections (incident cases) in the numerator and the sum of follow-up times in the denominator.

Joinpoint regression models were fitted to analyse changes in trends of HIV and viral hepatitis over time. These models evaluate changes that are produced on a logarithmic scale with a binomial distribution for the prevalence of infection and a Poisson distribution for the incidence of infection.

Descriptive analyses of the data were performed with STATA, version 8.0 (Stata Corp., College Station, TX, USA). For the Joinpoint regression models, we used the US National Cancer Institute's Joinpoint Regression Program software [28].

P values less than 0.05 ($p<0.05$) were considered statistically significant.

3. Results

3.1. Characteristics of the study population

Between January 1997 and December 2006 there were 3,318 admissions corresponding to 2,488 patients, of which 2,432 were eligible. Median age at admission was 34 years (IQR: 29 - 40 years) and 78.7% were men. A total of 925 (38%) patients were non-IDUs and 1,507 (62%) were current or past IDUs.

The baseline characteristics of the patients according to the antecedent of IDU/non-IDU are presented in Table 1. The majority of non-IDUs cases were patients with alcohol use disorders.

The main drug of abuse in IDUs patients was opiates (57.8%) and the median duration of drug abuse was 12 years (IQR:5 – 17 years); 28.9% of them were receiving methadone at admission. Non-IDU patients were significantly older (37 years, IQR 30 – 45 years) than in IDU (32 years, IQR 28 – 37 years) ($p<0.05$). The non-IDU were admitted mostly (65.1%) during the 2002 – 2006 period, whereas IDUs were admitted mostly (63%) during the 1997 – 2001 period ($p<0.05$). As expected, the prevalence of HCV infection was significantly higher in IDUs (86.6%) than in non-IDUs (9.7%) ($p< 0.05$). In this sense, the prevalence of hepatitis B virus infection (HBcAb-positive) was significantly higher in IDUs (56.8%) than in non-IDUs (17.7%) ($p<0.05$) (Table 1).

	Non-IDU	**IDU**	p-value
	N=925	N=1507	
	N (%)	*n (%)*	
Male	726 (78.5)	1188 (78.8)	0.840
Age *median [IQR]*	37 [30-45]	32 [28-37]	<0.05
Year of admission*median [IQR]*	2003 [2000-2005]	2000 [1998-2003]	<0.05
Period of admission			
1997-2001	323 (34.9)	949 (63.0)	
2002-2006	602 (65.1)	558 (37.0)	<0.05
Duration of drug abuse, years (n=1888) *median [IQR]*	10 [5-18]	12 [5-17]	0.079
HIV positive	26 (2.8)	636 (42.2)	<0.05
HCV positive (n=2394)	88 (9.7)	1284 (86.6)	<0.05
HBcAb positive (n=1890)	136 (17.7)	636 (56.8)	<0.05
Main drug of abuse (n=2421)			
Opiates	231 (25.1)	867 (57.8)	
Alcohol	432 (46.9)	124 (8.3)	
Other	258 (28.0)	509 (33.9)	<0.05
Antecedent of imprisonment (n=2291)	168 (19.4)	716 (50.2)	<0.05
Methadone* (n=1499)	46 (7.7)	261 (28.9)	<0.05

* Available in two hospitals

Table 1. Characteristics of IDU and non-IDU patients admitted to substance abuse treatment programmes in the Barcelona area, Spain, 1997-2006.

3.2. HIV infection

Table 2 shows the prevalence and incidence of HIV infection in non-IDUs according to the year of admission. Regarding HIV prevalence, 2.8% (95% CI: 1.8-4.1) of patients were HIV-positive at admission with the highest prevalence of infection observed in 1999 (8.3%).

Among the 899 non-IDU, HIV-negative patients, 364 (40.5%) were followed-up for a median of 2.3 years (IQR: 0.9 – 4.1 years; 1060 p-y); only five patients acquired HIV infection during follow-up (incidence rate 0.47 x 100 p-y; 95% CI: 0.2-1.1).

The prevalence of HIV in IDUs was 42.2% (636/1507). The highest prevalence was observed in 1997 (45.1%) and the lowest in 2006 (32.1%).

Among the 871 IDUs, HIV-negative patients, 47.1% were followed for a median of 2.7 years (IQR: 1.2 - 5.2 years, 1415.5 p-y) and 36 acquired HIV infection (incidence rate 2.54 x 100 p-y (95% CI: 1.8-3.5); the highest rate of infection was observed in 1999 (3.7 x 100p-y). Patients followed-up were similar to those not followed regarding the proportion of male/female, the main drug of abuse and the prevalence of HCV infection and HBV (HBcAb) infection.

	HIV PREVALENCE		HIV INCIDENCE					
			Patients at risk	Patients followed	P-Y	Incident cases	Incident rate	
	n (%)	*95% CI*		*n (%)*			*x100 p-y*	*95% CI*
1997	0 (0.0)	--	51	24 (47.1)	13.7	0	0.00	--
1998	2 (3.3)	(0.4-11.3)	59	30 (50.8)	37.8	1	2.65	(0.4-18.8)
1999	5 (8.3)	(2.8-18.4)	55	25 (45.5)	52.1	0	0.00	--
2000	2 (2.7)	(0.3-9.4)	72	24 (33.3)	71.1	0	0.00	--
2001	1 (1.3)	(0.03-7.0)	76	34 (44.7)	93.9	0	0.00	--
2002	4 (3.9)	(1.1-9.6)	99	44 (44.4)	112.8	0	0.00	--
2003	2 (1.7)	(0.2-6.0)	116	50 (43.1)	138.3	1	0.72	(0.1-5.1)
2004	3 (2.5)	(0.5-7.0)	119	50 (42.0)	170.1	1	0.59	(0.1-4.2)
2005	3 (2.5)	(0.5-7.0)	118	35 (29.7)	184.9	1	0.54	(0.1-3.8)
2006	4 (2.9)	(0.8-7.2)	134	48 (35.8)	185.3	1	0.54	(0.1-3.8)
1997-2006	26 (2.8)	(1.8-4.1)	899	364 (40.5)	1060	5	0.47	(0.2-1.1)

Table 2. HIV serial prevalence and HIV serial incidence among non-IDUs by year of admission to substance abuse treatment programmes in the Barcelona area, Spain, 1997-2006.

http://dx.doi.org/10.5772/53074

Table 3 shows the prevalence and incidence of HIV infection in IDUs according to the year of admission, ultimately showing values slightly lower than the rates registered since 1999.

Trends of HIV prevalence in non-IDUs is shown in the upper part of Figure 2 (Graphic A). Overall, changes in HIV prevalence were not statistically significant, in spite of the model indicating a decrease in prevalence over time (p=0.24).

In terms of HIV incidence (Figure 2, Graphic B), the model shows statistically significant differences over time (p=0.004).

The trend of HIV prevalence in IDUs showed a significant (p=0.01) decline between 1997 and 2006 (Figure 3, Graphic A). With respect to HIV incidence among IDUs, no changes in the trends of infection rate were detected after adjusting the regression model (p=0.944) (Figure 3, Graphic B).

	HIV PREVALENCE		**HIV INCIDENCE**					
			Patients at risk	**Patients followed**	**P-Y**	**Incident cases**	**Incident rate**	
	n (%)	*95% CI*		*n (%)*			*x100 p-y*	*95% CI*
1997	124 (45.1)	(39.1-51.2)	151	84 (55.6)	45.3	1	2.21	(0.3-15.7)
1998	84 (43.5)	(36.4-50.8)	109	63 (57.8)	102.4	2	1.95	(0.5-7.8)
1999	83 (44.4)	(37.1-51.8)	104	52 (50.0)	133.3	5	3.75	(1.6-9.0)
2000	71 (41.8)	(34.3-59.6)	99	47 (47.5)	153.5	3	1.95	(0.6-6.1)
2001	53 (42.7)	(33.9-51.9)	71	29 (40.8)	163.3	4	2.45	(0.9-6.5)
2002	59 (38.6)	(30.8-46.8)	94	35 (37.2)	168.9	3	1.77	(0.6-5.5)
2003	50 (42.7)	(33.6-52.2)	67	31 (46.3)	174.0	6	3.45	(1.5-7.7)
2004	53 (42.7)	(33.9-51.9)	71	31 (43.7)	175.6	5	2.85	(1.2-6.8)
2005	34 (39.5)	(29.1-50.7)	52	21 (40.4)	160.4	4	2.49	(0.9-6.6)
2006	25 (32.1)	(21.9-43.6)	53	17 (32.1)	138.8	3	2.16	(0.7-6.7)
1997-2006	636 (42.2)	(39.7-44.7)	871	410 (47.1)	1415.5	36	2.54	(1.8-3.5)

Table 3. HIV serial prevalence and HIV serial incidence in IDUs by year of admission to substance abuse treatment programmes in the Barcelona area, Spain, 1997-2006.

In sensitivity analysis, the rate of HIV infection among non-IDUs was 0.19x100 p-y (95% CI: 0.07-0.45) and 1.08 x100p-y (95% CI: 0.5-1.5) among IDUs.

In sensitivity analysis, trends of HIV incidence for non-IDU patients remained unchanged with respect to the direct method. However, HIV incidence for IDUs significantly decreased over time in the best scenario (no new infections among those lost to follow-up, p=0.04).

3.3. Viral hepatitis

The prevalence of HCV infection and HBV (HBcAb) infection in non-IDUs was 9.7%, and 17.7%, respectively. The prevalence of HCV in the years analysed oscillated between 6.8% and 15.6%, but differences were not statistically significant (p=0.589) (Figure 4, Graphic A). As expected, the prevalence of HCV infection in IDUs was high (86.6%) and changes over the years analysed were negligible (p=0.240) (Figure 5, Graphic A).

The prevalence of HBV (HBcAb) infection in non-IDUs oscillated between 8.3% and 22.9%, and changes over time were not statistically significant (p=0.696) (Figure 4, Graphic B). HBV (HBcAb) infection was observed in 56.8% of IDUs, which oscillated between 48.8% and 64.3% in the years analysed. Analysis of the trend did not show statistically significant differences during the period analysed (p=0.218) (Figure 5, Graphic B).

Graphic A

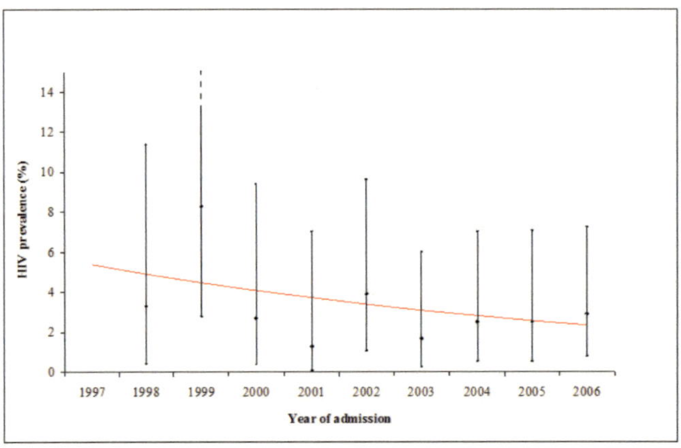

Graphic B

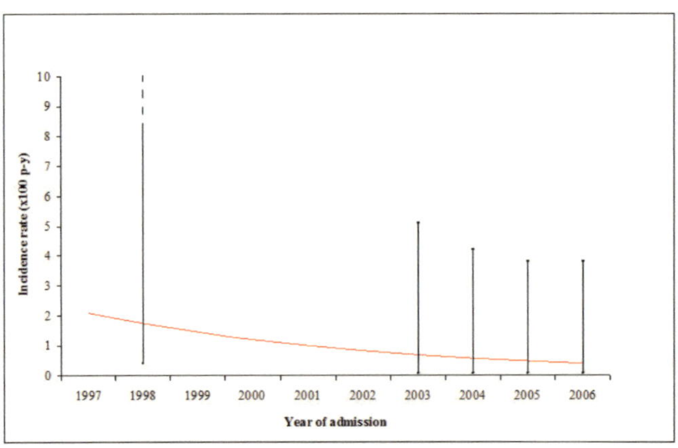

Figure 2. Trends in HIV prevalence (Graphic A) and HIV incidence (Graphic B) in non-IDU patients admitted to substance abuse treatment programmes in the Barcelona area, Spain, 1997- 2006.

http://dx.doi.org/10.5772/53074

Graphic A

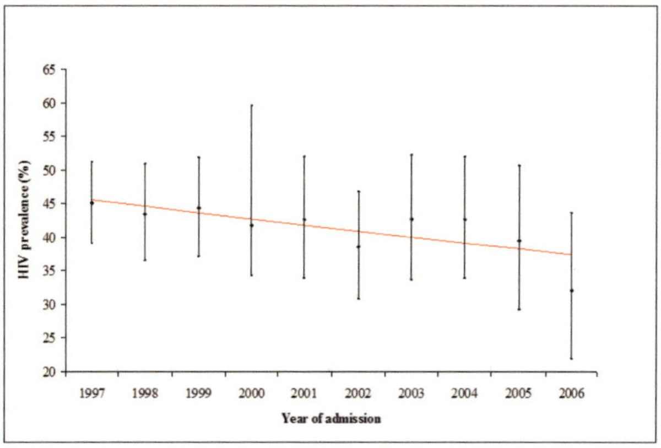

Graphic B

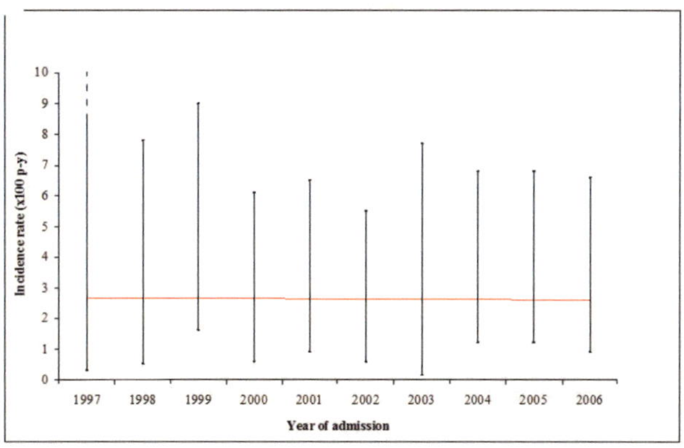

Figure 3. Trends in HIV prevalence (Graphic A) and HIV incidence (Graphic B) in IDUs admitted to substance abuse treatment programmes in the Barcelona area, Spain, 1997- 2006.

Graphic A

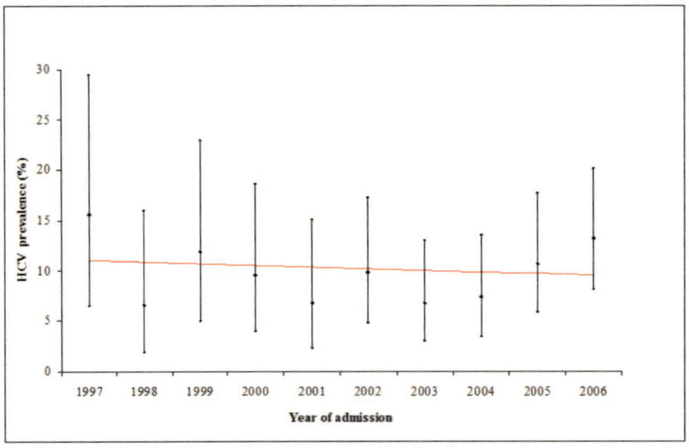

Graphic B

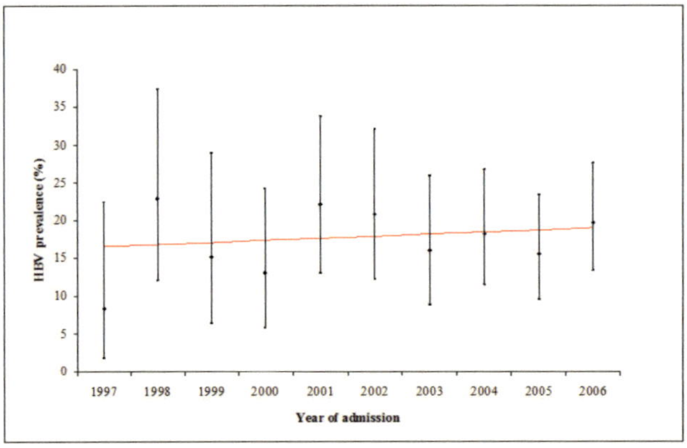

Figure 4. Prevalence of HCV infection (Graphic A) and HBV infection (Graphic B) in non-IDUs admitted to treatment programmes in the Barcelona area, Spain, 1997- 2006.

http://dx.doi.org/10.5772/53074

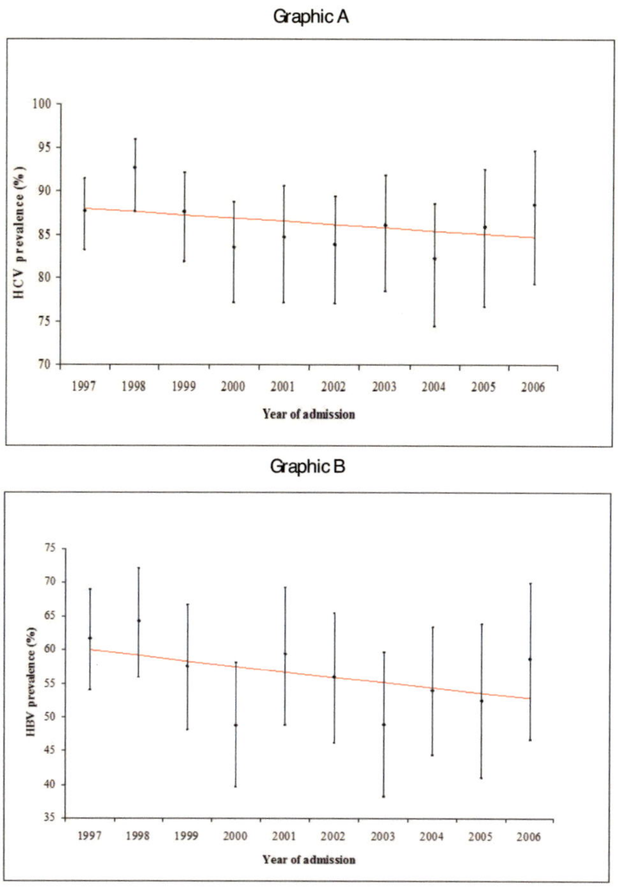

Figure 5. Prevalence of HCV infection (Graphic A) and HBV infection (Graphic B) in IDUs admitted to treatment programmes in the Barcelona area, Spain, 1997- 2006.

4. Discussion

Results from this cohort of patients seeking substance abuse treatment indicate that drug users, irrespective of the main route of drug administration, are at increased risk of HIV infection and viral hepatitis. In fact, the prevalence of HIV infection and HCV infection in non-IDU patients is 2.8% and 9.7%, respectively. Several studies analysing risky sexual behaviour of drug and alcohol abusers suggest an association between cocaine, amphetamines or alcohol abuse and the sexual transmission of HIV [19-24], which could explain the relatively high prevalence of HIV infection among non-IDU patients from this study [29-34]. Despite the relatively high prevalence of HIV infection, there was a trend in the decline of HIV incidence among the non-IDUs. To some extent, the incidence of HIV infection was low (0.47 per 100 p-y) and the results shown here indicate that non-IDUs have a fivefold lower risk of HIV than the IDUs, as shown in a previous study [35].

The observed decline in the prevalence of HIV infection among IDUs is likely the result of some preventive interventions introduced in Spain at the beginning of 1990s. Harm-reduction interventions to reduce the impact of the HIV epidemic associated with heroin dependence included the access to opioid substitution therapy with methadone and the needle exchange programmes, among other interventions. Our findings indicate that HIV infection among IDUs from metropolitan Barcelona has stabilized and that rates of new infections are moderate with respect to reports from other cities [36-38]. In addition, our results agree with those reported nationally, indicating that sexual transmission now represents 80% of new HIV infections in Spain [39]. Further, our results show that the proportion of IDUs being admitted for substance abuse treatment is declining, suggesting a decrease in the number of IDUs in Spain [40].

Data from European countries show tendencies toward a low rate of HIV infection in drug users. For example, Poland, Finland and Germany have considerably reduced the rates of infection to two cases per million inhabitants in 2007 [41]. In this study, we determined an overall rate of infection of 2.54 per 100 p-y between 1997 and 2006, which is similar to that observed in other studies [6].

In contrast, the decline in the prevalence of HIV infection is not accompanied by a decline in HCV prevalence [42,43]. This observation suggests that IDUs still maintain non-sterile injection practices. The HIV and hepatitis C virus are transmitted primarily by large or repeated direct percutaneous exposures to contaminated blood. In Spain, IDU is a factor in 28% of all contemporary AIDS cases and it accounts for more than 60% of new hepatitis C infections in Europe and the USA [1,44].

It is well known that the majority of IDUs become infected with hepatitis C during their first year of injecting and that because of its infectivity HCV spreads more rapidly than HIV [45,46,47].

In this study, the prevalence of HBV is high. A recent systematic review suggests that worldwide around 1.2 million IDUs are chronic carriers of HBV infection and that the pat-

http://dx.doi.org/10.5772/53074

tern of infection shows clear geographical differences [17]. In fact, rates of HBcAb-positive varied widely between countries from 4.2% in Slovenia to 85.0% in Mexico [17].

Because of the high rate of both HCV and HBV infection, the probability of coinfection in IDUs is high. In this sense, vaccination against HBV must be prioritized for all susceptible drug users.

There are several limitations to this study that need to be mentioned. First of all, a proportion of patients, HIV-seronegative, were not re-tested for HIV infection during follow-up despite the fact that many of them were regularly visited in their primary care centres; in this sense, assessment of risk behaviour and awareness of drug use disorders by health care professionals are key components for developing preventive interventions. Second, in this study assessment of HBV infection was limited to one marker of infection; in other words, more accurate estimation of chronic carriers of HBV infection, susceptibility to infection or immunization due to HBV vaccination was not available. For the HCV pattern of infection we only analysed antibodies against HCV and RNA-HCV was not available; it is well known that a minority (10-15%) of the individuals infected with HCV clear the virus during the natural history of the disease. Third, in this study we did not analyse the impact of sexual transmission of HIV and viral hepatitis on the results shown here. In this sense, drug-addicted women have been reported to have a higher risk of HIV infection than drug-addicted men [48].

In contrast, the strength of this cross-sectional and longitudinal study is based on data collected at three centres that provide clinical care and treatment for the majority of severe drug addicts in Barcelona and its metropolitan area. Having data from the three hospitals adds external validity to the results and may reflect changes in the epidemiology of HIV and viral hepatitis in young adults seeking treatment for substance abuse in an urban area.

In summary, since 1997 we observed a significant decline in the prevalence of HIV infection in IDUs, however, background prevalence of HIV and viral hepatitis is still high thus suggesting that prevention efforts and treatment of substance abuse are necessary to further reduce transmission of blood-borne infections in this population.

Nomenclature

HIV= Human Immunodeficiency Virus.

IDU= Injecting Drug User.

AIDS= Acquired Immunodeficiency Syndrome.

HAART= Highly Active Antiretroviral Therapy.

HCV= Hepatitis C virus.

HBV= Hepatitis B virus.

HBsAg= Surface Antigen of Hepatitis B Virus.

HBcAb= Hepatitis B core Antibody.

EIA= Enzyme Immunoassay.

IQR= Interquartile Range.

CI= Confidence Interval.

RNA= Ribonucleic Acid

Acknowledgments

This work was partially funded by grants from the Ministry of Science and Innovation, Spain (grants RD06/001, RD06/006 and PI07/0342), Ministry of Health (grant EC11-042) and Ministry of Education (grant 2010-0945).

Author details

Arantza Sanvisens[1], Ferran Bolao[2], Gabriel Vallecillo[3], Marta Torrens[4], Daniel Fuster[5,8], Santiago Pérez-Hoyos[6], Jordi Tor[5], Inmaculada Rivas[7] and Robert Muga[1*]

*Address all correspondence to: rmuga.germanstrias@gencat.cat

1 Department of Internal Medicine and AIDS Vaccine Research Project – HIVACAT. Hospital Universitari Germans Trias i Pujol, Badalona, Universitat Autònoma Barcelona, Spain

2 Department of Internal Medicine. Hospital Universitari de Bellvitge, L'Hospitalet de Llobregat, Universitat de Barcelona, Spain

3 Department of Internal Medicine and Institute of Neuropsychiatry & Addictions. Parc de Salut Mar, Barcelona, Universitat Autònoma Barcelona, Spain

4 Institute of Neuropsychiatry & Addictions. Parc de Salut Mar, Barcelona, Universitat Autònoma Barcelona, Spain

5 Department of Internal Medicine. Hospital Universitari Germans Trias i Pujol, Badalona, Universitat Autònoma Barcelona, Spain

6 Department of Preventive Medicine and Public Health. Vall d'Hebrón Institut de Recerca. Universitat Autònoma Barcelona, Spain

7 Municipal Centre for Substance Abuse Treatment (Centro Delta). IMSP Badalona, Spain

8 Section of General Internal Medicine. Boston Medical Center, Boston University School of Medicine; Boston (MA), U.S.A.

References

[1] Vigilancia epidemiológica del VIH en España. Nuevos diagnósticos de VIH en España. Periodo 2003-2009. Ministerio de Sanidad, Política Social e Igualdad, Ministerio de Ciencia e Innovación; 2010.

[2] Hernandez-Aguado I, Avino MJ, Perez-Hoyos S, Gonzalez-Aracil J, Ruiz-Perez I, Torrella A, et al. Human immunodeficiency virus (HIV) infection in parenteral drug users: evolution of the epidemic over 10 years. Valencian Epidemiology and Prevention of HIV Disease Study Group. Int J Epidemiol 1999;28(2):335-340.

[3] Castilla J, Lorenzo JM, Izquierdo A, Lezaun ME, Lopez I, Moreno-Iribas C, et al. Characteristics and trends of newly diagnosed HIV-infections, 2000-2004. Gac Sanit 2006;20(6):442-448.

[4] European Monitoring Centre for Drugs and Drug Addiction. Annual report 2011: The state of the drug problems in Europe. EMCDDA, Lisbon, November 2011. http://www.emcdda.europa.eu/attachements.cfm/att_143743_EN_EMCDDA_AR2011_EN.pdf (accessed 30 July 2012)

[5] Muga R, Sanvisens A, Bolao F, Tor J, Santesmases J, Pujol R, et al. Significant reductions of HIV prevalence but not of hepatitis C virus infections in injection drug users from metropolitan Barcelona: 1987-2001. Drug Alcohol Depend 2006;82 Suppl 1:S29-33.

[6] Hurtado I, Alastrue I, Ferreros I, del Amo J, Santos C, Tasa T, et al. Trends in HIV testing, serial HIV prevalence and HIV incidence among people attending a Center for AIDS Prevention from 1988 to 2003. Sex Transm Infect 2007;83(1):23-28. DOI: 10.1136/sti.2005.019299.

[7] Celentano DD, Latimore AD, Mehta SH. Variations in sexual risks in drug users: emerging themes in a behavioral context. Curr HIV/AIDS Rep 2008;5(4):212-218.

[8] Nelson KE, Galai N, Safaeian M, Strathdee SA, Celentano DD, Vlahov D. Temporal trends in the incidence of human immunodeficiency virus infection and risk behavior among injection drug users in Baltimore, Maryland, 1988-1998. Am J Epidemiol 2002;156(7):641-653.

[9] Chitwood DD, Comerford M, Sanchez J. Prevalence and risk factors for HIV among sniffers, short-term injectors, and long-term injectors of heroin. J Psychoactive Drugs 2003;35(4):445-453.

[10] Miller CL, Wood E, Spittal PM, Li K, Frankish JC, Braitstein P, et al. The future face of coinfection: prevalence and incidence of HIV and hepatitis C virus coinfection among young injection drug users. J Acquir Immune Defic Syndr 2004;36(2):743-749.

[11] Jenness SM, Neaigus A, Hagan H, Murrill CS, Wendel T. Heterosexual HIV and sexual partnerships between injection drug users and noninjection drug users. AIDS Patient Care STDS 2010;24(3):175-181. DOI:10.1089/apc.2009.0227.

[12] Strathdee SA, Sherman SG. The role of sexual transmission of HIV infection among injection and non-injection drug users. J Urban Health 2003;80(4 Suppl 3):iii7-14.

[13] Howe CJ, Cole SR, Ostrow DG, Mehta SH, Kirk GD. A prospective study of alcohol consumption and HIV acquisition among injection drug users. AIDS 2011;25(2): 221-228. DOI:10.1097/QAD.0b013e328340fee2.

[14] Zakhari S, Li TK. Determinants of alcohol use and abuse: Impact of quantity and frequency patterns on liver disease. Hepatology 2007;46(6):2032-2039. DOI:10.1002/hep. 22010.

[15] Shuper PA, Neuman M, Kanteres F, Baliunas D, Joharchi N, Rehm J. Causal considerations on alcohol and HIV/AIDS--a systematic review. Alcohol Alcohol 2010;45(2): 159-166. DOI:10.1093/alcalc/agp091.

[16] Te HS, Jensen DM. Epidemiology of hepatitis B and C viruses: a global overview. Clin Liver Dis 2010;14(1):1-21, vii. DOI:10.1016/j.cld.2009.11.009.

[17] Nelson PK, Mathers BM, Cowie B, Hagan H, Des Jarlais D, Horyniak D, et al. Global epidemiology of hepatitis B and hepatitis C in people who inject drugs: results of systematic reviews. Lancet 2011;378(9791):571-583. DOI:10.1016/S0140-6736(11)61097-0.

[18] Mast EE, Weinbaum CM, Fiore AE, Alter MJ, Bell BP, Finelli L, et al. A comprehensive immunization strategy to eliminate transmission of hepatitis B virus infection in the United States: recommendations of the Advisory Committee on Immunization Practices (ACIP) Part II: immunization of adults. MMWR Recomm Rep 2006;55(RR-16):1-33; quiz CE1-4.

[19] Kuo I, Sherman SG, Thomas DL, Strathdee SA. Hepatitis B virus infection and vaccination among young injection and non-injection drug users: missed opportunities to prevent infection. Drug Alcohol Depend 2004;73(1):69-78.

[20] Alter MJ. Epidemiology and prevention of hepatitis B. Semin Liver Dis 2003;23(1): 39-46. DOI:10.1055/s-2003-37583.

[21] Goldstein ST, Alter MJ, Williams IT, Moyer LA, Judson FN, Mottram K, et al. Incidence and risk factors for acute hepatitis B in the United States, 1982-1998: implications for vaccination programs. J Infect Dis 2002;185(6):713-719. DOI:10.1086/339192.

[22] Garfein RS, Vlahov D, Galai N, Doherty MC, Nelson KE. Viral infections in short-term injection drug users: the prevalence of the hepatitis C, hepatitis B, human immunodeficiency, and human T-lymphotropic viruses. Am J Public Health 1996;86(5): 655-661.

[23] Levine OS, Vlahov D, Koehler J, Cohn S, Spronk AM, Nelson KE. Seroepidemiology of hepatitis B virus in a population of injecting drug users. Association with drug injection patterns. Am J Epidemiol 1995;142(3):331-341.

[24] Burt RD, Hagan H, Garfein RS, Sabin K, Weinbaum C, Thiede H. Trends in hepatitis B virus, hepatitis C virus, and human immunodeficiency virus prevalence, risk be-

haviors, and preventive measures among Seattle injection drug users aged 18-30 years, 1994-2004. J Urban Health 2007;84(3):436-454. DOI:10.1007/s11524-007-9178-2.

[25] Salleras L, Bruguera M, Taberner JL, Dominguez A, Batalla J, Buti M, et al. Effectiveness of the mass antihepatitis B program in preadolescents in Catalonia. Med Clin (Barc) 2003;121 Suppl 1:79-82.

[26] Muga R, Roca J, Egea JM, Tor J, Sirera G, Rey-Joly C, et al. Mortality of HIV-positive and HIV-negative heroin abusers as a function of duration of injecting drug use. J Acquir Immune Defic Syndr 2000;23(4):332-338.

[27] Rivas I, Martinez E, Sanvisens A, Bolao F, Tor J, Torrens M, et al. Hepatitis B virus serum profiles in injection drug users and rates of immunization over time in Barcelona: 1987-2006. Drug Alcohol Depend 2010;110(3):234-9. DOI:10.1016/j.drugalcdep.2010.03.005.

[28] US National Cancer Institute Software. Jointpoint Regression Program. 2010;3.4.3.

[29] Wang B, Li X, Stanton B, Zhang L, Fang X. Alcohol Use, Unprotected Sex, and Sexually Transmitted Infections Among Female Sex Workers in China. Sex Transm Dis 2010;37(10):629-36. DOI:10.1097/OLQ.0b013e3181e2118a.

[30] Baliunas D, Rehm J, Irving H, Shuper P. Alcohol consumption and risk of incident human immunodeficiency virus infection: a meta-analysis. Int J Public Health 2010;55(3):159-166. DOI:10.1007/s00038-009-0095-x.

[31] Booth RE, Kwiatkowski CF, Chitwood DD. Sex related HIV risk behaviors: differential risks among injection drug users, crack smokers, and injection drug users who smoke crack. Drug Alcohol Depend 2000;58(3):219-226.

[32] de Azevedo RC, Botega NJ, Guimaraes LA. Crack users, sexual behavior and risk of HIV infection. Rev Bras Psiquiatr 2007;29(1):26-30.

[33] Colfax G, Santos GM, Chu P, Vittinghoff E, Pluddemann A, Kumar S, et al. Amphetamine-group substances and HIV. Lancet 2010;376(9739):458-474. DOI:10.1016/S0140-6736(10)60753-2.

[34] Van Tieu H, Koblin BA. HIV, alcohol, and noninjection drug use. Curr Opin HIV AIDS 2009;4(4):314-318. DOI:10.1097/COH.0b013e32832aa902.

[35] Kellogg TA, McFarland W, Perlman JL, Weinstock H, Bock S, Katz MH, et al. HIV incidence among repeat HIV testers at a county hospital, San Francisco, California, USA. J Acquir Immune Defic Syndr 2001;28(1):59-64.

[36] Kozlov AP, Shaboltas AV, Toussova OV, Verevochkin SV, Masse BR, Perdue T, et al. HIV incidence and factors associated with HIV acquisition among injection drug users in St Petersburg, Russia. AIDS 2006;20(6):901-906. DOI:10.1097/01.aids.0000218555.36661.9c.

[37] Duan S, Xiang LF, Yang YC, Ye RH, Jia MH, Luo HB, et al. Incidence and risk factors on HIV infection among injection drug users in Dehong prefecture area of Yunnan province. Zhonghua Liu Xing Bing Xue Za Zhi 2009;30(12):1226-1229.

[38] Hurtado Navarro I, Alastrue I, Del Amo J, Santos C, Ferreros I, Tasa T, et al. Differences between women and men in serial HIV prevalence and incidence trends. Eur J Epidemiol 2008;23(6):435-440. DOI:10.1007/s10654-008-9246-2.

[39] Valoración de los nuevos diagnósticos de VIH en España a partir de los sistemas de notificación de casos de las CCAA. Periodo 2003-2008. Ministerio de Sanidad y Política Social, Ministerio de Ciencia e Innovación;2009. http://www.isciii.es/htdocs/pdf/nuevos_diagnosticos_ccaa.pdf. (accessed 30 july 2012)

[40] Sanchez-Niubo A, Domingo-Salvany A, Melis GG, Brugal MT, Scalia-Tomba G. Two methods to analyze trends in the incidence of heroin and cocaine use in Barcelona [Spain]. Gac Sanit 2007;21(5):397-403.

[41] European Monitoring centre for Drugs and Drug Addiction. Drug-related infectious diseases and drug-related deaths. http://www.emcdda.europa.eu/situation/diseases-and-deaths/1 (accessed 30 july 2012).

[42] Somaini B, Wang J, Perozo M, Kuhn F, Meili D, Grob P, et al. A continuing concern: HIV and hepatitis testing and prevalence among drug users in substitution programmes in Zurich, Switzerland. AIDS Care 2000;12(4):449-460. DOI: 10.1080/09540120050123855.

[43] van Beek I, Dwyer R, Dore GJ, Luo K, Kaldor JM. Infection with HIV and hepatitis C virus among injecting drug users in a prevention setting: retrospective cohort study. BMJ 1998;317(7156):433-437.

[44] Centers for Disease Control and Prevention (CDC). HIV Infection Among Injection-Drug Users --- 34 States, 2004--2007. MMWR 2009;58:1291-1295.

[45] Thorpe LE, Ouellet LJ, Levy JR, Williams IT, Monterroso ER. Hepatitis C virus infection: prevalence, risk factors, and prevention opportunities among young injection drug users in Chicago, 1997-1999. J Infect Dis 2000;182(6):1588-1594. DOI: 10.1086/317607.

[46] Garfein RS, Vlahov D, Galai N, Doherty MC, Nelson KE. Viral infections in short-term injection drug users: the prevalence of the hepatitis C, hepatitis B, human immunodeficiency, and human T-lymphotropic viruses. Am J Public Health 1996;86(5):655-661.

[47] Hagan H, Des Jarlais DC. HIV and HCV infection among injecting drug users. Mt Sinai J Med 2000;67(5-6):423-428.

[48] Evans JL, Hahn JA, Page-Shafer K, Lum PJ, Stein ES, Davidson PJ, et al. Gender differences in sexual and injection risk behavior among active young injection drug users in San Francisco (the UFO Study). J Urban Health 2003;80(1):137-146. DOI: 10.1093/jurban/jtg137.

Chapter 17

Prevention of Sexually Transmitted HIV Infection

Jose G. Castro and Maria L. Alcaide

Additional information is available at the end of the chapter

http://dx.doi.org/10.5772/54168

1. Introduction

Bio-medical prevention of sexually transmitted HIV infection is an evolving area in the field of HIV. In recent years, multiple studies have demonstrated the efficacy of diverse biomedical interventions to prevent the sexual acquisition of HIV infection in specific populations. The major developments in the field of prevention of sexual transmission of HIV include male circumcision, HIV viral suppression of HIV infected individuals (Treatment of positives), use of antiretrovirals before exposure to HIV (Pre-exposure prophylaxis), and use of microbicides. Some of these highly controlled studies demonstrated high levels of protection ranging from 55 to more than 90% when a single intervention has been studied. However, in real world situations, it is foreseeable that individuals will have the opportunity and option to choose, and ideally to combine, appropriate interventions according to their background, attitudes, preferences and availability of methods.

Male circumcision: Male circumcision effectively decreases rates of heterosexual transmission of HIV: There is now ample scientific evidence that male circumcision reduces the risk of acquiring HIV through heterosexual intercourse in males by approximately 51 to 60%, thus exceeding the 30 percent risk reduction set as a target for an AIDS vaccine. This level of protection is similar to the 67.5% relative reduction in the risk of maternal-infant transmission of HIV with the use of zidovudine in HIV infected pregnant women; currently one of the most successful strategies to prevent HIV infection in a selected population, newborns. The evidence of the effectiveness of male circumcision in decreasing the risk of HIV infection in males is so compelling that in March 2007, the World Health Organization and the Joint United Nations Programme on HIV/AIDS held a technical consultation on male circumcision and produced a document that stated that male circumcision should be recognized as an efficacious intervention for the prevention of heterosexually acquired HIV infection in men. Male circumcision (MC) has been proven to be a potent HIV prevention strategy, reducing risk of HIV acquisition in heterosexual men by 50-60%. One of the most successful interventions to prevent the acquisition of HIV infection in heterosexual men is circumcision, which has reduced HIV risk by 50-60% among heterosexual men in sub-Saharan Africa. The uptake of male circumcision in traditionally non-circumcision communities have been varied and influenced by different factor. In the US males from racial and ethnic minorities are less likely to be circumcised and also more likely to become infected with HIV so a recently published analyses showed that newborn circumcision resulted in lower expected HIV-related treatment costs and a slight increase in quality-adjusted life years.

Treatment of Positives: Since the early years of the epidemic, it was demonstrated that the use of antiretrovirals in infected pregnant women decreased the likelihood of HIV infection in the new born. Additional studies demonstrated that the key factor in the transmission of the infection from the mother to the newborn was the maternal HIV viral load; and then the suppression of HIV by the administration of antiretrovirals became the standard of care in the management of HIV infected pregnant women. This practice led to the almost eradication of congenital HIV infection in communities with access to medications. Circumstantial evidence suggested that the same principle could be applied to the sexual transmission of HIV as in general there is correlation between the HIV viral load in blood and genital secretions. In 2011 a breakthrough study proved that treatment of HIV positive decreased the likelihood of sexual transmission in more than 96% in discordant heterosexual couples.

Pre-exposure prophylaxis (PrEP) in MSM and heterosexual men and women: PrEP involves the use of antiretroviral medications before potential HIV exposure to prevent infection. In recent years several studies suggested the possible efficacy of the use of TDF/FTC as PrEP; but in the last six months, several controlled studies have provided definitive proof of its efficacy in certain populations: iPrEx was a study that randomized 2499 HIV-negative MSM or transgender women who have sex with men to take oral daily tenofovir and emtricitabine (FTC/TDF) or placebo. Overall, 100 subjects became infected during the study (36 in the FTC/TDF group and 64 in the placebo group), indicating a 44% reduction in the HIV incidence. The Partners PrEP Study was a phase III, randomized, double blind, placebo-controlled, three arm trial of oral daily (FTC/TDF) PrEP for the prevention of HIV acquisition by HIV seronegative partner in HIV serodiscordant partnerships. The independent DSMB recommended that the results of the study be publically reported, nearly 2 years earlier than expected, and the placebo arm discontinued, because clear demonstration of HIV protection due to PrEP. The TDF2A was a double-blind, randomized, trial of daily oral FTC/TDF or placebo for prevention of HIV acquisition in young (18-39) women and men in Bostwana. A total of 1219 individuals were randomized, about 30% of the study population did not complete follow up. Adherence to PrEP overall was estimated to be approximately 84%. Overall 9 HIV infections occurred among those assigned to FTC/TDF compared to 24 among those assigned to placebo, translating to an efficacy for HIV protection of 63%. All these studies shown that PrEP is a viable biomedical intervention that can be use for the prevention of sexually transmitted HIV infection in both heterosexual and male who have sex with men populations but is highly dependent of the adherence to the medications. There are few promising agents that could be use over extended periods of time decreasing the need for daily medication.

Microbicides: Given the theoretical advantages of a microbicide (controlled by women, no need for male cooperation) the search for an effective product was elusive until investigators from CAPRISA 004 study reported at the World AIDS conference in 2010 in Vienna, that 1% tenofovir gel used with coitus reduced HIV risk by 39% among 889 South African women. Sub-analyses of the data showed that protection was more pronounced (54%) in women with higher adherence to the gel. Several studies are under way with other products and with alternative delivery systems that will alleviate the need for strict adherence to its use before and after sex.

2. Bio-medical interventions to prevent hiv sexually transmitted infection

2.1. Male circumcision

Male circumcision is the surgical procedure that consists in the removal of some or all the foreskin of the penis [1]. The word "circumcision" comes from the Latin circum (meaning "around") and caedere (meaning "to cut") [2]. The foreskin is a continuation of the skin from the shaft of the penis, which covers the glans penis and the urethral meatus. The foreskin is attached to the glans by the frenulum, a highly vascularized tissue of the penis. Male circumcision is one of the oldest surgical procedures known, traditionally undertaken as a mark of cultural identity or religious importance [3]. Rates of male circumcision are different around the word and related to cultural and religious beliefs [4]. Historically, male circumcision has been associated with religious practice and ethnic identity. Circumcision was practiced among ancient Semitic peoples including Egyptians and Jews, with the earliest records depicting the practice coming from Egyptian tomb artwork (from the Sixth Dynasty, 2345-2181 B.C.) and wall paintings dating from around 2300 BC [3]. Muslims are the largest religious group to practice male circumcision. As an Abrahamic faith, Muslims practice circumcision, as a confirmation of their relationship with God, and the practice is also known as tahera, meaning purification [3]. With the global spread of Islam from the 7th century AD, circumcision was widely adopted among previously non-circumcising peoples. In some regions, male circumcision was already a cultural tradition prior to the arrival of Islam (for example among the Poro in West Africa, and in Timor in SE Asia). [5-7] Circumcision has also been practice for non-religious reasons for many thousand of years in sub-Saharan Africa, and in many ethnic groups around the world, including aboriginal Australasians, the Aztecs and Mayans in the Americas, inhabitants of the Philippines and eastern Indonesia and various pacific Islands, including Fiji and the Polynesian islands [3]. In the majority of these cultures, circumcision is an integral part of a rite of passage to manhood, although originally it may have been a test of bravery and endurance. Male circumcision traditionally has been done for medical and non medical reasons (including religious or cultural reasons). When it is practiced for non-medical reasons it is typically performed in the neonatal period or just before the adolescence. The practice of circumcision, in particular of neonatal circumcision remains highly controversial despite recent evidence of the medical benefits, including decreased risk of heterosexual acquisition of HIV infection by men, decreased risk of acquisition of several sexually transmitted infections, decreased risk of urinary tract infection and recent evidence of decreased risk of prostate cancer [8-10]. There are no reliable data of the rate of circumcision in many areas of the world in particular in regions where is not commonly practiced; but in general it is believed that rates of circumcision are very low in Latin-America including the Caribbean region, China, India and Europe [2], Fig 1.

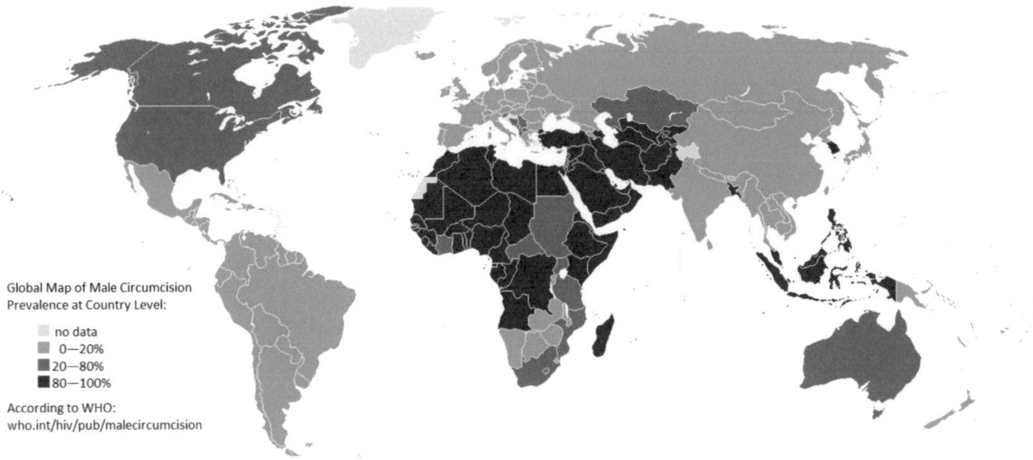

Global map of male circumcision prevalence at country level, as of December 2006.

Figure 1. Worldwide prevalence of Male Circumcision.

2.1.1. Studies addressing MC in the field of HIV prevention

2.1.1.1. Cohort studies

The first paper suggesting a protective effect of MC against HIV infection was published in 1986 [11]. Since then, many observational studies have been published, some of which have observed that most men living in East and southern Africa, the regions with the highest prevalence of HIV are not circumcised [12-14]. More than 30 cross-sectional studies found the prevalence of HIV to be significantly higher in uncircumcised men than in those who are circumcised [15] and 14 prospective studies all showed a protective effect, ranging from 48% to 88% [16-18]. A systematic review and meta analyses of studies from sub-Saharan Africa reported an adjusted relative risk of 042 (95% CI 0.34-0.54) in all circumcised men, with a stronger adjusted relative risk of 0.29 (0.20 – 0.41) in circumcised men who were at higher risk of acquiring HIV [19].

2.1.1.2. Randomized studies

Given the compelling observational data of the potential protective role of male circumcision in the acquisition of heterosexually transmitted HIV infection and the growing crisis of HIV infection in sub-Saharan Africa; it was clear that only randomized studies could provide unequivocally evidence of this protection. Under the sponsorship of the National Institutes of

Health (NIH) and the ARNS (French National Research Agency), three independent but similar randomized control trials were launched in three different communities in South Africa in 2002-2003 to address this question. The studies were performed in South Africa, Kenya, and Uganda, within peri-urban, urban, and rural communities respectively [20-22]. The study conducted in South Africa (Orange farm, bordering Johannesburg) included 3,128 men 18 to 24 years old. Eligible men were randomly allocated to undergo immediate or delayed (offered at the end of the follow up period) circumcision. Men were assessed at 3, 12 and 24 months for HIV acquisition, sexually transmitted infections, and changes in sexual behaviors. Interim analysis in 2004 revealed a 0.4 relative risk of HIV acquisition (95% CI, 0.24%-0.68%.; $P < 0.001$) among the circumcised compared to uncircumcised participants. This finding corresponds to a protective effect of circumcision of 60%, which is a level of protection similar many used vaccines. Given these striking results, the safety and monitoring board discontinued the trial early, and circumcision was offered to the control arm. The Orange Farm study results prompted ethical concerns about continuation of the two remaining studies. The World Health Organization (WHO) recommended continuation but mandated a previously unplanned, earlier interim evaluation. At the interim evaluation, the studies in Kenya and Uganda provided evidence of protection against HIV infection of 50% to 60%, remarkably similar to the results from the Orange Farm trial. These two trials were discontinued prematurely on December 12, 2006. Together, the three studies demonstrated a 50% to 60% reduction in HIV acquisition by medicalized circumcision. [20-22] In total, 10,908 uncircumcised, HIV-negative adult men were randomly assigned to intervention or control arms, and followed for up to 2 years. Overall retention rates were high (86-92% at the end of follow up, when men in the control arm were offered circumcision). Recent findings support the long-term benefit conveyed by MC, with the Kisumu, Kenya cohort maintaining/modestly increasing the earlier level of protection (60% to 64%) at 54 month follow up [23]. These studies, among others, provide "unequivocal evidence that circumcision plays a causal role in reducing the risk of HIV infection among men" [24].

On the basis of the findings from the three clinical trials, a WHO and UNAIDS consultation in March 2007, recommended that circumcision should be recognized as an effective intervention for HIV prevention of heterosexual HIV acquisition in men [24]. WHO and UNAIDS also recommended that male circumcision should be offered HIV-negative men in addition, but not as a substitute, to other HIV risk-reduction strategies. The public-health effect of male circumcision will be largest in generalized epidemics. As such, WHO and UNAIDS recommend that countries with hyperendemic and generalized epidemics and low prevalence of male circumcision expand access to safe male circumcision services within the context of ensuring universal access to comprehensive HIV prevention, treatment, care, and support. [25]

2.2. Acceptability of MC as a tool for HIV prevention

The public health benefit of MC as a tool for HIV prevention, will depend of many factors. One of the most important is the acceptability and uptake of circumcision in traditionally non-circumcising societies. It can be expected that the benefit can spread beyond circumcised men because if sufficient number of males are circumcised, circumcision in the long range will also protect women; effect similar to herd immunity [26]. In addition to the proportion of males who will become circumcised, the age at circumcision will be also a determinant of how rapidly the intervention results in reduction of HIV prevalence in the population. For example, if boys and young men before sexual debut are targeted, the measurable impact it is not likely to be realized for over 10 years; if older boys and men up to 30 years are prioritized a more rapid effect can be expected. On the other hand, circumcision of neonates, in whom the procedure is simpler and less risky, the impact of the strategy on HIV incidence would not be expected for at least 20 years. [25] Because acceptance of male circumcision by men and by parents of males in traditionally non-circumcising communities will be crucial to the success of a MC intervention for reducing HIV prevalence a significant number of studies have been conducted in different non-circumcising communities with high or increasing rates of HIV infection across the globe [26-29]. Across most of these studies, the most common barriers to the acceptability of male circumcision include the following factors: pain (apprehension about pain during and after the procedure has been reported to be the major barrier to MC acceptability; culture and religion have also factors that have been consistently brought up in the discussions about acceptability of MC in diverse groups; cost of the procedure has been named as a significant barrier to MC acceptability and safety (potential for complications and adverse effects). Other potential barriers named in some but not in all studies include: lack of access to health care, required time away from work, the concern about loss of penile sensitivity, reduction in penis size, decreased ability to satisfy women, excessive sexual desire, increased promiscuity and the perception of circumcision as old-fashioned [28-29]. On the other hand, the most consistently named facilitators of MC include the following factors: hygiene, which has universally been recognized as a major benefit of MC; protection from sexually transmitted diseases and HIV (linked through hygiene) and improved sexual pleasure.

In summary, the protective effect of adult male circumcision on HIV acquisition has been reported in a review of epidemiological studies and demonstrated by three randomized controlled trials conducted in Southern and Eastern Africa, which found that the risk of HIV acquisition among circumcised men was reduced by about 60%. Based on this evidence, in 2007 WHO/UNAIDS recommended adult male circumcision as an important, additional intervention which should be delivered as part of a comprehensive HIV prevention package in communities with generalized HIV epidemics and low male circumcision rates. Since then, a number of initiatives have taken place in different countries to role out adult male circumcision services as an additional scientifically proven biomedical strategy to prevent HIV acquisition.

3. Treatment of positives

The idea to use antiretrovirals to prevent the acquisition and transmission of the Human Immunodeficiency virus was tested early in the 90's after animal models of retroviral infection demonstrated that zidovudine could prevent or alter the course of maternally transmitted HIV infection [30 – 33]. The results of this initial US Pediatric AIDS Clinical Trials Group Protocol (PACTG) 076 clinical trial were announced in 1994, which showed that giving pregnant women infected with HIV oral zidovudine from 14 weeks, intravenously at labor and delivery, and followed by six weeks of zidovudine prophylaxis to their newborns, could reduce transmission by 67.5% (95 percent confidence interval, 40.7 to 82.1 percent) [30]. Since this pivotal study proved the concept that antiretrovirals could be use to prevent HIV infection, significant progress has been accomplished in the prevention of mother to child transmission, to the point that current transmission rates are estimated at less than 2 percent with the use of triple antiretroviral drugs during pregnancy. [34, 35], Figure 2. Despite these major advances in the prevention of mother to child transmission of HIV-1, it was not until several years later that these ideas were extrapolated to the prevention of sexual transmission of HIV-1. A central idea was that the quantity of HIV-1 in plasma was a primary determinant of the risk of HIV-1 transmission [36]. By then it was already clear that antiretroviral therapy could reduce plasma HIV-1 to undetectable concentrations within 6 months of initiation in most patients [37, 38] and seminal and cervicovaginal HIV-1 concentrations could also be reduced to undetectable levels in most people on ART [39 – 41]. A meta-analyses of data from five studies reported only five cases of HIV-1 transmission from patients receiving antiretroviral therapy to sexual partners during 1098 person-years of follow up, which is consistent with an infection rate of 0.19 – 1.09 per 100 person-years [42]. Additional evidence was obtained from a pos-hoc analysis of the Partners in Prevention HSV/HIV Transmission study of acyclovir HSV-2 suppressive therapy versus placebo [43]. In this analysis of almost 3,400 HIV-1 serodiscordant heterosexual couples from seven African countries, ART use by the infected person was accompanied by a 92% reduction in the risk of HIV-1 transmission to their partner. Several other observational and some ecological studies added to the evidence and set the need for a randomized study to test the hypothesis if index individuals taking ART are less likely to transmit HIV infection than individuals not on ART. In 2007 the HIV Prevention Trials Network (HPTN) started to enroll participants in a multi-continent, randomized, controlled trial, called HPTN 052, to compare early versus delayed antiretroviral therapy for patients with HIV-1 infection who had CD4 counts between 350 and 550 cells per cubic millimeter and who were in a stable heterosexual relationship with a partner who was not infected [44]. A total of 1763 HIV-1 serodiscordant couples were enrolled (886 couples were randomly assigned to the early therapy group and 877 to the delayed-therapy group). The study was slated to end in 2015, but an interim data review on April 26 2011, by an independent data and safety monitoring board (DSMB) found that of the total 28 cases of HIV infection among the previously uninfected partners, only one case occurred among those couples where the HIV-infected partner began immediate antiretroviral therapy. The DSMB, therefore, called for immediate public release of the study's findings on the basis of data collection through February 21, 2011. At that time, 90% of couples remained enrolled in the study, with a median follow up of 1.7 years. This study demonstrated the power of early antiretroviral treatment (ART) for almost completely preventing onward sexual HIV transmission in the clinical trial setting. This study offered proof of the concept that reduction of viral load through treatment could prevent HIV transmission, a concept that has served as the foundation for multiple modeling studies on treatment-as-prevention and one which was already held to be true by many. The data are incontrovertible, and although they resolve the question of whether this approach can prevent HIV transmission, they also lead to a more fully informed discussion of how ART might actually be used to prevent transmission in communities. The magnitude of protection against HIV infection demonstrated in HPTN 052 has made the successful strategy of the clinical trial a key component of public health policies recently discussed by federal officials and others saying that achieving an end to the HIV/AIDS pandemic is now feasible with additional research and implementation efforts. Given the profound implications of HPTN 052's for the future response to the AIDS epidemic, the journal Science choose this study as its Breakthrough of the Year [45].

In summary, in 2011 it was scientifically demonstrated that treating individuals with HIV infection will prevent the transmission of HIV infection. However, the use of this strategy to the population level it is still not ready to fully achieve its potential because there are resource constraints and logistical hurdles, that limit its implementation.

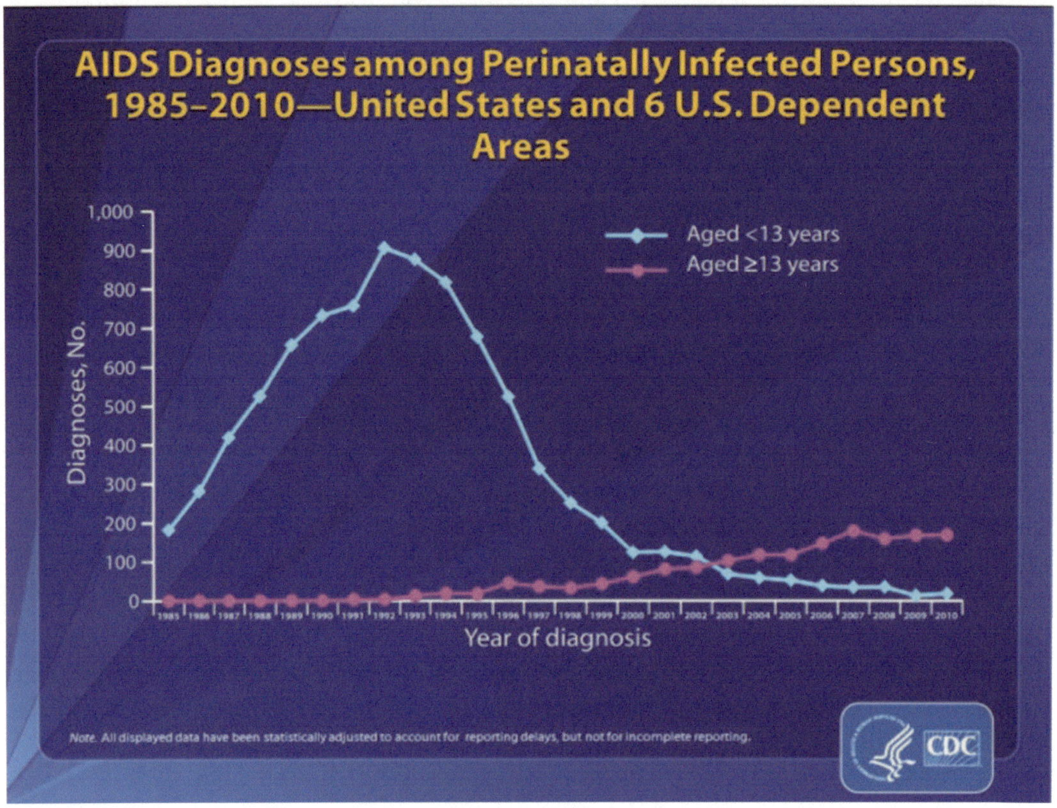

Figure 2. AIDS Diagnoses among perinatally infected persons, 1985-2010. United States and 6 U.S. dependent areas.

This slide from the CDC presents trends from 1985 through 2010 in the estimated numbers of AIDS diagnoses among persons who were perinatally infected in the U.S. The blue line shows the annual numbers of perinatally infected children who were diagnosed with AIDS when they were less than 13 years of age; the pink line shows the annual numbers of persons who were infected with HIV perinatally and were diagnosed with AIDS at the age of 13 or older.

http://dx.doi.org/10.5772/54168

This graphic provides evidence of the impact at the population of an effective bio-medical intervention to prevent HIV infection.

4. Pre-exposure prophylaxis

Pre-exposure prophylaxis (PrEP) involves the use of antiretroviral medications by HIV negative individuals before exposure to the HIV virus, to prevent HIV acquisition. The principle behind the use of antiretrovirals (ART) to prevent sexually acquisition of HIV lies on the success of HIV prevention in mother to Child transmission (PMTCT) and accidental exposure in healthcare workers. Early in the HIV epidemics, two large prevention trials (HIV Prevention Network Trial, HPTN 076 and HIVNET 012) showed that providing ART to infants born to HIV positive mothers significantly decreased the rates of HIV infection in newborns [30,46]. This is one of the greatest accomplishments in the field of HIV prevention, has been incorporated to PMTCT guidelines, and provided a starting ground for PrEP [30,46, 47]. In the area of health care related exposure to HIV, primarily needle sticks, the use of ART by the negative individual during the weeks after exposure reduces HIV acquisition by 80% [48, 49].

Following the human studies assessing PMTCT and prevention in the healthcare setting, animal studies to address PrEP demostrated that the administration of ART to macaque monkeys exposed to HIV prevented HIV infection [50,51]. All this data provided basis for designing clinical trials to test PrEP in humans.

In recent years, tremendous advances in the field of PrEP in individuals at risk for HIV acquisition have led to landmark large randomized controlled studies using oral or topical agents. Results of the initial major studies addressing PrEP were somehow controversial, but recent data provides evidence that PrEP is an effective and safe alternative to prevent HIV infection.

A major benefit of PrEP is its use by the individual at risk without involvement of sexual partners. Men who have sex with men (MSM) and women are especially vulnerable to HIV infection due to cultural, social and biological factors. Stigma associated with homosexuality, gender disparities, inability for women to negotiate condom use and fidelity, as well as frangibility of vaginal and rectal mucosa, predispose these populations to HIV infection and make them ideal candidates for such preventive method. PrEP is therefore emerging as a new powerful prevention method of especial importance in those populations at higher risk.

To date, most studies regarding PrEP have focused on two main modes of delivery: oral agents or topical microbidides. The two delivery modes will be presented separate in this chapter. Other forms of delivery such as subcutaneous or vaginal implants are under investigation and will be briefly mentioned.

While some studies addressing PrEP yielded important and relevant results, other studies are still undergoing and some are in the early stages of development. PrEP is therefore an evolving area in the field of HIV prevention and emerging data is likely to change the way we prevent sexually acquired HIV infection in the near future.

Table 1 summarizes the results of clinical trials on oral and topical agents addressing PrEP.

Study name	Sponsor	Country	Participants	Design	Results
iPREX (Grant 2010)	NIAID Gates Foundation	South America Thailand USA	2,499 MSM	FTC/TDF vs placebo	42% reduction (CI=6-60)
TDF2 (Thigpen 2012)	CDC NIH	Bostwana	1,219 heterosexual men and women	FTC/TDF vs placebo	62% reduction (CI=21-83)
Partners PrEP (Baeten 2012)	Gates Foundation	Sub Saharan African countries	4,758 serodiscordant couples	TDF vs placebo FTC/TDF vs placebo	TDF: 76% reduction (CI=42-81) FTC/TDF: 75% reduction (55-87)
FemPrEP (van Damme 2012)	US Agency for International Development	Kenia, Tanzania South Africa	2,210 women	FTC/TDF vs placebo	Study discontinued due to futility (2011)
VOICE	Microbicides Trial Network NIH	South Africa Uganda, Zambia Zimbabwe	5,000 women	TDF vs placebo FTC vs placebo TDF gel vs placebo	TDF oral and gel discontinued due to futility (2011) FTC/TDF ongoing
CAPRISA (Abdoul Karim 2010)	Multiple agencies	South Africa	1,341 women	TDF gel vs placebo	39% reduction

Table 1. Summary of randomized controlled studies addressing the use of PrEP to prevent sexually transmitted HIV infection.

4.1. PrEP using oral agents to prevent HIV infection in MSM and heterosexual men and women

The oral agents evaluated or under evaluation for PrEP include anti HIV drugs currently approved for treatment of HIV infection. Such drugs are tenofovir (TDF) and a combination of emtricitabine/tenofovir FTC/ TDF.

Tenofovir is a nucleoside analog approved in combination with other ART for the treatment of HIV infection. As a nucleoside analog, the mechanism of action of TDF is to blocking HIV reverse transcriptase, which prevents HIV virus from replicating. In HIV infected individuals, as a result, TDF lowers HIV viral load in the blood. Tenofovir is a drug that achieves good drug levels in plasma as well as in female lower genital tract mucosa and rectal mucosa [52]. TDF is used orally and once a day, and is normally well tolerated, but as most drugs, could have potential side effects. The most common side effects of TDF are gastrointestinal (nausea and vomiting), rash or headaches, and occur in about 10% of the patients. The most serious risk factors of TDF are acute liver and kidney toxicity. Chronic risk factors of TDF, relevant to the chronic use of TDF for PrEP, include decline in kidney function and decrease in bone density [52].

Emtricitabine/tenofovir is a combination of nucleoside analogs approved for treatment of HIV. FTC/TDF is formulated as single day pill and is taken in combination with other agents for the treatment of HIV infection. Orally administered emtricitabine achieves good levels in plasma, lower female genital tract, and especially in the rectum making this combination a promise for PrEP [52]. The combination of FTC/TDF can cause those side effects listed above as well as those associated with FTC. Emtricitabine common side effects include nausea, vomiting, headaches, rash, abdominal pain, dizziness or abnormal dreams and occur in about 10% of the cases. Emtricitabine can also be associated with fatal lactic acidosis, liver or kidney toxicity.

4.1.1. Studies addressing oral PrEP

Five studies have evaluated the use of oral agents to prevent HIV infection and will be described in this section. One study included only MSM (iPrEX), 2 included men and women (TDF2, PIP), and 2 included exclusively women (FEM-PrEP and VOICE). Two of these studies have validated the use of PrEP for HIV prevention, two have been prematurely stopped due to futility, and others are undergoing. Important to say is that all of these studies have addressed the use of PrEP in combination with intensive safer sex practices counseling.

4.1.1.1. iPREX (pre exposure prophylaxis initiative)

iPREX was a randomized controlled study to evaluate the efficacy in reduction of new HIV infections using a daily tablet of fixed dose of FTC/TDF when compared to placebo. iPREX was funded by the National Institute of Allergy and Infectious Diseases and by the Bill and Melinda Gates Foundation. The study included 2499 young high-risk MSM in South America, Thailand and the US. The preliminary results of this study were released in 2010 and the study was the landmark for the use of oral PrEP. Results suggested for the first time that oral ART in combination with safe sex and condom use counseling could be used to reduce new HIV infections in MSM. The use of oral FTC/TDF was associated with a 42% reduction in HIV acquisition over 3 years (CI: 6%-60%). The study also analyzed the results according to self-reported adherence and reveal the importance of adhere to the prescribed drug. The incidence of new HIV cases was reduced to 68% when adherence was high (more than 90% of pills taken), to 50% if adherence was between 50% and 90%, and to 32% if adherence was low (less than 50%). In order to clarify if detectable drug levels were associated with protection against HIV infection a case control design was used to compare rates of infection in individuals with detectable blood levels with those without detectable levels. A relative risk reduction of 92% (CI: 40%-99%) in individuals with detectable study drug levels was found. This finding provided evidence that protection was directly related with drug levels, an indirect measurement of adherence. In addition, this study showed that FTC/TDF had a good safety profile with minimal gastrointestinal side effects. A minimal decrease in bone density in individuals taking the drug was also observed. Among the individuals that seroconvert, most of them were in the process of HIV seroconversion at enrollment and some developed a virus with resistant mutations. This finding reinforced the importance of excluding HIV infection when using FTC/

TDF for PrEP. The study results were published in the New England Journal of Medicine in 2010 [53]

4.1.1.2. TDF2

TDF2 was a randomized controlled study to evaluate the efficacy to reduce new HIV infection of a daily fixed dose of an oral combination pill of TDF/FTC when compared to placebo. This study was funded by the Centers for Disease Control and Prevention (CDC) and the division of AIDS at the National Institutes of Health. The study was conducted in Bostwana and included 1219 males and females, unmarried adults. This study had high rates of loss of follow up (30%) and due to low retention, enrollment was prematurely stopped and study closed. Enrolled participants were followed as planned and the last participant was followed until 2011. The results offered 62% (CI: 21%-83%) protection against HIV infection overall. This study also evaluated drug levels in individuals receiving the drug and revealed that plasma concentration were lower among the participants who seroconverted to HIV. Reported adherence was high and similar in the two groups (above 80%), although detectable drug levels in the drug arm suggested that adherence was lower that reported. Risky sexual behaviors were similar and did not change in the two groups during the study. Among the participants receiving the study drugs, there was and increase number of gastrointestinal side effects (nausea and vomiting) and dizziness as well as a significant decline in bone density. One participant was enrolled with unrecognized acute HIV infection and developed a resistant virus [54].

4.1.1.3. Partners PrEP (partners in prevention)

Partners in Prevention study is the largest trial evaluating PrEP in heterosexual discordant couples. It is an ongoing study with 3 study arms: daily TDF, daily TDF/FTC, and placebo. This study is supported by the Bill and Melinda Gates Foundation. The study enrolled 4758 serodiscordant couples in which the HIV infected partner was not eligible for ART according to country guidelines. This study in being conducted in sub Saharan Africa (Bostwana, Kenya, Rwanda, South Africa, Tanzania, Uganda and Zambia). Extensive counseling in safe sex and condom use was additionally provided to enrolled participants. TDF conferred a 67% (CI: 44%-81%) and FTC/TDF a 75% (CI: 55%-87%) reduction in new HIV infections. The difference in rates of HIV seroconversion among the two treatment groups was not statistically different. In July 2011 the DSMB recommended that the placebo group discontinued since the predetermined criteria for stopping had already been made and a benefit in the treatment arms was achieved [55]. The study results followed iPREX in supporting the use of PrEP in high risk individuals.

4.1.1.4. FEM-PrEP

The FEM-PrEP study was a randomized controlled trial that included women in sub Saharan Africa (Kenya, South Africa and Tanzania). This study was supported by US Agency for International Development. Women were randomized to receive either oral daily FTC/TDF or placebo. This study evaluated 2120 women and was the first one designed to address the effectiveness and safety of PrEP by gender. Incidence of new HIV infections was 4.7% person-years in the treatment group and 5% person-years in the placebo group and this different was not statistically significant. This study was the first large study discontinued based on recommendations from the Data Safety Monitoring Board after interim results were unable to demonstrate efficacy of PrEP. In April of 2011 the study was stopped. As in prior studies, gastrointestinal side effects occurred more commonly in the treatment arm (nausea, vomiting and elevation of ALT) as well as renal laboratory abnormalities. Despite extensive counseling on adherence, less than 40% of the women in the treatment arm enrolled in the study had detectable drug levels raising once again the importance of adherence to the prescribed regimen, perhaps lower in women [56].

4.1.1.5. VOICE (vaginal and oral interventions to control the epidemic)

VOICE is the largest clinical trial being conducted evaluating efficacy of PrEP in women. The study is sponsored by the Microbicide Trials Network and the National Institutes of Health. It enrolled over 5000 women in South Africa, Uganda, Zambia and Zimbabwe. Women were randomized to 3 arms: daily oral TDF, daily oral TDF/FTC, or topical TDF. Results of this trial resulted in the discontinuation of the oral TDF arm in September 2011 and the topical TDF arm in November 2011 because of inability to demonstrate efficacy. The topical arm of the study will be discussed under the microbicide section below and results of the TDF/FTC arm are expected to be reported in 2013 [57].

4.1.1.6. Bangkok TDF trial

The Bangkok tenofovir study is an ongoing trial evaluating the efficacy of oral TDF in male injection drug users receiving direct observation therapy. Enrollment for this study is complete but no results are available at the time of this publication.

Studies addressing oral PrEP have yielded conflicting results and although the use of oral PrEP appears to be beneficial in high risk MSM, the use in women still is under debate. Partners PrEP, TDF2 and iPrEx provided a proof of concepts for the use of oral antiretrovirals for HIV prevention. However, the results from VOICE and Fem-PrEP and other ongoing studies will provide further information on the efficacy and safety of oral PrEP, especially in women.

Efficacy of PrEP seems to be directly related to adherence, and detectable blood levels is a better marker of protection than self-reported adherence or pill count. Although in most studies, adherence measured by self reporting or by pill count was high, detectable blood drug levels were found only in 50% of participants in the treatment arm of iPREX [53].

The highest levels of adherence were reported in Partner PrEP, where serodiscordant couples were enrolled and received extensive counseling. Tenofovir was detected in over 80% of participants in the treatment group and PrEP reduced by 70% new HIV infections. The results of Partner PrEP suggest that partner involvement is important, especially when addressing HIV prevention in women [58,59].

In regards to decrease efficacy of PrEP in women the question of availability of drug at the exposure site has been raised. However, high drug levels are found in cervicovaginal lavages, and even higher than in plasma or rectal mucosa, what would dispute this hypothesis [52,60]. Another possibility is a decrease of drug levels in women receiving hormonal contraceptives and it is under evaluation by the study team.

Nevertheless, the possibility of low efficacy of oral PrEP in women suggest that microbicides or other delivery methods may be a better option in this population.

Following the positive results of daily ART use for HIV prevention, especially in MSM, newer studies are undergoing to evaluate the use of intermittent PrEP. These intermittent regimens could be more feasible in certain setting such as in non stable relationships. A large study in Kenia (ADAPT, Alternative Dosing to Augment PrEP Pill-Taking) is evaluating the safety and adherence to daily oral TDF/FTC versus intermittent TDF/FTC (Monday, Friday and within 2 hours after sex) or placebo. Another study (HPTN 067) is a study including MSM and heterosexual women aiming to identify dosing regiments in people at high risk for HIV infection. Preliminary data demonstrated that although adherence may be decreased in intermittent dosing, it may still be appropriate for PrEP.

4.1.2. Potential problems associated with oral PrEP

In July 2012, and based on the results of the mentioned trials, especially iPREX and Partners PrEP, the United States Food and Drug administration (US FDA) approved the use of daily TDF/FTC or Truvada® for prevention of sexually acquired HIV in individuals at risk for HIV infection. However, even if approval was granted, serious concerns have been raised by experts in the field of HIV prevention. The issues that need to be addressed before recommending PrEP as a generalized HIV prevention strategy are: development of drug resistance viruses, long term side effects, increase in sexual risk behaviors, cost, and incorporating PrEP as part of primary care prevention.

4.1.2.1. Development of drug resistant viruses

Development of drug resistance was identified in some of the participants who seroconvert in the mentioned studies but in most cases, occurred in individuals that enrolled with a new non identified HIV infection. Addressing this potential problem is difficult, since individuals at risk may have an early infection missed by routine antibody testing and routine viral load may not be easily available in high risk settings.

4.1.2.2. Long term side toxicity

As both TDF and FTC have potential serious long term side effects, it is important to determine if long use of FTC/TDF in HIV negative individuals will increase the risk of kidney failure or osteoporosis. In order to evaluate long term side effects, long term follow up is necessary to address if decline in renal function or bone density are clinically significant. However, as in HIV positive individuals using those agents, side effects may take many years to develop.

4.1.2.3. Increased of high risk sexual behavior

In regards to increase of risky sexual risk behaviors, both iPREX and Partners PrEP revealed that all participants increased condom use, decrease number in sexual partners, unprotected anal intercourse, and reduced rates for syphilis. This was likely due to the extensive counseling that both drug and placebo groups received and sustainability of sexual risk behavior needs to be further examined.

4.1.2.4. Cost

The cost of providing PrEP to individuals at risk is of course under great debate due to both economical and ethical issues. ART are expensive medications and not available for all HIV infected patients in need for their own health. PrEP is an expensive approach and cost effectiveness will need to be justified prior to generalization to the population at risk. A cost-effectiveness analysis of PrEP for HIV prevention in MSM published in 2012 in Annals of Internal Medicine revealed that although PrEP could have an important impact in the HIV epidemics, it will be an extremely expensive approach [63]. In a modeling analysis, Juusola recently showed that providing PrEp to all high-risk MSM for 20 years will cost $75 billion in health care related cost, a non-insignificant amount [61]. An ethical concern is whether providing them to those HIV uninfected individuals will interfere with the treatment of HIV infected patient in need for treatment, especially in poor resource settings.

4.1.3. Feasibility of generalizing the use of oral PrEP to the population at risk.

The use of PrEP includes identification of high risk individuals, extensive risk counseling, provision of a drug and follow up risk assessments, HIV and laboratory tests. If PrEp is incorporated as part of primary care prevention activities, the primary care physician will need to become familiar with drugs normally prescribed for highly specialized physicians and will need to be aware of new research data and changes in the recommendations as they become available [63].

As summary, oral PrEP has demonstrated efficacy in certain populations at risk for HIV infection, especially in MSM. Studies assessing acceptability, long term efficacy, toxicity, risk of HIV resistance, cost and use in women are needed before including oral PrEP as part of HIV prevention tools in the population at risk.

4.2. Microbicides to prevent HIV infection in women and MSM

Women are more vulnerable than men to acquire HIV during sex due to biological factors as well as difficulties in negotiating barrier methods and fidelity. Women can rarely negotiate condom use or faithfulness with their sexual partners and could greatly benefit of controlling their own risk of HIV infection without involvement of male partners. Studies addressing oral PrEP suggested lower efficacy of oral agents in women, which make microbicides an attractive alternative for HIV prevention in women at risk.

Microbicides are topical products applied to the rectum or the vagina to prevent HIV infection in HIV negative individuals. Research on microbicides has included primarily women but studies addressing several rectal formulations in MSM are currently undergoing. Unfortunately, results on microbicide research have been conflicting and further research is needed. Topical vaginally applied TDF showed promising results in the CAPRISA trial. However, other agents have not been efficacious and research in this area is ongoing.

In order for a microbicide to be successful it must fulfill the following characteristics: be biologically active, safe, and acceptable by the individual at risk. The principals mechanisms of action evaluated in microbide development are: buffer agents, surfactants, blockers and antiretrovirals.

4.2.1. Buffers

Buffers are supplements to the natural immune defenses of the vagina. Buffers maintain the vaginal pH favoring the persistence of the naturally protective vaginal lactobacilli. Alterations of the vaginal pH due to exposure to semen or vaginal infections such as bacterial vaginosis damage the vaginal microbiota and facilitate HIV infection. Buffergel ®, a buffer designed to maintain vaginal pH was tested in animals and in a phase III effectiveness trial; but unfortunately, did not prevent new HIV infections [63].

4.2.2. Surfactants

Surfactants act by inactivating infectious agents. Noxynol-9, a wide available microbicide with known activity against several infectious agents has been tested in multiple forms (film, sponge and gel) and was not effective in preventing new HIV infections [64]. SAVVY® (C31G) was a surfactant in a gel form tested in Ghana and Nigeria between 2004-2006 and not found to be effective [65]. Surfactants are no longer being considered as potential agents for microbicide use.

4.2.3. Blockers

Blockers inhibit the fusion of the HIV virus to the cell membrane. Four compounds in this category have been tested to date: PRO2000®, Carrguard®, cellulose sulfate and dextrin 2-sulfate and have not demonstrated activity in clinical trials [66].

4.2.4. Drugs with anti HIV activity

Antiretroviral agents act by inhibiting the HIV replication cycle in the vaginal mucosa have been tested in two major clinical trials (CAPRISA and VOICE). Other agents acting as co-receptor blockers binding to chemokine co-receptors such as VVR5 or CxCR4 are also under investigation.

4.2.4.1. CAPRISA

The landmark study suggesting that the potential of microbicides as HIV prevention tools is CAPRISA, a two-arm randomized double blind placebo controlled trial conducted in South Africa between 2007 and 2010. The study evaluated the efficacy in HIV reduction of a coitally (before and after sex) related application of TDF vaginal gel when compared to placebo. 1341 women were enrolled. The incidence of HIV infections in the tenofovir arm was 5.6 (CI: 4.0-7.7) per 100 women-years and 9.1 (CI: 6.9-11.7) in the placebo arm. (IRR: 0.61; CI:0.4-0.94,p=0.017). Tenofovir gel reduced HIV acquisition by an estimate of 39% overall and by 54% in women with high adherence to the gel. This study did not find major side effects associated with the use of TDF and no TDF resistant virus were found in women who seroconverted. The results of this study were released in the International AIDS conference in Vienna in 2010 and provided a potential armamentum for women unable to negotiate fidelity and condom use. Caprisa also provided a reduction in HSV acquisition [67].

4.2.4.2. VOICE

VOICE as described in the oral PrEP section included one arm evaluating daily use of vaginal TDF gel. The gel arm enrolled approximately 1000 women. In September of 2011 this arm was discontinued as a recommendation from the DSMB due to no efficacy. No safety issues were identified [68]. In order to clarify if the differences between CAPRISA (39% reduction on new HIV infections) was found and VOICE (no effect of TDF gel), a new study will replicate CAPRISA (FACTS 001) and its results will help to clarify if TDF gel is useful and can be incorporated to the field of HIV prevention.

4.2.5. Agents under development

4.2.5.1. Vaginal rings

The use of vaginal rings for prevention of HIV acquisition is under evaluation in several studies. Vaginal rings with antivirals could potentially be used in combination with contraceptives, and will release antiviral agent long term and independent of sexual intercourse. Dapivirine (TMC120) vaginal ring is currently evaluated under phase III studies as ASPIRE – A Study to Prevent Infection with a Ring for Extended study [69]. A combination of Dapivirine and Maraviroc is currently undergoing a phase 1 safety and pharmacokinetic study [70]. Other vaginal rings with maraviroc alone or in combination with tenofovir are also being developed.

4.2.5.2. Long acting injectables

The use of a long acting injectable agent that will provide protection for 3-9 months is a potential method that will increase adherence. Rilpivirine is under development for this purpose [71].

PrEP using oral or topical agents is a promising strategy in the field of HIV prevention. However, as single intervention may not be successful in controlling the HIV epidemics and the results obtained in controlled clinical trials are unlikely to persist overtime. The CDC recently published interim guidance for clinicians considering the use of PrEP for the prevention of HIV infection in heterosexually active adults [72]. This report addresses the remaining gap in knowledge regarding PrEP but provides a comprehensive evaluation of the available data and guidance to health care providers regarding the use of PrEP. However, HIV prevention guidelines are under development and 30 years of the history of HIV have shown the scientific community that a single intervention is unlikely to succeed.

In summary, the science of HIV prevention has seen significant progress in recent years. After decades of frustration and lagging behind the spectacular progress brought up in the control of HIV disease by the use of antiretrovirals, the field of biomedical prevention of HIV has been revolutionized and energized by the scientific evidence produced in the last few years that supports the use of the four strategies discussed above: adult male circumcision, treatment of HIV infected people, pre-exposure prophylaxis and microbicides (Figure 3). However, although the foundations for successful HIV prevention programs are being laid out, there are still significant challenges ahead that will need to be solved before all these strategies can be fully scaled up, combined and delivered to the at risk individuals and communities. The field is also confident that the still elusive vaccine to prevent HIV infection can be unveiled in a not distant future.

Figure 3 lists currently proven biomedical interventions that prevent sexually transmitted HIV infection by gender.

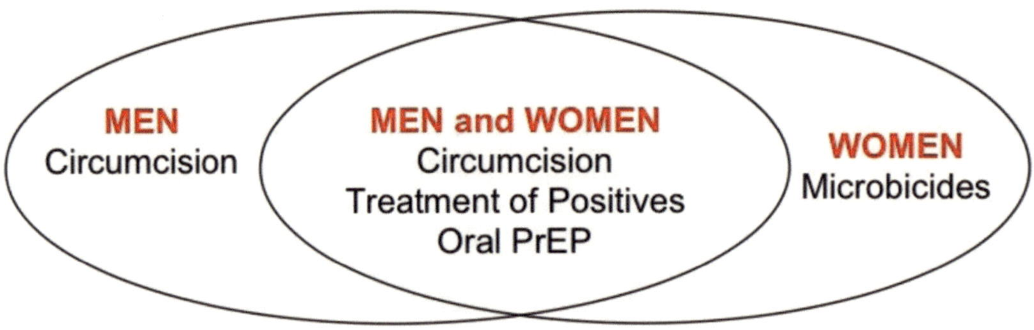

Figure 3. Interventions to Prevent Sexually Transmited HIV Infection by Gender

Author details

Jose G. Castro* and Maria L. Alcaide

*Address all correspondence to: Jcastro2@med.miami.edu

Division of Infectious Disease, Department of Medicine, Miller School of Medicine of the University of Miami, Miami, Florida, USA

References

[1] Alanis, M. C, & Lucidi, R. S. Neonatal circumcision: a review of the world's oldest and most controversial operation. Obstet Gynecol Surv. (2004). May; , 59(5), 379-95.

[2] Johnson, P. Israelities, in A History of the jews. (1993). Phoenix Press. , 37.

[3] Dunsmuir, W. D, & Gordon, E. M. The history of circumcision. BJU International ((1999). Suppl. , 1, 1-12.

[4] UNAIDSMale circumcision: Global trends and determinants of prevalence, safety and acceptability. (2007).

[5] Thomas, A. Circumcision: an ethnomedical study. (2003). The Gilgal Society.

[6] Hull, T. H, & Budiharsana, M. Male circumcision and penis enhacement in Southeast Asia: matters of pain and pleasure. Reprod Health Matters. (2001). , 9(18), 60-7.

[7] Mcwilliam, A. Case studies in dual classification as process: childbirth, headhunting and circumcision in West Timor, Oceania. (1994). , 65, 59-74.

[8] Siegfried, N, Muller, M, & Volmink, J. Male circumcision for prevention of heterosexual acquisition of HIV in men. Cochrane Database Sust Rev. (2003). CD003362.

[9] Benatar, M, & Benatar, D. Between prophylaxis and child abuse: the ethics of neonatal male circumcision. Am J Bioeth. (2003). Spring; , 3(2), 35-48.

[10] Wright, J. L, Lin, D. W, & Stanford, J. L. Circumcision and the risk of prostate cancer. Cancer, (2012). published on line; doicncr.26653.

[11] Fink, A. J. A possible explanation for heterosexual male infection with AIDS. N Engl J Med. (1986).

[12] Bongaarts, J, Reining, P, Way, P, & Conant, F. The relationship between male circumcision and HIV infection in Africa population. AIDS (1989). , 3, 373-377.

[13] Caldwell, J. C, & Caldwell, P. The African AIDS epidemic. 1996 Sci Am (1996).

[14] Moses, S, Bradley, J. E, Nagelkerke, N. J, Ronald, A. R, et al. Geographical patterns of male circumcision practices in Africa: Association with HIV seroprevalence. Int J Epidemiol (1990). , 19, 693-697.

[15] Bailey, R. C, Plummer, F. A, & Moses, S. Male circumcision and HIV prevention: current knowledge and future research directions. Lancet Infect Dis (2001). , 1, 223-31.

[16] Buchbinder, S. P, Vittinghoff, E, & Heagerty, P. J. Sexual risk, nitrite inhalant use and lack of circumcision associated with HIV seroconversion in men who have sex with men in the United States. J Acquir Immune Def Syndr (2005). , 39, 82-89.

[17] MacDonald KSMalonza I, Chen DK. Vitamin A and risk of HIV-1 seroconversion among Kenyan men with genital ulcers. AIDS (2001). , 15, 635-39.

[18] Reynolds, S. J, Shepherd, M. E, & Risbud, A. R. Male circumcision and risk of HIV-1 and other sexually transmitted infections in India. Lancet (2004). , 363, 1039-40.

[19] Weiss, H. A, Quigley, M. A, & Hayes, R. J. Male circumcision and risk of HIV infection in sub-Saharan Africa: a systematic review and meta-analysis. AIDS (2000). , 14, 2361-70.

[20] Bailey, R. C, Moses, S, Parker, C. B, Agot, K, Maclean, I, Krieger, J. N, et al. Male circumcision for HIV prevention in young men in Kisumu, Kenya: a randomized controlled trial. Lancet (2007). , 369, 643-656.

[21] Gray, R. H, Kigozi, G, Serwadda, D, Makumbi, F, Watya, S, Nalugoda, F, et al. Male circumcision for HIV prevention in men in Rikai, Uganda: a randomized trial. Lancet (2007). , 369, 657-666.

[22] Auvert, B, Taljaard, D, Lagarde, E, Sobngwi-tambekou, J, Sitta, R, & Puren, A. Randomized, controlled intervention trial of male circumcision for reduction of HIV infection risk: the ANRS 1265 trial. PLoS Med (2005). e298.

[23] Riess, T. H, Achieng, M. M, Otieno, S, Ndinya-achola, J. O, & Bailey, R. C. (2010). When I Was Circumcised I Was Taught Certain Things": Risk Compensation and Protective Sexual Behavior among Circumcised Men in Kisumu, Kenya. PLoS ONE 5(8): e12366. doi:10.1371/journal.pone.0012366.

[24] Byakika-TusiimeJayne. Circumcision and HIV Infection: Assessment of Causality. AIDS and Behavior (2008). DOI:s10461-008-9453-6., 12(6)

[25] UNAIDS and WHONew data on male circumcision and HIV prevention: policy and programme implications; WHO/UNAIDS technical consultation male circumcision and HIV prevention: research implications for policy and programming Montreaux, Geneva: Joint United Nations Programme on HIV/AIDS and World Health Organization, (2007).

[26] Westercamp, N, & Bailet, R. C. Acceptability of male circumcision for prevention of HIV/AIDS in sub-Saharan Africa: A review. AIDS Behav (2007). , 11, 341-355.

[27] Castro, J. G, Jones, D. L, Lopez, M, Barradas, I, & Weiss, S. Making the case for circumcision as a public health strategy: opening the dialogue. AIDS Patient Care and STDs. (2010). , 24(6), 367-372.

[28] Madhivanan, P, Krupp, K, & Chandrasekaran, V. Acceptability of male circumcision among mothers with male children in Mysore, India. AIDS (2008). , 22, 983-988.

[29] Castro, J. G, Jones, D. L, Lopez, M, Deeb, K, Barradas, I, & Weiss, S. Acceptability of neonatal circumcision by Hispanics in southern Florida. Journal of STD & AIDS (2010). , 21, 591-4.

[30] Connor, E. M, Sperling, R. S, Gelber, R, Kiselev, P, & Scott, W. Reduction of maternal-infant transmission of human immunodeficiency virus type 1 with zidovudine treatment. N Eng J Med (1994). , 331, 1173-1180.

[31] Shih, C-C, Kaneshima, H, & Rabin, L. Post exposure prophylaxis with zidovudine suppresses human immunodeficiency virus type 1 infection in SCID-hu mice in a time-dependent manner. J Infect Dis (1991). , 163, 625-627.

[32] Sharpe, A. H, Jaenisch, R, & Ruprecht, R. M. Retroviruses and mouse embryos: a rapid model for neurovirulence and transplacental antiviral therapy. Science (1987). , 236, 1671-4.

[33] Sharpe, A. H, Hunter, J. J, Ruprecht, R. M, & Jaenisch, R. Maternal transmission of retroviral disease: transgenic mice as a rapid test system for evaluating perinatal and transplacental antiretroviral therapy. Proc Natl Acad U S A (1988). , 85, 9792-6.

[34] Dorenbaum, A, Cunningham, C. K, & Gelber, R. Two-dose intrapartum/newborn nevirapine and standard antiretroviral therapy to reduce perinatal HIV transmission: a randomized trial. JAMA (2002). , 288(2), 189-98.

[35] Cooper, E. R, Charurat, M, & Mofenson, L. Combination antiretroviral strategies for the treatment of pregnant HIV-1 infected women and prevention of perinatal HIV-1 transmission. J Acquir Immune Defic Syndr (2002). , 29(5), 484-94.

[36] Quinn, T. C, Wawer, M. J, & Sewankambo, N. Viral load and heterosexual transmission of human immunodeficiency virus type 1. Rakai Project Study Group. N Eng J Med (2000). , 342, 921-929.

[37] Chaisson, R. E, Keruly, J. C, & Moore, R. D. Association of initial CD4 cell count and viral load with response to highly active antiretroviral therapy. JAMA (2000). , 284, 3128-29.

[38] Phillips, A. N, Staszewski, S, & Weber, R. HIV viral load response to antiretroviral therapy according to the baseline CD4 cell count and viral load. JAMA (2001). , 286, 2560-67.

[39] Graham, S. M, Holte, S. E, & Peshu, N. M. Initiation of antiretroviral therapy leads to a rapid decline in cervical and vaginal HIV-1 shedding. AIDS (2007). , 21, 501-07.

[40] Gupta, P, Mellors, J, & Kingsley, L. High viral load in semen of human immodeficiency virus type 1-infected men at all stages of disease and its reduction by therapy with protease and nonnucleoside reverse transcriptase inhibitors. J Virol (1997). , 71, 6271-75.

[41] Marcelin, A. G, & Tubiana, R. Lambert-Niclot. Detection of HIV-1 RNA in seminal plasma samples from treated patients with undetectable HIV-1 RNA in blood plasma. AIDS (2008).

[42] Attia, S, Egger, M, & Muller, M. Sexual transmission of HIV according to viral load and antiretroviral therapy: systematic review and meta-analysis. AIDS (2009). , 23, 1397-404.

[43] Celum, C, Wald, A, & Lingappa, J. R. Acyclovir and transmission of HIV-1 from persons infected with HIV-1 and HSV-2. N Engl J Med (2010). , 362, 427-39.

[44] Cohen, M. S, Chen, Y. Q, & Mccauley, M. Prevention of HIV-1 infection with early antiretroviral therapy. N Engl J Med (2011). , 365, 493-505.

[45] Cohen, J. Breakthrough of the year. HIV treatment as prevention, Science 23 December (2011). , 334(6063), 1628.

[46] Guay, L. A, Musoke, P, Fleming, T, Bagenda, D, Allen, M, Nakabiito, C, et al. Intrapartum and neonatal single-dose nevirapine compared with zidovudine for prevention of mother-to-child transmission of HIV-1 in Kampala, Uganda: HIVNET 012 randomised trial. Lancet. (1999). Sep 4; , 354(9181), 795-802.

[47] World Health OrganizationUse of Antiretroviral Medication for Treating Pregnant Women and Preventing HIV infection in Infants (2012). Available from: http://www.who.int/hiv/PMTCT_update.pdf

[48] Cardo, D, Culver, D. H, & Ciesielski, C. A. study of HIV seroconversion in health care worker after percutaneous exposure. New Eng J Med., , 337, 1485-90.

[49] Garcia-lerma, J. G, Otten, R. A, & Qari, S. H. (2008). Prevention of rectal SHIV transmission in macaques by daily or intermittent prophylaxis with emtricitabine and tenofovir. PLOS medicine, e , 28, 0291-0299.

[50] Van Rompay, K. K, Mcchesney, M. B, & Aguirre, N. L. (2001). Two low doses of tenofovir protect new-born macaques against oral simian immunodeficiency virus infection. J Infect Dis. 2001; , 184, 429-438.

[51] Anderson, P. L, Kiser, J. J, Gardner, E. M, Rower, J. E, Meditz, A, & Grant, R. M. Pharmacological considerations for tenofovir and emtricitabine to prevent HIV infection. J Antimicrob Chemother. (2011). , 66(2), 240-50.

[52] Gilead laboratoriesTenofovir disoproxil fumarate. Updated August (2012). Available from: http://www.gilead.com/pdf/viread_pi.pdf.

[53] Gant, R, Lama, J, Anderson, P, Mcmahan, V, Liu, A, & Vargas, L. el al. IPrEX study team. Peexposure Chemoprophylaxis for HIV Prevention in Men Who Have Sex with Men. NEngl J Med (2010). , 363(27), 2587-2599.

[54] Thigpen, M. C, Kebaabetswe, P. M, Paxton, L. A, Smith, D. K, Rose, C. E, Segolodi, T. M, et al. TDF2 Study Group. Antiretroviral preexposure prophylaxis for heterosexual HIV transmission in Botswana. N Engl J Med. (2012). , 367(5), 423-34.

[55] Baeten, J. M, Donnell, D, Ndase, P, Mugo, N. R, Campbell, J. D, Wangisi, J, et al. Antiretroviral prophylaxis for HIV prevention in heterosexual men and women. N Engl J Med. (2012). , 367(5), 399-410.

[56] Van Damme, L, Corneli, A, Ahmed, K, Agot, K, Lombaard, J, Kapiga, S, et al. Preexposure prophylaxis for HIV infection among African women. N Engl J Med. (2012). Aug 2; , 367(5), 411-22.

[57] Microbicide Trials NetworkVOICE (MTN-003) study. Available from:http://www.mtnstopshiv.org/news/studies/mtn003.

[58] Montgomery, E. T, Van Der Straten, A, Chidanyika, A, Chipato, T, Jaffar, S, & Padian, N. The importance of male partner involvement for women's acceptability and adherence to female initiated HIV prevention methods in Zimbabwe. AIDS Behav (2011). , 15, 959-969.

[59] Montgomrery, E. T, Van Der Straten, A, & Torjesen, K. Male involvement in womens and children's HIV prevention: challenges in definition and interpretation. J Acqui Immune Defic Syndr (2011). e , 114-116.

[60] Patterson, K, Prince, H, Kraft, E, Jenkings, A, Shaheen, N. J, Rooney, J. F, et al. Penetration of tenofovir and emtricitabine in mucosal tissues: implications for prevention of HIV-1 transmission, Sci Transl Med (2011).

[61] Juusola, J, Brandeau, M, Owens, D, & Bendavid, E. The Cost-Effectiveness of Preexposure Prophylaxis for HIV Prevention in the United States in Men Who Have Sex With Men. Ann Intern Med (2012). , 156, 541-550.

[62] Krakower, D, & Mayer, K. H. What Primary Care Providers Need to Know About Preexposure Prophylaxis for HIV Prevention: A Narrative Review. (2012). epub ahead of print].

[63] Abdool Karim SSRichardson B, Ramjee G. Safety and effectiveness of BufferGel and 0.5% PRO2000 gel for the prevention of HIV infection in women. AIDS (2010). , 25, 957-966.

[64] Van Damme, L, Ramjee, G, & Alary, M. Effectiveness of COL-1492, a nonoxynol-9 vaginal gel, on HIV-1 transmission in female sex workers: a randomized controlled trial. Lancet (2002). , 360, 971-977.

[65] Van Damme, L, Govinden, R, & Mirembe, F. M. Lack of Effectiveness of Cellulose Sulfate Gel for the Prevention of Vaginal HIV TransmissionInternational Partnership for Microbicides (2012). Available from: http://www.ipmglobal.org/our-work/ipm-product-pipeline/maraviroc.

[66] 66. Skoler-karpoff, S, Ramjee, G, & Ahmed, K. Efficacy of Carraguard for prevention of HIV infection in women in South Africa: a randomised, double-blind, placebo-controlled trial. The Lancet (2008). , 372, 1977-1987.

[67] Abdool Karim QAbdool Karim S, Frohlich J, Grobler A, Baxter C, Mansoor L et al. Effectiveness and safety of tenofovir gel, an antiretroviral microbicide, for the prevention of HIV infection in women. Science; , 329(5996), 1168-1174.

[68] Microbicide Trials NetworkVOICE (MTN-003) study. Available from: http://www.mtnstopshiv.org/node/3909.Accessed September 10th (2012).

[69] International Partnership for Microbicides (2012). Available from: http://ipmglobal.org/node/532

[70] International Partnership for Microbicides (2012). Available from: http://www.ipmglobal.org/our-work/ipm-product-pipeline/maraviroc.

[71] Van'Klooster, t, Hoeben, G, Borghys, E, Looszova, H, Bouche, A, Van Velsen, M, et al. Pharmacokinetics and disposition of rilpivirine (TMC 278) nanosuspension as a long-acting injectable antiretroviral formulation. Antimicrob Agents Chemother (2010). , 54, 2042-2050.

[72] Smith, D, Thigpen, M, Nesheim, S, Lampe, M, Pazton, L, Fenton, M, et al. Interim Guidance for Clinicians Considering the Use of Preexposure Prophylaxis for the Prevention of HIV Infection in Heterosexually Active Adults. MMWR (2012). Available from: http://www.cdc.gov/mmwr/preview/mmwrhtml/mm6131a2.htm?s_cid=mm6131a2_w , 586-589.

Section 6

Recent Advances

Chapter 18

HIV-2 Interaction with Target Cell Receptors, or Why HIV-2 is Less Pathogenic than HIV-1

José Miguel Azevedo-Pereira

Additional information is available at the end of the chapter

http://dx.doi.org/10.5772/53201

1. Introduction

Although sharing identical transmission routes as well as structural and genomic properties, human immunodeficiency viruses 1 and 2 (HIV-1 and HIV-2, respectively) show different pathogenic abilities in human host. Despite both HIV-1 and HIV-2 lead to immunological failure and Acquired Immunodeficiency Syndrome (AIDS), a slower rate of disease progression with a longer asymptomatic period and lower levels of viremia in general characterize HIV-2 infection (Table 1). Comparative studies measuring the progression rates of both HIV-1 and HIV-2 infections provided clear evidence that the majority of HIV-2 infected individuals fit in a definition of long-term non-progressors [1-3].

	HIV-1	*HIV-2*
Geographic distribution	Worldwide	Restricted to West African countries and to countries sharing economical-social links with them
Viral load	Usually moderate to high	Usually undetectable
Transmission	By sexual route is usually inefficient, requiring multiple exposures	Scarce data but less efficiently transmitted than HIV-1
Duration of asymptomatic stage	Usually less than 10 years	Usually decades
Treatment	Plenty of data regarding viral susceptibility to all anti-retroviral drugs. Resistance-conferring mutations well established and defined	Naturally resistant to non-nucleoside analogous targeting reverse transcriptase. Scarce and sometimes conflicting results regarding susceptibility to other anti-retroviral drugs

Table 1. Comparison between epidemiologic and clinical data of HIV-1 and HIV-2 infections

All these findings support the notion that in HIV-2 infected individuals several factors (e.g. virologic and immunologic) should account for a best fitted response that ultimately leads to a better control of HIV-2 infection compared to HIV-1. Deciphering these factors should provide crucial information about the mechanisms underlying the delayed disease progression and may help explain how a retroviruses infection could be coped for such a long time without causing disease. This knowledge is important to clarify AIDS pathogenesis and to identify the correlates of protection crucial to develop an efficient HIV vaccine.

Despite the potential importance of HIV-2 as a model to address those issues, it has been mostly neglected and very few data exists regarding HIV-2 interaction with target cells. In this chapter I will focus on these interactions, particularly those concerning early events. Distinguishing features between HIV-1 and HIV-2 will be highlighted and their implications in viral fitness and pathogenic differences between the two viruses will be discussed.

2. Origin of HIV-2

HIV-2, as HIV-1, belongs to Family *Retroviridae*, Subfamily *Orthoretrovirinae*, Genus *Lentivirus* [4]. It was first isolated from a symptomatic patient from Guinea-Bissau [5] and subsequently associated with immunological failure and clinical manifestations typically observed in AIDS patients infected with HIV-1 [6].

HIV-1 and HIV-2 were introduced into human population as a consequence of multiple cross-species transmissions from simian immunodeficiency virus (SIV)-infected non-human primates. The genetic relatedness between HIV-1, HIV-2 and SIV strains, and the coincidence of natural habitats of specific simian species and geographic regions where HIV-1 and HIV-2 had probably emerged, allowed the identification of SIVcpz (infecting the chimpanzee subspecies *Pan troglodytes troglodytes*) and SIVsm (infecting sooty mangabey subspecies *Cercocebus atys*) as viral ancestors of HIV-1 and HIV-2, respectively [7-9]. Through a combination of phylogenetic and molecular clock analysis it was estimated that the date of the most recent common ancestor of HIV-1 group M was 1930 ± 15, and that of "HIV-2 group A was 1940 ± 16 [8, 10]. These cross-species transmission events was then fuelled-up by social, sexual and iatrogenic factors during colonial period in Africa [11], converting a restricted zoonotic disease into an epidemic (HIV-2) and pandemic (HIV-1) infections.

3. Genomic organization of HIV-2

The genomic information of HIV-2 is comprised in two identical copies of 9.2 kb single strand RNA. HIV-2 genome encodes nine open reading frames (i.e. *gag, pol, vif, vpr, tat, rev, vpx, env* and *nef*), flanked by two long terminal repeats (5'LTR and 3'LTR). Soon after entry into target cell the genomic RNA is converted to a double-stranded DNA molecule, a reaction catalized by reverse transcriptase (RT) enzyme, that occurs in a cytoplasmic complex, named reverse transcriptase complex (RTC). The RTC transforms

http://dx.doi.org/10.5772/53201

to the preintegration complex (PIC) composed by several cellular and viral components, e.g. viral DNA, RT, integrase (IN), matrix (MA) and Vpr proteins (reviewed in [12]). This PIC allows the reverse transcribed viral DNA to enter the nucleus through the nuclear pore and to be integrated into the genome of target cell.

After integration, the HIV-2 proviral DNA is transcribed into several mRNAs by cellular RNA polymerase II, a process initiated through the binding of cellular activation factors to the viral LTR, culminating in the synthesis of viral proteins and in the production of new progeny virions. The function of each HIV-2 protein has been inferred from HIV-1 counterparts and reviewed in [13].

Compared to HIV-1, HIV-2 lacks the *vpu* gene while has the *vpx* gene. The Vpu protein has been associated with two main functions in HIV-1 replication: induces a rapid degradation of CD4 molecules (see below the role of CD4 as viral receptor) in endoplasmic reticulum through the ubiquitin-proteasome system [14]; and enhancing the budding and release of viral particles [15] by counteracting the activity of Tetherin/BST2, a cellular factor that restricts the egress of enveloped viruses (e.g. HIV, Ebola virus), thereby reducing viral production and cell-free virus propagation [16, 17]. In HIV-2, this latter role in viral replication seems to be assumed by the membrane-anchored subunit and the extracellular domain of transmembrane (TM) envelope glycoprotein [18, 19].

Vpx is a protein only present in HIV-2 and SIVsm lineage. Sequence analysis suggests that the *vpx* gene is a duplication of *vpr* gene but despite amino acid sequence similarities between both proteins, their functions are clearly distinct. While Vpr is mainly involved in cell cycle arrest in G2/M phase [20], the Vpx protein has been recently linked to the enhancement of HIV-1 infection of dendritic cells and an essential factor in innate response to HIV infection [21]. The obvious importance of Vpx in the pathogenesis of human lentiviral infection will be further discussed in subchapters 4 and 5.

4. HIV-2 as a limited spreading virus

As in all zoonosis, the emergence of HIV-1 and HIV-2, as successful new human pathogens, involved not only a close contact with animal reservoirs but also the capability of the cross-species viruses to: encounter and efficiently infect human host cells, and to be able to be effectively transmitted within the human population.

Although HIV-1 and HIV-2 shared common transmission routes, they show a clear distinct epidemiology. While HIV-1, particularly group M, has spread literally worldwide, HIV-2 infection reveal a much more confined geographic distribution: West Africa and countries that maintained social-economic links to this region (e.g. Portugal, France and their former colonies). Since both viruses had begun to spread nearly at the same time, somewhere between 1950 and 1970, this limited expansion of HIV-2 indicates a less efficient human transmission. Heterosexual spread of HIV-2 is remarkably lower than in HIV-1: it seems that HIV-2 is five to nine times less efficiently transmitted than HIV-1 by sexual route [22]. Likewise, mother-to-child transmission rate of HIV-2 is 0-4%, while in HIV-1 this transmission occurs in 15-40% of untreated pregnancies [23].

This poor capability to infect new hosts could lead HIV-2 to a dead end. Viral ecology imposes two ideal conditions: maintain the host alive as long as possible while being efficiently transmitted within host population. HIV-2 only fulfils the first condition leading to a decline in HIV-2 prevalence even in regions (i.e. West Africa) where, in the early stages of AIDS epidemic, a clear predominance of HIV-2 infections existed compared to HIV-1 [24].

4.1. Viral load and transmission

Many different factors account for a successful transmission of HIV by sexual route. One of the most critical is the amount of infectious viral particles present in the transmitting body fluid (e.g. blood, semen or cervicovaginal secretion). Higher concentrations are more likely associated with transmission events. Apparently, in HIV-1, the cutoff of 1500 copies of viral RNA per ml of plasma is required for efficient transmission [25].

Not surprisingly, plasma and semen viral loads are significantly lower in patients infected with HIV-2 compared to those infected with HIV-1 [26, 27], providing a likely explanation for the reduced transmission rate and spread within human population. This lower viral load is observed throughout the infection and persists until late in the course of the disease, but is remarkably important during asymptomatic stage. During this stage, which in HIV-2 could last for several decades, an undetectable viremia is a hallmark of almost every HIV-2 patients. However, a similar proviral burden is detected in both HIV-1 and HIV-2-infected individuals [28, 29]. This apparent paradox suggests that the lower plasma viral load observed in HIV-2 infection may be due to lower levels of infectious virus production, or a better host-driven suppression of viral replication, or both.

4.2. The mucosal barrier

Besides viral load, numerous barriers decrease the efficiency of mucosal transmission. The foundations of this important notion emanates from studies of couples discordant for HIV-1 infection, which demonstrated that heterosexual transmission is very inefficient requiring multiple exposures for a successful transmission [30, 31]. A detailed understanding of the events surrounding transmission should provide important clues how HIV establishes a new infection and what additional vulnerabilities HIV-2 has, at this stage, that can help explain its lower spread.

Although HIV-1 and HIV-2 (as well as SIV) are commonly referred as "lentivirus" based on the long incubation period and slow onset of disease, it is now clear from data using rhesus macaque model infected with SIV, that initial virus-host interactions, crucial to establishing systemic infection, take place in a rapid succession of related events, soon after mucosal transmission (recently reviewed in [32]). In sexual transmission, the most common form of HIV transmission, these events involve the interactions with cells present in cervical/vaginal mucosa epithelial surfaces. To establish infection, HIV present in semen must go through mucus that covers female genital epithelia and penetrate through the epithelial layer to access susceptible cells such as T lymphocytes, macrophages, Langerhans cells and dendritic cells. Mucus, particularly abundant in upper female genital tract, provides the first barrier to HIV infection. Mucus protective role of underlying epithelial cells is provided by the presence of soluble factors (e.g. chemokines produced by epithelial cells) that decrease viral infectivity and by mechanical trapping of virions in the dense protein mesh that constitutes the cervical mucus [33]. By slowing viral diffusion, mucus reduces the probability of infectious virus reach the surface of underlying cells.

Virions that successfully crossed the mucus encounters the epithelial cells layer that line the different compartments of the female genital tract. These different compartments show remarkable differences in the structure of epithelial layer. The mucosa from the lower female genital tract (i.e. exocervix and vagina) consists of stratified squamous epithelium, several layers thick. In contrast, in the upper reproductive compartment (i.e. endocervix and endometrium) the mucosal lining is composed of a single layer of columnar epithelium over the basement membrane and is characterized by the presence of tight junctions between cells.

As expected by their different composition, the lower female genital epithelium is much more robust and provides a more effective physical barrier than the fragile single columnar layer of upper genital epithelium. Furthermore, the junction between the exocervix and the endocervix, where the structure of the epithelium abruptly changes from stratified to single layer (called the transitional or transformational zone), is characterized by an intense immunologic activity and thus enriched with abundant lymphocytes and antigen presenting cells (e.g. dendritic cells and macrophages), particularly during inflammatory processes [34]. The physical vulnerability and the presence of abundant target cells in transitional zone, make this region highly susceptible to HIV entry and infection [35].

Even the thicker vaginal epithelial barrier could quickly expose susceptible cells in the submucosa to HIV. In fact, the stratified squamous epithelium changes markedly through the menstrual cycle, in response to progesterone [36], leading to a thinning of this physical barrier. Additionally, breaches could occur because of microulcerations and breaks in the epithelium due to sexual intercourse, inflammatory processes, sexually transmitted infections, and other genital infections, increasing the likelihood of establishing an HIV infection [37-39].

Additionally, the mere exposure of genital mucosa to semen induces local alterations that could potentiate the transmission of HIV-1 and (probably) HIV-2. These include the neutralization of the acidic pH of the cervicovaginal secretions, the regulation of inflammatory cytokines in genital tract epithelial cells, and the promotion of leukocyte infiltration and the attraction of Langerhans cells in cervical and vaginal mucosae [40, 41]. Semen could also directly promote HIV infection of epithelial target cells through the formation of amyloid fibrils that capture HIV particles and enhances virus-cell attachment and fusion [42]. This amyloidogenic activity of human semen seems to be related with fragments of prostatic acidic phosphatase [42]. Apparently this enhancement is semen donor-dependent but independent of HIV strain or cell type used [43].

In contrast to female genital tract, HIV transmission through male genital tract is poorly understood. Despite the presence of CD4+ T lymphocytes, Langerhans cells, dendritic cells and macrophages in the foreskin and glans of the penis [44, 45], the mechanisms underlying the transmission across these mucosae are not completed elucidated. Foreskin seems to play a crucial role in female-to-male transmission of HIV-1, since several randomized controlled clinical trials have shown that circumcision reduce this route of transmission by approximately 60% [46]. One plausible mechanism for greater susceptibility to HIV-1 infection in uncircumcised men could be the increased risk for sexually transmitted infections and consequent inflammation of the foreskin (reviewed in [47]). This predisposition to local infection and inflammatory reactions will lead to the recruitment of activated target cells that facilitates the early events of HIV transmission and provides a local environment suitable for productive HIV systemic infection.

The vaginal flora could in some circumstances also favour female-to-male HIV transmission. The predominance of potential pathogenic bacteria instead of normal *Lactobacillus* species, observed during bacterial vaginosis, seems to be related not only with increased risk of HIV-1 acquisition by women (as referred above) but also with higher concentrations of HIV-1 in cervicovaginal secretions, due to a bacterial-driven augmentation of HIV-1 replication and shedding [48-50]. Thus, women with bacterial vaginosis are more infectious and the probability of female-to-male HIV-1 transmission during sexual intercourse is greater than in women with normal vaginal flora [51].

4.3. Crossing the intact mucosal barrier

Although infection of mucosal epithelial cells could happen, HIV must gain access to permissive host cells present in underlying submucosa tissue (e.g. dendritic cells macrophages and CD4+ T-lymphocytes) to facilitate virus production and dissemination. The mechanisms for crossing intact stratified squamous epithelium of the vagina or the simple columnar epithelium of the cervix could be one (or more) of the following: (i) transcytosis by a vesicular pathway [52] – an apparently rare but possible event [53]; (ii) capture or infection of dendritic cells resident in the stratified squamous epithelium of the vaginal mucosa and in the underlying tissues of the vagina and cervix [54]; and (iii) direct infection of intraepithelial lymphocytes in the endocervical mucosa [55].

Regardless the pathway used by cell-free HIV virions to penetrate the epithelial cell barrier, they ultimately lead to viral exposure of dendritic cells, macrophages and CD4+ T-lymphocytes present in underlying submucosal tissues, allowing the initiation of infection. Dendritic cells can capture HIV virions through C-type lectin receptors (CLRs) present at cell membrane (e.g. DC-SIGN, DCIR), and internalize the captured virus without being infected. This internalized virus, as well as those bound to dendritic cell membrane, remains full infectious and able to be transmitted to surrounding CD4+ T-lymphocytes through a structure analogous to the immunological synapse, named "virological synapse". This tight adhesive junction between an HIV-exposed dendritic cell and an uninfected CD4+ T-lymphocyte allows the virus to be efficiently transferred from one cell to the other, in a process named *trans*-infection (for a review in HIV interactions with dendritic cells see [56]). Besides trans-infection through virological synapse, dendritic cells could also transfer HIV to CD4+ T lymphocytes by cell-free exosomes. These endosomal multivesicular bodies (MVB), containing endocytosed HIV particles, could be released to extracellular milieu and fuse with target-cell membranes allowing the transfer of HIV to them [57].

Alternatively, HIV can directly infect the dendritic cell subset, present in submucosal tissues (*cis*-infection), using the natural expression of the main HIV cellular receptors (i.e. CD4 and CCR5; see bellow) at dendritic cell surface [56, 58, 59]. Despite the susceptibility of dendritic cells, conferred by the presence of these major receptors, HIV replication in dendritic cells is in general less productive, compared with CD4+ T lymphocytes [60]. The reasons for the decreased viral production in dendritic cells include: (i) lower expression levels of HIV receptors; (ii) degradation of internalized virions, soon after infection; and (iii) presence of intracellular restriction factors that inhibited post-entry events of replication cycle.

Interestingly, although HIV can infect dendritic cells, extensive viral replication only takes place after dendritic cells come into contact with CD4+ T lymphocytes in lymphoid tissue [61]. The dendritic cell-T lymphocyte interaction provides activation signaling to the latter, allowing HIV to be presented to a population of highly activated and susceptible T-lymphocytes. This further indicates that the infection of dendritic cells by HIV-1 is a double-edged sword: dendritic cells must deliver appropriate signals to T lymphocytes in order to induce an HIV-specific immune response; however, this interaction imposes a close contact between dendritic cells and T lymphocytes (immunological synapse) leaving the latter susceptible to infection by the HIV-1 carried by dendritic cells.

In conclusion, dendritic cell-mediated virus transfer occurs in two distinct phases: in the first phase (*trans*-infection), dendritic cell capture and internalize virus within endosomal compartments which are relocated at the dendritic cell/CD4+ T-lymphocyte contact zone (virological synapse); alternatively, a fraction of the endocytosed particles may be targeted for exocytosis, associated with exosomes [62]. Both processes occur without dendritic cell productive infection. In the second phase, the direct infection of dendritic cell (*cis*-infection) contributes to the spread of newly synthesized progeny virus to CD4+ T-lymphocytes [63]. In this regard, several studies have provided important data defining entry-enhancement factors on dendritic cells, such as DC-SIGN, and other C-type lectins receptors (mannose receptor, langerin, syndecan-3, and dendritic cell immunoreceptor - DCIR) [63]. The role of C-type lectin receptors seems to be crucial in both *trans*- and *cis*-infection modes. For example, HIV-1 bound to DC-SIGN is rapidly taken up within endolysosomal vacuoles and protected from degradation while remaining infectious for 1–3 days [64]. Interestingly, suppression of DC-SIGN expression has been shown to impair the viral synapse formation, and to inhibit *trans*-infection of HIV-1 to CD4+ T-lymphocytes [65].

All the data reviewed until now was obtained almost exclusively using HIV-1 model (and in some instances SIV). As referred earlier in this chapter, HIV-2 is a lentivirus that shows a decreased capacity to spread between humans, and probably with additional vulnerabilities during transmission, compared with HIV-1. Besides the lower viral load both in plasma and semen referred previously, little is know about HIV-2 interaction with mucosal cells and how the described physical barriers counteract effective HIV-2 transmission to a new host. For example, very few data exists about HIV-2 interaction with DC-SIGN or the way HIV-2 uses *trans*-infection mechanisms to spread to T-lymphocytes. Apparently the T-cell line adapted strain HIV-2_{ROD} is able to bind to DC-SIGN [66], however data from primary isolates (more closely related to circulating viral variants) are still missing.

Early reports referred that dendritic cells derived from hematopoietic progenitor cells or from peripheral blood monocytes are less susceptible to productive infection by HIV-2 compared with HIV-1 [67, 68]. Paradoxically, recent data have disclosed a cellular protein (SAMHD1) that inhibits HIV-1 replication in immature monocytes-derived dendritic cells, in dendritic cells derived from PMA-differentiated THP-1 monocytic cell line [69] and in macrophages [70]. This restriction factor affects the efficiency of reverse transcription leading to a reduced amount of viral cDNA [71]. SAMHD1 is counteracted by the HIV-2/SIV Vpx protein and its inhibitory mechanism, in the absence of Vpx, helps to explain the different permissivity of these non-dividing cells to lentiviral infection [21]. In this scenario, the non-permissiveness of dendritic cells to HIV-1 infection favours viral dissemination by *trans*-infection pathway, enabling more virions being delivered to CD4+ T-lymphocytes through virological synapse and eventually enhancing the depletion of these latter cells [72]. More importantly, HIV-2 avoiding the effect of SAMHD1 is more prone to trigger host innate immune responses through type I interferon, mediated by viral DNA-exposed dendritic cells [73, 74]. Also, productive infection of dendritic cells by HIV-2 may lead to a different spectrum of presented antigens that ultimately could lead to a different adaptive immune response [74].

5. HIV-2 chronic infection in human host: a natural long-term non progressive infection

The long-term non-progressive infection that characterizes the HIV-2 infection in humans is determined by several host-virus interactions that, in contrast to HIV-1, enable the control and the confinement of HIV-2 pathogenic potential.

As referred above, the different pathogenic outcome observed in HIV-2 infection compared to HIV-1 seems to be dictated as early as the initial interactions with dendritic cells and macrophages present at mucosae surfaces. The expression of Vpx by HIV-2, allowing the bypass of SAMHD1 restriction and the consequent productive infection of dendritic cells and macrophages (*cis*-infection), may result in reduced *trans*-infection to CD4+ T-lymphocytes, a more appropriate innate and adaptive immune response and thus to a more limited infection.

Noteworthy, and despite the described mechanisms that could lead to a hindrance in HIV-2 dissemination at early stages during acute infection, a similar proviral load is observed in HIV-2 and HIV-1 infected patients. These observations suggest that HIV-2, like HIV-1, is able to disseminate and an equal number of target cells are infected during acute and chronic phase or, alternatively, that in HIV-1 a greater number of infected CD4+ T-cells are destroyed in the course of the disease, leading to a similar number of cells containing integrated HIV-1 or HIV-2 genomes.

Typically, infection with HIV-1 is characterized by a gradual and irreversible depletion of CD4+ T-lymphocytes, leading to severe immune dysfunction and the development of AIDS

http://dx.doi.org/10.5772/53201

within a median time of 10 years. However, in contrast to the aforementioned typical progression, virtually all HIV-2 and a small percentage [75] of HIV-1 infections (appropriately referred as "long-term nonprogressors" or "elite controllers") remain healthy for several decades without any antiretroviral therapy, with undetectable plasma viral load and CD4+ cell counts above 500 cells/μL.

A longer asymptomatic phase and slower progression to AIDS are indeed hallmarks of the natural course of HIV-2 infection [1-3]. A clear demonstration of both features was provided by a prospective study conducted with untreated Senegalese sex workers, where 67% of HIV-1-infected women remain AIDS-free 5 years after seroconversion, in contrast with 100% for HIV-2-infected women [3]. The rate of developing CD4+ lymphocyte counts bellow 400 cells/μl was also reduced in HIV-2 participants [3]. Thus, as a rule, HIV-2-infection has no effect on survival in adults [2].

The mechanisms responsible for this less pathogenic course of HIV-2 infection are still poorly understood but surely result from a combination of distinct factors involving the virus, the infected cell and the equilibrium established between viral replication and host immunologic response. This equilibrium is clearly much well preserved in HIV-2 than in HIV-1 infection and it is paradoxical that the study of HIV-2 interaction with host cells remains poorly explored and sometimes neglected. Interestingly, a recent report indicates that a pre-existing infection by HIV-2 appears to inhibit the rate of HIV-1 disease progression [76], together with higher CD4+ T-cell counts and lower viral diversity of HIV-1. This apparent protective effect of HIV-2 may be explained by several viral and immunological mechanisms, namely the higher immunosupression of surface glycoprotein of HIV-2 compared to HIV-1 counterpart [77], or the ability of HIV-2 Nef protein to promote the downmodulation of TCR-CD3 from the surface of CD4+ T-cells [78] and thus the impairment of immunological synapse, established between these lymphocytes and antigen presenting cells (i.e. dendritic cells and macrophages). Both mechanisms have direct impact on immune activation and may help explain the better outcome of HIV-2 infection alone or after superinfection with HIV-1.

5.1. HIV-2 entry into target cells — Early events

HIV replication cycle begins by a specific interaction between viral envelope glycoproteins and cellular receptors allowing the binding of virion to target cell. Further sequential interactions eventually lead to viral envelope and cell membrane fusion. The cellular receptors involved in these early events are the CD4 molecule [79, 80] and a member of seven-transmembrane, G-protein-coupled, receptors' family (GPCRs), referred as coreceptor. According to the proposed model, the specific binding of SU envelope glycoprotein to CD4 induces structural changes in this glycoprotein that expose, create or stabilize the coreceptor-binding regions, enabling the SU to engage the coreceptor molecule. This second binding event causes further conformational changes in SU that allows the disclosure of an amino-terminal hydrophobic region (fusion peptide) of the TM envelope glycoprotein subunit. The insertion of the fusion peptide in the cell surface leads to the fusion of viral envelope with the cell membrane and the release of viral nucleocapside into the cell cytoplasm (reviewed in [81, 82]). This fusion process as long been assumed to occur at the cell surface through a direct fusion mechanism independent of the pH [83]. However, more recent data describe HIV-1 entry and fusion occurs following endocytosis [84, 85].

After the initial identification of CXCR4 and CCR5 in 1996 [86, 87], several other GPCRs have been described as being able to act as coreceptors for HIV-1, HIV-2 and SIV: CCR1, CCR2b, CCR3, CCR4, CCR5, CCR8, CCR9, CCR10, CXCR2, CXCR4, CXCR5, CXCR6, CX3CR1, XCR1, FPRL1, GPR1, GPR15, APJ, ChemR23, CXCR7/ RDC1, D6, BLTR and US28 [88-92]. Despite this extensive array of potential HIV entry coreceptors, only CCR5 and CXCR4 have been considered important for HIV-1 infection *in vivo* [93, 94]. This notion stems from studies reporting: (i) the apparent selection of CCR5-using (R5) variants during mucosal transmission; (ii) the predominance of R5 population during asymptomatic stage of infection; and (iii) the arise and eventual predominance of CXCR4-using (X4) variants in late stages of HIV-1 infection. However, several exceptions to this simplistic R5/X4 dichotomy have been reported [89, 91, 95-104], revealing that some HIV-1 and HIV-2 isolates can exploit other coreceptors *in vitro*, raising the possibility that these alternate molecules can *in vivo* contribute to HIV infection of natural target cells, at least under certain circumstances.

Genetic studies of HIV-1 variants present soon after sexual transmission have shown that only R5, and occasionally dual tropic R5X4, are transmitted regardless the diversity of viral population present in initial inoculum. During chronic infection HIV genetic diversity increases due to viral replication based on an error-prone reverse transcriptase. The resulting viral population (or *quasiespecies*) provides the substrate for natural selection exerted by host immune response and local environment, leading to continuous viral adaptation and persistence within HIV infected patient. However, during mucosal transmission this diversity is severely reduced suggesting a "bottleneck" or "gatekeeper" effect (reviewed in [105]), probably as a result of the biology of mucosal transmission and the kind of cells encountered by HIV (discussed above).

The analysis by single-genome amplification, together with full-length cloning of transmitted/ founder variants, has provided remarkable data on HIV transmission and viral evolution during acute infection. Based on this data, the selection of transmitted/founder viruses encompasses three main signatures: usage of CCR5, high replication rate in CD4+ T-lymphocytes and lack of macrophage tropism (reviewed in [106]). The deficient replication in monocyte-derived macrophages observed in HIV-1 transmitted viruses, although requiring confirmation using tissue macrophages, is consistent with data obtained in nonhuman primates infected with SIV, indicating that CD4+ T-lymphocytes are the predominant cellular substrate for viral replication soon after transmission.

However, a recent and unprecedented observation, regarding HIV coreceptor usage and transmission, revealed that a transmitted/founder HIV-1 was unable to efficiently use either CCR5 or CXCR4 to infect CD4+ cell lines or peripheral blood mononuclear cells [95]. Alternate GPCRs (GPR15, APJ, and FPRL-1) were efficiently used, further emphasizing the notion that "rare" coreceptors could be used *in vivo* in some circumstances or in some cell populations by HIV-1 and HIV-2 alike. Additionally, Chalmet *et al.* [107] have recently provided important data showing that the transmitted viruses could be X4 or R5X4. Considering the established concept, stating that during mucosal transmission the R5 variants present in initial inoculum population of transmitted viruses are favored, these two reports support the idea that non-R5 viruses could indeed be transmitted. This warrants reconsidering the dogma of exclusive R5 variants transmission and should lead us to the following question: is there actually any biological filter at mucosae environment (including physical or chemical barriers, epithelial cells and immune cells present at mucosal surface or in the submucosal layer) that suppresses the invasion and/or dissemination of non-R5 variants; and why in these cases (and other cases?) they were not selected? In other words, are there sufficient and conclusive data to discard the hypothesis of random transmission in favor of a gatekeeper or bottleneck theory [108]? Perhaps the preferential transmission of R5 variants are solely a consequence of their higher proportion in body fluids involved in transmission, either in acute or during most of chronic infection. Further studies are warranted in order to elucidate if X4 or R5X4 variants (and other biotypes, including CCR8-using viruses) are less transmissible.

In HIV-2 no data exists regarding transmitted/founder viruses, or the characteristics or the viral evolution during primary infection. The mechanisms described for HIV-1 and SIV should also be present in HIV-2 infection. However, the identification of HIV-2 isolates unable to infect target cells using the CCR5 or CXCR4 coreceptors [96, 109] obtained from individuals at asymptomatic stage of infection and immunologically competent [96], raises the possibility that, at least in some patients, CCR5 usage is acquired *in vivo* as a result of HIV-2 evolution from an initial population of CCR5- and CXCR4-independent viruses.

5.2. Molecular determinants of coreceptor usage

Identification of the biochemical processes required for HIV fusion and the engagement of chemokine receptors as critical step for HIV entry, has also unveiled several important aspects on envelope glycoproteins structure crucial to the fusion process. HIV-1 and HIV-2 SU glycoprotein contain five conserved regions (C1 to C5), separated by an equal number of variable regions (V1 to V5). The variable regions are limited by cysteine residues forming flexible loops on the outer domain of SU glycoprotein [110-112]. HIV coreceptor usage seems to be largely determined by variable regions of the SU subunit. In HIV-1, the most studied model, the third variable (V3) region has been referred as the major determinant of coreceptor engagement [113-117]. Higher positive net charge (above +5) in V3 region of HIV-1 has been associated with CXCR4 usage (or usage of both CXCR4 and CCR5) [118, 119]. Structural models of SU bound to CD4 and chemokine receptor have provided further information about the functional roles played by several regions of SU, revealing that the V1V2 region is also involved in coreceptor binding, by a direct cooperation with the V3 region [120-124].

In HIV-2, structural and functional studies of the envelope glycoproteins regions are much more scarce and in some aspects contradictory. The genetic characterization of HIV-2 SU has revealed a limited variability, probably as a result of the lower replication rate within the infected individual. Noteworthy, in contrast to HIV-1, the V3 region of HIV-2 SU glycoprotein appears to be highly conserved. Conversely, the V1V2 region is much more prone to genetic variation [125], suggesting that either this region is more exposed and under a stronger selective pressure, or that the lack of V3 loop variation is related to some functional constraints that impairs its evolution. Accordingly, the role of HIV-2 V3 region as a target for neutralizing antibodies has been controversial [126-132].

Similar to neutralization data, molecular determinants of coreceptor usage by HIV-2 is also controversial. Some studies had claimed an association between V3 loop sequence and CCR5 or CXCR4 usage [133-137], while others had found no genetic signature underlying coreceptors usage [138-140]. Particularly, the C-terminal region of the V3 loop, a global net charge above +6 and the presence of mutations in amino acids 18 and 19, appear to dictate the ability to use CXCR4 alone or in addition to CCR5 [134, 137]. However, those studies have some limitations due to the low number of X4 or R5X4 strains and because they restricted the coreceptors usage to the dichotomy R5 vs. X4, without considering the concomitant or alternative use of other coreceptors. We have shown in the molecular characterization of the *env* gene of two CCR5/CXCR4-independent isolates that, although this phenotype is determined by the SU glycoprotein [125], no genetic signature could be clearly found in the V3 region of those strains [125]. Noteworthy and considering that the ability to use a certain coreceptor is solely determined by the V3 loop, the absence of a significant variability in this region is hardly concealed with the broad and "exotic" coreceptor usage observed in HIV-2. Obviously, different regions beside V3 cooperate during envelope glycoproteins interaction with cellular receptors, playing a role in coreceptor choice by a particular virus. One of the strongest candidates is the V1V2 region, where an outstanding genetic variability was observed [140], including length variation and loss of potential glycosilation sites. Moreover, some unique sequence signatures were also founded in the central ectodomain and in the second heptad repeat (HR2) of the TM glycoprotein [140]. All these mutations may affect the conformation of the envelope glycoproteins complex, leading to a more open structure. This will affect not only the dynamics of HIV-2 interaction with cellular receptors, but also the way neutralizing epitopes are exposed and recognized by host immune response, leading to decreased viral fitness, lower replication rate and increased susceptibility to neutralization.

5.3. Evolution of coreceptor usage during HIV-2 chronic infection

Earlier studies addressing the correlation between HIV infection stages (i.e. acute/primary infection, asymptomatic stage and AIDS) and *in vitro* biological characteristics of HIV, gave rise to three distinct classifications according to: (i) the efficiency of replication (rapid/high, slow/low); (ii) the capacity to induce syncytia formation in T-cells (syncytium-inducing/non syncytium-inducing; SI/NSI); and (iii) the ability to replicate in primary macrophages vs. T-cell lines (M-tropic/T-tropic). From these earlier studies it was also clear that, during the course of infection, selection might occur for variants more cytopathic (i.e. able to induce syncytia), with faster replication kinetics (rapid/high) and with tropism for T-cell lines (T-tropic).

Identification of the biochemical processes required for HIV fusion and the engagement of chemokine receptors, clarified the determinants of HIV tropism. Consistent with the proposed model, HIV cell tropism is largely determined by the expression patterns of the appropriate coreceptor molecule at the target-cell membrane. T-tropic viruses (in general with rapid/high and SI phenotype) required the presence of CXCR4 coreceptor (X4 strains) while M-tropic (associated generally with slow/low and NSI phenotype) use CCR5 as coreceptor (R5 strains).

The evolution that was observed in viral phenotype has now an explanation based on the coreceptors used: isolates obtained during asymptomatic stage are R5 (formerly NSI, M-tropic and slow/low) while in later stages of infection, coincident with immunodeficiency and opportunistic infections, the predominant variants are X4 (formerly SI, T-tropic and rapid/high). This shift from predominance of R5 variants to X4, during disease progression, occurs in about 40% of the patients and could be seen as an additional consequence of an already deteriorated immune response, which contributes to an accelerated depletion of T-lymphocytes and disease progression.

In HIV-2, the usage of cell receptors seems to be much more complex and the correlation between disease stage and receptors usage is apparently less clear-cut than in HIV-1. The key notions about cell receptors engagement by HIV-2 are: (i) non-usage of CCR5 or CXCR4 as coreceptors; (ii) a broader coreceptor usage compared to HIV-1; and (iii) the CD4-independent infection of target cells.

5.3.1. Non-usage of CCR5 or CXCR4 as coreceptors

Although CCR5 or CXCR4 usage seems to be an absolute requirement for HIV to fuse its envelope with target-cell membrane, we and others have identified HIV-2 variants that *in vitro* do not use those chemokine receptors (or use it inefficiently) as cofactors for viral entry. These reports indicate that other coreceptors could replace CCR5 and CXCR4 as key players in HIV infection, not just "in addition to" but also "instead of" these coreceptors, clearly suggesting that they have an important role in HIV-2 infection and pathogenesis. Furthermore, we demonstrated that these variants have lower replicative capacity *in vitro* [96, 125], an observation later confirmed by others [141].

The main inference made from studies addressing coreceptors usage by HIV is that the acquisition of CCR5 usage is crucial for HIV pathogenesis. And why CCR5 usage is so important and provides a clear selective advantage *in vivo*? One of the reasons is because CCR5 usage confers HIV the ability to infect stimulated, full-permissive cells, leading to the production of a significantly more infectious viral population. While CXCR4 is expressed in both resting and stimulated T-lymphocytes [142], CCR5 expression is higher in memory CD4+ T-cells (CD45RO+) than in naïve (non-activated) CD4+ T-lymphocyte subset (CD45RA+) [143, 144]. Remarkably, the former are highly permissive to HIV replication, while productive infection of CD45RA+ lymphocytes requires cellular activation soon after viral entry; otherwise, an abortive infection is observed [145].

In addition, the persistence of R5 viruses throughout the asymptomatic stage and in some cases even in individuals with clinical symptoms, suggests that they may escape immune surveillance mechanisms (e.g. neutralization by specific antibodies) or that they could infect long-lived cell reservoirs, such as macrophages and dendritic cells, thus providing long-lasting R5 viruses production.

Interestingly, the described CCR5/CXCR4-independent HIV-2 variants were obtained during asymptomatic stage of infection [96, 109]. As referred, HIV-1 and HIV-2 infections are strikingly different during this period: a longer asymptomatic period with higher CD4+ T-cell counts and undetectable viremia is observed in HIV-2. The host and viral factors that contributes for this high level of control remain poorly understood, but we hypothesized that one of the viral factors that could be involved is the existence of a less fitted viral population, during a variable period of the asymptomatic stage. This population has lower replicative capacity and, at least in some cases, they do not efficiently use CCR5 and/or CXCR4 coreceptors.

5.3.2. Broad coreceptor usage

A hallmark of earlier studies addressing the coreceptors usage by HIV-2 primary isolates was that HIV-2 entry into target cells could be mediated by an array of different GPCRs *in vitro* (reviewed in [146, 147]). In contrast, HIV-1 isolates with coreceptor usage biotype other than R5 and/or X4 have been rarely described. Furthermore, HIV-2 isolates can exploit these alternative coreceptors as efficiently as they use CCR5 or CXCR4, even those rarely used by HIV-1. However, it should be noted that most of the viruses used in these studies were obtained from patients in advanced disease stages, were more pathogenic variants could be present, presumably leading to a bias in the viral population that was preferentially isolated.

The ability to use a larger set of coreceptors should constitute an advantage for HIV-2, since it contributes to a potentially broader cell tropism, with the inherent ability to infect different cell types in different compartments [98, 135, 148]. Yet, as referred in R5-to-X4 evolution (see above) this could lead to the infection of non-activated cells, and thus to abortive cycles. Moreover, the engagement of alternative GPCRs, although being sufficient to mediate HIV-2 entry, could be inadequate to trigger appropriate intracellular signaling required for productive infection. Several studies have shown a direct correlation between the capacity of envelope glycoproteins to elicit appropriate signaling and the ability to perform a productive infection in several cell types (reviewed in [149]). Such signalling events affect multiple intracellular pathways (in a process mimicking chemokine signaling through binding to their receptors) and include: actin depolymerization, cytoskeleton rearrangement, migration of cells and activation of kinases and transcription factors associated with cell activation (Table 2). Although the relevance of coreceptor signaling in HIV pathogenesis has not been clearly defined, it seems that HIV takes advantage of the chemokine signaling network to create an intracellular environment suitable to accomplish a productive infection [149].

Another factor that may account for the apparent paradox of HIV-2 broad coreceptor usage and low virus production *in vivo*, could be the relative concentration of appropriate viral receptors and their co-localization in plasma membrane of specific cell types [150-153]. Moreover, their expression levels could change during activation/differentiation of T lymphocytes and macrophages, as referred for CD4, CCR5 and CXCR4 [144, 154, 155]. Thus, the availability of target cells expressing CD4 and the appropriate coreceptor *in vivo* could be a limiting factor for HIV-2 infection and spread.

Recently we have studied the contribution of CCR8 as an effective coreceptor for HIV-1 and HIV-2 primary isolates [89]. A major and interesting finding arise from this report: a minor coreceptor such as CCR8 was used much more frequently by HIV-1 than by HIV-2 primary isolates, regardless the clinical stage, the plasma viral load or the CD4+ T-cell counts of patients. The rationale for revisiting CCR8 as coreceptor was based on our earlier findings, revealing the existence of HIV-2 unable to use CCR5 or CXCR4 as coreceptors to infect primary CD4+ lymphocytes or CD4-expressing cell lines [96, 125]. CCR8, formerly known as TER1, ChemR1 and CKR-L1, is the receptor for the chemokine CCL1/I-309 [156, 157]. It is expressed in a wide range of cells; some of them are primary targets for HIV infection *in vivo*, e.g. monocytes, thymocytes and peripheral blood CD4+ T-lymphocytes [157-159]. Its tissue distribution and the significant proportion of HIV-1 isolates able to use CCR8, deserves a deeper discussion. If in HIV-2, due to the well-known promiscuous usage of chemokine receptors as coreceptors, the usage of this GPCR was expected, in HIV-1, this was completely unpredicted. As I pointed before, identification of viruses able to use other coreceptors besides CCR5 and CXCR4 seems to be an abnormality in HIV-1. Yet, the findings presented in the cited report [89] together with previous data [91, 100, 103, 160], indicating the efficient use of CCR8 as coreceptor by distinct HIV-1 isolates, either in indicator cell lines or in primary cells, highlight the potential relevance of this molecule for viral transmission and pathogenesis, including HIV-1.

Chemokine interaction with CXCR4* or CCR5** receptors		***HIV interaction*** with CCR5 or CXCR4 coreceptors***	
Primary activation	**Downstream outcome**	**Primary activation**	**Downstream outcome**
Activation of phospholipase C-γ	Transcriptional activation. Cell migration (chemotaxis)	Activation of phospholipase C-γ	Transcriptional activation. Cell migration
Activation of lipid kinase PI3K	Transcriptional activation. Cell adhesion. Cell survival	Activation of lipid kinase PI3K	Cell adhesion. Cell survival
Activation of guanine nucleotide exchange factors specific for Rho family GTPases	Modulation of cytoskeleton: actin rearrangement; myosin light-chain phosphorilation and microtubule rearrangement	Activation of guanine nucleotide exchange factors specific for Rho family GTPases	Modulation of cytoskeleton: actin rearrangement

* Ligand: SDF-1α; ** Ligands: MIP-1α, MIP-1β, and RANTES; *** by the surface envelope glycoprotein

Table 2. Major chemokine receptor signalling pathways triggered after binding of chemokines or HIV envelope surface glycoprotein (for more details see [149])

It is widely recognized that during later stages of HIV-1 infection, a significant proportion of viral variants that constitute the *quasispecies* within an infected individual, evolve in order to efficiently use CXCR4 (and probably other chemokine receptors) in addition to, or instead of, CCR5-using variants, which predominate during early stages of infection [161]. These X4 variants are characterized by increased replicative capacity, a more cytopathic phenotype and the ability to infect a broader range of cells [162]. Accordingly, the emergence of X4 variants is associated with accelerated disease progression and increased CD4+ T-lymphocytes depletion [161]. The infection of naive T-cells by X4 strains is likely to occur early in T-lymphocyte ontogeny and may thus contribute to the described enhancement of T-cells depletion by X4 strains. Studies of thymocyte development demonstrated that CXCR4 is highly expressed on immature T-cell progenitors resident to thymic cortex. As a result, infection of immature thymocytes by X4 strains may disrupt thymopoiesis leading to an impairment of T-cell development and to an accelerated T-cell depletion [163-165].

However, in HIV-2 the correlation between disease progression and coreceptor usage was not consistently observed and a clear pattern of R5-to-X4 evolution, along with disease progression, has been difficult to establish. Even so, R5 viruses are mainly observed in asymptomatic or early symptomatic patients, and strains showing a restricted CXCR4 usage are only observed in late symptomatic individuals [96, 166-168]. In a study comparing CCR5, CXCR4 and CCR8 usage by HIV-1 and HIV-2, an interesting observation was withdrawn pointing to a more frequent usage of CXCR4 by HIV-1 than by HIV-2 primary isolates [89]. Conversely, CCR5 use was significantly more common in HIV-2 isolates than in HIV-1. According to the described enhancement of T-cell depletion by X4 variants, the predominance of a non-X4 viral population, mostly observed in HIV-2 cohort, may contribute to better preserve CD4+ lymphocyte repertoire and immune system functionality and help explain the slower disease progression, generally observed in HIV-2 infected patients compared with HIV-1.

5.3.3. CD4-independent infection

Despite the potential advantage of broader cell tropism associated with lower CD4 dependency, CD4-independent HIV-1 variants, although readily derived *in vitro* [169-172], have been rarely described *in vivo* [173-175]. In contrast, several primary HIV-2 and SIV isolates have been shown to enter cells in a CD4-independent way [81, 148, 168, 176-179].

The ability to entry cells through direct interaction with the coreceptor molecule, bypassing the requirement of prior CD4 engagement, may enable viruses to infect a broader range of cells CD4 negative/coreceptor positive, or cells where CD4 expression is lower and thus limiting. This notion is consistent with studies showing that neutopathogenic HIV-1 variants show reduced CD4 dependence and the ability to infect CD4-negative cells. Viruses with a CD4-independent phenotype could infect cells in different tissue compartments within an infected individual, besides haematopoietic CD4+ cells, such as the brain, testes, lymphoid tissue, kidneys or lungs, further suggesting that CD4-independence could constitute an advantage and might play an important role in some particular tissue settings [148, 173-175, 180, 181]. Interestingly, the CD4-independent phenotype not only appears to be a potential advantage but it can be easily acquired as a consequence of very few amino acids changes in viral envelope glycoproteins [169-172, 182, 183]. Therefore, a central question may arise: why CD4-independent HIV-1 variants are so rare, or why the occurrence of such variants in HIV-2 is not associated with an increased pathogenic outcome?

The infrequent detection of CD4-independent HIV-1 isolates should reflect the selective advantage of CD4 interaction prior to coreceptor engagement. One of the reasons could be the high affinity of CD4-SU envelope glycoprotein binding, stabilizing virion attachment to target cell. However, many other surface molecules have been described to interact with HIV-1 (reviewed in [184]) and thus capable of mediate a stabilizing interaction with virions. Another possible explanation for CD4 dependency could be the shielding of coreceptor binding sites from neutralizing antibodies [170, 182, 185-189]. Considering the proposed mechanism for HIV fusion, the CD4-independent infection imposes that the coreceptor-binding site is already formed or exposed allowing the virus to circumvent the need for prior CD4 interaction. The conformation of envelope glycoproteins allowing the direct interaction with coreceptor (as well as the interaction with different coreceptors) might elicit neutralizing antibodies targeting these critical regions, favoring the host immunological control in HIV-2 infection. Consistent with this notion, sera from HIV-2 infected individuals have higher and broader neutralizing capacity compared to those of HIV-1 [126, 190].

Studies conducted with HIV-2 CD4-independent strains clearly demonstrated a less fitted interaction and a reduced replication rate *in vitro*. This suggests that the coreceptor-binding site is only partially formed (or exposed) affecting the stability/affinity of the complex formed between coreceptor and the envelope glycoproteins. In turn, this may also indicate that prior CD4 interaction is important to assure the infection of more permissive cells, enabling a more productive infection. The intracellular factors that dictate this "friendly" environment for viral replication in CD4+ cells remain unknown but may be related to some unidentified restriction factors that could be present in CD4 negative cells. Conversely, the interaction with CD4 may induce cell-signaling events that could account for optimal viral replication conditions, as I discussed earlier about coreceptor engagement by envelope glycoproteins.

6. Concluding remarks

Two lentiviruses infect humans with different outcomes. HIV-1 and HIV-2, both a result of cross-species transmission, have similar genomic and structural characteristics, and yet they distinctively affect human host. While HIV-1 infection leads to severe immune dysfunction and the development of AIDS within a median time of 10 years, HIV-2 usually takes decades to accomplish that.

Through this chapter, I have provided several data that help to explain this different pathogenic potential of HIV-1 and HIV-2 (see Table 3 for a brief summary). I have focused on those viral characteristics that determines different virus-host interactions and outcomes:

- Lower viral load in body fluids directly involved in HIV-2 transmission.
- Avoidance of SAMHD1 degradation of viral cDNA during infection of dendritic cells, leading to sensing and stronger innate immune response by HIV-2.
- Inability to use CCR5 or CXCR4 that severely affects viral fitness during asymptomatic phase of infection.
- A less common acquisition of CXCR4 usage during the course of infection and the consequent maintenance of a predominant less cytopathic R5 population, which may help to better preserve CD4+ lymphocyte repertoire and immune system functionality in HIV-2 infected individuals.
- Usage of alternate coreceptors that ultimately could lead to inappropriate cell signalling and/or infection of cell populations unable to fully support the HIV-2 replication cycle.

- CD4-independent infection of target cells, providing the potential to infect cells in different compartments but also exposing critical regions of coreceptor binding site to host neutralizing immune response.
- A more relaxed envelope glycoproteins structure that could modulate HIV-2 interaction with cellular receptors, helping explaining the exotic coreceptor usage and CD4-independency but also a less fitted interaction with those receptors and thus to an inappropriate cell signalling.

Much more data is needed to fully comprehend the way human host is able to cope with HIV-2 but not with HIV-1 infection. Further studies addressing HIV-2-cell interactions are warranted as they could reveal undisclosed mechanisms and pathways that may help to clarify the underlying causes for the different pathogenic potential observed between HIV-2 and HIV-1, en route to assist in HIV vaccine development and new therapeutic strategies.

	HIV-1	*HIV-2*
Infection of dendritic cells	Conflicting results. Susceptible to antiviral activity of cellular factor SAMHD1	Conflicting results. Resistant to antiviral activity of cellular factor SAMHD1 (by Vpx protein)
Innate immune response	Less efficiently triggered due to several factors, namely to the restricted infection of dendritic cells	More robust than in HIV-1 namely because infection of dendritic cells could trigger IFN-I mediated response
Coreceptor usage	Generally described has only being able to efficiently use CCR5 and CXCR4	Generally described has being able to efficiently use other coreceptors besides CCR5 and CXCR4
CD4-independent infection	Rarely described	Several primary isolates reported
Molecular determinants of coreceptor usage	Mostly the V3 region of SU envelope glycoprotein	Conflicting data. Probably V1/V2 region and, to a lesser extend, V3 region
Neutralization capacity of serum antibodies	Reduced	Higher and broader

Table 3. Differences between HIV-1 and HIV-2 regarding virus-host interaction (see text for further details)

Acknowledgements

The author wish to acknowledge bioMérieux Portugal for the financial support in the article processing charge of this chapter.

Author details

José Miguel Azevedo-Pereira

Molecular Pathogenesis Centre, Retrovirus and Related Infections Unit (CPM-URIA), Faculty of Pharmacy, University of Lisbon (FFUL), Lisbon, Portugal

References

[1] Whittle, H, Morris, J, Todd, J, Corrah, T, Sabally, S, Bangali, J, et al. HIV-2-infected patients survive longer than HIV-1-infected patients. AIDS. (1994). , 8(11), 1617-1620.

[2] Poulsen, A. G, Aaby, P, Larsen, O, Jensen, H, Naucler, A, Lisse, I. M, et al. year HIV-2-associated mortality in an urban community in Bissau, west Africa. Lancet. (1997). , 349(9056), 911-914.

[3] Marlink, R, Kanki, P, Thior, I, Travers, K, Eisen, G, Siby, T, et al. Reduced rate of disease development after HIV-2 infection as compared to HIV-1. Science. (1994). , 265(5178), 1587-1590.

[4] Virus Taxonomy: (2009). Release [database on the Internet]International Comittee on Taxonomy of Viruses (ICTV). [cited 19 June 2012]. Available from: http://ictvonline.org/virusTaxonomy.asp?version=2009&bhcp=1.

[5] Clavel, F, Guetard, D, Brun-vezinet, F, Chamaret, S, Rey, M. A, Santos-ferreira, M. O, et al. Isolation of a new human retrovirus from West African patients with AIDS. Science. (1986). , 233(4761), 343-346.

[6] Clavel, F, Mansinho, K, Chamaret, S, Guetard, D, Favier, V, Nina, J, et al. Human immunodeficiency virus type 2 infection associated with AIDS in West Africa. New England Journal of Medicine. (1987). , 316(19), 1180-1185.

[7] Keele, B. F, Van Heuverswyn, F, Li, Y, Bailes, E, Takehisa, J, Santiago, M. L, et al. Chimpanzee reservoirs of pandemic and nonpandemic HIV-1. Science. (2006). , 313(5786), 523-526.

[8] Lemey, P, Pybus, O. G, Wang, B, Saksena, N. K, Salemi, M, & Vandamme, A. M. Tracing the origin and history of the HIV-2 epidemic. Proceedings of the National Academy of Sciences of the United States of America. (2003). , 100(11), 6588-6592.

[9] Hahn, B. H, Shaw, G. M, De Cock, K. M, & Sharp, P. M. AIDS as a zoonosis: scientific and public health implications. Science. (2000). , 287(5453), 607-614.

[10] Korber, B, Muldoon, M, Theiler, J, Gao, F, Gupta, R, Lapedes, A, et al. Timing the ancestor of the HIV-1 pandemic strains. Science. (2000). , 288(5472), 1789-1796.

[11] Sharp, P. M, & Hahn, B. H. The evolution of HIV-1 and the origin of AIDS. Philosophical Transactions of the Royal Society of London Series B, Biological sciences. (2010). , 365(1552), 2487-2494.

[12] Suzuki, Y, & Craigie, R. The road to chromatin- nuclear entry of retroviruses. Nature Reviews Microbiology. (2007). , 5(3), 187-196.

[13] Frankel, A. D, & Young, J. A. HIV-1: fifteen proteins and an RNA. Annual Review of Biochemistry. (1998). , 67-1.

[14] Schubert, U, Anton, L. C, Bacik, I, Cox, J. H, Bour, S, Bennink, J. R, et al. CD4 glycoprotein degradation induced by human immunodeficiency virus type 1 Vpu protein requires the function of proteasomes and the ubiquitin-conjugating pathway. Journal of Virology. (1998). , 72(3), 2280-2288.

[15] Varthakavi, V, Smith, R. M, Bour, S. P, Strebel, K, & Spearman, P. Viral protein U counteracts a human host cell restriction that inhibits HIV-1 particle production. Proceedings of the National Academy of Sciences of the United States of America. (2003). , 100(25), 15154-15159.

[16] Perez-caballero, D, Zang, T, Ebrahimi, A, Mcnatt, M. W, Gregory, D. A, Johnson, M. C, et al. Tetherin inhibits HIV-1 release by directly tethering virions to cells. Cell. (2009). , 139(3), 499-511.

[17] Neil, S. J, Zang, T, & Bieniasz, P. D. Tetherin inhibits retrovirus release and is antagonized by HIV-1 Vpu. Nature. (2008). , 451(7177), 425-430.

[18] Abada, P, Noble, B, & Cannon, P. M. Functional domains within the human immunodeficiency virus type 2 envelope protein required to enhance virus production. Journal of Virology. (2005). , 79(6), 3627-3638.

[19] Bour, S. P, Schubert, U, Peden, K, & Strebel, K. The envelope glycoprotein of human immunodeficiency virus type 2 enhances viral particle release: a Vpu-like factor? Journal of Virology. (1996). , 70(2), 820-829.

[20] Andersen, J. L, & Planelles, V. The role of Vpr in HIV-1 pathogenesis. Current HIV Research. (2005). , 3(1), 43-51.

[21] Goujon, C, Rivière, L, Jarrosson-wuilleme, L, Bernaud, J, Rigal, D, Darlix, J-L, et al. SIVSM/HIV-2 Vpx proteins promote retroviral escape from a proteasome-dependent restriction pathway present in human dendritic cells. Retrovirology. (2007).

[22] Kanki, P, Boup, M, Marlink, S, Travers, R, Hsieh, K, & Gueye, C. C. A, et al. Prevalence and risk determinants of human immunodeficiency virus type 2 (HIV-2) and human immunodeficiency virus type 1 (HIV-1) in west African female prostitutes. American Journal of Epidemiology. (1992). , 136(7), 895-907.

[23] Burgard, M, Jasseron, C, Matheron, S, Damond, F, Hamrene, K, Blanche, S, et al. Mother-to-child transmission of HIV-2 infection from 1986 to 2007 in the ANRS

French Perinatal Cohort EPF-CO1. Clinical Infectious Diseases. (2010). , 51(7), 833-843.

[24] Van Tienen, C, Van Der Loeff, M. S, Zaman, S. M, Vincent, T, Sarge-njie, R, Peterson, I, et al. Two Distinct Epidemics: The Rise of HIV-1 and Decline of HIV-2 Infection Between 1990 and 2007 in Rural Guinea-Bissau. Journal of Acquired Immune Deficiency Syndromes. (2009). , 53(5), 640-647.

[25] Quinn, T. C, Wawer, M. J, Sewankambo, N, Serwadda, D, Li, C, Wabwire-mangen, F, et al. Viral load and heterosexual transmission of human immunodeficiency virus type 1. Rakai Project Study Group. New England Journal of Medicine. (2000). , 342(13), 921-929.

[26] Gottlieb, G. S, Hawes, S. E, Agne, H. D, Stern, J. E, Critchlow, C. W, Kiviat, N. B, et al. Lower levels of HIV RNA in semen in HIV-2 compared with HIV-1 infection: implications for differences in transmission. AIDS. (2006). , 20(6), 895-900.

[27] Popper, S. J, Sarr, A. D, Travers, K. U, Gueye-ndiaye, A, Mboup, S, Essex, M. E, et al. Lower human immunodeficiency virus (HIV) type 2 viral load reflects the difference in pathogenicity of HIV-1 and HIV-2. Journal of Infectious Diseases. (1999). , 180(4), 1116-1121.

[28] Gomes, P, Taveira, N. C, Pereira, J. M, Antunes, F, Ferreira, M. O, & Lourenco, M. H. Quantitation of human immunodeficiency virus type 2 DNA in peripheral blood mononuclear cells by using a quantitative-competitive PCR assay. Journal of Clinical Microbiology. (1999). , 37(2), 453-456.

[29] Popper, S. J, Sarr, A. D, Gueye-ndiaye, A, Mboup, S, Essex, M. E, & Kanki, P. J. Low plasma human immunodeficiency virus type 2 viral load is independent of proviral load: low virus production in vivo. Journal of Virology. (2000). , 74(3), 1554-1557.

[30] Wawer, M. J, Gray, R. H, Sewankambo, N. K, Serwadda, D, Li, X, Laeyendecker, O, et al. Rates of HIV-1 transmission per coital act, by stage of HIV-1 infection, in Rakai, Uganda. Journal of Infectious Diseases. (2005). , 191(9), 1403-1409.

[31] Gray, R. H, Wawer, M. J, Brookmeyer, R, Sewankambo, N. K, Serwadda, D, Wabwire-mangen, F, et al. Probability of HIV-1 transmission per coital act in monogamous, heterosexual, HIV-1-discordant couples in Rakai, Uganda. Lancet. (2001). , 357(9263), 1149-1153.

[32] Haase, A. T. Early events in sexual transmission of HIV and SIV and opportunities for interventions. Annual Review of Medicine. (2011). , 62-127.

[33] Lai, S. K, Hida, K, Shukair, S, Wang, Y. Y, Figueiredo, A, Cone, R, et al. Human immunodeficiency virus type 1 is trapped by acidic but not by neutralized human cervicovaginal mucus. Journal of Virology. (2009). , 83(21), 11196-11200.

[34] Pudney, J, Quayle, A. J, & Anderson, D. J. Immunological microenvironments in the human vagina and cervix: mediators of cellular immunity are concentrated in the cervical transformation zone. Biology of Reproduction. (2005). , 73(6), 1253-1263.

[35] Moss, G. B, Clemetson, D, Costa, D, Plummer, L, Ndinya-achola, F. A, & Reilly, J. O. M, et al. Association of cervical ectopy with heterosexual transmission of human immunodeficiency virus: results of a study of couples in Nairobi, Kenya. Journal of Infectious Diseases. (1991). , 164(3), 588-591.

[36] Marx, P. A, Spira, A. I, Gettie, A, Dailey, P. J, Veazey, R. S, Lackner, A. A, et al. Progesterone implants enhance SIV vaginal transmission and early virus load. Nature Medicine. (1996). , 2(10), 1084-1089.

[37] Norvell, M. K, Benrubi, G. I, & Thompson, R. J. Investigation of microtrauma after sexual intercourse. Journal of Reproductive Medicine. (1984). , 29(4), 269-271.

[38] Sewankambo, N, Gray, R. H, Wawer, M. J, Paxton, L, Mcnaim, D, Wabwire-mangen, F, et al. HIV-1 infection associated with abnormal vaginal flora morphology and bacterial vaginosis. Lancet. (1997). , 350(9077), 546-550.

[39] Cohn, M. A, Frankel, S. S, Rugpao, S, Young, M. A, Willett, G, Tovanabutra, S, et al. Chronic inflammation with increased human immunodeficiency virus (HIV) RNA expression in the vaginal epithelium of HIV-infected Thai women. Journal of Infectious Diseases. (2001). , 184(4), 410-417.

[40] Sharkey, D. J, Macpherson, A. M, Tremellen, K. P, & Robertson, S. A. Seminal plasma differentially regulates inflammatory cytokine gene expression in human cervical and vaginal epithelial cells. Molecular Human Reproduction. (2007). , 13(7), 491-501.

[41] Berlier, W, Cremel, M, Hamzeh, H, Levy, R, Lucht, F, Bourlet, T, et al. Seminal plasma promotes the attraction of Langerhans cells via the secretion of CCL20 by vaginal epithelial cells: involvement in the sexual transmission of HIV. Human Reproduction. (2006). , 21(5), 1135-1142.

[42] Münch, J, Rücker, E, Ständker, L, Adermann, K, Goffinet, C, Schindler, M, et al. Semen-derived amyloid fibrils drastically enhance HIV infection. Cell. (2007). , 131(6), 1059-1071.

[43] Kim, K-A, Yolamanova, M, Zirafi, O, Roan, N. R, Staendker, L, Forssmann, W-G, et al. Semen-mediated enhancement of HIV infection is donor-dependent and correlates with the levels of SEVI. Retrovirology. (2010).

[44] Mccoombe, S. G, & Short, R. V. Potential HIV-1 target cells in the human penis. AIDS. (2006). , 20(11), 1491-1495.

[45] Patterson, B. K, Landay, A, Siegel, J. N, Flener, Z, Pessis, D, Chaviano, A, et al. Susceptibility to human immunodeficiency virus-1 infection of human foreskin and cervical tissue grown in explant culture. American Journal of Pathology. (2002). , 161(3), 867-873.

[46] Auvert, B, Taljaard, D, Lagarde, E, Sobngwi-tambekou, J, Sitta, R, & Puren, A. Randomized, controlled intervention trial of male circumcision for reduction of HIV infection risk: the ANRS 1265 Trial. PLoS Medicine. (2005). e298.

[47] Edwards, S. Balanitis and balanoposthitis: a review. Genitourinary Medicine. (1996)., 72(3), 155-159.

[48] Sha, B. E, Zariffard, M. R, Wang, Q. J, Chen, H. Y, Bremer, J, Cohen, M. H, et al. Female genital-tract HIV load correlates inversely with Lactobacillus species but positively with bacterial vaginosis and Mycoplasma hominis. Journal of Infectious Diseases. (2005)., 191(1), 25-32.

[49] Hashemi, F. B, Ghassemi, M, Faro, S, Aroutcheva, A, & Spear, G. T. Induction of human immunodeficiency virus type 1 expression by anaerobes associated with bacterial vaginosis. Journal of Infectious Diseases. (2000)., 181(5), 1574-1580.

[50] Simoes, J. A, Hashemi, F. B, Aroutcheva, A. A, Heimler, I, Spear, G. T, Shott, S, et al. Human immunodeficiency virus type 1 stimulatory activity by Gardnerella vaginalis: relationship to biotypes and other pathogenic characteristics. Journal of Infectious Diseases. (2001)., 184(1), 22-27.

[51] Cohen, C. R, Lingappa, J. R, Baeten, J. M, Ngayo, M. O, Spiegel, C. A, Hong, T, et al. Bacterial Vaginosis Associated with Increased Risk of Female-to-Male HIV-1 Transmission: A Prospective Cohort Analysis among African Couples. PLoS Medicine. (2012). e1001251.

[52] Bomsel, M. Transcytosis of infectious human immunodeficiency virus across a tight human epithelial cell line barrier. Nature Medicine. (1997)., 3(1), 42-47.

[53] Bobardt, M. D, Chatterji, U, Selvarajah, S, Van Der Schueren, B, David, G, Kahn, B, et al. Cell-free human immunodeficiency virus type 1 transcytosis through primary genital epithelial cells. Journal of Virology. (2007)., 81(1), 395-405.

[54] Frank, I, & Pope, M. The enigma of dendritic cell-immunodeficiency virus interplay. Current Molecular Medicine. (2002)., 2(3), 229-248.

[55] Zhang, Z, Schuler, T, Zupancic, M, Wietgrefe, S, Staskus, K. A, Reimann, K. A, et al. Sexual transmission and propagation of SIV and HIV in resting and activated CD4+ T cells. Science. (1999)., 286(5443), 1353-1357.

[56] Wu, L. KewalRamani VN. Dendritic-cell interactions with HIV: infection and viral dissemination. Nature Reviews Immunology. (2006)., 6(11), 859-868.

[57] Wiley, R. D, & Gummuluru, S. Immature dendritic cell-derived exosomes can mediate HIV-1 trans infection. Proceedings of the National Academy of Sciences of the United States of America. (2006)., 103(3), 738-743.

[58] Rubbert, A, Combadiere, C, Ostrowski, M, Arthos, J, Dybul, M, Machado, E, et al. Dendritic cells express multiple chemokine receptors used as coreceptors for HIV entry. Journal of Immunology. (1998). , 160(8), 3933-3941.

[59] Granelli-piperno, A, Moser, B, Pope, M, Chen, D, Wei, Y, Isdell, F, et al. Efficient interaction of HIV-1 with purified dendritic cells via multiple chemokine coreceptors. Journal of Experimental Medicine. (1996). , 184(6), 2433-2438.

[60] Canque, B, Bakri, Y, Camus, S, Yagello, M, Benjouad, A, & Gluckman, J. C. The susceptibility to X4 and R5 human immunodeficiency virus-1 strains of dendritic cells derived in vitro from CD34(+) hematopoietic progenitor cells is primarily determined by their maturation stage. Blood. (1999). , 93(11), 3866-3875.

[61] Granelli-piperno, A, Finkel, V, Delgado, E, & Steinman, R. M. Virus replication begins in dendritic cells during the transmission of HIV-1 from mature dendritic cells to T cells. Current Biology. (1999). , 9(1), 21-29.

[62] Izquierdo-useros, N, Naranjo-gómez, M, Erkizia, I, Puertas, M. C, Borràs, F. E, Blanco, J, et al. HIV and mature dendritic cells: Trojan exosomes riding the Trojan horse? PLoS Pathogens. (2010). e1000740.

[63] Turville, S, Wilkinson, J, Cameron, P, Dable, J, & Cunningham, A. L. The role of dendritic cell C-type lectin receptors in HIV pathogenesis. Journal of Leukocyte Biology. (2003). , 74(5), 710-718.

[64] Freer, G, & Matteucci, D. Influence of dendritic cells on viral pathogenicity. PLoS Pathogens. (2009). e1000384.

[65] Arrighi, J. F, Pion, M, Wiznerowicz, M, Geijtenbeek, T. B, Garcia, E, Abraham, S, et al. Lentivirus-mediated RNA interference of DC-SIGN expression inhibits human immunodeficiency virus transmission from dendritic cells to T cells. Journal of Virology. (2004). , 78(20), 10848-10855.

[66] Pohlmann, S, Baribaud, F, Lee, B, Leslie, G. J, Sanchez, M. D, Hiebenthal-millow, K, et al. DC-SIGN interactions with human immunodeficiency virus type 1 and 2 and simian immunodeficiency virus. Journal of Virology. (2001). , 75(10), 4664-4672.

[67] Vanham, G, Van Tendeloo, V, Willems, B, Penne, L, Kestens, L, Beirnaert, E, et al. The HIV-2 genotype and the HIV-1 syncytium-inducing phenotype are associated with a lower virus replication in dendritic cells. Journal of Medical Virology. (2000). , 60(3), 300-312.

[68] Duvall, M. G, Loré, K, Blaak, H, Ambrozak, D. A, Adams, W. C, Santos, K, et al. Dendritic cells are less susceptible to human immunodeficiency virus type 2 (HIV-2) infection than to HIV-1 infection. Journal of Virology. (2007). , 81(24), 13486-13498.

[69] Laguette, N, Sobhian, B, Casartelli, N, Ringeard, M, Chable-bessia, C, Ségéral, E, et al. SAMHD1 is the dendritic- and myeloid-cell-specific HIV-1 restriction factor counteracted by Vpx. Nature. (2011). , 474(7353), 654-657.

[70] Hrecka, K, Hao, C, Gierszewska, M, Swanson, S. K, Kesik-brodacka, M, Srivastava, S, et al. Vpx relieves inhibition of HIV-1 infection of macrophages mediated by the SAMHD1 protein. Nature. (2011). , 474(7353), 658-661.

[71] Goldstone, D. C, Ennis-adeniran, V, Hedden, J. J, Groom, H. C, Rice, G. I, Christodoulou, E, et al. HIV-1 restriction factor SAMHD1 is a deoxynucleoside triphosphate triphosphohydrolase. Nature. (2011). , 480(7377), 379-382.

[72] Altfeld, M, Fadda, L, Frleta, D, & Bhardwaj, N. DCs and NK cells: critical effectors in the immune response to HIV-1. Nature Reviews Immunology. (2011). , 11(3), 176-186.

[73] Manel, N, Hogstad, B, Wang, Y, Levy, D. E, Unutmaz, D, & Littman, D. R. A cryptic sensor for HIV-1 activates antiviral innate immunity in dendritic cells. Nature. (2010). , 467(7312), 214-217.

[74] Manel, N, & Littman, D. R. Hiding in plain sight: how HIV evades innate immune responses. Cell. (2011). , 147(2), 271-274.

[75] Lambotte, O, Boufassa, F, Madec, Y, Nguyen, A, Goujard, C, Meyer, L, et al. HIV controllers: a homogeneous group of HIV-1-infected patients with spontaneous control of viral replication. Clinical Infectious Diseases. (2005). , 41(7), 1053-1056.

[76] Esbjornsson, J, Mansson, F, Kvist, A, Isberg, P-E, Nowroozalizadeh, S, Biague, A. J, et al. Inhibition of HIV-1 disease progression by contemporaneous HIV-2 infection. The New England journal of medicine. (2012). , 367(3), 224-232.

[77] Cavaleiro, R, Sousa, A. E, Loureiro, A, & Victorino, R. M. Marked immunosuppressive effects of the HIV-2 envelope protein in spite of the lower HIV-2 pathogenicity. AIDS. (2000). , 14(17), 2679-2686.

[78] Arhel, N, Lehmann, M, Clau, K, Nienhaus, G. U, Piguet, V, & Kirchhoff, F. The inability to disrupt the immunological synapse between infected human T cells and APCs distinguishes HIV-1 from most other primate lentiviruses. Journal of Clinical Investigation. (2009). , 119(10), 2965-2975.

[79] Dalgleish, A. G, Beverley, P. C, Clapham, P. R, Crawford, D. H, Greaves, M. F, Weiss, R. A, & The, C. D. T4) antigen is an essential component of the receptor for the AIDS retrovirus. Nature. (1984). , 312(5996), 763-767.

[80] Klatzmann, D, Champagne, E, Chamaret, S, Gruest, J, Guetard, D, Hercend, T, et al. T-lymphocyte T4 molecule behaves as the receptor for human retrovirus LAV. Nature. (1984). , 312(5996), 767-768.

[81] Clapham, P. R, & Mcknight, A. Cell surface receptors, virus entry and tropism of primate lentiviruses. Journal of General Virology. (2002). Pt 8) 1809-1829.

[82] Doms, R. W, & Trono, D. The plasma membrane as a combat zone in the HIV battlefield. Genes and Development. (2000). , 14(21), 2677-2688.

[83] Marsh, M, & Helenius, A. Virus entry: open sesame. Cell. (2006). , 124(4), 729-740.

[84] Daecke, J, Fackler, O. T, Dittmar, M. T, & Krausslich, H. G. Involvement of clathrin-mediated endocytosis in human immunodeficiency virus type 1 entry. Journal of Virology. (2005)., 79(3), 1581-1594.

[85] Miyauchi, K, Kim, Y, Latinovic, O, Morozov, V, & Melikyan, G. B. HIV enters cells via endocytosis and dynamin-dependent fusion with endosomes. Cell. (2009)., 137(3), 433-444.

[86] Alkhatib, G, Combadiere, C, Broder, C. C, Feng, Y, Kennedy, P. E, Murphy, P. M, et al. CC CKR5: a RANTES, MIP-1alpha, MIP-1beta receptor as a fusion cofactor for macrophage-tropic HIV-1. Science. (1996)., 272(5270), 1955-1958.

[87] Feng, Y, Broder, C. C, Kennedy, P. E, & Berger, E. A. HIV-1 entry cofactor: functional cDNA cloning of a seven-transmembrane, G protein-coupled receptor. Science. (1996)., 272(5263), 872-877.

[88] Broder, C. C, & Jones-trower, A. Coreceptor use by primate Lentiviruses. In: Kuiken C, Foley BT, Hahn B, Korber B, McCutchan F, Marx PA, et al., (eds.) Human Retroviruses and AIDS: A Compilation and Analysis of Nucleic Acid and Amino Acid Sequences. Los Alamos, NM: Theoretical Biology and Biophysics Group, Los Alamos National Laboratory; (1999)., 517-541.

[89] Calado, M, Matoso, P, Santos-costa, Q, Espirito-santo, M, Machado, J, Rosado, L, et al. Coreceptor usage by HIV-1 and HIV-2 primary isolates: the relevance of CCR8 chemokine receptor as an alternative coreceptor. Virology. (2010)., 408(2), 174-182.

[90] Neil, S. J, Aasa-chapman, M. M, Clapham, P. R, Nibbs, R. J, Mcknight, A, & Weiss, R. A. The promiscuous CC chemokine receptor D6 is a functional coreceptor for primary isolates of human immunodeficiency virus type 1 (HIV-1) and HIV-2 on astrocytes. Journal of Virology. (2005)., 79(15), 9618-9624.

[91] Shimizu, N, Tanaka, A, Oue, A, Mori, T, Ohtsuki, T, Apichartpiyakul, C, et al. Broad usage spectrum of G protein-coupled receptors as coreceptors by primary isolates of HIV. AIDS. (2009)., 27(7), 761-769.

[92] Simmons, G, Reeves, J, Hibbitts, S, Stine, J, Gray, P, Proudfoot, A, et al. Co-receptor use by HIV and inhibition of HIV infection by chemokine receptor ligands. Immunological Reviews. (2000)., 177-112.

[93] Zhang, Y. J, Dragic, T, Cao, Y, Kostrikis, L, Kwon, D. S, Littman, D. R, et al. Use of coreceptors other than CCR5 by non-syncytium-inducing adult and pediatric isolates of human immunodeficiency virus type 1 is rare in vitro. Journal of Virology. (1998)., 72(11), 9337-9344.

[94] Moore, J. P, Kitchen, S. G, Pugach, P, & Zack, J. A. The CCR5 and CXCR4 coreceptors--central to understanding the transmission and pathogenesis of human immunodeficiency virus type 1 infection. AIDS Research and Human Retroviruses. (2004)., 20(1), 111-126.

[95] Jiang, C, Parrish, N. F, Wilen, C. B, Li, H, Chen, Y, Pavlicek, J. W, et al. Primary infection by a human immunodeficiency virus with atypical coreceptor tropism. Journal of Virology. (2011). , 85(20), 10669-10681.

[96] Azevedo-pereira, J. M, Santos-costa, Q, Mansinho, K, & Moniz-pereira, J. Identification and characterization of HIV-2 strains obtained from asymptomatic patients that do not use CCR5 or CXCR4 coreceptors. Virology. (2003). , 313(1), 136-146.

[97] Xiao, L, Rudolph, D. L, Owen, S. M, Spira, T. J, & Lal, R. B. Adaptation to promiscuous usage of CC and CXC-chemokine coreceptors in vivo correlates with HIV-1 disease progression. AIDS. (1998). F, 137-143.

[98] Willey, S. J, Reeves, J. D, Hudson, R, Miyake, K, Dejucq, N, Schols, D, et al. Identification of a subset of human immunodeficiency virus type 1 (HIV-1), HIV-2, and simian immunodeficiency virus strains able to exploit an alternative coreceptor on untransformed human brain and lymphoid cells. Journal of Virology. (2003). , 77(11), 6138-6152.

[99] Pohlmann, S, Krumbiegel, M, & Kirchhoff, F. Coreceptor usage of BOB/GPR15 and Bonzo/STRL33 by primary isolates of human immunodeficiency virus type 1. Journal of General Virology. (1999). Pt 5) 1241-1251.

[100] Lee, S, Tiffany, H. L, King, L, Murphy, P. M, Golding, H, & Zaitseva, M. B. CCR8 on human thymocytes functions as a human immunodeficiency virus type 1 coreceptor. Journal of Virology. (2000). , 74(15), 6946-6952.

[101] Edinger, A. L, Hoffman, T. L, Sharron, M, Lee, B, Dowd, O, & Doms, B. RW. Use of GPR1, GPR15, and STRL33 as coreceptors by diverse human immunodeficiency virus type 1 and simian immunodeficiency virus envelope proteins. Virology. (1998). , 249(2), 367-378.

[102] Deng, H. K, & Unutmaz, D. KewalRamani VN, Littman DR. Expression cloning of new receptors used by simian and human immunodeficiency viruses. Nature. (1997). , 388(6639), 296-300.

[103] Cilliers, T, Willey, S, Sullivan, W. M, Patience, T, Pugach, P, Coetzer, M, et al. Use of alternate coreceptors on primary cells by two HIV-1 isolates. Virology. (2005). , 339(1), 136-144.

[104] Gharu, L, Ringe, R, & Bhattacharya, J. Evidence of extended alternate coreceptor usage by HIV-1 clade C envelope obtained from an Indian patient. Virus Research. (2012). , 163(1), 410-414.

[105] Grivel, J-C, Shattock, R. J, & Margolis, L. B. Selective transmission of R5 HIV-1 variants: where is the gatekeeper? Journal of Translational Medicine. (2011). Suppl 1 S6.

[106] Keele, B. F, & Estes, J. D. Barriers to mucosal transmission of immunodeficiency viruses. Blood. (2011). , 118(4), 839-846.

[107] Chalmet, K, Dauwe, K, Foquet, L, Baatz, F, Seguin-devaux, C, Van Der Gucht, B, et al. Presence of CXCR4-Using HIV-1 in Patients With Recently Diagnosed Infection: Correlates and Evidence for Transmission. Journal of Infectious Diseases. (2012). , 205(2), 174-184.

[108] Hedskog, C, Mild, M, & Albert, J. Transmission of the X4 Phenotype of HIV-1: Is There Evidence Against the "Random Transmission" Hypothesis? Journal of Infectious Diseases. (2012). , 205(2), 163-165.

[109] Sol, N, Ferchal, F, Braun, J, Pleskoff, O, Treboute, C, Ansart, I, et al. Usage of the coreceptors CCR-5, CCR-3, and CXCR-4 by primary and cell line-adapted human immunodeficiency virus type 2. Journal of Virology. (1997). , 71(11), 8237-8244.

[110] Mcknight, A, Shotton, C, Cordell, J, Jones, I, Simmons, G, & Clapham, P. R. Location, exposure, and conservation of neutralizing and nonneutralizing epitopes on human immunodeficiency virus type 2 SU glycoprotein. Journal of Virology. (1996). , 70(7), 4598-4606.

[111] Starcich, B. R, Hahn, B. H, Shaw, G. M, Mcneely, P. D, Modrow, S, Wolf, H, et al. Identification and characterization of conserved and variable regions in the envelope gene of HTLV-III/LAV, the retrovirus of AIDS. Cell. (1986). , 45(5), 637-648.

[112] Willey, R. L, Rutledge, R. A, Dias, S, Folks, T, Theodore, T, Buckler, C. E, et al. Identification of conserved and divergent domains within the envelope gene of the acquired immunodeficiency syndrome retrovirus. Proceedings of the National Academy of Sciences of the United States of America. (1986). , 83(14), 5038-5042.

[113] Cho, M. W, Lee, M. K, Carney, M. C, Berson, J. F, Doms, R. W, & Martin, M. A. Identification of determinants on a dualtropic human immunodeficiency virus type 1 envelope glycoprotein that confer usage of CXCR4. Journal of Virology. (1998). , 72(3), 2509-2515.

[114] Hoffman, T. L, & Doms, R. W. HIV-1 envelope determinants for cell tropism and chemokine receptor use. Molecular Membrane Biology. (1999). , 16(1), 57-65.

[115] Hoffman, T. L, Stephens, E. B, Narayan, O, & Doms, R. W. HIV type I envelope determinants for use of the CCR2b, CCR3, STRL33, and APJ coreceptors. Proceedings of the National Academy of Sciences of the United States of America. (1998). , 95(19), 11360-11365.

[116] Hu, Q, Trent, J. O, Tomaras, G. D, Wang, Z, Murray, J. L, Conolly, S. M, et al. Identification of ENV determinants in that influence the molecular anatomy of CCR5 utilization. Journal of Molecular Biology. (2000). , 3

[117] Smyth, R. J, Yi, Y, Singh, A, & Collman, R. G. Determinants of entry cofactor utilization and tropism in a dualtropic human immunodeficiency virus type 1 primary isolate. Journal of Virology. (1998). , 72(5), 4478-4484.

[118] Briggs, D. R, Tuttle, D. L, Sleasman, J. W, Goodenow, M. M, & Envelope, V. amino acid sequence predicts HIV-1 phenotype (co-receptor usage and tropism for macrophages). AIDS. (2000). , 14(18), 2937-2939.

[119] Delobel, P, Nugeyre, M. T, Cazabat, M, Pasquier, C, Marchou, B, Massip, P, et al. Population-based sequencing of the region of env for predicting the coreceptor usage of human immunodeficiency virus type 1 quasispecies. Journal of Clinical Microbiology. (2007). , 3

[120] Kwong, P. D, Wyatt, R, Robinson, J, Sweet, R. W, Sodroski, J, & Hendrickson, W. A. Structure of an HIV gp120 envelope glycoprotein in complex with the CD4 receptor and a neutralizing human antibody. Nature. (1998). , 393(6686), 648-659.

[121] Labrosse, B, Treboute, C, Brelot, A, & Alizon, M. Cooperation of the V2 and V3 domains of human immunodeficiency virus type 1 gp120 for interaction with the CXCR4 receptor. Journal of Virology. (2001). , 1

[122] Nabatov, A. A, Pollakis, G, Linnemann, T, Kliphius, A, Chalaby, M. I, & Paxton, W. A. Intrapatient alterations in the human immunodeficiency virus type 1 gp120 and V3 regions differentially modulate coreceptor usage, virus inhibition by CC/CXC chemokines, soluble CD4, and the b12 and 2G12 monoclonal antibodies. Journal of Virology. (2004). , 1V2

[123] Pollakis, G, Kang, S, Kliphuis, A, Chalaby, M. I, & Goudsmit, J. Paxton WA. N-linked glycosylation of the HIV type-1 gp120 envelope glycoprotein as a major determinant of CCR5 and CXCR4 coreceptor utilization. Journal of Biological Chemistry. (2001). , 276(16), 13433-13441.

[124] Wyatt, R, Moore, J, Accola, M, Desjardin, E, Robinson, J, & Sodroski, J. Involvement of the V2 variable loop structure in the exposure of human immunodeficiency virus type 1 gp120 epitopes induced by receptor binding. Journal of Virology. (1995). , 1

[125] Santos-costa, Q, Mansinho, K, Moniz-pereira, J, & Azevedo-pereira, J. M. Characterization of HIV-2 chimeric viruses unable to use CCR5 and CXCR4 coreceptors. Virus Research. (2009).

[126] De Silva, T. I, Aasa-chapman, M, Cotten, M, Hué, S, Robinson, J, Bibollet-ruche, F, et al. Potent Autologous and Heterologous Neutralizing Antibody Responses Occur in HIV-2 Infection across a Broad Range of Infection Outcomes. Journal of Virology. (2012). , 86(2), 930-946.

[127] Kong, R, Li, H, Bibollet-ruche, F, Decker, J. M, Zheng, N. N, Gottlieb, G. S, et al. Broad and Potent Neutralizing Antibody Responses Elicited in Natural HIV-2 Infection. Journal of Virology. (2012). , 86(2), 947-960.

[128] Marcelino, J. M, Borrego, P, Rocha, C, Barroso, H, Quintas, A, Novo, C, et al. Potent and Broadly Reactive HIV-2 Neutralizing Antibodies Elicited by a Vaccinia Virus

Vector Prime-C2Polypeptide Boost Immunization Strategy. Journal of Virology. (2010). , 3C3

[129] Ozkaya Sahin GHolmgren B, da Silva Z, Nielsen J, Nowroozalizadeh S, Esbjörnsson J, et al. Potent Intratype Neutralizing Activity Distinguishes Human Immunodeficiency Virus Type 2 (HIV-2) from HIV-1. Journal of Virology. (2012). , 86(2), 961-971.

[130] Bjorling, E, Broliden, K, Bernardi, D, Utter, G, Thorstensson, R, Chiodi, F, et al. Hyperimmune antisera against synthetic peptides representing the glycoprotein of human immunodeficiency virus type 2 can mediate neutralization and antibody-dependent cytotoxic activity. Proceedings of the National Academy of Sciences of the United States of America. (1991). , 88(14), 6082-6086.

[131] Bjorling, E, Chiodi, F, Utter, G, & Norrby, E. Two neutralizing domains in the region in the envelope glycoprotein gp125 of HIV type 2. Journal of Immunology. (1994). , 3

[132] Matsushita, S, Matsumi, S, Yoshimura, K, Morikita, T, Murakami, T, & Takatsuki, K. Neutralizing monoclonal antibodies against human immunodeficiency virus type 2 gp120. Journal of Virology. (1995). , 69(6), 3333-3340.

[133] Albert, J, Stalhandske, P, Marquina, S, Karis, J, Fouchier, R. A, Norrby, E, et al. Biological phenotype of HIV type 2 isolates correlates with genotype. AIDS Research and Human Retroviruses. (1996). , 3

[134] Isaka, Y, Sato, A, Miki, S, Kawauchi, S, Sakaida, H, Hori, T, et al. Small amino acid changes in the loop of human immunodeficiency virus type 2 determines the coreceptor usage for CXCR4 and CCR5. Virology. (1999). , 3

[135] Morner, A, Thomas, J. A, Bjorling, E, Munson, P. J, Lucas, S. B, & Mcknight, A. Productive HIV-2 infection in the brain is restricted to macrophages/microglia. AIDS. (2003). , 17(10), 1451-1455.

[136] Shi, Y, Brandin, E, Vincic, E, Jansson, M, Blaxhult, A, Gyllensten, K, et al. Evolution of human immunodeficiency virus type 2 coreceptor usage, autologous neutralization, envelope sequence and glycosylation. Journal of General Virology. (2005). Pt 12) 3385-3396.

[137] Visseaux, B, Hurtado-nedelec, M, Charpentier, C, Collin, G, Storto, A, Matheron, S, et al. Molecular Determinants of HIV-2 R5-X4 Tropism in the Loop: Development of a New Genotypic Tool. Journal of Infectious Diseases. (2012). , 3

[138] Kulkarni, S, Tripathy, S, Agnihotri, K, Jatkar, N, Jadhav, S, Umakanth, W, et al. Indian primary HIV-2 isolates and relationship between genotype, biological phenotype and coreceptor usage. Virology. (2005). , 3

[139] Owen, S. M, Ellenberger, D, Rayfield, M, Wiktor, S, Michel, P, Grieco, M. H, et al. Genetically divergent strains of human immunodeficiency virus type 2 use multiple coreceptors for viral entry. Journal of Virology. (1998). , 72(7), 5425-5432.

[140] Santos-costa, Q, Parreira, R, Moniz-pereira, J, & Azevedo-pereira, J. M. Molecular characterization of the env gene of two CCR5/CXCR4-independent human immunodeficiency 2 primary isolates. Journal of Medical Virology. (2009). , 81(11), 1869-1881.

[141] Blaak, H, Van Der Ende, M. E, Boers, P. H, Schuitemaker, H, & Osterhaus, A. D. In vitro replication capacity of HIV-2 variants from long-term aviremic individuals. Virology. (2006). , 353(1), 144-154.

[142] Baggiolini, M, Dewald, B, & Moser, B. Human chemokines: an update. Annual Review of Immunology. (1997). , 15-675.

[143] Bleul, C. C, Wu, L, Hoxie, J. A, Springer, T. A, & Mackay, C. R. The HIV coreceptors CXCR4 and CCR5 are differentially expressed and regulated on human T lymphocytes. Proceedings of the National Academy of Sciences of the United States of America. (1997). , 94(5), 1925-1930.

[144] Wu, L, Paxton, W. A, Kassam, N, Ruffing, N, Rottman, J. B, Sullivan, N, et al. CCR5 levels and expression pattern correlate with infectability by macrophage-tropic HIV-1, in vitro. Journal of Experimental Medicine. (1997). , 185(9), 1681-1691.

[145] Woods, T. C, Roberts, B. D, Butera, S. T, & Folks, T. M. Loss of inducible virus in CD45RA naive cells after human immunodeficiency virus-1 entry accounts for preferential viral replication in CD45RO memory cells. Blood. (1997). , 89(5), 1635-1641.

[146] Azevedo-pereira, J. M, Santos-costa, Q, & Moniz-pereira, J. HIV-2 infection and chemokine receptors usage- clues to reduced virulence of HIV-2. Current HIV Research. (2005). , 3(1), 3-16.

[147] Reeves, J. D, & Doms, R. W. Human immunodeficiency virus type 2. Journal of General Virology. (2002). Pt 6) 1253-1265.

[148] Willey, S, Roulet, V, Reeves, J. D, Kergadallan, M. L, Thomas, E, Mcknight, A, et al. Human Leydig cells are productively infected by some HIV-2 and SIV strains but not by HIV-1. AIDS. (2003). , 17(2), 183-188.

[149] Wu, Y, & Yoder, A. Chemokine coreceptor signaling in HIV-1 infection and pathogenesis. PLoS Pathogens. (2009). e1000520.

[150] Kozak, S. L, Platt, E. J, Madani, N, & Ferro, F. E. Jr, Peden K, Kabat D. CD4, CXCR-4, and CCR-5 dependencies for infections by primary patient and laboratory-adapted isolates of human immunodeficiency virus type 1. Journal of Virology. (1997). , 71(2), 873-882.

[151] Kuhmann, S. E, Platt, E. J, Kozak, S. L, & Kabat, D. Cooperation of multiple CCR5 coreceptors is required for infections by human immunodeficiency virus type 1. Journal of Virology. (2000). , 74(15), 7005-7015.

[152] Lee, B, Sharron, M, Montaner, L. J, Weissman, D, & Doms, R. W. Quantification of CD4, CCR5, and CXCR4 levels on lymphocyte subsets, dendritic cells, and differen-

tially conditioned monocyte-derived macrophages. Proceedings of the National Academy of Sciences of the United States of America. (1999). , 96(9), 5215-5220.

[153] Platt, E. J, Wehrly, K, Kuhmann, S. E, Chesebro, B, & Kabat, D. Effects of CCR5 and CD4 cell surface concentrations on infections by macrophagetropic isolates of human immunodeficiency virus type 1. Journal of Virology. (1998). , 72(4), 2855-2864.

[154] Naif, H. M, Li, S, Alali, M, Sloane, A, Wu, L, Kelly, M, et al. CCR5 expression correlates with susceptibility of maturing monocytes to human immunodeficiency virus type 1 infection. Journal of Virology. (1998). , 72(1), 830-836.

[155] Tuttle, D. L, Harrison, J. K, Anders, C, Sleasman, J. W, & Goodenow, M. M. Expression of CCR5 increases during monocyte differentiation and directly mediates macrophage susceptibility to infection by human immunodeficiency virus type 1. Journal of Virology. (1998). , 72(6), 4962-4969.

[156] Roos, R. S, Loetscher, M, Legler, D. F, Clark-lewis, I, Baggiolini, M, & Moser, B. Identification of CCR8, the receptor for the human CC chemokine I-309. Journal of Biological Chemistry. (1997). , 272(28), 17251-17254.

[157] Tiffany, H. L, Lautens, L. L, Gao, J. L, Pease, J, Locati, M, Combadiere, C, et al. Identification of CCR8: a human monocyte and thymus receptor for the CC chemokine I-309. Journal of Experimental Medicine. (1997). , 186(1), 165-170.

[158] Ambrosio, D, Iellem, D, Bonecchi, A, Mazzeo, R, Sozzani, D, & Mantovani, S. A, et al. Selective up-regulation of chemokine receptors CCR4 and CCR8 upon activation of polarized human type 2 Th cells. Journal of Immunology. (1998). , 161(10), 5111-5115.

[159] Zingoni, A, Soto, H, Hedrick, J. A, Stoppacciaro, A, Storlazzi, C. T, Sinigaglia, F, et al. The chemokine receptor CCR8 is preferentially expressed in Th2 but not Th1 cells. Journal of Immunology. (1998). , 161(2), 547-551.

[160] Horuk, R, Hesselgesser, J, Zhou, Y, Faulds, D, Halks-miller, M, Harvey, S, et al. The CC chemokine I-309 inhibits CCR8-dependent infection by diverse HIV-1 strains. Journal of Biological Chemistry. (1998). , 273(1), 386-391.

[161] Connor, R. I, Sheridan, K. E, Ceradini, D, Choe, S, & Landau, N. R. Change in coreceptor use coreceptor use correlates with disease progression in HIV-1--infected individuals. Journal of Experimental Medicine. (1997). , 185(4), 621-628.

[162] van'Wout, t, Blaak, A. B, Ran, H, Brouwer, L. J, Kuiken, M, & Schuitemaker, C. H. Evolution of syncytium-inducing and non-syncytium-inducing biological virus clones in relation to replication kinetics during the course of human immunodeficiency virus type 1 infection. Journal of Virology. (1998). , 72(6), 5099-5107.

[163] Berkowitz, R. D, Beckerman, K. P, Schall, T. J, & Mccune, J. M. CXCR4 and CCR5 expression delineates targets for HIV-1 disruption of T cell differentiation. Journal of Immunology. (1998). , 161(7), 3702-3710.

[164] Kitchen, S. G, & Zack, J. A. CXCR4 expression during lymphopoiesis: implications for human immunodeficiency virus type 1 infection of the thymus. Journal of Virology. (1997). , 71(9), 6928-6934.

[165] Taylor, J. R. Jr., Kimbrell KC, Scoggins R, Delaney M, Wu L, Camerini D. Expression and function of chemokine receptors on human thymocytes: implications for infection by human immunodeficiency virus type 1. Journal of Virology. (2001). , 75(18), 8752-8760.

[166] Guillon, C, Van Der Ende, M. E, Boers, P. H, Gruters, R. A, Schutten, M, & Osterhaus, A. D. Coreceptor usage of human immunodeficiency virus type 2 primary isolates and biological clones is broad and does not correlate with their syncytium-inducing capacities. Journal of Virology. (1998). , 72(7), 6260-6263.

[167] Mcknight, A, Dittmar, M. T, Moniz-periera, J, Ariyoshi, K, Reeves, J. D, Hibbitts, S, et al. A broad range of chemokine receptors are used by primary isolates of human immunodeficiency virus type 2 as coreceptors with CD4. Journal of Virology. (1998). , 72(5), 4065-4071.

[168] Reeves, J. D, Hibbitts, S, Simmons, G, Mcknight, A, Azevedo-pereira, J. M, Moniz-pereira, J, et al. Primary human immunodeficiency virus type 2 (HIV-2) isolates infect CD4-negative cells via CCR5 and CXCR4: comparison with HIV-1 and simian immunodeficiency virus and relevance to cell tropism in vivo. Journal of Virology. (1999). , 73(9), 7795-7804.

[169] Dumonceaux, J, Nisole, S, Chanel, C, Quivet, L, Amara, A, Baleux, F, et al. Spontaneous mutations in the env gene of the human immunodeficiency virus type 1 NDK isolate are associated with a CD4-independent entry phenotype. Journal of Virology. (1998). , 72(1), 512-519.

[170] Hoffman, T. L. LaBranche CC, Zhang W, Canziani G, Robinson J, Chaiken I, et al. Stable exposure of the coreceptor-binding site in a CD4-independent HIV- 1 envelope protein. Proceedings of the National Academy of Sciences of the United States of America. (1999). , 96(11), 6359-6364.

[171] Kolchinsky, P, Mirzabekov, T, Farzan, M, Kiprilov, E, Cayabyab, M, Mooney, L. J, et al. Adaptation of a CCR5-using, primary human immunodeficiency virus type 1 isolate for CD4-independent replication. Journal of Virology. (1999). , 73(10), 8120-8126.

[172] LaBranche CCHoffman TL, Romano J, Haggarty BS, Edwards TG, Matthews TJ, et al. Determinants of CD4 independence for a human immunodeficiency virus type 1 variant map outside regions required for coreceptor specificity. Journal of Virology. (1999). , 73(12), 10310-10319.

[173] Xiao, P, Usami, O, Suzuki, Y, Ling, H, Shimizu, N, Hoshino, H, et al. Characterization of a CD4-independent clinical HIV-1 that can efficiently infect human hepatocytes through chemokine (C-X-C motif) receptor 4. AIDS. (2008). , 22(14), 1749-1757.

[174] Zerhouni, B, Nelson, J. A, & Saha, K. Isolation of CD4-independent primary human immunodeficiency virus type 1 isolates that are syncytium inducing and acutely cytopathic for CD8+ lymphocytes. Journal of Virology. (2004). , 78(3), 1243-1255.

[175] Saha, K, Zhang, J, Gupta, A, Dave, R, Yimen, M, & Zerhouni, B. Isolation of primary HIV-1 that target CD8+ T lymphocytes using CD8 as a receptor. Nature Medicine. (2001). , 7(1), 65-72.

[176] Azevedo-pereira, J. M, Santos-costa, Q, Taveira, N, Verissimo, F, & Moniz-pereira, J. Construction and characterization of CD4-independent infectious recombinant HIV-2 molecular clones. Virus Research. (2003). , 97(2), 159-163.

[177] Edinger, A. L, Mankowski, J. L, Doranz, B. J, Margulies, B. J, Lee, B, Rucker, J, et al. CD4-independent, CCR5-dependent infection of brain capillary endothelial cells by a neurovirulent simian immunodeficiency virus strain. Proceedings of the National Academy of Sciences of the United States of America. (1997). , 94(26), 14742-14747.

[178] Endres, M. J, Clapham, P. R, Marsh, M, Ahuja, M, Turner, J. D, Mcknight, A, et al. CD4-independent infection by HIV-2 is mediated by fusin/CXCR4. Cell. (1996). , 87(4), 745-756.

[179] Liu, H. Y, Soda, Y, Shimizu, N, Haraguchi, Y, Jinno, A, Takeuchi, Y, et al. CD4-Dependent and CD4-independent utilization of coreceptors by human immunodeficiency viruses type 2 and simian immunodeficiency viruses. Virology. (2000). , 278(1), 276-288.

[180] Gorry, P. R, Taylor, J, Holm, G. H, Mehle, A, Morgan, T, Cayabyab, M, et al. Increased CCR5 affinity and reduced CCR5/CD4 dependence of a neurovirulent primary human immunodeficiency virus type 1 isolate. Journal of Virology. (2002). , 76(12), 6277-6292.

[181] Marras, D, Bruggeman, L. A, Gao, F, Tanji, N, Mansukhani, M. M, Cara, A, et al. Replication and compartmentalization of HIV-1 in kidney epithelium of patients with HIV-associated nephropathy. Nature Medicine. (2002). , 8(5), 522-526.

[182] Edwards, T. G, Hoffman, T. L, Baribaud, F, & Wyss, S. LaBranche CC, Romano J, et al. Relationships between CD4 independence, neutralization sensitivity, and exposure of a CD4-induced epitope in a human immunodeficiency virus type 1 envelope protein. Journal of Virology. (2001). , 75(11), 5230-5239.

[183] Reeves, J. D, Schulz, T. F, & The, C. D. independent tropism of human immunodeficiency virus type 2 involves several regions of the envelope protein and correlates with a reduced activation threshold for envelope-mediated fusion. Journal of Virology. (1997). , 71(2), 1453-1465.

[184] Ugolini, S, Mondor, I, & Sattentau, Q. J. HIV-1 attachment: another look. Trends in Microbiology. (1999). , 7(4), 144-149.

[185] Bhattacharya, J, Peters, P. J, & Clapham, P. R. CDindependent infection of HIV and SIV: implications for envelope conformation and cell tropism in vivo. AIDS. (2003). Suppl 4 S35-43., 4.

[186] Kolchinsky, P, Kiprilov, E, & Sodroski, J. Increased neutralization sensitivity of CD4-independent human immunodeficiency virus variants. Journal of Virology. (2001). , 75(5), 2041-2050.

[187] Puffer, B. A, Pohlmann, S, Edinger, A. L, Carlin, D, Sanchez, M. D, Reitter, J, et al. CD4 independence of simian immunodeficiency virus Envs is associated with macrophage tropism, neutralization sensitivity, and attenuated pathogenicity. Journal of Virology. (2002). , 76(6), 2595-2605.

[188] Thomas, E. R, Shotton, C, Weiss, R. A, Clapham, P. R, Mcknight, A, & Hiv-2, C. D4-d. e. p. e. n. d. e. n. t a. n. d C. D4-i. n. d. e. p. e. n. d. e. n. t. consequences for neutralization. AIDS. (2003). , 17(3), 291-300.

[189] Zhang, P. F, Bouma, P, Park, E. J, Margolick, J. B, Robinson, J. E, Zolla-pazner, S, et al. A variable region 3 (mutation determines a global neutralization phenotype and CD4-independent infectivity of a human immunodeficiency virus type 1 envelope associated with a broadly cross-reactive, primary virus-neutralizing antibody response. Journal of Virology. (2002). , 3

[190] Bjorling, E, Scarlatti, G, Von Gegerfelt, A, Albert, J, Biberfeld, G, Chiodi, F, et al. Autologous neutralizing antibodies prevail in HIV-2 but not in HIV-1 infection. Virology. (1993). , 193(1), 528-530.

Chapter 19

Interaction of FIV with Heterologous Microbes in the Feline AIDS Model

Joseph Ongrádi, Stercz Balázs, Kövesdi Valéria,
Nagy Károly and Pistello Mauro

Additional information is available at the end of the chapter

http://dx.doi.org/10.5772/52767

1. Introduction

Since the emergence of the acquired immune deficiency syndrome (AIDS), there has been a great deal of interest in identifying cofactors that accelerate progression of the disease elicited by human immunodeficiency virus types 1 or 2 (HIV-1, HIV-2). Beside inherent factors and environmental agents, speculations led to the conclusion that infectious diseases frequently occur in HIV infected persons, might augment HIV replication, and consequently facilitate AIDS progression. HIV infection is followed by a long disease-free period, during which a low number of CD4+ immune cells contains transcriptionally silent provirus. Activation of CD4+ cells by external factors, including heterologous viruses, terminates latency forcing towards a productive HIV infection. Transactivation of the HIV long terminal repeat (LTR) by cellular, nuclear transcriptional factors (e.g. NF-κB, Sp1) induced by mitogens, cytokines, chemokines, simultaneous virus infections is followed by gene expression including the synthesis of the HIV transactivator protein (TAT), which binds to the transactivating response (TAR) element of the genome, ultimately leading to large scale production of HIV and death of infected cells through apoptosis [1,2]. *In vitro* studies showed that products of immediate early (IE) or early (E) genes of several DNA viruses such as human herpesviruses (HHV) -1, 2, 3, 4, 5, 6A, 8, adenoviruses, as well as hepatitis B virus (HBV) X gene, human T lymphotropic virus type I (HTLV-I) *tax* gene upregulated production of these transcriptional factors and activate HIV-1 or HIV-2 in the same cells. Simultaneous infection in a single cell is relatively rare event *in vivo*; therefore such type of biological effects in nature could be minimal. On the contrary, cross-talk between immune cells carrying different viruses via cytokines, chemokines is more common. Heterologous viruses infect many types of cells, which are not targets of HIV, but release several immunomodulatory mediators, usually in an abnormal pattern. High level of tumour necrosis factor (TNF)-α, interleukin (IL)-6, IL-10, and low level of IL-2, IL-12 were frequently observed in the blood of AIDS patients, only to mention the most important ones. Abundant pro-inflammatory cytokines bind to HIV carrier cells and through consequently activated secondary messenger systems activate the same transcriptional factors for HIV activation. This category of interaction has a more significant impact on HIV infection. This phenomenon called as transcellular transactivation can last lifetime, its intensity may vary depending on the host, the other transiently or chronically coinfecting microbes, etc. [3]. These external confounding factors act in a pleiotropic manner, which is impossible to study *in vitro*. Animal studies are ideal to establish their role in AIDS progression [4].

2. The feline AIDS model

Feline AIDS (FAIDS) induced by feline immunodeficiency virus (FIV) is the only natural small animal model of human AIDS [4,5-8]. FIV shares many genetic, structural and biological characteristics with HIV. FIV also shows tropism for CD4+ immune cells, but its receptor is the CD134 molecule with the CXCR4 coreceptor. FIV LTR accommodates multiple enhancer or promoter protein-binding sites (e.g. NF-κB, AP-1). Although FIV lacks TAT and the TAR element, its Orf-2 (also designated as Orf-A) acts as a transactivator gene to some degree and is necessary for productive FIV replication [7,9]. The similarities in the clinical course of infection between HIV and FIV are striking [6,8,10]. Male gender and adult age are known risk factors for both HIV and FIV transmission [6,7,11,12]. Domestic cats infected with FIV develop progressive immune dysfunction characterised by depletion of CD4+ T cells, wasting, cachexia, gingivostomatitis, neuropathological disorders, opportunistic infections, unusual malignancies such as B cell lymphomas, fibrosarcomas [13]. CD4+CD25+hi-FoxP3+ immunosuppressive regulatory T (Treg) cells have been implicated as a possible cause of immune dysfunction during FIV and HIV-1 infection, as they are capable of modulating virus-specific and inflammatory immune responses. Influence of Treg cell suppression during FIV and HIV pathogenesis is most prominent after Treg cells are activated in the environment of established FIV infection [10]. It is important to remember that increased activity of Treg cells promotes immunosenescence in the normal elderly, and AIDS is regarded as an extremely rapid ageing process [14]. Disease progression occurs over a similar time scale to HIV-1 infection in humans [6]. FIV is distributed worldwide; it has several subtypes similarly to HIV [12,15]. Species-specific strains of FIV circulate in many members of *Felidae* family, including endangered big cats in which also induce AIDS-like illnesses [6,12]. Some opportunistic infections in cats also occur worldwide such as feline leukaemia virus (FeLV), feline herpesvirus type 1 (FHV-1), *Toxoplasma gondii* (TG), feline coronavirus (FCoV), *Bartonella henselae* (BH), canine distemper virus (CDV), fungal pathogens or mycoplasmas. Their incidence depends on geographical regions, cat subpopulations (pet, indoor, stray, feral, free-roaming, etc.), gender and age [11,12,16-28]. Incidence of other opportunistic microbes depends on endemic geographical areas and local vectors (e.g. haemoplasma or Leishmania species, different helminths) [16,18,29-33]. Some of these microbes establish coinfection in a

http://dx.doi.org/10.5772/52767

particular felid species that carries a specific strain of FIV. Typical examples have been reported recently. A highly virulent FeLV outbreak in FIV_{Pco} infected free ranging Florida pumas (*Puma concolor coryi*) threatened this endangered species [12]. In another outbreak in the Serengeti, FIV_{Ple} B infected lions (*Panthera leo*) were twice as likely to survive CDV infection compared to lions infected with FIV_{Ple} A or FIV_{Ple} C [34]. These cases clearly demonstrate that specificities of both microbes might express increased risk for severe synergistic pathogenicity. Recent surveys on coinfections mentioned above were carried out for descriptive epidemiological purposes. In the majority of studies, occurrence of heterologous microbes were judged as opportunistic infections, but some of the investigators have come to the conclusion that FIV and heterologous microbes might mutually aggravate immunosuppression at the level of the organism [12,17]. Both FIV and FeLV independently might predispose animals for toxoplasma infection [21]. In spite of similar clinical manifestations by FIV or FeLV, they might specifically predispose the host for different heterologous microbial pathogens: FIV predisposes to Leishmania [12,16], mycoplasma [25,27,33,35], fungal [26], FCoV [12] infections, while FeLVsensitises the organism to BH infection [36]. Others found that the rate of toxoplasma [16,30,32] or FCV [24] infections occur independently of FIV status. These result, even some of them are contradictory, clearly show that each retrovirus must have its specific way to interact with other microbes at molecular or immunological level. It is conceivable that HIV and human microbes have similar ways for interactions. Both direct transactivation of FIV in the simultaneously infected cells (Figure 1) or cross-talk between cells infected by FIV, and other cells infected by heterologous microbes (Figure 2) can take place in the body of cats.

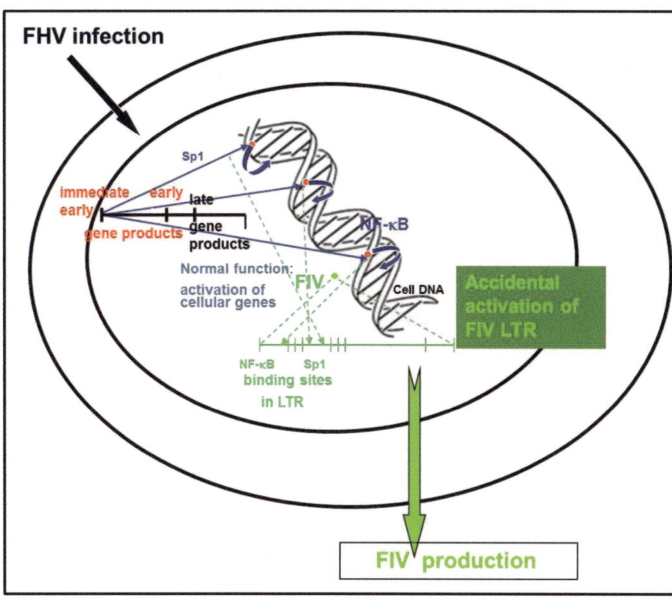

Figure 1. Scheme of intracellular virus transactivation

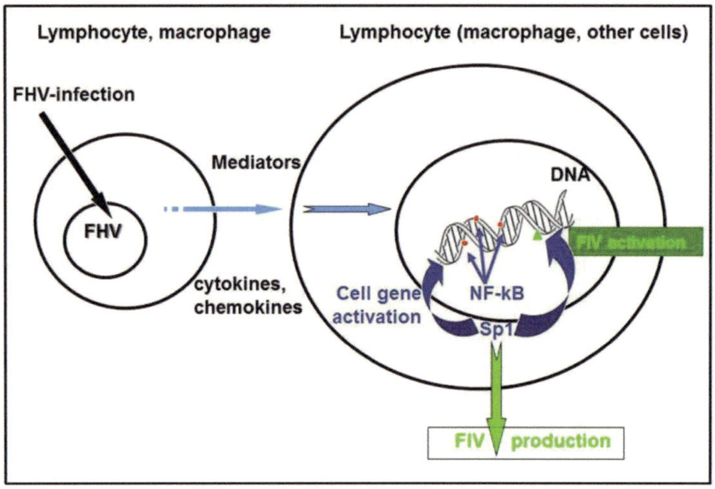

Figure 2. Scheme of transcellular transactivation

Comparison of human clinical observations on opportunistic infections in HIV infected patients and *in vitro* transactivation studies unambiguously demonstrate that several viruses can cause both opportunistic infection and transactivate HIV. The domestic cat is afflicted with multiple microbes that also induce human diseases (e.g. TG, Leishmania, fungi, mycobacteria). Furthermore, domestic cats harbour several feline virus species that are homologous to human viruses: FIV, FeLV, FHV, FCV, FCoV, as well as feline sarcoma virus, feline parvovirus, feline morbillivirus [12]. These feline microbe species provide a panoply of infectious disease models for many devastating human diseases including for studies on the possible interaction between retroviruses and heterologous microbes among natural conditions of FAIDS at molecular, immunological, cellular level in any organ or the whole body of infected cats by any available methodology.

3. Simultaneous infections: Both opportunists and transactivators

3.1. Feline herpesvirus

Simultaneous infection by retroviruses and heterogenous microbes and their association with a variety of diseases have come into focus recently. The very sensitive methods to detect nucleic acids of microbes have promoted our understanding that microbial interaction may result in the synergistic induction of more severe disease course. Retroviruses and herpesviruses might be associated with a variety of diseases in animals. Coinfection of chickens with Marek's disease virus (*Gammaherpesvirinae*) and retrovirus (avian leukosis virus) increase the incidence of retrovirus associated tumours [37]. As several species of human herpesviruses have been implicated as cofactors for AIDS progression, possible interaction of feline herpesvirus 1 (FHV-1, subfamily *Betaherpesvirinae,* a homologue of human cytomegalovirus /CMV/), with FIV has been studied *in vivo* and *in vitro*. FHV-1 might spread in some captive felids with higher frequency than in their free-ranging counterparts demonstrating the importance of human intervention in natural epidemiology [11,29,38]. Single or simultaneous infection by FHV-1 and TG or BH have been implicated as causative agents of feline uveitis [20]. It is of note, that FHV-1 homologue human CMV induces very severe retinitis in HIV infected humans [12], and human CMV was found one of the clinically most frequent and strongest transactivator of HIV. On the contrary to human experience with HSV-1 and adenoviruses [39], FHV-1 could not be implicated in the multifactorial aetiology of gingivitis [24]. FHV-1 also infects T lymphocytes. FHV-1 is a significant pathogen limited to the family *Felidae,* causing an upper respiratory disease in cats. Interaction of acute FHV-1 infection in chronically, experimentally FIV infected specific pathogen-free (SPF) animals results in several immunological abnormalities. FIV infected cats produce less FHV-1 neutralising IgM antibodies during the first 3 weeks of infection than non-FIV infected animals, whereas the IgG antibody response remains unaffected. The ongoing IgG antibody response to FIV is not affected by FHV-1 infection. Lymphocyte blastogenic response to concanavalin A (Con-A) is depressed in FIV-infected and non-infected cats, but response to pokeweed mitogen (PWM) takes longer to return to normal in FIV infected animals. Lymphocytes from FIV infected cats have a greater and more sustained proliferative response to FHV-1 antigen than non-infected cats [40]. Cats with pre-existing FIV infection have more severe signs of disease after exposure to FHV-1 or TG, than FIV-free counterparts. Primary immune responses to all heterologous pathogens are delayed or diminished in FIV infected compared with non-FIV-infected animals. Repeated infections have no significant effect on the level of FIV-specific antibodies or on the production of peripheral blood mononuclear cells (PBMC) containing FIV proviral DNA. FIV infected cats exposed to cofactors have normal levels of IL-2R and major histocompatibility complex (MHC)-II antigen expression on PBMCs, while only-FIV-infected animals have upregulated IL-2R and down-regulated MHC-II expression [41]. By transfection of a recombinant plasmid containing the FIV LTR linked to the chloramphenicol acetyltransferase (CAT) gene, followed by infection of FHV-1 into Crandell feline kidney (CrFK) or *Felis catus* whole fetus 4 (fcwf-4) cells enhancement of CAT activity was demonstrated. Both immunofluorescence and electron microscopy showed productive coinfection of individual T lymphocytes [42]. A series of FIV LTR deletion mutants were constructed and cotransfected with FHV-1 to identify the regions that are responsible for transactivation. It was demonstrated that sequences between -124 and -79, and between -21 and -32 (relative to the cap site) are essential of FIV replication in fcwf-4 cells and that the sequence between -63 and -23 responds to transactivation of FIV LTR by FHV-1 [43]. FHV-1 infected-cell-protein 4 (ICP4) was found to down-regulate FIV LTR directed gene expression via the C/EBP site in the LTR, but after introduction of a site-specific mutation of this site, ICP4 significantly stimulated LTR. These results indicate that FHV-1 ICP4 possesses both abilities to transactivate or down-regulate FIV-directed gene expression. C/EBP and AP-1 regulatory sequences are known to act as both positive and negative regulators [44]. Interestingly enough, plasmids expressing ICP4 homologues of Alphaherpesviruses, namely pseudorabies virus (PRV) and equine herpesvirus type 1 (EHV-1) could significantly inhibit FIV LTR-directed gene expression in CrFK and fcwf-4 cells. Moreover, the ICP4 homologues also exhibited a marked suppressive effect on FIV replication in CrFK cells cotransfected with an infectious clone of FIV [45]. These experiments drow attention to the role of other herpesviruses, among them Roseoloviruses [46], which might exist in cats. Similarities and differences between the human or feline AIDS could help elucidating their devastating role in human and feline patients.

3.2. Feline adenovirus

Among other DNA viruses, adenovirus (AdV) also might enhance AIDS progression in cats. So far, the only feline adenovirus (FeAdV) isolate (also the first one from the family *Felidae*) was obtained from a fecal sample of a cat with AdV PCR positivity [47] and unknown FIV serostatus [48]. Its hexon [49], fiber [50], and nucleotide sequences published so far suggest that it might be related to human AdV type 1 (HAdV-1). Similar nucleotide sequences have been shown in the feces of a small child suffering with gastroenteritis and her cat in Japan [51], and in one nasopharyngeal aspirate sample of a 468 member cohort of children presenting acute respiratory disease in Brazil [52]. This virus might be widespread all over the world and one can speculate that it could transactivate both HIV and FIV, e.g. in pet owners. Seroepidemiological studies show that approx. 10-20% of free roaming cats are seropositive in Hungary and Europe [53,54]. In a series of consecutive transfer of FIV by intravenous inoculation of experimental SPF casts, four were AdV seropositive, but their serostatus before FIV inoculation remained unknown. One can speculate that accidental transfer of AdV along with FIV occurred [55]. FeAdV would be ideal to compare its unique clinical and molecular effects in the human and the cat both *in vivo* and *in vitro* similarly to studies on the interaction of HHV-6 and SIV in humans and pig-tailed macaques [56,57]. As it was isolated from cat feces, one could use FeAdV and FIV to model intestinal molecular interaction of HAdVs and HIV.

3.3. Feline leukaemia virus

Another common interaction in nature is between FIV infection and FeLV. FeLV is of particular significance because it can also induce immunodeficiency [58]. FeLV is a homologue of human T lymphotropic virus (HTLV). It displays a prevalence of 1-8% worldwide [16,24,33,38], but in some geographical areas much higher prevalence of FeLV antigen has been detected (14.2% in Iran, [21], 24.5% in Thailand, [18], 26% in Portugal, [28]). In catteries its prevalence could be much lower or up to zero [17,26,30,32]. Its prevalence has been decreasing in most countries and is regarded as a less important deadly infectious agent in the last 20 years compared to FIV [19]. In confined geographical regions or among captive animals in different facilities, simultaneous decline in the seroprevalence of both FeLV and FIV has also been observed [29,33]. Seroprevalence is higher in intact males than females, and increases with age [17,18]. Transmission is usually by direct contact or saliva wounds. FeLV infection among non-domestic cats of the *Felidae* family is rare, but FeLV has been shown to cross species barriers, especially in case of prior or simultaneous microbial immunosuppression [12,28]. There are four naturally occurring exogenous FeLV strains: FeLV-A, -B, -C, and –T. FeLV-A is the predominant subgroup circulating in feral cats. Its integrated proviral sequences are transmitted vertically through the germ line. Recombination might occur between FeLV-A and other subgroups. The outcome after exposure depends on several host and environmental factors, but the clinical course is more aggressive than seen with FIV. In approximately one third of exposed cats, viraemia is persistent and eventually results in clinical disorders such as immunosuppression, bone marrow suppression (mainly anaemia), and neoplasm (mainly lymphoma) [12,19]. Like FIV, FeLV infection alone also renders the animals more susceptible to infection, persistence and disease elicited by heterologous microbes [19,28,33] such as TG [21] or BH [36]. Mortality among persistently FeLV infected cats is high as 83% die within 3.5 years [references in 12]. About 10 to 15% of the cats that are clinically ill with FIV infection are coinfected with FeLV worldwide [59,60]. Upon superinfection with FIV, asymptomatic cats with persistent FeLV infection manifest a more accelerate and exacerbated FIV disease, anticipated death and show a higher FIV load in lymphoid tissues than did naive cats under both natural and experimental conditions, while the blood level of FeLV p27 antigen was not elevated. Interestingly, the synergy between FIV and FeLV is bidirectional: doubly infected cats develop FeLV induced tumours more frequently than did cats infected with either virus alone [61]. Dually infected cats remain more leukopenic than cats infected with FIV or FeLV alone, and their CD4+/CD8+ T lymphocyte ratios become rapidly inverted [62]. This interrelationship is similar to what has been described for HIV and HTLV-I [63].

3.4. Simultaneous Listeria and FIV infection

Scarce data are available on the possible effect on FIV and FAIDS exerted by feline bacterial infections. *Listeria monocytogenes* (LM) can infect both humans and cats, and its profound immunomodulatory capabilities are well known. Beside HIV, both FIV and LM impair the innate immune response that fails to gain control of their replication prior to the adaptive immune response. These effects might be additive or synergistic in simultaneously infected individuals. In a series of recent experiments, chronically FIV infected and SPF control cats were challenged with LM, then their whole blood and lymph nodes were collected 3 days after challenge. The number and functions of natural killer (NK) cells (CD3-CD56+), NKT cells (CD3+CD56+), CD4 (CD3+CD4+), CD8 (CD3+CD8+), regulatory T cells (CD4+CD25+Fox3+) and Langerhans cells (CD1a) were evaluated. NK, NKT, CD4+ and CD8+ T cells in the LM challenged lymph node of FIV-infected cats did not increase in number, NK cells did not increase their proliferation, apoptosis was elevated, and perforin expression was not upregulated when compared to SPF control animals. No difference in Treg cell number was found. Delayed control and clearance of opportunistic LM was also observed. In the blood compartment of LM challenged cats, CD4+ T cell proliferation did not differ in SPF-control and FIV positive cats, while CD8+ T cell proliferation increased in FIV-positive animals. The number of Langerhans cells did not decrease in FIV and LM infected animals, but their ability to produce NK-activating IL-15 and other mediators became impaired. Although it is concluded that FIV-infected cats are more vulnerable to LM superinfection [2], it is conceivable that precedent or ongoing Listeria infection diminishes the activity of NK cells, helps promote FIV replication and dissemination in the body of animals. In HIV-infected patients, dysfunction of NK cells with low perforin expression, anergy, furthermore, abnormal antigen presentation and low level of IL-15, IL-12 levels are also known [2]. In humans, infection by LM or other bacteria with immunosuppressive potential might augment impaired immunosurveillance, consequently increase HIV load, and ultimately facilitate AIDS progression.

3.5. Feline haemotropic mycoplasmas (haemoplasmas)

Epidemiological surveys on simultaneous infections by FIV and feline haemophilic mycoplasmas suggest that opportunistic infections also promote FIV progression. Feline haemophilic mycoplasmas (*Mycoplasma haemofelis, Candidatus Mycoplasma haemominutus*) collectively called haemoplasmas can cause anaemia and severe clinical disease of affected cats. *Candidatus Mycoplasma haemominutus* (CMH) is usually not associated with clinical disease, but typically causes anaemia in cats carrying pre-existing FIV or FeLV infection [29,64,65]. Chronic FIV infection appears to modify the acute phase response to feline haemotropic mycoplasmas, which varies with the infecting haemoplasma species, namely CMH and *M. haemofelis* (MH), respectively [64]. A recent study in a Canadian feral cat population found that CMH positive cats were significantly more likely to be concurrently retrovirus positive than were CMH negative animals [33]. Another recent study in Spain found that, FIV seropositivity and male sex were significantly associated with MH, CMH and *Ca. M. turicensis* infection [27]. It is of note, that mycoplasmas in HIV infected patients have been regarded as AIDS promoting factors for a long time, and this phenomenon was proved *in vitro*, either [66]. A meta-analysis of former studies unambiguously demonstrated that genital infection by *M. genitalium* poses high risk for acquisition of HIV. Testing and treatment of *M. genitalium*-positive individuals in high risk groups is recommended as a potential HIV prevention strategy [67]. Bacterial vaginosis-associated microflora in the female genital tract also predisposes for HIV infection. Among flora members, *M. hominis* was shown to activate NF-κB and AP-1. Through mediation of a soluble HIV inducing factor (HIF), these transcriptional factors may subsequently increase genital tract viral load and potentially contribute to HIV transmission [68]. MH infection along with BH infection has been verified by PCR in an HIV infected person [69]. The 34 year old man owned several cats. Haemoplasma DNA is present in saliva and feces of cats, which suggests that aggressive interactions among cats and humans involving biting may lead to transmission of the organism. So far, haemotropic mycoplasma infections have been reported in a patient with systemic lupus erythematosus (SLE) and in an anaemic patient showing that some forms of immunosuppression are required for acquisition of an unusual pathogen [70]. Increasing number of human patients with compromised immune systems living near cats increases the possibility that haemoplasma infections may emerge in this population [69]. Haemoplasma positive cats like mycoplasma positive humans ought to be regarded at increased risk for retrovirus infection. Testing would also be appropriate prior to relocation of felids [29]. Feline mycoplasmas could provide a unique model to clarify the exact role of mycoplasmas in AIDS progression.

http://dx.doi.org/10.5772/52767

3.6. Feline mycobacteria

Mycobacteria are important opportunistic infections in HIV infected patients worldwide. Especially in Sub-Saharan Africa very aggressive forms of tuberculosis occur in the immunocompromised population induced by several mycobacterium species. Mycobacteria severely suppress activities of the cellular immune reactions but due to the difficulties in their cultivation and the chronic nature of the disease, it is extremely difficult to study their mutual effects on the immune system. Several mycobacterium species that infect the human and are prevalent in HIV infected patients (*e.g. M. bovis, M. avium, M. microti*), induce disease in cats [23]. This finding raises the idea that FAIDS would be an appropriate model to study intimate relationship between mycobacteria and feline retroviruses *in vivo*.

Repeated exposure of FIV positive cats to bacterial lipopolysaccharide endotoxin (LPS) resulted in lower plasma and brain viremia. In HIV infected humans and FIV infected cats, macrophages produce elevated amount of specific chemokine CXCL10, which in turn damages brain cells. LPS treatment of infected macrophages release IL-10 counteracting CXCL10 expression of brain cells. Suppressed CXCL10 level in the brain of FIV-positive cats and ensuing T cell infiltration is concomitant with reduction in neurovirulence [71]. This observation is in correlation with earlier results, namely that LPS treatment of HHV-6A infected lymphoid cells decrease expression of such soluble mediators that transactivate HIV-1 in other lymphoid cultures [3].

3.7. Fungal and parasitic infections in FIV infected cats

Humans and cats can be infected by several common fungal pathogens, such as Cryptococcus [22], Malassezia, Microsporum [26] and others [28]. Dermatophyte fungi were isolated in 29.4% from stray cats in Portugal [28]. *Microsporum gypseum* and, occasionally, *M. canis* were found in an equal ratio of FIV negative and positive cats (8 and 8.5%, respectively). In contrast, Malassezia species were more frequently isolated from FIV infected cats than FIV-uninfected cats (84% vs. 28.6%) thus showing a closer biological relationship in the effect of FIV and certain fungal species. The CD4:CD8 ratio for FIV infected cats with cutaneous overall fungal infection was significantly lower than the CD4:CD8 ratio in the FIV infected cats but without cutaneous fungal infection. It is obvious that worsening cellular immunity represents a risk factor to cutaneous fungal colonisation in cats [26], but existence of a cutaneous or systematic fungal infection due to insufficient activity of the cellular immunity acquired by inherent or environmental effects might also make easier to acquire FIV infection. Damaged local immunity in the skin in case of wound FIV infection could be one of the most frequent examples. Cats having human or human homologues of fungal species would be ideal models to study such aspects.

Cats having access to the outdoor world, very easily acquire parasitic infections. Feral cats can serve as a direct or indirect source of infectious diseases for pet cats. Contact with animals of other species, conditions of breeding, food supply and age are considered significant for infections. A recent study conducted in a Brazilian cat colony free from FIV, FeLV and *Neospora caninum* infection, clearly showed these differences. Of cats from urban and rural areas, 10.4% and 27.2% were seropositive for TG, respectively. Cats having access to streets

(17.1%), cats cohabiting with rats (19.6%), and cats feeding on homemade food and raw milk (27.2%) were positive for this protozoon. In addition, 4.2% of cats were positive for *Leishmania spp.* [30]. In several countries, parasitic infections, especially intestinal parasites, of cats are more frequent than infections with FIV or FeLV. In Italy, comparison of FIV, FeLV and TG IgG seropositivity resulted in the same ratio: 6.6%, 3.8% and 30.5%, respectively [11]. Epidemiological studies in Portugal found 24.2% TG seropositivity, 31% carrier state of intestinal parasites (*Toxocara cati, Isospora felis, Ankylostoma stenocephala, Toxascaris leonina*) as compared to FIV and FeLV infection (10.2% and 7.1%, respectively) in the same stray cat population [28]. In a confined region of Canada, 29.8% of cats had TG antibodies, 1.3% excreted oocysts in their feces, while FIV and FeLV seropositivity was significantly lower (5.2% and 3.1%, respectively [33]. In Thailand, although the ratio between retroviral and parasitic infections were different (FIV, FeLV, heartworm (*Dirofilaria immitis*) and TG IgG (20.1%, 24.5%, 4.6% and 10.1%, respectively) from the other data mentioned above, of the 348 cats sampled for all four pathogens, 3.1%, 2.8% and 0.28% were positive for TG antibodies and FIV antibodies, FeLV antigen or *D. immitis* antigen, respectively. Of the 35 TG seropositive cats, 42.9% were coinfected with at least one of the other three pathogens [18]. Feral cats from Cairo, Egypt exhibited an extremely high ratio of TG infestation as compared to FIV, FeLV of heartworm seroprevalence: 95.5%, 33.9%, 4.6% and 3.4%, respectively. It is of interest that 57.4% of TG positive cats had very high antibody titre (>1:640) [31]. Oocyst shedding was found to be accompanied by high level antibodies: cats shedding TG had high antibody level (>1:256). In the same cat cohort, *Toxocara cati* eggs were identified in 37%, *Cystoisospora felis* oocysts in 14%, *Taenia sp.* segments in 15% of animals. Most of the fecal samples showed evidence of at least one intestinal parasite, while many samples contained evidence of multiple intestinal parasites. High prevalence of antibodies reflects latent infections. However, it must be emphasized that cats with latent infection can pose a considerable zoonotic risk with respect to the shedding of intestinal parasites in their feces. Stress conditions induce shedding. Intercurrent retroviral infections (FIV or FeLV or both) with consequent declination in systemic and mucosal immunity are regarded as important stress factors [33]. Result of the multivariate logistic regression analysis of another recent survey on simultaneous virus and parasite seropositivity (FIV, FeLV and TG was 19.2%, 14.2% and 32.1%, respectively) in Iran showed that retroviral-associated immunosuppression is a risk factor for activation of toxoplasmosis in cats [21]. Beside toxoplasmosis, Leishmania infection is frequent in many countries. Cellular immunity of normal cats effectively controls *Leishmania infantum* (syn. *L. chagasi*). However, feline immunosuppressive diseases such as FIV and FeLV infection impair the normal response to infection and expose cats to reactivation or new infections by other pathogens, among them Leishmania. Although no statistical evidence of association between TG and Leishmania was found, but in cats coinfected with FIV, a strong statistical association for the triple coinfection was found [16]. One can conclude from these epidemiological surveys, that parasites cause not only opportunistic infections in retrovirus infected cats, but activation of their latent infection by retroviruses suggests existence of a closer relationship between phylogenetically distant two groups of foreign agents at molecular or immunological level.

http://dx.doi.org/10.5772/52767

Following infection of FIV carrier cats with a secondary pathogen, cytokine dysregulation is more pronounced. TG increases both IFN-γ and IL-10, but fails to increase IL-2, IL-12, while TG infected FIV negative cats show an increase in IFN-γ, IL-2 and IL-12 [72]. A similar dysregulation has been reported in cats challenged with LM [73]. The increase in IL-10 to IL-12 ratio predicts the loss of cellular immunity in FIV infected cats [72,74]. These *in vivo* studies are in good correlation with *in vitro* experiments. Latent infection in HIV or FIV infected lymphocytes and macrophages can be reactivated and virus production can be increased by chemical immune activators such as phorbol myristate acetate [75], concanavalin A [5], granulocyte macrophage-colony stimulating factor [76]. Both HIV and FIV induce apoptosis not only in the infected cells, but in the vicinity of infected cells as well. Programmed cell death of infected cells is mediated mainly by TNF-α released from infected cells [77]. Cytokine dysregulation affects not only the FIV carrier animal, but damages the fetus by causing a pro-inflammatory placental microenvironment at early pregnancy: increased expression of IL-6, IL-12, decreased expression of IL-1β, SDF-1α. Similarly to AIDS patients, IL-6 expression correlated with FIV load [78]. The exact role of cytokines and chemokines in the process of simultaneous infections waits for clarification.

4. Diagnosis, treatment and prevention of simultaneous infections

Preventing exposure of healthy cats to FIV or FeLV infected cats by tests and removal or isolation is an important measure, and is not alternative to vaccination. The most common method for diagnosis of FIV infection is screening for antibodies (typically against p24 and p15) using an ELISA. Several commercial kits are available worldwide. Confirmatory testing for cats with positive results is strongly recommended, Western-blot and immunofluorescent antibody assays (IFA) are used. Infection from queens can be transmitted to kittens, testing for newly acquired cats and kittens is strongly recommended. Vaccinated cats also produce antibodies that cannot be distinguished, by any commercially available antibody test [79], from antibodies due to natural infection, and queens might transmit these antibodies to the litter via colostrum. FIV vaccine induces fewer antibodies for non-structural proteins compared to natural infection. There are tests to discriminate this pattern, but these are unsuitable for routine use. Polymerase chain reaction (PCR) has promoted by some commercial laboratories as a method to determine a cat's true infection status. The test detects FIV RNA or proviral DNA. A real-time PCR assay for FIV quantification of proviral DNA in PBMC has high sensitivity and specificity. This and reverse transcriptase (RT)-PCR are methods to quantitate viral load and dissemination in the body after activation of latent FIV infection. Due to genetically heterologous nature of FIV, tests with concurrent determination of subtype differentiation are recommended. Serological diagnosis of FeLV relies on detection of the core antigen p27 in PBMC using an ELISA. IFA test is also used but discordant results might occur. PCR is offered by a number of commercial laboratories, it can be performed on blood, saliva, bone marrow and tissues. Kittens can be tested for FeLV at any age, as passively acquired maternal antibody does not interfere with testing for viral antigen.

Compliance of cat owners with FIV and FeLV testing is low, in spite of using combined test kits, and professional recommendations by veterinarians (Table 1).

At risk of infection	
	cats access to outdoors
	known exposure to retrovirus infected cats
	multicat environment
	bite wounds
	oral disease
Sick cats	
Cats entering new homes, shelters	
Newly acquired cats and kittens about to be vaccinated for FIV or FeLV	
Cats used for blood or tissue donation	

Table 1. Major recommendations for FIV and FeLV testing of cats

The owner must also consider the cost of immunisation, fecal parasite testing, de-worming, or blood screening to reveal and eliminate concomitant infections [17]. Further commercially available kits for serological screening, and/or antigen detection including FHV-1 and the most pathogens are widely available for domestic and large cats. These kits used separately depending on the clinical course of the animal can be combined in definitively. Well established, cheap but somewhat laborious and time consuming classical methods have been used for direct detection of common bacteria, fungi and parasites (cultivation, biochemistry, microscopy, etc.). For feline pathogens causing infection in humans, the same methods and kits can be used as in human medicine. With technological advances quantitative real-time or RT-PCR assays have been used subsequently their products are sequenced to determine species or variants. Load of viruses in body fluids can be determined by quantitative molecular methods [5,7,24,36]. Simultaneous detection of nucleic acids of coinfecting microbes would be ideal by using multiple PCR [20, 29]. Development of easily available panels is a financial interest of biotechnology companies. Gene arrays capable of detecting even hundreds of microbes at nucleic acid level could also be marketed in near future.

Aims of detecting simultaneous infection in cats and large felids are very variable. As retroviral infection might represent a considerable risk factor to several bacterial, fungal and parasitic opportunistic infections and activating potential of their latency, demonstration of retroviruses ought to be followed by screening for other pathogens [21]. Vice versa, cats living in endemic areas of certain parasites are significantly more likely to be co-infected with FIV and/or FeLV, which may present confounding clinical signs and therefore cats in such areas should be always carefully screened for coinfections [16]. Occasionally, knowing the cat's geographical location can be helpful, while the nature of the clinical presentation might be less informative [23]. Informations concerning risk assessment of viral pathogens to other animal populations are currently an important issue [28]. Screening for multiple infections is appropriate prior to relocation of cats and other felids to prevent introduction of pathogens in host colonies (households, catteries, zoos, national parks, etc.) [29]. As with HIV, careful consideration should also be given to systematic testing and treatment of individuals in high-risk populations, and this may prove to be a potential strategy to prevent FIV transmission [67]. Preventive measures are important, because transmission of pathogens in cluster conditions may occur between asymptomatic cats and immunocompromised animals [25,32]. Furthermore, certain FIV or FeLV strains are able to emerge in new host species. Domestic cat strains of viruses can cross species barriers with potentially devastating consequences to fragile populations of large felids [12]. As seen with feline haemoplasma, it could infect even the immunocompromised human cat owner [69] so; cat owners ought to be protected from common zoonotic infections.

While testing and identification of infected cats is necessary for prevention and transmission, vaccination is also an important tool. Various independent bodies, including the International Vaccination Guidelines Group (IVGG), the European Advisory Board on Cat Diseases (ABCD), the World Small Animal Veterinary Association (WSAVA), or the American Association of Feline Practitioners (AAFP) have developed and regularly issues recommendations for vaccination protocols for cats and kittens. The guidelines encompass the types of antigens used, the types of vaccines available, the frequency of vaccination and the anatomical site used for administration. These guidelines differ from each other and also from the manufacturer's datasheets or recommendations of national authorities. General aspects and details of vaccination of cats are far beyond the scope of recent review; in this regard see a recent publication by Dean et al. 2012. Core vaccines are defined as those vaccines which all cats, regardless of circumstances, should receive to protect animals from severe, life threatening diseases which have global distribution. Only to emphasize those in context with microbes with transactivating and opportunistic potential, FHV-1 vaccination of kittens seems to be important. Vaccination against FCV, FPV also belongs to core vaccines. These vaccinations are recommended to start as early as vaccination with FeLV, applying revaccinations up to 16-20 weeks of age. Most practices routinely give the commonly used antigens annually, although with the exception of the FHV, the FCV and FIV vaccination is recommended every 3 years [80]. Non-core vaccines are those that are required by only those animals whose geographic location, local environment or lifestyle place them at risk of contracting specific infections. This moment, both FIV and FeLV vaccines are regarded as non-core. FIV vaccine development was initiated as a model for HIV vaccination. Vaccination against HIV started with experiments to trigger a specific, potent and long-lasting immunity in a surrogate animal model. Later, several novel approaches were tested in the feline model. Although the quest for a truly effective AIDS vaccine is years away [81], vaccination against FIV became available [82]. This vaccine (Fel-O-Vax FIV®) is marketed in many countries, but it might not protect cats against all field strains of subtypes A or B. Lifespan of infected cats appears similar to that of uninfected cats, but exposure to other infectious diseases drastically reduces survival of FIV positive animals [17]. Historically, FeLV vaccination has been used for decades, well before FIV vaccination. The combined use of testing and vaccination programs is assumed to have decreased the prevalence of FeLV over the last 20 years [17,19]. Administering the first vaccine to kittens is at 8-10 weeks of age, with regular revaccinations usually every year. Several practitioners stopped revaccinating indoor and older cats, once they reached a certain age (≥ 6 years) assuming that they would not have close contact with a persistently infected cat, or elder cats are less easily infected with FeLV than younger animals. As persistently infected cats have been diagnosed at all ages, due to the decreased susceptibility to FeLV infection, vaccinating at 2-3 years intervals rather than annually seems to be acceptable. For free-roaming cats, annual FeLV vaccination is recommended. To increase revaccination interval assuming the presence of high level antibodies is not feasible because quantitative assays to measure serum FeLV antibodies are commercially available in few countries [80]. A marked difference in vaccination efficacy exists, and suggests that only inactivated whole virus or canarypox-vectored recombinant vaccines should be used. Cats with access to outdoors should be vaccinated, but should have at least one negative FeLV ELISA test before vaccination. Several studies showed that the mean survival time of FeLV positive cats are significantly shorter than that of FeLV-negative cats including vaccinated ones (references in 17). Aspecific measures to prevent FIV and FeLV transmission were set according to the biological characteristics of these viruses. Although retroviruses become inactivated within a few hours on dry surfaces, they may remain viable in dried biological deposits for more than a week. Both viruses are inactivated by common detergents and hospital disinfectants. Spreading via body fluids is best prevented by single set of instruments in clinical practice. To prevent infections by other microbes, including those with transactivation or opportunistic potential, hospitalised cats should not be allowed to have direct contact with one another. It is important not to keep retrovirus-infected cats in contagious disease ward as they are potentially immunosuppressed and carry or acquire other pathogens [17]. A recent survey in the UK showed that several veterinarians are not aware of the guidelines, or they do not adhere to them. Similarly to guidelines in human healthcare, other barriers included lack of agreement or lack of ability to follow guidelines, lack of motivation to follow them, and lack to perceive benefits to patients. The frequency, combination and selection of antigens routinely given to cats by veterinarians remain unknown, as are the anatomical sites to inject cats. Therefore, the impact of the published guidelines on practitioners working also remains unknown [80]. Further work is required to elicit why following guidelines may reduce occurrence and severity of both opportunistic infections and halt onset and slow progression of FAIDS by eliminating infection by other microbes.

The FIV/cat model has provided a unique opportunity to test novel therapeutic interventions aimed at eradicating latent virus, but the use of antiretroviral drugs in FIV infected cats and other felids has not gained grounds in the routine veterinary practice [7,8]. Several conventional microbial coinfections are treated with routine medication.

5. Conclusions

Descriptive epidemiological surveys on the simultaneous infection by feline retroviruses, namely FIV and/or FeLV, and heterologous microbes clearly show that progression of FAIDS is facilitated by certain viruses, bacteria and other parasites that also induce opportunistic infections in a vicious circle. Scarce experimental data suggest that FIV transactivating potential of heterologous microbes might increase FIV load, facilitate FAIDS course, and help induce malignancies resulting in considerably impaired quality of life and shorter life span of afflicted domestic cats. Simultaneous cross-species transmission of infection by particular FIV and FeLV strains in endangered big cats may also occur. Emerging infections by FIV transactivating and opportunistic feline microbes in immunocompromised humans have already been described. Additive or synergistic impairing effects on the native immune reactions, activation of negatively affecting Treg cells, depression of cytotoxic T cell activities, and abnormal cytokine pattern exerted by heterologous microbes demonstrate striking similarities between AIDS and FAIDS. Regular vaccination against transactivating microbes (e.g. FeLV, FHV-1) and transactivated microbe (FIV) starting at early age prevents and disrupts deleterious microbial interactions. These result in a complete halt or a significant slowdown of acquired immunodeficiency states. Experience verified in the feline model enables us to continue studying microbial interactions at molecular, cellular, immunological or clinical levels. Further experiments are warranted to better delineate the role of putative cofactors in FIV infection. Further studies should examine concurrent infections as contributing factors in the development and progression of neoplasia in FIV-positive cats. Determination of viral cooperative mechanisms that promote cancer during co-infection would be highly relevant to both FIV- and HIV-related diseases.

Author details

Joseph Ongrádi[1*], Stercz Balázs[1], Kövesdi Valéria[1], Nagy Károly[1] and Pistello Mauro[2]

*Address all correspondence to: ongjos@hotmail.com

1 Institute of Medical Microbiology, Semmelweis University, Budapest, Hungary

2 Retrovirus Centre, University of Pisa, Pisa, Italy

References

[1] Folkl A, Wen X, Kuczynski E, Clark ME, Bienzle D. Feline programmed death and its ligand: characterization and changes with feline immunodeficiency virus infection. The Veterinary Immunology and Immunopathology 2010;134(1-2) 107-114.

[2] Simões RD, Howard KE, Dean GA. In Vivo assessment of natural killer cell responses during chronic feline immunodeficiency virus infection. PLoS One 2012;7(5) 3760-3766.

[3] Ongrádi J, Ceccherini-Nelli L, Soldaini E , Bendinelli M, Conaldi PG, Specter S, Friedman H. Endotoxin suppresses indirect activation of HIV-1 by human herpesvirus 6. In: Nowotny A, Spitzer J J, Ziegler EJ. (eds.) Cellular and molecular aspects of endotoxin reactions. Amsterdam: Elsevier Science Publishers B.V; 1990. p387-394.

[4] Ongrádi J, Kövesdi V, Nagy K, Matteoli B, Ceccherini-Nelli L, Ablashi D. In vitro and in vivo transactivation of HIV by HHV-6. In: Chang TL. (ed.) HIV-Host Interactions. Vienna: InTech; 2011. p257-298. ISBN: 978-953-307-442-9. Available from www.intechopen.com/books/hiv-host-interactions/in-vitro-and-in-vivo-transactivation-of-hiv-1-by-human-herpesvirus-6 (accessed 1 October 2012)

[5] Murphy B, Vapniarsky N, Hillman C, Castillo D, McDonnel S, Moore P, Luciw PA, Sparger EE. FIV establishes a latent infection in feline peripheral blood CD4+ T lymphocytes in vivo during the asymptomatic phase of infection. Retrovirology 2012; 9(12) doi10.1186/1742-4690-9-12

[6] Kenyon JC, Lever AM. The molecular biology of feline immunodeficiency virus (FIV). Viruses 2011;3(11) 2192-2193.

[7] Elder JH, Lin YC, Fink E, Grant CK. Feline immunodeficiency virus (FIV) as a model for study of lentivirus infections: parallels with HIV. Current HIV Research 2010; 8(1) 73-80.

[8] McDonnel SJ, Sparger EE, Luciw PA, Murphy BG. Transcriptional regulation of latent feline immunodeficiency virus in peripheral CD4+ T-lymphocytes. Viruses 2012;4(5) 878-888.

[9] Gemeniano MC, Sawai ET, Leutenegger CM, Sparger EE. Feline immunodeficiency virus ORF-A is required for virus particle formation and virus infectivity. The Journal of Virology 2003;77(16) 8819-8830.

[10] Mikkelsen SR, Long JM, Zhang L, Galemore ER, VandeWoude S, Dean GA. Partial regulatory T cell depletion prior to acute feline immunodeficiency virus infection does not alter disease pathogenesis. PLoS One 2011;6(2) 17181723.

[11] Spada E, Proverbio D, della Pepa A, Perego R, Baggiani L, DeGiorgi GB, Domenichini G, Ferro E, Cremonesi F. Seroprevalence of feline immunodeficiency virus, feline leukaemia virus and Toxoplasma gondii in stray cat colonies in Northern Italy and correlation with clinical and laboratory data. Journal of Feline Medicine and Surgery 2012;14(6) 369-377.

[12] O'Brien SJ, Troyer JL, Brown MA, Johnson WE, Antunes A, Roelke ME, Pecon-Slattery J. Emerging viruses in the Felidae: shifting paradigms. Viruses 2012;4(2) 236-257.

[13] Magden, E, Quackenbush SL, VandeWou de S. FIV associated neoplasms: a mini-review. The Veterinary Immunology and Immunopathology 2011; 143(3-4) 227-234.

[14] Ongrádi J, Stercz B, Kövesdi V, Vértes L. Immunosenescence and vaccination of the elderly. Part I. Age-related immune impairment. Acta Microbiologica et Immunologica Hungarica 2009;56(3) 199-210.

[15] Steinrigl A, Ertl R, Langbei, I, Klein D. Phylogenetic analysis suggests independent introduction of feline immunodeficiency virus clades A and B to Central Europe and identifies diverse variants of clade B. The Veterinary Immunology and Immunopathology 2010;134(1-2) 82-89.

[16] Sobrinho LS, Rossi CN. Vides JP, Braga ET, Gomes AA, de Lima VM, Perri SH, Generoso D, Langoni H, Leutenegger C, Biondo AW, Laurenti MD, Marcondes M. Coinfection of Leishmania chagasi with Toxoplasma gondii, Feline Immunodeficiency Virus (FIV) and Feline Leukemia Virus (FeLV) in cats from an endemic area of zoonotic visceral leishmaniasis. Veterinary Parasitology 2012;187(1-2) 302-306.

[17] Little S, Bienzle D, Carioto L, Chisholm H, O'Brien E, Scherk M. Feline leukemia virus and feline immunodeficiency virus in Canada: recommendations for testing and management. The Canadian Veterinary Journal 2011;52(8), 849-855.

[18] Sukhumavasi W, Bellosa ML, Lucio-Forster A, Liotta JL, Lee AC, Pornmingmas P, Chungpivat S., Mohammed HO, Lorentzen L, Dubey JP, Bowman DD. Serological survey of Toxoplasma gondii, Dirofilaria immitis, Feline Immunodeficiency Virus (FIV) and Feline Leukemia Virus (FeLV) infections in pet cats in Bangkok and vicinities, Thailand. Veterinary Parasitology,2012;188(1-2) 25-30.

[19] Hartmann K. Clinical aspects of feline immunodeficiency and feline leukemia virus infection. Veterinary Immunology and Immunopathology2011;143(3-4) 190-201.

[20] Powell CC, McInni, CL, Fontenelle JP, Lappin MR. Bartonella species, feline herpesvirus-1, and Toxoplasma gondii PCR assay results from blood and aqueous humor samples from 104 cats with naturally occurring endogenous uveitis. Journal of Feline Medicine and Surgery 210;12(12) 923-928.

[21] Akhtardanesh B, Ziaal, N, Sharifi H, Rezaei S. Feline immunodeficiency virus, feline leukemia virus and Toxoplasma gondii in stray and household cats in Kerman-Iran: seroprevalence and correlation with clinical and laboratory findings. Research in Veterinary Science 2010;89(2) 306-310.

[22] Sykes JE. Immunodeficiencies caused by infectious diseases. Veterinary Clinics of North America: Small Animal Practice 2010; 40(3) 409-423.

[23] Gunn-Moore DA, McFarland SE, Brewer JI, Crawshaw TR, Clifton-Hadley RS, Kovalik M, Shaw DJ. Mycobacterial disease in cats in Great Britain: I. Culture results, geographical distribution and clinical presentation of 339 cases. Journal of Feline Medicine and Surgery 2011;12(12) 934-944.

[24] Belgard S, Truyen U, Thibault JC, Sauter-Louis C, Hartmann K. Relevance of feline calicivirus, feline immunodeficiency virus, feline leukemia virus, feline herpesvirus

and Bartonella henselae in cats with chronic gingivostomatitis. Berliner und Münchener Tierärztliche Wochenschrift 2010;123(9-10) 369-376.

[25] Tanahara M, Miyamoto S, Nishio T, Yoshii Y, Sakuma M, Sakata Y, Nishigaki K, Tsujimoto H, Setoguchi A, Endo Y. An epidemiological survey of feline hemoplasma infection in Japan. Journal of Veterinary Medical Science 2010;72(12) 1575-1581.

[26] Reche A Jr, Daniel AG, Lazaro Strauss TC, Taborda CP, Vieira Marques SA, Haipek K, Oliveira LJ, Monteiro JM, Kfoury JR Jr. Cutaneous mycoflora and CD4:CD8 ratio of cats infected with feline immunodeficiency virus. Journal of Feline Medicine and Surgery 2010;12(4) 355-358.

[27] Roura X, Peter, IR, Alte, L, Tabar MD, Barker EN, Planellas M, Helps CR, Francino O, Shaw SE, Tasker S. Prevalence of hemotropic mycoplasmas in healthy and unhealthy cats and dogs in Spain. Journal of Veterinary Diagnostic Investigation 2010;22(2) 270-274.

[28] Duarte A, Castr, I, Pereira da Fonseca IM, Almeida V, Madeira de Carvalho LM, Meireles J, Fazendeiro MI, Tavares L, Vaz Y. Survey of infectious and parasitic diseases in stray cats at the Lisbon Metropolitan Area, Portugal. Journal of Feline Medicine and Surgery 2010;12(6) 441-446.

[29] Filoni C, Catão-Dias JL, Cattori V, Willi B, Meli ML, Corrêa SH, Marques MC,Adania CH, Silva JC, Marvulo MF, Ferreira Neto JS, Durigon EL, de Carvalho VM,Coutinh, SD, Lutz H, Hofmann-Lehmann R. Surveillance using serological and molecular methods for the detection of infectious agents in captive Brazilian neotropic and exotic felids. Journal of Veterinary Diagnostic Investigation 2012;24(1)166-173.

[30] Coelho WM, do Amarante AF, Apolinário Jde C, Coelho NM, de Lima VM, Perri SH, Bresciani, KD. Seroepidemiology of Toxoplasma gondii, Neospora caninum, and Leishmania spp. infections and risk factors for cats from Brazil. Parasitology Research 2011;109(4) 1009-1013.

[31] Al-Kappany YM, Lappin MR, Kwok OC, Abu-Elwafa SA, Hilali M, Dubey JP. Seroprevalence of Toxoplasma gondii and concurrent Bartonella spp., feline immunodeficiency virus, feline leukemia virus, and Dirofilaria immitis infections in Egyptian cats. Journal of Parasitology 2011;97(2) 256-258.

[32] Miró G, Hernández, Montoya A, Arranz-Solís D, Dado D, Rojo-Montejo S, Mendoza-Ibarra JA, Ortega-Mora LM, Pedraza-Díaz S. First description of naturally acquired Tritrichomonas foetus infection in a Persian cattery in Spain. Parasitology Research 2011;109(4) 1151-1154.

[33] Stojanovic V, Foley P. Infectious disease prevalence in a feral cat population on Prince Edward Island, Canada. The Canadian Veterinary Journal 2011;52(9) 979-982.

[34] Troyer JL, Roelke ME, Jespersen JM, Baggett N, Buckley-Beason V, MacNulty D,Craft M, Packer C, Pecon-Slattery J, O'Brien SJ. FIV diversity: FIV_{Ple} subtype composition

may influence disease outcome in African lions. The Veterinary Immunology and Immunopathology 2011;143(3-4) 338-346.

[35] Korman RM, Cerón JJ, Knowles TG, Barker EN, Eckersall PD, Tasker S. Acute phase response to Mycoplasma haemofelis and 'Candidatus Mycoplasma haemominutum' infection in FIV-infected and non-FIV-infected cats. The Veterinary Journal 2012; http://dx.doi.org/10.1016/j.tvjl.2011.12.009

[36] Buchmann AU, Kershaw O, Kempf VA, Gruber AD. Does a feline leukemia virus infection pave the way for Bartonella henselae infection in cats? Journal of Clinical Microbiology 2010;48(9) 3295-3300.

[37] Bacon LD, Witter RL, FadlyAM. Augmentation of retrovirus-induced lymphoid leukosis by Marek's disease herpesviruses in White Leghorn chickens. Journal of Virology 1989;63(2) 504-512.

[38] Thalwitzer S, Wachter B, Robert N, Wibbelt G, Müller T, Lonzer J, Meli ML, Bay G, Hofer H. Lutz H. Seroprevalences to viral pathogens in free-ranging and captive cheetahs (Acinonyx jubatus) on Namibian Farmland. Clinical and Vaccine Immunology, 2010;7(2) 232-238.

[39] Ongrádi J, Sallay K, Kulcsár G. The decreased antibacterial activity of oral polymorphonuclear leukocytes coincides with the occurence of virus-carrying oral lymphocytes and epithelial cells. Folia microbiologica 1987;32(5) 438-447.

[40] Reubel GH, George JW, Barlough JE, Higgins J, Grant CK, Pedersen NC. Interaction of acute feline herpesvirus-1 and chronic feline immunodeficiency virus infections in experimentally infected specific pathogen free cats. The Veterinary Immunology and Immunpathology 1992;35(1-2) 95-119.

[41] Reubel GH, Dean GA, George JW, Barlough, JE, Pedersen NC. Effects of incidental infections and immune activation on disease progression in experimentally feline immunodeficiency virus-infected cats. Journal of Acquired Immune Deficiency Syndromes, 1994;7(10) 1003-1015.

[42] Kawaguchi Y, Miyazawa T, Horimoto T, Itagaki S, Fukasawa M, Takahashi E, Mikami T. Activation of feline immunodeficiency virus long terminal repeat by feline herpesvirus type 1. Virology 1991;184(1) 449-454.

[43] Kawaguchi Y, Norimine J, Miyazawa T, Kai C, Mikami T. Sequences within the feline immunodeficiency virus long terminal repeat that regulate gene expression and respond to activation by feline herpesvirus type 1. Virology 1992;190(1) 465-468.

[44] Kawaguchi Y, Maeda K, Pecoraro MR, Inoshima Y, Jang HK, Kohmoto M, Iwatsuki K, Ikeda Y, Shimojima M, Tohya Y, et al. The feline herpesvirus type 1 ICP4 downregulates feline immunodeficiency virus long terminal repeat (LTR)-directed gene expression via the C/EBP site in the LTR. Journal of Veterinary Medical Science 1995;57(6) 1129-1131.

[45] Kawaguchi Y, Maeda K, Miyazawa T, Ono M, Tsubota K, Tomonaga K, Mikami T. Inhibition of feline immunodeficiency virus gene expression and replication by alphaherpesvirus ICP4 homologues. Journal of General Virology 1994;75(10) 2783-2787.

[46] Ongrádi J, Maródi CL, Nagy K., Csiszár A, Bánhegyi D, Horváth A. HHV-6A primary infections at risk and recurrent infections during the course of AIDS. Journal of Acquired Immune Deficiency Syndrome and Human Retroviruses 1999;22(3) 311-312.

[47] Lakatos B, Farkas J, Egberink HF, Vennema H, Horzinek MC, van Vliet A, Rossen, J, Benkő M, Ongrádi J. PCR detection of adenovirus in a cat. Hungarian Veterinary Journal 1997;119, 517-519.

[48] Ongrádi J. Identification of a feline adenovirus isolate that replicates in monkey and human cells in vitro American Journal of Veterinary Research 1999;60(12) 1463.

[49] Pring-Akerblom P, Ongrádi J. Feline adenovirus hexon. GenBank Accession Number AY512566

[50] Pring-Akerblom P, Ongrádi J. Feline adenovirus fiber. GenBank Accession Number AY 518270

[51] Phan TG, Shimizu H, Nishimura S, Okitsu S, Maneekarn N, Ushijima H. Human adenovirus type 1 related to feline adenovirus: evidence of interspecies transmission. Clinical Laboratory 2006;52(9-10) 515-518.

[52] Luiz LN, Leite JP, Yokosawa J, Carneiro BM, Pereira Filho E, Oliveira TF, Freitas GR, Costa LF, Paula NT, Silveira HL, Nepomuceno JC, Queiróz DA. Molecular characterization of adenoviruses from children presenting with acute respiratory disease in Uberlândia, Minas Gerais, Brazil, and detection of an isolate genetically related to feline adenovirus. Memórias do Instituto Oswaldo Cruz 2010;105(5) 712-716.

[53] Lakatos B, Farkas J, Ádám É, Jarrett O, Egberink HF, Bendinelli M, Nász I, Ongrádi J. Data to the adenovirus infection of European cats. Hungarian Veterinary Journal 1996; 51,543-545.

[54] Lakatos B, Farkas J, Ádám É, Dobay O, Jeney Cs, Nász I, Ongrádi J. Serological evidence of adenovirus infection in cats. Archieves of Virology 2000;145(5) 1029-1033.

[55] Ongrádi J, Pistello M, Mazzetti P, Bendinelli M. The effect of cytokines on the early events of feline immunodeficiency virus (FIV) infection of macrophages Annual Meeting of the International Society for Interferon and Cytokine Research, Budapest, Hungary, 2-7 October, 1994. Journal of Interferon Research 14 (Suppl.1), 137, 1994.

[56] Biancotto A, Grivel JC, Lisco A, Vanpouille C, Markham PD, Gallo RC, Margolis LB, Lusso P. Evolution of SIV toward RANTES resistance in macaques rapidly progressing to AIDS upon coinfection with HHV-6A. Retrovirology 2009;2(6), 61.

[57] Lusso P, Crowley RW, Malnati MS, Di Serio C, Ponzoni M, Biancotto A, Markham PD, Gallo RC. Human herpesvirus 6A accelerates AIDS progression in macaques.

Proceedings of National Academy of Sciences of the United States of America 2007;104(12) 5067-5072.

[58] Rojko JL, Olsen RG. The immunobiology of the feline leukemia virus. The Veterinary Immunology and Immunpathology 1984; 6(1-2) 107-165.

[59] Ishida T, Washizu T, Toriyabe K, Motoyoshi S, Tomoda I, Pedersen NC. Feline immunodeficiency virus infection in cats of Japan. Journal of theAmerican Veterinary Medical Association 1989;194(2) 221-225.

[60] Yamamoto JK, Hansen H, Ho EW, Morishita TY, Okuda T, Sawa TR, Nakamura RM. Pedersen NC. Epidemiologic and clinical aspects of feline immunodeficiency virus infection in cats from the continental United States and Canada and possible mode of transmission. Journal of the American Veterinary Medical Association 1989; 194(2) 213-210.

[61] Shelton GH, Grant CK, Cotter SM, Gardner MB, Hardy WD Jr. DiGiacomo RF. Feline immunodeficiency virus and feline leukemia virus infections and their relationships to lymphoid malignancies in cats: a retrospective study (1968-1988). Journal of Acquired Immune Deficiency Syndromes 1990;3(6) 623-630.

[62] Pedersen NC, Torten M, Rideout B, Sparger E, Tonachini T, Luciw PA, Ackley C, Levy N, Yamamoto J. Feline leukemia virus infection as a potentiating cofactor for the primary and secondary stages of experimentally induced feline immunodeficiency virus infection. Journal of Virology 1990;64(2) 598-606.

[63] Levy JA. Pathogenesis of human immunodeficiency virus infection. Microbiol Review 1993;57(1) 183-289.

[64] Korman RM, Cerón JJ, Knowles TG, Barker EN, Eckersall PD, Tasker S. Acute phase response to Mycoplasma haemofelis and 'Candidatus Mycoplasma haemominutum' infection in FIV-infected and non-FIV-infected cats. The Veterinary Journal 2012; 193(2) 433-438.

[65] George JW, DVM, PhD Bruce A, Rideout, DVM, PhD Stephen M. Griffey, DVM, PhD Niels C. Pedersen, DVM, PhD Effect of preexisting FeLV infection or FeLV and feline immunodeficiency virus coinfection on pathogenicity of the small variant of Haemobartonella felis in cats. American Journal of Veterinary Research 2002;63(8) 1172-1178.

[66] Chowdhury MI, Munakata T, Koyanagi Y, Arai S, Yamamoto N. Mycoplasmastimulates HIV-1 expression from acutely- and dormantly-infected promonocyte/monoblastoid cell lines. Archives of Virology 1994;139(3-4) 431-438.

[67] Mavedzenge SN, Van Der Pol B, Weiss HA, Kwok C, Mambo F, Chipato T, Van derStraten A, Salata R, Morrison C. The association between Mycoplasma genitalium and HIV-1 acquisition in African women. AIDS 2012;26(5) 617-24.

[68] Al-Harthi L, Spear GT, Hashemi FB, Landay A, Sha BE, Roebuck KA. A human immunodeficiency virus (HIV)-inducing factor from the female genital tract activates

HIV-1 gene expression through the kappaB enhancer. Journal of Infectious Diseases. 1998;178(5) 1343-1351.

[69] dos Santos AP, dos Santos RP, Biondo AW, Dora JM, Goldani LZ, de Oliveira ST, de Sá Guimarães AM, Timenetsky J, de Morais HA, González FH, Messick JB.Hemoplasma infection in HIV-positive patient, Brazil. Emerging Infectious Diseases 2008;14(12) 1922-1924.

[70] Kallick CA, Levin S, Reddi KT, Landau WL. Systemic lupus erythematosus associated with haemobartonella-like organisms. Nature New Biology 1972;236(66) 145-146.

[71] Maingat F, Viappiani S, Zhu Y, Vivithanapor, P, Ellestad KK, Holden J, Silva, C, Power C. Regulation of lentivirus neurovirulence by lipopolysaccharide conditioning: suppression of CXCL10 in the brain by IL-10. Journal of Immunology2010;184(3) 1566-1574.

[72] Levy JA, Hsueh F, Blackbourn DJ, Wara D, Weintrub PS. CD8 cell noncytotoxic antiviral activity in human immunodeficiency virus-infected and -uninfected children. Journal of Infectious Diseases. 1998;177(2) 470-472.

[73] Dean GA, Higgins J, LaVoy A, Fan Z, Pedersen NC. Measurement of feline cytokine gene expression by quantitative-competitive RT-PCR. The Veterinary Immunology and Immunpathology 1998;63(1-2) 73-82.

[74] Dean GA, Pedersen NC. Cytokine response in multiple lymphoid tissues during the primary phase of feline immunodeficiency virus infection. Journal of Virology 1998;72,(12) 9436-9440.

[75] Tochikura, TS, Naito Y, Kozutsumi Y, Hohdatsu T. Induction of feline immunodeficiency virus from a chronically infected feline T-lymphocyte cell line. Research in Veterinary Science 2012;92(2) 327-332.

[76] Ongrádi, J.Report on the feline AIDS model study of the University of Pisa. Medical Journal/OrvosiHetilap 1993;134(47) 2621-2622.

[77] Ongrádi J, Sheikh JM, Austen B, Pistello M, Bendinelli M, Dalgleish AG. Programmed cell death of cultured immune cells induced by HIV-1 or FIV. Acta Microbiologica et Immunologica Hungarica 1997;44(1) 48-49.

[78] Scott VL, Boudreaux CE, Lockett NN, Clay BT, Coats KS. Cytokine dysregulation in early- and late-term placentas from feline immunodeficiency virus (FIV)-infected cats. American Journal of Reproductive Immunology 2011;65(5) 480-491.

[79] Levy J, Crawford C, Hartmann K, Hofmann-Lehmann R, Little S, Sundahl E, Thayer V. 2008 American Association of Feline Practitioners' feline retrovirus management guidelines. Journal of Feline Medicine and Surgery 2008;10(3) 300-316.

[80] Dean RS, Pfeiffer DU, Adams VJ. Feline vaccination practices and protocols used by veterinarians in the United Kingdom. The Veterinary Journal. 2012; http://dx.doi.org/10.1016/j.tvjl.2012.02.024

[81] Pistello M, Conti F,Vannucci L, Freer G. Novel approaches to vaccination against the feline immunodeficiency virus. Veterinary Immunology and Immunopathology 2010;134(1-2) 48-53.

[82] Yamamoto JK, Pu R, Sato E, Hohdatsu T. Feline immunodeficiency virus pathogenesis and development of a dual-subtype feline-immunodeficiency-virus vaccine. AIDS 2007;21(5) 547-563.